Tinnitus Handbook

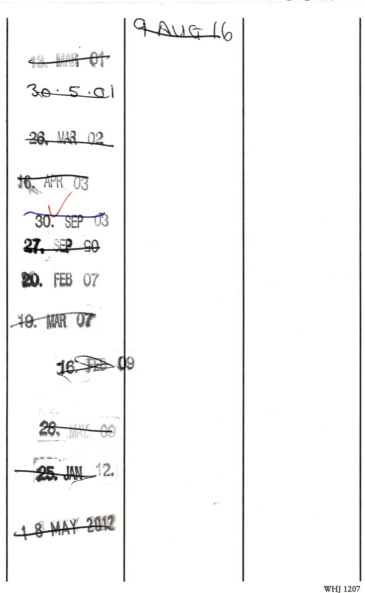
Books should be returned to the SDH Library on or before
the date stamped above unless a renewal has been arranged.

Salisbury District Hospital Library

Telephone: Salisbury (01722) 336262   extn. 4432 / 33
Out of hours answer machine in operation

Tinnitus Handbook

Edited by

Richard Tyler, Ph.D.
Professor and Director of Audiology
Department of Otolaryngology
The University of Iowa
Iowa City, Iowa

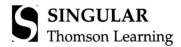 **SINGULAR**
Thomson Learning

Africa • Australia • Canada • Denmark • Japan • Mexico • New Zealand • Philippines
Puerto Rico • Singapore • Spain • United Kingdom • United States

NOTICE TO THE READER

COPYRIGHT © 2000
Singular Publishing Group is a division of Thomson Learning. The Thomson Learning logo is a registered trademark used herein under license.

Printed in the United States of America
2 3 4 5 6 7 8 9 10 XXX 05 04 03 02 01 00

For more information, contact Singular Publishing Group, 401 West "A" Street, Suite 325 San Diego, CA 92101-7904; or find us on the World Wide Web at http://www.singpub.com

Library of Congress Cataloging-in-Publication Data:

Tinnitus handbook / edited by Richard Tyler
    p. ; cm. – (A Singular audiology textbook)
  Includes bibliographical references and index.
  ISBN 1-56593-922-0 (soft cover : alk. paper)
  1. Tinnitus—Handbooks, manuals, etc. I. Tyler, Richard S. II. Singular audiology text
[DNLM: 1. Tinnitus, WV 272 T591235 2000]
RF293.8 .T565 2000
617.8—do21   99-057052

CONTENTS

CONTRIBUTORS

Robert Burkard, Ph.D.
University Of Buffalo
Department of Communicative
    Disorders & Science
Department of Otolaryngology
Buffalo, New York

Ross Coles, FRCP (Ed.)
Institute Of Hearing Research
Nottingham, United Kingdom

Rene Dauman, M.D.
Department Of Audiology
Hopital Pellegrin
Bordeaux, France

Adrian Davis, Ph.D.
Medical Research Council
Institute Of Hearing Research
Nottingham, United Kingdom

Jos J. Eggermont, Ph.D.
University Of Calgary
Department Of Psychology
Calgary, Canada

Amr El Refaie, M.D.
Medical Research Council
Institute Of Hearing Research
Nottingham, United Kingdom

Soly Erlandsson, Ph.D.
Goteborg Universitet
Department Of Psychology
Goteberg, Sweden

Bruce Gantz, M.D.
University Of Iowa
Department of Otolaryngology—
    Head And Neck Surgery
Iowa City, Iowa

Joseph Hegarty, M.D.
San Francisco General Hospital
University of California
San Francisco, California

Jane L. Henry, Ph.D.
School Of Psychology
University Of New South Wales
Sydney, Australia

Gary Jacobson, Ph.D.
Henry Ford Hospital
Department of Otolaryngology—
    Head And Neck Surgery
Detroit, Michigan

Pawel Jastreboff, Ph.D.
Tinnitus & Hyperacusis Center
Department of Otolaryngology
Emory University School of Medicine
Atlanta, Georgia

Alan Lockwood, M.D.
Department Of Communicative
    Disorders & Sciences
Department Of Neurology
Department Of Nuclear Medicine
VA Medical Center
Buffalo, New York

Laurence McKenna, Ph.D.
Institute Of Laryngology And Otology
Royal National Throat, Nose,
    And Ear Hospital
London, England

Mary B. Meikle, Ph.D.
Oregon Hearing Research Center
Oregon Health Sciences University
Portland, Oregon

M. J. (Lynn) Penner, Ph.D.
University Of California At San Diego
Department Of Psychology
La Jolla, California

Brian P. Perry, M.D.
The Otology Group of Texas
San Antonio, Texas

Gloria Reich, Ph.D.
American Tinnitus Association
Portland, Oregon

Richard J. Salvi, Ph.D.
State University of New York at Buffalo
Department Of Communicative Disorders
   & Sciences
Department of Neurology
Buffalo, New York

Richard Smith, M.D.
University Of Iowa
Department of Otolaryngology—
   Head And Neck Surgery
Iowa City, Iowa

Dafydd Stephens, M.D.
Welsh Hearing Institute
University Hospital Of Wales
United Kingdom

Robert Sweetow, Ph.D.
University Of California at San Francisco
Department Of Audiology
San Francisco, California

Richard S. Tyler, Ph.D.
Department of Otolaryngology—
   Head & Neck Surgery
Department Of Speech Pathology And
   Audiology
University Of Iowa
Iowa City, Iowa

Jack Vernon, Ph.D.
Emeritus Professor Of Otolaryngology
Oregon Health Sciences University
Portland, Oregon

Peter Wilson, Ph.D.
Flinders University Of South Australia
School Of Social Sciences
Adelaide, Australia

David Young, M.A.
University Of Iowa
Department Of Family Practice
Iowa City, Iowa

To
Kathleen Tyler
(For a lifetime of hard work and love for her family)

PREFACE

Tinnitus remains one of the most difficult hearing disorders to treat. First, tinnitus has numerous causes and many neurophysiological mechanisms are likely to be involved. Second, there are inherent differences among individuals in their ability to cope with novel situations and stress. Therefore, a uniform therapy for all is unlikely. In addition, the "subjective" nature of tinnitus renders it very difficult to develop good animal models. This is fundamental to many avenues of scientific investigations. It is no wonder many clinicians have chosen to avoid tinnitus patients instead of helping them.

However, we can help tinnitus patients. And we are obligated to do so.

This book attempts to organize current knowledge and treatments for tinnitus. It is intended as a handbook for clinicians and students to facilitate the consideration of all treatment options and to provide some familiarity with details about different treatments. Many of the topics originated from our annual Management of the Tinnitus Patient conference held at The University of Iowa.

Many thanks to all the authors for their scholarly contributions.

Rich Tyler
Iowa City
January 3, 2000

CHAPTER 1

Epidemiology of Tinnitus

Adrian Davis
El Amr Rafaie

SCOPE

In this chapter, the prevalence of tinnitus in different populations will be reviewed together with those demographic, systemic, and environmental factors that influence the prevalence. The public health and clinical implications are derived from these data, showing that tinnitus is a widespread problem that causes considerable disability or handicap for which systematic considered intervention should have a high priority.

DEFINITION

Many people, especially when in a quiet room or after listening to loud music, report that they can hear sound in their ears or in their head. These sounds or noises are referred to as tinnitus. There is considerable variation in tinnitus expression, its etiology, and its effect on patients' lives. Tinnitus may be triggered or originate from within the auditory system or from para-auditory structures, and it may be a pointer to underlying pathological conditions. It can impair the quality of life of individuals and their

family, leading to social and psychological complications. A clear definition of what we mean by tinnitus is needed to allow uniform comparisons about the condition to be made, whether for descriptive or intervention studies.

McFadden (1982) suggested that "Tinnitus is the conscious expression of a sound that originates in an involuntary manner in the head of its owner, or may appear to him to do so."

At present, it is too early to preempt universal agreement on a definition of tinnitus. However, it is important that an operational definition of tinnitus is made, adapting certain standard and uniform criteria, for instance, to distinguish clinically significant tinnitus from temporary insignificant tinnitus. Such operational definitions are required for rigorous epidemiological studies, and also in treatment trials, although in practice they may differ for different purposes. The National Study of Hearing (Coles, 1984a, b) used the concept of prolonged spontaneous tinnitus to differentiate between significant and insignificant tinnitus. In subsequent studies (Davis, 1995) suggested that the tinnitus must last for five minutes or more. However, not all tinnitus is the same severity; some may not disturb or annoy at all while some may totally affect quality of life; some may be continuously present while some may be intermittent (for example, occurring at night time). Therefore, an estimate of tinnitus severity is also needed. In addition, there are other classification systems that can be useful for other purposes.

CLASSIFICATION

Classification of tinnitus could play a constructive role in research and treatment. However, the lack of a clear understanding of a mechanism of generation and perception makes a single classification difficult to envisage.

Dauman and Tyler (1992) suggested that several classification systems are needed. They first distinguished between *normal* and *pathological* tinnitus. *Normal tinnitus* is experienced by most people without hearing loss, lasting for less than five minutes less than once a week. *Pathological tinnitus* lasts more than five minutes more than once a week and is usually experienced by people having hearing loss. They further divided pathological tinnitus into *acceptable* or *unacceptable tinnitus* and *temporary* or *permanent tinnitus*. *Acceptable tinnitus* does not bother the person (nonclinical), while *unacceptable tinnitus* is disturbing to the patient. Accept-

ability of tinnitus depends on the physiological mechanism and psychological factors related to the patient. *Temporary tinnitus* is short-term, probably due to temporary dysfunction of the auditory system, such as after noise at work, noise in a club, or drug exposure, while *permanent tinnitus* may be either constant or intermittent (when tinnitus returns after a period of disappearance). They also classified tinnitus by determining the site of dysfunction (middle ear or sensorineural [peripheral or central]), or the etiology (noise-induced, Ménière's disease, ototoxicity, presbyacusis, unknown causes, and so on). Table 1-1 summarizes the classifications they proposed.

While the above classification concentrated on causative and descriptive aspects of tinnitus, Stephens and Hetu (1991) concentrated on the effect tinnitus causes on the patient's abilities and quality of life. They followed the WHO classification of diseases into impairment, disability, and handicap (1980) to classify tinnitus. Impairment is the physiological/psychophysical defect measurable in the clinic or laboratory (tinnitus loudness, tinnitus frequency, hearing sensitivity). Disability is the effect of this defect in terms of the auditory difficulties experienced by the patient in real life, while handicap describes the nonauditory effects of the disability (annoyance, effort to overcome social withdrawal, occupational effects). Regardless of which definitions or classifi-

Table 1-1. Classification of Tinnitus. *Dauman and Tyler (1992)*

Pathology	Severity	Duration	Site	Etiology
• Normal	• Acceptable	• Temporary	• Middle ear	• Noise-induced
• Pathological	• Unacceptable	• Permanent	• Peripheral neural	• Ménière's disease
				• Ototoxicity
			• Central neural	• Presbyacusis
				• Unknown etiology

cations are used, any demographic study should include *at least* two elements:

1. Tinnitus that lasts for five minutes or more (additionally whether it is present some or all of the time).
2. An assessment of the impact of the tinnitus (for example, severity or annoyance).

EPIDEMIOLOGICAL STUDIES

A basic understanding of the difference between prevalence and incidence is essential for the purpose of this chapter. The prevalence of tinnitus is the number of people who suffer from tinnitus at a given time. This can also be expressed as a prevalence rate or percentage. For example, if there are twenty-five adult tinnitus patients in a population of one hundred people, of whom there are fifty adults and fifty children, then the population prevalence rate is 25 percent, while the adult population prevalence rate is 50 percent. Incidence is the number of new cases arising per given time period (usually a year). Very few data have been collected on the incidence. We have restricted our discussion to prevalence in this chapter.

In order to generalize estimates of the prevalence of tinnitus we have to make several assumptions for those generalizations to be relevant.

Four of the most important assumptions are:

1. The risk factors (for example, hearing impairment) are known and can be accounted for in some way in the estimate.
2. That there is cultural independence of the self-report assessment of tinnitus and the risk factors.
3. That mortality is not affected by tinnitus.
4. Co-morbidity is not changing between the sample and the population being estimated.

Most of the epidemiological studies (Hinchcliffe, 1961; Leske, 1981; Office of Population Census and Surveys, 1983; Davis, 1995; Axelsson and Ringdahl, 1989; Brown, 1990) have used a questionnaire, sent by mail, or asked during an interview, to a random sample of the population. The main question was whether or not the person had experienced noises in the ear or head. Table 1-2 shows the main question used in six different studies. The data were analyzed and an estimate of the prevalence in the population was made, together with

Table 1-2. Questions about tinnitus used in six different epidemiological studies

Study	Questions Asked
Hinchcliffe (1961)	Have you at one time or another, noticed noises in your ears or head?
The Office of Population Census and Surveys (1983)	Did you hear noises in your head or ears such as ringing or buzzing sounds?
Leske (1981)	At any time over the past few years, have you ever noticed ringing (tinnitus) in your ears or have you been bothered by other funny noises?
The National Study of Hearing (1984)	Have you ever had noises in your head or ears? Nowadays do you get noises in your head or ears?
Axelsson and Ringdahl (1989)	Do you suffer from tinnitus?
Brown (1990)	Does anyone in the family now have tinnitus or ringing in the ear?

the effect of different factors like age, sex, noise exposure, and socioeconomic conditions among others.

One of the earliest studies concerned with the epidemiology of hearing problems including tinnitus was the one by Hinchcliffe (1961), where two random samples of adults between eighteen and seventy-four years of age, were drawn from a rural population in the United Kingdom (South Wales and Southwest Scotland). Both samples were stratified for age and sex and examined directly by mobile units. The examination involved an interview, audiometry and clinical otolarygology examination as well as radiological and bacteriological tests. The prevalence of tinnitus was determined in response to a question whether individuals have experienced noises in their ears or their head. The prevalence varied from 21 percent in the eighteen to twenty-four age group to 39 percent in the fifty-five to sixty-four age group. In another study, The Office of Population Census and Surveys published a report (1983) estimating the prevalence of tinnitus in adults in the United Kingdom population as part of a general household survey. Twenty-two percent of adults interviewed said that they had heard noises in their head or ears such as ringing or buzzing sounds. The percentage decreased to 15 percent after excluding those experiencing tinnitus due to external stimulation only (loud noises, cold, catarrh). One in seven of this 15 percent (2 percent of the total adult sample) had tinnitus all the time.

Leske (1981) published a report on the prevalence of communicative disorders in the United States for the Food and Drug Administration. There were 6,672 respondents to the survey aged eighteen to seventy-nine who were part of a probability sample representing the civilian, noninstitutionalized population of the United States between 1960 to 1962. They were asked: "At any time over the past few years, have you ever noticed ringing (tinnitus) in your ears or have you been bothered by other funny

noises?" Leske concluded that 32.4 percent of the adult population of the United States have experienced some form of tinnitus, which means that around 70 million people from the population over seventeen years of age at this time experienced tinnitus.

The National Study of Hearing, conducted by the Medical Research Council, Institute of Hearing Research provides prevalence data for planning purposes and control data for other studies by suitable matching such important variables as age, gender, noise exposure, socioeconomic group, and other demographic variables (Coles, 1984 a and b; Smith and Coles, 1987; Davis, 1989; Coles, 1995; Davis, 1995). The study had two parts, tier A and tier B (see Davis, 1989 for more [or specific methods] details) and three main phases (phase I, II, and III) after a prepilot and pilot studies. Tier A consisted of a postal questionnaire sent out to a random sample of adults on the electoral register of four United Kingdom cities: Cardiff, Glasgow, Nottingham, and Southampton. In this random sample, 48,313 people were sent questionnaires and the response rate after two further reminders when necessary was just over 80 percent. Tier B amounted to an in-clinic examination comprising further questionnaires and a detailed medical and occupational history, ear examination, and a range of audiological and blood tests. The numbers were far too large to examine all of the respondents, so sampling was necessary. The sampling was stratified on the tier A response in order to examine large proportions of those with hearing disorders and tinnitus, and 3,234 people were examined. Respondents were asked several questions concerning their tinnitus. The answers from three questions were combined to produce the operational concept of prolonged spontaneous tinnitus. These were:

1. "Have you ever had noises in your head or ears?"
2. "Nowadays do you get noises in your head or ears?"

3. "Do these noises usually last for longer than 5 minutes?", with answers: No; Yes, some of the time; and Yes, most of the time. (Davis, 1995).

Results varied slightly between phase to phase and city to city, but an overall conclusion on the prevalence of self-reported prolonged spontaneous tinnitus was derived. From tier A data, about 10.1 percent of adults experience prolonged spontaneous tinnitus: 5.1 percent reported unilateral tinnitus, and 5 percent bilateral tinnitus.

The major indicator used in this study for tinnitus severity was tinnitus annoyance. The study showed that about 5 percent had tinnitus which is moderately or severely annoying. Another indicator of tinnitus severity is sleep disturbance. Again 5 percent reported sleep disturbing tinnitus. There was considerable overlap with tinnitus annoyance such that 6 percent suffered either sleep disturbance or moderate-severe annoyance or both. The impact of tinnitus on the individual quality of life was examined by asking directly how tinnitus had affected their quality of life or their ability to lead a normal life. Not surprisingly the prevalence rate for a severe effect on quality of life was lower than those who had moderate-severely annoying tinnitus at about 1 percent. The prevalence of those who reported a severe effect on their ability to lead a "normal" life was even less at 0.5 percent. While this latter figure may seem small, it represents a large number of people: 200 to 250,000 in the United Kingdom and in excess of one million in the United States.

The questionnaire data from tier A showed three main determinants of prolonged spontaneous tinnitus. Age was important, the prevalence rising from 4.3 percent in the seventeen to thirty years age group to 15.8 percent in the sixty-one to seventy years age group. The effect of age, gender, noise, and socioeconomic group will be discussed later in this chapter.

Analysis of tier B results (clinical examination and detailed questionnaire) showed high correlation between the hearing threshold levels at high frequencies and the prevalence of prolonged spontaneous tinnitus. The odds ratio of having moderate or severely annoying tinnitus increases as the hearing threshold at high frequencies increases. The odds ratio was about 2 for those with threshold of 10 to 19 dBHL, as compared with hearing threshold levels of less than 10 dB, while in the group with threshold of more than 80 dBHL, the odds ratio was 27 (Coles, 1995). The prevalence of prolonged spontaneous tinnitus in adults detected by clinical examination was 10.1 percent, equal to that detected by postal questionnaire.

Axelsson and Ringdahl (1989) examined a random sample of 3,600 people, stratified for age and sex, between twenty and eighty years of age. They were drawn from the register of the city of Gothenburg. The participants were asked to return a questionnaire by mail. The main question asked was "Do you suffer from tinnitus?", and the respondent had to choose between never, seldom, often, and always, after a brief definition of tinnitus. The response rate was 71 percent, among them only 66 percent could be analyzed, with the rest being incompatible answers, return with no answers, or other similar causes. Analysis of the results showed that 14.2 percent suffered from tinnitus "often" or "always" with 2.4 percent of the whole population suffering from continuous tinnitus all day. There was no significant relationship between the occurrence of tinnitus and the degree of subjective hearing loss, although tinnitus was generally more common with coexistent hearing loss.

Brown (1990) conducted a study for the Center of Assessment and Demographic Studies, Gallaudet Research Institute, to explore the prevalence of tinnitus in the older American population and the effect of some demographic factors on this prevalence. He used data from the 1982–1987 Health Interview Surveys, the supplement on Aging to the 1984 Health Interview Surveys, and the First Health and Nutrition

Examination Survey 1971–1975. The health interview survey data were weighted to represent the entire United States population by gender, race, and five-year age groups up to seventy-five years of age and over. Participants were asked to respond to three questions. The first two were related to the hearing status. The third was "Does anyone in the family now have tinnitus or ringing in the ear?". The supplement on Aging to the 1984 Health Interview Survey examined a sample of one-half of the persons fifty-five to sixty-four years of age (4,651 people) and virtually all persons sixty-five years of age and over (11,497 people) using the same questions. The First Health and Nutrition Examination Survey studied people between twenty-five and seventy-five years of age (6,913), using more detailed questions involving the frequency and the annoyance of tinnitus, as well as audiometry. The variables employed in this study included age, gender, race, region and place, level of education, participation or nonparticipation in the labor force, poverty and family income, hearing status, running or discharging ears, health, activity limitation, functional limitation, and the presence of general diseases (such as arthritis, hypertension). The study concluded a prevalence rate

for tinnitus in the general population of 4.5 percent, rising to 12.3 percent of persons 55 years of age and over. The effect of various demographic factors will be discussed later.

Quaranta et al. (1996) studied the prevalence of self-reported hearing disability and tinnitus in the adult population in Italy. The study was conducted in five big cities using questionnaires and audiological assessment. The results showed that 14.5 percent experienced prolonged spontaneous tinnitus. Table 1-3 shows the prevalence estimate of tinnitus as a function of age groups in six different studies.

These studies show that the prevalence of tinnitus in adults ranged between 10.1 percent and 14.5 percent, which are fairly comparable figures between three studies in three countries, and the prevalence can be up to 22 to 32 percent if the criteria of tinnitus were relaxed to include occasional tinnitus following noise exposure or common cold. These data show about 3 to 4 percent of adults consulting the family doctor about tinnitus at least once in a lifetime, with a similar percentage consulting about a hearing problem and tinnitus, an indication of the magnitude of the problem and the considerable implication for the health services needed.

Table 1-3. Prevalence of tinnitus as a function of age. Data from six epidemiological studies

I		II		III		IV		V		VI	
Age	%	Age	%	Age	%	Age	%	Age	%	Age	%
18–24	21	18–24	26.6	16–44	12	17–30	4.3	20–29	7.5	18–44	1.6
25–34	27	25–34	27.4								
35–44	24	35–44	30.5			31–40	4.9	30–39	5.8		
45–54	27	45–54	32.5	45–64	16	41–50	7.9	40–49	8.9		
55–64	39	55–64	37.5			51–60	12.4	50–59	18.6	45–64	4.9
65–74	37	65–74	44.5	> 65	20	61–70	15.8	60–69	20.3	65–74	8.9
		75–79	41.2			71–80	14.3	70–79	21.3	> 75	7.5

Source: I: Hinchcliffe (1961); II: Leske (1981); III: The Office of Population Census and Surveys (1983); IV: The National Study of Hearing (1984–1995); V: Axelsson and Ringdahl (1989); VI: Brown (1990).

TINNITUS IN CLINICAL PRACTICE

As tinnitus is a common symptom in a wide range of otological pathologies, it is not surprising to find its prevalence high in clinic population. Fowler (1944) estimated 86 percent of people had tinnitus complaints in a consecutive 2,000 patients in the otology clinic. Spoendlin (1987) gave figures of 50 percent in patients with sudden sensorineural hearing loss, 70 percent in those with presbyacusis, 30 to 90 percent in ototoxicity patients, 50 to 90 percent in chronic acoustic trauma patients and 100 percent (by definition) in patients suffering from Ménière's disease (Table 1-4).

The National Study of Hearing tried to estimate the percentage of people seeking medical/audiological help for tinnitus or hearing difficulties. Seven point one percent of the respondents indicated that they had consulted their doctor, and 2.5 percent had furthermore attended hospitals on this account. They also found that 37 percent of the tinnitus complaints were referred to hospitals by general practitioners, compared with 48 percent of those complaining of hearing difficulties. The results show that fewer patients consult their doctor about tinnitus compared to hearing problems, and the consequent referral also was less. More public education through leaflets and self-support groups, combined with making information and training available for general practitioners are needed. Table 1-5 shows the prevalence of clinical tinnitus in

Table 1-4. The main entities of pathological conditions of the inner ear frequently associated with tinnitus, with frequency of occurrence (%) and degree of tinnitus (+.....+++)   *Spoendlin (1987)*

Pathology	Frequency of occurrence	Degree of tinnitus
Sudden deafness	50%	+
Acoustic neurinomas	70%	+
Presbyacusis	70%	+/–
Intoxications	30–90%	+/– ..... ++
Chronic noise trauma	50–90%	+/– ..... ++
Acute acoustic trauma	100%	+++
Ménière's attack	100%	++ ..... +++
(Normal hearing)	15–35%	+/– ..... +++ (1%)

Table 1-5. Prevalence of clinical tinnitus and hearing difficulty in different occupational and gender groups. Results from Phase III, respondents to the questionnaire of the National Study of Hearing (Davis, 1995).

	Manual	Nonmanual	Female	Male	Overall
Tinnitus					
–been to doctor	9.1%	5.2%	8.3%	5.9%	7.1%
–been to hospital	3.3%	1.7%	2.6%	2.5%	2.5%
Hearing					
–been to doctor	16.0%	10.7%	11.8%	15.2%	13.4%
–been to hospital	7.3%	4.7%	5.6%	6.6%	6.1%

different occupational and gender groups from phase III of the National Study of Hearing (Davis, 1995). It shows that more people from different gender or occupational groups sought help regarding hearing than for tinnitus, in the meantime, more manual workers than nonmanual workers sought help for tinnitus, and more females than males.

TINNITUS AND HEARING IMPAIRMENT

The National Study of Hearing showed that hearing impairment is the dominant factor in predicting the occurrence of prolonged spontaneous tinnitus (Coles, Smith, and Davis, 1988). The major predictor for tinnitus was high frequency hearing impairment on the worse ear, while other major factors reported are history of "runny ears," history of childhood otitis media, chronic serous otitis media, and reported difficulty with speech in noise (Davis, 1995). Brown (1990) also concluded that persons who have had discharge or running in the ear are more likely to report tinnitus than those who have not. Figure 1-1 shows the prevalence of prolonged spontaneous tinnitus, either unilateral or bilateral, as a function of chronic suppurative otitis media and history of runny ears from the National Study

of Hearing study. It shows that when a patient had chronic suppurative otitis media and a history of runny ears, he/she was most likely to have unilateral tinnitus, while when both conditions were absent, the percentage of unilateral and bilateral tinnitus were almost the same. The study showed that the prevalence and severity of tinnitus correlate with the degree of hearing difficulty. Slight hearing difficulty most commonly goes with slight tinnitus annoyance, and no hearing at all with severe tinnitus annoyance. Figure 1-2 shows that for a given degree of tinnitus annoyance, people are more likely to have greater hearing loss across all frequencies, but particularly at high frequencies in the worse ear. There was no significant difference in the percentage of people suffering from prolonged spontaneous tinnitus or severe tinnitus between conductive, mixed, and sensorineural types of impairment.

Similar results were reported by Brown (1990). He found that the prevalence of tinnitus is associated with the degree of hearing loss, and this association increases the more high frequencies hearing threshold increases or when hearing loss is asymmetrical, although in case of asymmetrical hearing loss, the difference in the means across frequencies is small, but consistent. Among the elderly, persons with impaired hearing report tinnitus prevalence rates about three

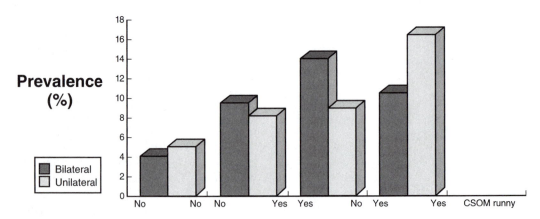

Figure 1-1. Prevalence of Prolonged Spontaneous Tinnitus, as a function of chronic suppurtive otitis media and history of runny ears (e.g., No, No indicates 'No' CSOM and 'No' runny ears)

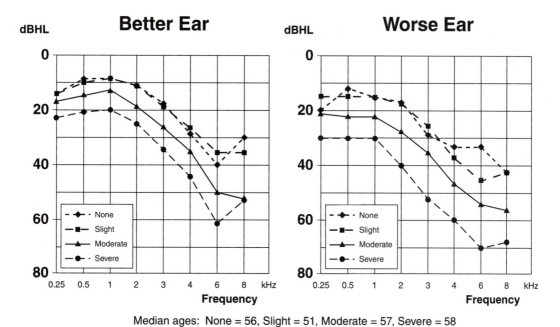

FIGURE 1-2. Median hearing threshold level as a function of prolonged spontaneous tinnitus annoyance

times those reported by people without hearing impairment up to seventy-five years of age, when the gap narrows. Axelsson and Ringdahl (1989) data showed that only 28 percent of patients considered their hearing normal when they "often" complained of tinnitus, and only 19 percent among those patients "always" complain from tinnitus. They concluded that a relationship between subjective hearing loss and tinnitus exists, with tinnitus being more common and more severe in cases with hearing loss than in those without.

Stouffer and Tyler (1990) found that the most frequent etiological factor in their study was "unknown," with noise-induced hearing loss being the second most frequent. With regard to the severity and annoyance, patients with Ménière's disease showed the greater severity of tinnitus than any other etiological group. This data supports the clinical hypothesis that "Whatever caused the hearing loss, most probably caused the tinnitus too," but the role of the central auditory nervous system in perceiving, and sometimes generating tinnitus can

not be overlooked, even if most of the times peripheral disorder is present (Coles, 1995). One of the physiological evidences of a central site of lesion is the absence of any dramatic increase or decrease in the spontaneous activity of auditory nerve fibers after administration of agents that produce tinnitus in animal models. Also the ineffectiveness of auditory nerve sectioning in reducing tinnitus and the retrograde auditory nerve degeneration observed after peripheral auditory pathology and its effect on the cochlear nucleus cells are further evidences (Tyler, 1981). A considerable dose-response effect between the presence of small air-bone gap and tinnitus was reported by Davis (1995a), the bigger the air-bone gap, the higher the possibility of reported tinnitus for a given degree of hearing impairment. This might indicate that the prevalence of tinnitus in the adult population is related to the extent of the conductive pathology. The results also show that if a patient complains about unilateral tinnitus, it is at least twice as likely that there is the possible role of the middle ear compared to bilateral tinnitus. Figure 1-3 shows the prevalence of unilateral prolonged spontaneous tinnitus as a function of the presence or absence of air-bone gap for a given degree of hearing impairment. Further research is recommended to verify the importance of the presence of small air-bone gap in the etiology and effects of tinnitus.

Although tinnitus is related to hearing pathology most of the time, still some patients complain of tinnitus without obvious hearing loss. This is a highly important group, particularly when it comes to rehabilitation and what approach is taken. Several studies tried to explain the origin of tinnitus in those patients. Barnea et al. (1990) found that 8 percent of his tinnitus patients had within normal hearing thresholds (defined as thresholds better than or equal to 20 dB HL at each frequency examined in the range from 0.25 to 8 kHz). They used extended high frequency audiometry and brain stem response and found no obvious cochlear or central affection in comparison with the control group. Stouffer and Tyler (1990) found that the air conduction levels at 1,000 and 4,000 Hz were equal to or less than 25 dB for 18 percent of their study sample. McKee and Stephens (1992) found that otoacoustic emissions recording were worse from patients ears than a control group, judged by a numerical scale from 0 to 4 depending on the presence, strength, duration, and threshold of the waveform of the recorded emissions. They also found that neurotic personality traits were stronger in tinnitus patients with normal hearing than in the control group. This might be secondary to the otological condition, or may contribute to complaint behavior. Several studies working on the relation between spontaneous otoacoustic emissions and tinnitus found correlation in only a small number of patients (Tyler and Conrad-Armes, 1982; Penner, 1992). For further readings refer to Chapter 8. Mitchell et al. (1995) found evidence in the distortion-products otoacoustic emissions recording in a group of tinnitus sufferers with normal hearing thresholds suggesting possible damage to or loss of outer hair cells and perhaps detachment of the tectorial membrane without inner hair cells or nerve damage, while Duchamp et al. (1995) suggested possible dysfunction of medial olivo-cochlear efferent system. Further studies with larger

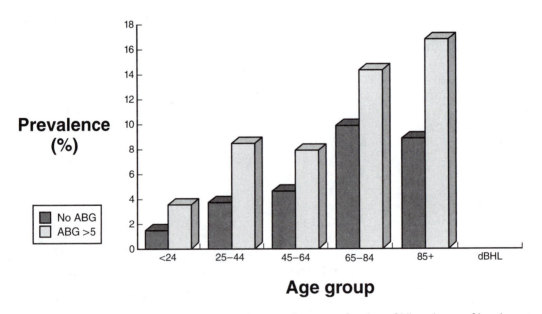

FIGURE 1-3. Unilateral prolonged spontaneous tinnitus prevalence as a function of HL and type of impairment. ABG = air-bone gap

samples are needed to establish a theory of causation, the extent of the condition, and expected benefits from different management techniques in this group of patients. Also widening the perspective of public education to reach patients with no hearing complaints is needed.

FACTORS RELATED TO THE PREVALENCE OF TINNITUS

Age

The prevalence of hearing impairment and tinnitus increases with age. Age-related changes affect the cochlear structures (Schuknecht, 1964), the cochlear nuclei, and the olivary complex (Gulya, 1991), as well as the temporal cortex (Brody, 1955). Figure 1-4 shows the prevalence of different levels of tinnitus annoyance as a function of age, with the tendency of moderate and severe annoyance to increase by age from the National Study of Hearing. In all the first three phases of the study, there was a significant increase with age in the prevalence of tinnitus, which was independent of the reported occupational noise history (Coles, 1984b). Chung (1984) also reported an increase of the incidence of tinnitus with

age, but because his population sample was from noise-exposed workers, he could not separate the age factor from noise exposure and hearing loss. Brown (1990) found the prevalence of tinnitus to increase with age, from 1.6 percent for persons eighteen to forty-four years of age to 4.9 percent for those forty-five to sixty-four and 8.9 percent for those sixty-five to seventy-four years of age. He suggested that the positive correlation is a function of the fact that both age and tinnitus are related to hearing and health variables.

Vernon and Press (1995) compared the characteristics of tinnitus in a group of elderly patients and a group of younger patients. The results showed that tinnitus pitch and loudness were lower in the elderly group and minimum masking level and residual inhibition were more favorable in the elderly group.

Gender

The effect of gender on different medical conditions is of considerable importance from the epidemiological point of view. It helps to increase our understanding of the etiology, as well as directing research and public health services to achieve maximum effectiveness. Factors related to internal

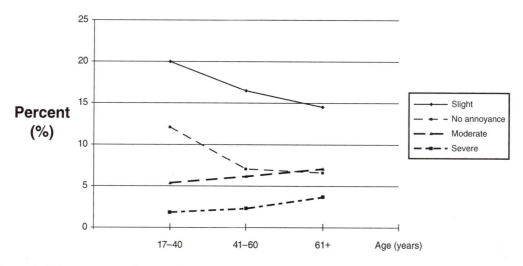

FIGURE 1-4. Annoyance as a function of age for tinnitus nowadays

physiological and anatomical differences, and external factors like occupational noise exposure and use of guns can affect the prevalence of the condition. The effect of gender on the prevalence of tinnitus was reported in several studies, after controlling for factors that might influence the prevalence of tinnitus such as age, history of noise exposure, and hearing loss.

Leske (1981) found that 30 percent of males reported tinnitus in comparison to 35 percent females. The Office of Population Census and Surveys study (1983) showed figures of 13 percent and 16 percent for males and females respectively. Chung et al (1984) did not find a significant difference and Axelsson and Ringdahl (1989) found a slight increase in the incidence of tinnitus in females compared to males under the age of fifty, but the percentage was nearly the same after fifty years of age. Stouffer and Tyler (1990) reported that 44 percent of males and 49 percent of females with tinnitus did not know what caused their tinnitus, but when noise-induced hearing loss was the cause, it constituted 30 percent of males while only 3 percent of females. Brown (1990) found that the relation of gender to the prevalence of tinnitus was not consistent. Quaranta (1996) found no significant

difference between males and females regarding the prevalence of tinnitus in his study group.

In the National Study of Hearing study, there was a small but significant trend for a higher prevalence of tinnitus among females, especially in the lower age group below forty to forty-five years of age. Davis (1983b) reported a much higher proportion of females complaining of tinnitus that was severely annoying or that interfered with going to sleep, which is in agreement with the results of Leske. Table 1-6 shows data from four studies about the effect of gender on the prevalence of tinnitus.

An interesting work by Gurr et al. (1993) studied the effect of the premenstrual period and pregnancy on tinnitus. They found a significant increase in the prevalence of tinnitus in pregnant women as compared with an age-matched nonpregnant control group, after excluding otological conditions. They hypothesized that it could be due to an increase in perilymphatic fluid pressure brought on by fluid retention due to hormonal changes during pregnancy, which is in agreement with a previous study by Reid et al. (1993). The later study found that the presence of tinnitus in young women is associated with an increased inner ear

Table 1-6. Data on gender difference in the prevalence of tinnitus from four studies

Study	Population	Number	Percent Tinnitus	
			Male	Female
Leske (1981)	Civilian non-institutionalized population	6,672	29.7	34.9
Office of Population Census and Survey (1983)	Sample of population in private households, United Kingdom	23,000	13	16
Chung et al. (1984)	Noise-exposed workers in the United Kingdom	30,000	6.6	5.6
National Study of Hearing Phase II 1981–1982. Davis (1995)	Random sample of adults in four big cities in the United Kingdom.	7,645	10.2	11.0

pressure, and was exacerbated in the premenstrual period. The other hypothesis is that the hyperdynamic circulatory changes cause venous hum and objective tinnitus.

In conclusion, it is clear that the effect of gender on the prevalence of tinnitus is inconsistent although many studies have shown females to be slightly more affected by tinnitus, but not reaching statistically significant values. More research is needed to verify the existence of a relation between tinnitus and pregnancy and hormonal changes during the premenstrual period.

Socioeconomic and Occupational Group

The effect of socioeconomic and occupational group on the epidemiology of tinnitus arises from the fact that it is a factor in the causation, as well as in perceiving the resulting handicap and effect on the quality of life. Factors other than noise exposure, like the stressful nature of some occupations, can contribute to tinnitus causation, increase the severity of existing tinnitus, and hinder coping mechanisms. This is possibly through its effect on the autonomic nervous system (Dauman and Tyler, 1992).

The National Study of Hearing showed a rise in the prevalence of tinnitus from the professional classes to the unskilled classes, which was fairly consistent during all the phases of the study. The fact that the male data in the groups where noise exposure is maximum do not climb to meet the female data suggests that the socioeconomic status conveys information about tinnitus additional to that of noise exposure (Coles, 1984b; Davis, 1983a).

Brown (1990) found that persons not in the labor force are more likely to report tinnitus than those who are, and this relation is clear and constant. He suggested that this association does not imply that nonparticipation causes tinnitus but the opposite. Most of the elderly population are outside the labor force and tinnitus may force some

to leave earlier than they otherwise would have, with obvious economic implications.

The Site of Tinnitus— Right Ear versus Left Ear

The comparison between left and right ears regarding the prevalence of tinnitus has been the focal point for several studies. The difference in the anatomical and physiological structures of the right and left central nervous system, as well as asymmetric noise exposure from gun shooting or occupational noise could suggest a cause. Hazell et al. (1981) reported that tinnitus affected the left ear more commonly than the right. Coles (1984b) reported marginal greater prevalence of tinnitus in the left ear in the pilot phase of the National Study of Hearing. He suggested that this could be mediated by handiness, but it becomes an insignificant factor after controlling for age further in the study, as handiness was found to be age dependent, with more people using the left hand in writing in the younger age group. Figure 1-5 shows the prevalence of tinnitus as a function of age, comparing prolonged spontaneous tinnitus in both ears and lateralization to one side from the National Study of Hearing. Another explanation suggested was asymmetrical noise exposure from shooting with a rifle or a shot gun, but further analysis proved it to be insignificant. It was clear that tinnitus laterality to the left increases beyond the under forty years age group, while under forty years of age, right-sided tinnitus was more prevalent in the female population, and left-sided tinnitus was more prevalent in males. Figure 1-6 shows the prevalence of prolonged spontaneous tinnitus side for left, right, and both ears as a function of the side of the better hearing ear from the National Study of Hearing. It shows that the percentage of left-sided tinnitus was greater than right-sided when the right ear threshold was better, and vice versa, while the percentage was almost equal when both ears had similar thresholds within 5 dB. In all

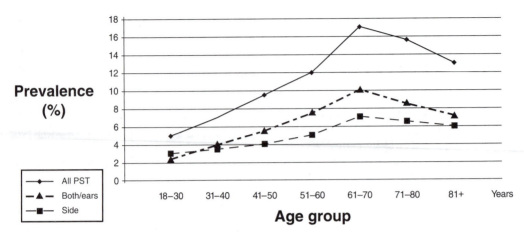

FIGURE 1-5. Prevalence of prolonged spontaneous tinnitus (PST) as a function of age and side of tinnitus

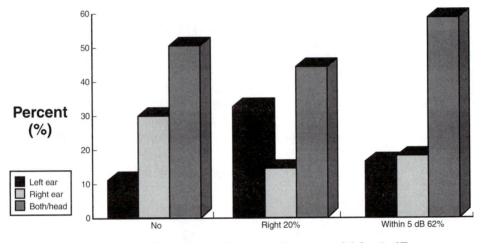

FIGURE 1-6. Prolonged spontaneous tinnitus side as a function of better ear side

situations, bilateral tinnitus or tinnitus perceived in the head was more prevalent. Stouffer and Tyler (1990) found that left ear tinnitus was more frequent than right ear in both males and females, with "left ear" as primary locus the most frequent response, followed by "both ears equally," "both ears—worse on the left side," then "right ear." Axelsson (1995) found that left-sided tinnitus was more common than right-sided, especially in females where it was the most common localization (26 percent), with right-sided tinnitus 21 percent and

bilateral tinnitus 23 percent. In males left-sided tinnitus was 21 percent, with right-sided and bilateral tinnitus at 13 percent and 31 percent respectively. The severity grading of tinnitus was considered worse for both males and females when the tinnitus was left-sided. However, Davis (1995) reported no significant differences in terms of the profile of tinnitus severity as indicated by tinnitus annoyance between left, right or bilateral tinnitus. Two point six percent of unilateral prolonged spontaneous tinnitus patients reporting moderate to severe annoyance, compared with 2.2 percent of the bilateral prolonged spontaneous tinnitus group.

The concept of left versus right ear differences needs more detailed research studies to establish a possible explanation, if a significant difference in the prevalence of tinnitus exists, whether it is related to peripheral factors, or mainly to central differences in the arrangement of the auditory cortex in both hemispheres and the neuronal pathways.

Noise

Excessive noise exposure is known to be one of the major factors that affects the auditory system at various levels, causing hearing loss and tinnitus. The increasing levels of noise pollution in our everyday life, from traffic noise to recreational noise, makes it even a more important contributor to the problem of tinnitus.

Noise is identified by its intensity, frequency spectrum and duration. It can be continuous, intermittent, fluctuating, impulsive or explosive. Pathologically, noise can lead to hair cell damage, especially the outer hair cells, through metabolic exhaustion or mechanical detachment from the basilar membrane. Biochemical changes in the cochlea and damage to the auditory nerve and central auditory system are also implicated. For more details refer to Alberti (1997) and Melnick (1996).

The National Study of Hearing found that noise is an important factor in tinnitus prevalence, although this importance is statistically marginalized by the limited number of people with large exposure to noise to be found in a random sample of the population, and the interaction of the age factor. Nevertheless, it was found that tinnitus prevalence was 7.5 percent in people with little or no noise exposure, compared to 20.7 percent for people with high lifetime noise exposure. Similar figures were obtained for shooting guns, people with little or no exposure to guns had a prevalence of 8.1 percent, while those who were exposed regularly to gun shots had a prevalence of 13.5 percent (Coles, 1995).

Axelsson, (1995) reported the results of a study involving 478 tinnitus patients relating the severity of tinnitus to different etiological factors. He found that noise-induced hearing loss was the main etiological factor, 37.8 percent of the study group with tinnitus. Patients who had never been exposed to occupational noise reported a mean severity grading of 22 points out of a maximum of 44 points, while those with a history of occupational noise exposure graded their tinnitus at 28 to 29 points.

The prevalence of tinnitus in noise-exposed workers was reported to be 58 percent by Alberti (1987), 17 to 20 percent by Griest (1995), and 6.6 percent after excluding those with hearing loss by Chung (1984). The prevalence will depend largely on the age of the study group, the degree of hearing loss, the detailed history of noise exposure and other factors like seeking compensation and change of work atmosphere.

It is clear from the previous studies that noise is a major factor affecting the prevalence of tinnitus, and noise must have a big role in determining priorities for public health resources.

Smoking

Experimental work on animals showed that nicotine can have degenerative effects on the cochlear structures. Maffei and Miani (1962) showed degeneration of the neuroepithelium in the cochlea of chronically intoxicated guinea pig. Zelman (1973) found an increase in the incidence of hearing loss among smokers than nonsmokers, especially in the high frequencies. The direct correlation between smoking and tinnitus, if any, still need to be studied on a larger sample of the population.

Coffee

Very little is written about the effect of coffee on the auditory system. Brown et al. (1981) categorized caffeine as a central nervous system stimulant with the potential of causing tinnitus without affecting the hearing status through its effect on biogenic amines. Kemp and George (1992) found no significant association between drinking coffee and any change in the nature of existing tinnitus. The role of caffeine, if any, is still unclear and further studies are required to clarify it.

Alcohol

Alcohol, if ingested in sufficient amounts, has the ability to cause an intracellular hyperosmolar state, owing to its low molecular weight and its accessibility to intracellular compartment, thus its potential to cause dysfunction (Robinson et al., 1971).

Quick (1973) considered alcohol as an ototoxic drug with the ability to cause structural damage to the inner ear. Spitzer and Ventry (1980) found a central auditory dysfunction at the level of the brain stem in patients with chronic alcoholism, but no effect on peripheral hearing. The data from studies on the effect of alcohol on tinnitus are contradictory and insufficient. McFadden (1982) noted that some patients reported that alcohol, in particular red wine, worsened the perceived loudness and pitch of tinnitus temporarily. Goodey (1981) reported that alcohol consumption in large quantities increased tinnitus sensation in almost all the patients in his study group, while small number of patients experienced actual improvement by alcohol consumption. Quaranta (1996) found that alcohol is a statistically significant risk factor for tinnitus if it is consumed on a daily basis. On the other hand, Kemp and George (1992) found only one patient out of nine reported adverse effects of alcohol on his tinnitus. Ronis (1984) showed that 80 percent of his sample reported no effect of alcohol on their tinnitus, 6 percent reported worsening and 13 percent said alcohol consumption improved their tinnitus. Pugh et al. (1995) found that 62 percent of his sample claimed that alcohol had no effect on their tinnitus,

22 percent reported worsening, and 16 percent improvement of their tinnitus. The question if alcohol consumption might have a direct effect on tinnitus, apart from the pathological central changes associated with chronic alcoholism, is still unclear.

TINNITUS IN CHILDREN

Tinnitus affecting children has been an underestimated problem for a long time. Teachers of the deaf and pediatricians accepted that "deaf children do not get tinnitus." Coles (1997) suggested some factors to explain why the problem was not apparent:

1. Children might consider tinnitus as "normal" if it is present since early in life.
2. Children are less prone to the anxiety suffered by adults regarding the medical implications.
3. Their complaints might be ignored by adults.

Although Nodar and LeZak (1984) concluded that for children tinnitus does not seem to have the debilitating effect it has on adults, many other reports suggest otherwise. Graham (1981a) found that the degree of annoyance was considered disturbing in 40 percent of children, causing confusion on audiometry, reluctance to wear hearing aids, and disturbance in coordination and behavior. Gabriels (1995) found that 42 percent of her sample suffered from sleep disturbance, 47 percent from concentration problems, and 33 percent reported sensitivity to sound from the direction of the ear affected by tinnitus. The earliest study concerned with the incidence of tinnitus in children was that by Nodar (1972). He examined all the children in grades 5 through 12 in three school systems in rural New York state between 1969 and 1972. Among the 2,000 children examined, the incidence of tinnitus was almost stable around 15 percent. Thirteen point three percent of children passing successfully the audiometric screen test complained of tinnitus, while 58.6 percent complained of tinnitus among children failing the test. The peak incidence was between thirteen and fifteen years of age.

Mills et al. (1986) reported an incidence of 29 percent in a smaller sample of healthy schoolchildren aged from five to sixteen years (9.6 percent found their tinnitus troublesome), compared to an incidence of 38.5 percent among a group of children of the same age with otological complaints. Graham (1981a), found an incidence of 49 percent of tinnitus among children attending partial hearing units and schools for the deaf, with only two children out of seventy-eight having continuous tinnitus, the rest having intermittent tinnitus. Forty-six percent complaining of accompanying dizziness, 23 percent of headache, and 73 percent of some degree of annoyance ranging between slight and always.

Mills and Cherry (1984) reported an incidence of 43.9 percent among a group of children with secretory otitis media, and 29.5 percent in children with sensorineural hearing loss. Stouffer et al. (1992) suggested that these figures might be a little bit exaggerated, a result of insufficiently clear questions or less rigorous study, they observed incidence figures of 24 to 29 percent among hearing-impaired children.

Martin and Snashall (1994) tried to follow the natural history of sixty-seven children complaining of tinnitus. Age of onset varied between infancy and sixteen years of age. 50 percent of those with tinnitus had normal hearing, with no specific relation to type or degree of hearing loss in the other 50 percent with hearing loss. Intermittent tinnitus was associated more with hearing loss, while continuous tinnitus was associated with normal hearing. Headache and dizziness were common associations. Twelve percent of the children reported disappearance of tinnitus during the study.

It is clear that tinnitus can be a common and serious problem in children. This has implications on the educational and social development of children warranting more research on how the problem is best tackled, and the availability of services for affected children. (For more reading, refer to Chapter 10).

IMPLICATIONS OF EPIDEMIOLOGICAL STUDIES

In order to establish a public health priority for tinnitus patients, four major elements are needed:

1. The prevalence of tinnitus in the appropriate population.
2. An understanding of the causes, risk factors, and the natural history.
3. A knowledge of the effects of tinnitus and how they compare with the effects of other chronic conditions.
4. A knowledge of which treatments and regimes are beneficial and cost-effective.

Understanding the natural history of tinnitus is of great importance. The first thing on the patient's mind, after being reassured about the cause of tinnitus, is how it will progress. Is it curable? Will it become worse in time? The lack of definite data from research until now tend to make these questions dependent on the clinician's personal experience of patients and general trends of the natural history of tinnitus.

Tyler and Baker (1983) found that tinnitus was associated with hearing difficulties in 53 percent of their study group and the severity of complaints decreased over time. Tinnitus had an effect on the lifestyle of 93 percent, an effect on general health in 56 percent and an effect on the emotional status in 70 percent of the study group. Hallam et al. (1984) proposed a habituation model for the effects of tinnitus on the patient, depending on epidemiological and clinical evidence that most of the people experiencing tinnitus do not complain about it. Also the annoyance from tinnitus tends to decrease over time and there is a lack of a relationship between complaint and the perceived loudness of tinnitus. The

National Study of Hearing results support the habituation model. Figures 1-7 and 1-8 show the natural history of tinnitus from onset to middle, and from middle to recent time. It shows the change over time of loudness and annoyance of tinnitus in both stages. In the first stage, loudness is mostly unchanged, but it increases in almost 26 percent of patients. Annoyance decreases in 31 percent of patients, and increases in only

9 percent. In the second stage, the figures are almost the same as the first stage for the loudness, with a slightly higher percentage decreasing, and for annoyance, the percentage decreasing falls to 10 percent.

The study concluded that tinnitus comes on suddenly. It subsequently alters little in loudness, although almost a third (28 percent) of the study sample for whom tinnitus came gradually tend to go on increasing in

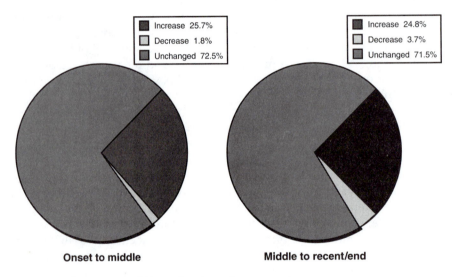

■ Increase 25.7%	■ Increase 24.8%
□ Decrease 1.8%	□ Decrease 3.7%
■ Unchanged 72.5%	■ Unchanged 71.5%

Onset to middle   **Middle to recent/end**

FIGURE 1-7. Tinnitus natural history, Loudness change over time

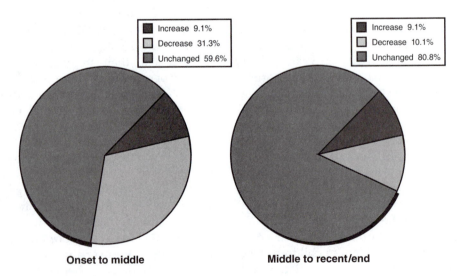

■ Increase 9.1%	■ Increase 9.1%
□ Decrease 31.3%	□ Decrease 10.1%
■ Unchanged 59.6%	■ Unchanged 80.8%

Onset to middle   **Middle to recent/end**

FIGURE 1-8. Tinnitus natural history, Annoyance change over time

loudness. On the other hand, there may be a slight tendency towards reduction of annoyance after the onset period, although there is little change after that. However, Stouffer and Tyler (1990) found that in two thirds of patients, tinnitus severity does not change, and when changes, severity usually increases.

It is becoming increasingly important to try to quantify the impact of particular condition on people's lives, and the potential gain from health care provision. Davis and Roberts (1995) studied the quality of life of tinnitus sufferers, using data from the Trent Life Style Survey (Roberts et al., 1995), the Glasgow and Manchester survey of hearing disability, and the Nottingham study of hearing in young adults. Figure 1-9 shows the prevalence of effect on quality of life as a function of tinnitus annoyance, from phase II of the National Study of Hearing. It shows that the more severe the annoyance from tinnitus, the more effect it had on the quality of life of the patient. Using a general outcome indicator, the study showed that tinnitus bears a significant effect on each subscale of the quality of life (general health, perception, physical function, social function, mental health, body pain, and energy and vitality), progressing from a

small effect for those reporting tinnitus some of the time, to much greater effects for those having tinnitus most of the time.

Patients complaining of tinnitus most of the time, or with severely annoying tinnitus have the least difference on health perception. It was also found that there is a significant and substantially raised risk of reported accidents among those who report tinnitus. For the 3 to 4 percent of people for whom tinnitus is a substantial problem, there is a substantial associated effect on general quality of life that may be mediated by the tinnitus, co-occurring pathology, or by a more general response bias.

COUNSELING IMPLICATIONS

Counseling is giving information, advice and support, to guide the opinion, attitude, and behavior of the patient (Hodgson, 1996). Epidemiological data are essential for the counselor to achieve these goals. Stouffer et al. (1991) recommended that three aspects of epidemiological data should be included in tinnitus counseling: conditions that affect severity, differences in tinnitus symptoms by etiology, and characteristics of tinnitus as a function of time since onset.

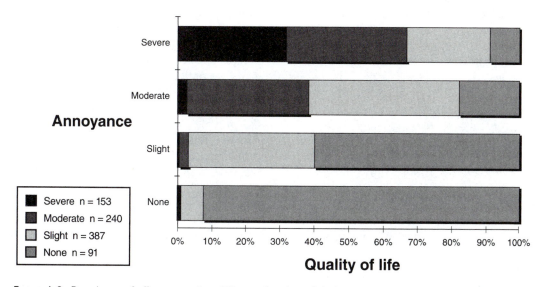

FIGURE 1-9. Prevalence of effect on quality of life as a function of tinnitus annoyance

It is beneficial in the beginning to alleviate a patient's fear that tinnitus is the symptom of a more dangerous condition, for example, a brain tumor. Patients often ask whether their tinnitus will improve or get worse. A realistic explanation, depending on the epidemiological data, must be given, which is not too bleak, but in the meantime avoiding inflating patients expectations without real base. Stouffer and Tyler (1990) found that 60 percent of their study group indicated concern that their tinnitus was a symptom of much worse disease, and 55 percent indicated that they were concerned about going deaf because of tinnitus.

Stouffer et al. (1991), in their study involving 528 tinnitus patients, proposed the following:

1. Patients need to be informed that tinnitus is a common problem most often associated with benign medical conditions.
2. Patients need to be carefully prepared for the fact that tinnitus loudness and severity may increase with time.
3. Patients can be informed that it is unlikely that tinnitus annoyance will change dramatically as a function of years since onset.
4. Have patients keep a record of activities and/or occasions when tinnitus is reduced or increased and attempt to maximize the amount of time spent in activities and/or conditions where tinnitus is reduced and minimize the amount of time spent in activities and/or conditions where tinnitus severity is increased.
5. Patients should be counseled regarding the importance and proper use of ear protection devices.
6. Because Ménière's syndrome patients experienced a louder tinnitus, more annoyance, depression and interference with sleep and speech from tinnitus than any of the other etiological groups, it is especially important to discuss tinnitus with Ménière's patients and point out ways in which other patients have successfully coped with the effects of tinnitus.

Other forms of counseling by using leaflets and through self-help groups are also additional means to provide important epidemiological information to tinnitus patients.

SUMMARY AND CONCLUSION:

It is complicated to find a single definition for tinnitus due to the obscurity of the mechanism of generation. Several classification systems can be used, depending on the cause and the effect of tinnitus on patients' lives.

Seven large studies from four different countries during the last 35 years have indicated that the prevalence of tinnitus in adults ranged between 10.1 percent and 14.5 percent for prolonged spontaneous tinnitus, and this figure can increase to 22 to 32 percent if the criteria of tinnitus includes occasional tinnitus. These figures give an impression of the magnitude of the problem we are facing and the urgency of allocating enough public health resources to manage it.

The relation between tinnitus and hearing impairment was found to be positive, with high-frequency hearing loss in the worst ear as the major predictor of tinnitus. Although hearing loss and tinnitus often originate from the same cause, tinnitus can occur in individuals without obvious peripheral hearing loss. There is a need to widen the perspective of public education to reach this group of patients outside the clinic or hospital environment.

Several factors that can have an effect on the prevalence of tinnitus were examined. Age was found to be strongly related to the prevalence of tinnitus. The effect of gender was not that clear, although some studies showed a slight increase in the proportion of females complaining of tinnitus. We explored the theory that hormonal differences might have a role. More research is needed to verify this explanation. The effect of the side of tinnitus was debatable. Although many studies showed marginal increase in the percentage of left-sided tinnitus, others did not find any significant difference.

The effect of socioeconomic and occupational group on the prevalence of tinnitus was found to be positive. Manual occupations with high noise exposure, not surprisingly, yielding higher prevalence figures, although noise was not enough to explain it all. The effect of noise on the auditory system is clearly related to the prevalence of tinnitus. Noise must have a big role in determining priorities for public health. The effect of smoking, coffee, and alcohol were discussed briefly and the data are inconclusive, partly because not enough detailed studies have addressed these aspects.

The prevalence of tinnitus in the children population was discussed. We reviewed several studies that estimated the prevalence of tinnitus in children around 15 to 29 percent in healthy children and up to 49 percent among children with otological problems. More services must be made available to manage affected children and help avoiding the negative effects tinnitus can have on their lives. There is a need for a more direct management plan for children with tinnitus.

The importance of understanding the natural history of tinnitus for counseling purposes can not be over emphasized. Tinnitus has an enormous impact on the patients lives and that of their families. The integration of epidemiological data into counseling is important. Patients need to be told about the causes, possible progression of the condition, and a realistic picture of the future.

REFERENCES

Alberti, P. W. (1987). Tinnitus in occupational hearing loss: Nosological aspects. *Journal of Otolaryngology*, 16, 34–35.

Alberti, P. W. (1997). Noise and the ear. In A. G. Kerr (Ed.), *Scott-Brown otolaryngology* (Vol 2, p. 11). London: Butterworth Heinemann.

Axelsson, A. (1995). Tinnitus epidemiology. In G. Reich, & J. Vernon (Eds.), *Proceedings of the Fifth International Tinnitus Seminar* (pp. 249–254). Portland, OR.: The American Tinnitus Association, .

Axelsson, A., & Ringdahl, A. (1989). Tinnitus: A study of its prevalence and characteristics. *British Journal of Audiology*, 23, 53–62.

Barnea, G., Attias, J., Gold, S., & Shahar, A. (1990). Tinnitus with normal hearing sensitivity: Extended high frequency audiometry and auditory-nerve brain stem-evoked response. *Audiology*, 29, 36–45.

Brody, H. (1955). Organization of the central cortex: Study of aging in human cerebral cortex. *Journal of Comparative Neurology*, 102, 511–556.

Brown, R. D., Penny, J. E., Henley, C. M., Hodges, K. B., Kupetz, S. A., Glenn, D. W., & Jobe, P. C. (1981). Ototoxic drugs and noise. In D. Evered & G. Lawrenson (Eds.), *Proceedings of the CIBA Foundation Symposium 85. Tinnitus* (pp. 151–165). London: Pitman.

Brown, S. C. (1990). Older Americans and tinnitus: A demographic study and chartbook. *GRI Monograph Series A*, No. 2, Johnson, R. C. and Hotto, S. A. (Eds.), Gallaudet Research Institute, Gallaudet University.

Chung, D., Gannon, R., & Mason, K. (1984). Factors affecting the prevalence of tinnitus. *Audiology*, 23, 441–452.

Coles, R. R. A. (1984a). Epidemiology of tinnitus: Prevalence. *Journal of Laryngology and Otology*, Suppl. 9, 7–15.

Coles, R. R. A. (1984b). Epidemiology of tinnitus: Demographic and clinical features. *Journal of Laryngology and Otology*, Suppl.9, 195–202.

Coles, R. R. A. (1995). Tinnitus: Epidemiology, Aetiology and Classification. In G. Reich & J. Vernon (Eds.), *Proceedings of the Fifth International Tinnitus Seminar* (pp. 25–29). Portland, OR: The American Tinnitus Association.

Coles, R. R. A. (1997). Tinnitus. In A. G. Kerr (Ed.), *Scott-Brown otolaryngology* (Vol. 2, Chap. 18). London: Butterworth Heinemann.

Coles, R. R. A., Smith, P., & Davis, A. C. (1988). The relationship between noise-induced hearing loss and tinnitus and its management. In B. Berglund, U. Berglund, J. Karlsson, & T. Lindvall (Eds.), *Noise as a public health problem* (Vol. 4).

Dauman, R., & Tyler, R. S. (1992). Some considerations on the classification of tinnitus. In J. M. Aran & R. Dauman (Eds.), *Proceedings of the Fourth International Tinnitus Seminar* (pp. 225–229). Bordeaux, France.

Davis, A. C. (1983b). Hearing disorders in the population: First phase findings of the MRC National Study of Hearing. In M.E. Lutman & M. P. Haggard (Eds.), *Hearing science and hearing disorders* (pp. 35–60). London: Academic Press.

Davis, A. C. (1989). The prevalence of hearing impairment and reported hearing disability among adults in Great Britain. *International Journal of Epidemiology, 18*(4), 911–917.

Davis, A. C. (1995). *Hearing in adults.* London: Whurr Publishers Ltd.

Davis, A. C. (1995a). The etiology of tinnitus: Risk factors for tinnitus in the UK population—A possible role for conductive pathology? In G. Reich & J. Vernon (Eds.), *Proceedings of the Fifth International Tinnitus Seminar.* (pp. 38–45). Portland, OR: The American Tinnitus Association.

Davis, A. C., & Roberts, H. (1995). Tinnitus and health status: SF-36 profile and accident prevalence. In G. Reich & J. Vernon, (Eds.), *Proceedings of the Fifth International Tinnitus Seminar* (pp. 257–265). Portland, OR: The American Tinnitus Association.

Duchamp, C., Morgon, A., & Chery-Croze, S. (1995). Data from functional investigations of tinnitus sufferers without hearing loss. In G. Reich & J. Vernon (Eds.), *Proceedings of the Fifth International Tinnitus Seminar* (pp. 266–269). Portland, OR: The American Tinnitus Association.

Fowler, E. P. (1944). Head noises in normal and in disordered ears: Significance, measurement, differentiation and treatment. *Archives of Otolaryngology, 39,* 498–503.

Gabriels, P. (1995). Children with tinnitus. In G. Reich & J. Vernon (Eds.), *Proceedings of the Fifth International Tinnitus Seminar* (pp. 270–275). Portland, OR: The American Tinnitus Association.

Goody, R. J. (1981). Drugs in the treatment of tinnitus. In D. Evered, & G. Lawrenson (Eds.), *Proceedings of the CIBA Foundation Symposium 85. Tinnitus* (pp. 263–273). London: Pitman.

Graham, J. M. (1981a). Pediatric tinnitus. *Journal of Laryngology and Otology, 95*(Suppl. 4), 117–120.

Griest, S. E., & Bishop, P. M. (1995). Evaluation of tinnitus and occupational hearing loss based on 20 years longitudinal data. In G. Reich & J. Vernon (Eds.), *Proceedings of the Fifth International Tinnitus Seminar* (pp. 381–394). Portland, OR: The American Tinnitus Association.

Gulya, J. (1991). Structural and physiological changes of the auditory and vestibular mechanisms with aging. In D. Ripich (Ed.), *Handbook of geriatric communication disorders.* Austin, TX.

Gurr, P., Owen, G., Reid, A., & Canter, R. (1993). Tinnitus in pregnancy. *Journal of Clinical Otolaryngology, 18,* 294–297.

Hallam, R. S., Rachman, S., & Hinchcliffe, R. (1984). Psychological aspects of tinnitus. In S. Rachman (Ed.), *Contributions to Medical Psychology* (Vol. 3, pp. 31–53). Oxford: Pergamon.

Hazell, J. W. P., William, G. R., & Sheldrake, J. B. (1981). Tinnitus maskers—Success and failures: A report on the state of the art. *Journal of Laryngology and Otology* (Suppl. 4), 80–87.

Hinchcliffe, R. (1961). Prevalence of the commoner ear, nose and throat conditions in the adult rural population of Great Britain. *British Journal of Preventive and Social Medicine, 15,* 128–140.

Hodgson, W. R. (1996). Audiologic counseling. In J. Katz (Ed.), *Handbook of Clinical Audiology,* (4th ed., pp. 616–623). Baltimore: Williams and Wilkins.

Kemp, S., & George, R. N. (1992). Diaries of tinnitus sufferers. *British Journal of Audiology, 26,* 381–386.

Leske, M. C. (1981). Prevalence estimates of communicative disorders in the U.S.: Language, learning and vestibular disorders. *The American Speech-Language and Hearing Association, 23,* 229–237.

Maffei, G., & Miani, P. (1962). Experimental tobacco poisoning. *Archives of Otolaryngology, 75,* 386–392.

Martin, K., & Snashall, S. (1994). Children presenting with tinnitus: A retrospective study. *British Journal of Audiology, 28*(2), 111–115.

McFadden, D. (1982). Tinnitus: Facts, theories and treatments. *Report of working group 89, Committee on Hearing Bioacoustics and Biomechanics,* Washington, DC: National Research Council National Academy Press.

McKee, G. J., & Stephens, S. D. G. (1992). An investigation of normally hearing subjects with tinnitus. *Audiology, 31,* 313–317.

Melnick, W. (1996). Industrial hearing conservation. In J. Katz (Ed.), *Handbook of Clinical Audiology.* (4th ed., pp. 534–552). Baltimore: Williams and Wilkins.

Mills, R. P., Albert, D., & Brain, C. (1986). Tinnitus in children. *Journal of Clinical Otolaryngology, 11.*

Mills, R. P., & Cherry, J. R. (1984). Subjective tinnitus in children with otological disorders. *International Journal of Pediatric Otolaryngology, 7,* 21–27.

Mitchell, C., Lilly, D., & Henry, J. (1995). Otoacoustic emissions in subjects with tinnitus and normal hearing. In G. Reich & J. Vernon (Eds.), *Proceedings of the Fifth International Tinnitus Seminar* (pp. 180–185). Portland, OR: The American Tinnitus Association.

Nodar, R. H. (1972). Tinnitus aurium in school age children. *Journal of Auditory Research, 12,* 133–135.

Nodar, R. H., & LeZak, M. H. W. (1984). Pediatric tinnitus (thesis revised). *Journal of Laryngology and Otology, 98*(Suppl. 9), 234–235.

Office of Population Census and Surveys (1983). General household survey: The prevalence of tinnitus 1981. *OPCS Monitor,* Reference GHS83/1.

Penner, M. J. (1992). Linking spontaneous otoacoustic emissions and tinnitus. *British Journal of Audiology, 26,* 115–123.

Pugh, R., Budd, R. J., & Stephens, S. D. G. (1995). Patients reports of the effect of alcohol on tinnitus. *British Journal of Audiology, 29,* 279–283.

Quaranta, A., Asennato, G., & Sallustio, V. (1996). Epidemiology of hearing problems among adults in Italy. *Scandinavian Audiology, 42* (Suppl. 25), 9–13.

Quick, C. A. (1973). Chemical and drug effects on the inner ear. In M. M. Paparella & D. A. Shumrick (Eds.), *Otolaryngology* (Vol. 2, p. 392). Philadelphia: Saunders.

Reid, A., Cottingham, C. A., & Marchbanks, R. J. (1993). The prevalence of perilymphatic hypertension in subjects with tinnitus: A pilot study. *Scandinavian Audiology, 22,* 61–63.

Roberts, H., Dengler, R., & Magowan, __. (1995). Trent health adult life style survey: 1992–1994. *Results. Department of Public Health Medicine and Epidemiology, University of Nottingham and NHS executive trent regional health authority.*

Robinson, A. G., & Loeb, J. N. (1971). Ethanol ingestion—Commonest cause of elevated plasma osmolarity? *New England Journal of Medicine, 284,* 1253–1255.

Ronis, M. L. (1984). Alcohol and dietary influences on tinnitus. *Journal of Laryngology and Otology, 98*(Suppl. 9), 242–246.

Schuknecht, H. (1964). Further observations on the pathology of presbyacusis. *Archives of Otolaryngology, 80,* 369–382.

Smith, P., & Coles, R. R. A. (1987). Epidemiology of tinnitus: An update. In H. Feldmann (Ed.), *Proceedings of the Third International Tinnitus Seminar* (pp. 147–153). Munster: Harsch Verlag Karlsruhe.

Spitzer, J. B., & Ventry, I. M. (1980). Central auditory dysfunction among chronic alcoholics. *Archives of Otolaryngology, 106,* 224–229.

Spoendlin, H. (1987). Inner ear pathology and tinnitus. In H. Feldmann (Ed.), *Proceedings of the Third International Tinnitus Seminar* (pp. 42–51). Munster: Harsch Verlag Karlsrehe.

Stephens, D., & Hetu, R. (1991). Impairment, disability and handicap in Audiology: Towards a consensus. *Audiology, 30,* 185–200.

Stouffer, J. L., & Tyler, R. S. (1990). Characterization of tinnitus by tinnitus patients. *Journal of Speech and Hearing Disorders, 55,* 439–453.

Stouffer, J. L., Tyler, R. S., Booth, J. C., & Buckrell, B. (1992). Tinnitus in normal hearing and hearing impaired children. In J. M. Aran & R. Dauman (Eds.), *Proceedings of the Fourth International Tinnitus Seminar* (pp. 255–258). Bordeaux, France.

Stouffer, J. L., Tyler, R. S., Kinley, P. R., & Dalzell, L. E. (1991). Tinnitus as a function of duration and etiology: Counseling implications. *The American Journal of Otology, 12* (3), 188–194.

Tyler, R. S. (1981). Animal models of tinnitus—Discussion. In *Proceedings of the CIBA Foundation Symposium 85. Tinnitus.* D. Evered (Ed.), London: Pitman, 136.

Tyler, R. S., & Baker, L. J. (1983). Difficulties experienced by tinnitus sufferers. *Journal of Speech and Hearing Disorders, 48,* 150–154.

Tyler, R. S., & Conrad-Armes, D. (1982). Spontaneous acoustic cochlear emissions and sensorineural tinnitus. *British Journal of Audiology, 16,* 193–194.

Vernon, J., & Press, L. (1995). Tinnitus in the elderly. In G. Reich & J. Vernon (Eds.), *Proceedings of the Fifth International Tinnitus Seminar* (pp. 289–297). Portland, OR: The American Tinnitus Association.

World Health Organization (WHO) (1980). International classification of impairments, disabilities, and handicaps. World Health Organization, Geneva.

Zelman, S. (1973). Correlation of smoking history with hearing loss. *Journal of the American Medical Association, 233,* 920.

CHAPTER 2

Psychological Profiles of Tinnitus Patients

Soly I. Erlandsson, Ph.D.

INTRODUCTION

The Relevance of Investigating Psychological Factors in Tinnitus Patients

Human life demands the capacity of the individual to select and sort out valuable information from the endless input of non-relevant stimuli from the surrounding environment. One example of such stimuli is the undesired, environmental noise that seems to increase in the modern world in an uncontrolled way.

Unpredictable, surrounding noise, operating without control, can easily become intrusive just like the tinnitus sound that is perceived as an internal source of aversive noise. How we react to undesired noise depends on individual differences in sensitivity (tolerance thresholds for physical and psychological stimuli) and exposure. A surprisingly strong coherence exists in the way individuals who experience a sudden onset of severe tinnitus describe their emotional reactions (Edgren-Sundin, 1993). Such descriptions are valuable material that can

give us insight into diagnostic, psychological aspects of the condition.

"A tremendous fear—that is what I remember. I was terribly afraid that it would become permanent."

"I was paralyzed with terror . . . I knew that something terrible had happened to me."

"Then the irritation concerned the fact that I, in many ways, was deprived of my freedom, that there were things that I could not do, for instance play the guitar."

"I think it is hopeless to have tinnitus, that's all. I must learn to accept it. If I could choose, I would like them to cut that piece off, but there is nothing that is physiologically wrong, they say."

"I used to sit there listening during the lecture, when it was quiet: Do I hear the sound now? I was scared of everything. If a child screamed, I became completely mad and tense in my whole body, my God, now it's getting worse."

Permanent, disabling tinnitus is a complication that often seems to resist the efforts that have been undertaken in terms of specialist treatment and handling of the patients who are in need of care. In spite of the fact that tinnitus has become an issue for interdisciplinary research and treatment teamwork, many patients continue to feel distressed and unhelped in the longer perspective. A great number of individuals with tinnitus are not going to end up as sufferers and do not become "patients" in need of professional help. This calls for refined strategies for the assessment of risk factors for prolonged distress reactions which most probably will lead to long-lasting suffering, as is the case in similar conditions, like chronic pain. Katon et al. (1993) reported improvements in patients' functional ability when depression was treated successfully.

Tinnitus has been characterized as the perception of internal noises, mainly originating involuntarily within the head, in the absence of external acoustic stimuli (Hallam, Rachman, & Hinchliffe, 1984; Chapter 1). It is a common medically defined problem most often associated with pathology of the auditory system. Besides tinnitus as a primary complaint related to different etiologies of hearing loss, tinnitus is also found in other disorders of both physiological and psychological origin. Some of them are mentioned in the following text. In medical terminology tinnitus is referred to as a *symptom,* however "symptom" is too narrow a concept and does not explain the severe affliction that in such a major way can influence the psychological health of the individual. McKenna, Hallam, and Hinchliffe (1991) reported that 45 percent of tinnitus patients, seen by a specialist at an ear, nose, and throat hospital, were diagnosed as requiring psychological treatment.

Patients for whom tinnitus becomes a chronic handicap often complain of the psychological problems that have come in the wake of the noises. They tend to mention emotional complications like irritation, annoyance, concentration and sleep difficulties, depression and despair (Tyler & Baker, 1983). These signs of psychological distress may indicate that, in addition to having tinnitus, the patient also suffers from

anxiety and depression (Sullivan et al., 1988; Collet, Moussu, Disant, Ahamai, & Morgan, 1990; Erlandsson, Rubinstein, Axelsson, & Carlsson, 1991). Beyond this, they often express disappointment over the lack of understanding they experience from others, and over the impact of their situation on their relationships to those near and dear to them. Somatic distress symptoms that patients with disabling tinnitus tend to report are headache, neck pain, temporomandibular problems (pain and tension in jaw muscles), dizziness, and hypersensitivity to sounds (Rubinstein & Erlandsson, 1991; Erlandsson, Hallberg, & Axelsson, 1992; Dineen, Doyle, & Bench, 1997). The different aspects of difficulties related to tinnitus are summarized in the following.

Emotional distress	Interpersonal complications	Somatic distress symptoms
irritation, annoyance, concentration and sleep difficulties, depression and despair	lack of understanding, negative impact on relationships (relatives, friends, colleagues)	headache, neck pain, pain/tension in jaw muscles, dizziness, hypersensitivity to sounds

In order to gain a thorough description, we need to conduct a relatively deep interview based on knowledge of personality factors seen from an interactionistic perspective. Trigger factors and external circumstances coinciding with the suffering need also to be considered. Hence it is not sufficient to make a medical examination of the patients' ears or to do an audiological test of their hearing and to measure the loudness and pitch of tinnitus. Most patients with annoying tinnitus who make an appointment at a medical or audiological department do so because they are uncertain about their symptoms—they do not know why their ears have started buzzing. The explanation that it is related to a hearing impairment seldom satisfies the anxious patient. He or she needs professional help in understanding the perceived distress, needs to be comforted and assured that there is hope for improvement.

Since chronic, disabling tinnitus seldom can be treated so successfully that it disappears entirely, somehow the individual will have to "learn to live with the noises." This kind of adaptation may be facilitated by the patient learning to process the thoughts and feelings that arise as reactions to tinnitus. It may be a long, demanding course of action, particularly for those who are already encumbered with psychological shortcomings. There is a great deal of clinical evidence that indicates that personality is an important factor in determining how the process of adaptation develops and how critical the situation will become. In the last two decades a large proportion of research contributions on tinnitus has focused on its relation to personality and psychopathology (House, 1981; Singerman, Riedner, & Folstein, 1980; Wood, Webb, Orschik, & Shea, 1983; Reich, & Johnson, 1984; Stephens, & Hallam, 1985; Harrop-Griffith, Katon, Dobie, Sakai, & Russo, 1987; Simpson, Nedzelski, Barber, & Thomas, 1988; Collet, Moussu, Disant, Ahamai, & Morgan, 1990; Halford &

Anderson, 1991; Erlandsson & Persson, 1996) and tinnitus severity; that is, the impact on the day-to-day living of the patients, including psychological distress symptoms, handicap and perceived social support (Hallam, Jakes, & Hinchcliffe, 1988; Kuk, Tyler, Russel, & Jordan, 1990; Wilson, Henry, Bowen, & Haralambous, 1991; Erlandsson et al., 1992; Hiller & Goebel, 1992; Budd & Pugh, 1996). It is clear that different perspectives are needed.

Comprehensive and well-defined psychological descriptors of tinnitus are a matter of great concern both for research and clinical purposes. The main issue to consider is: what do we need to know about the patients to be able to diagnose and treat them, and possibly ease their pain? We must understand the causes of the tinnitus complaint, and such causes cannot be generalized, but rather may be very different from one case to the next (see Figure 2-1). When patients seek help for distressing inner noises, there are always several reasons for them to do so, even when the reason they state (and consciously perceive) is tinnitus. Most often, what we observe in the clinical context is a complex interplay

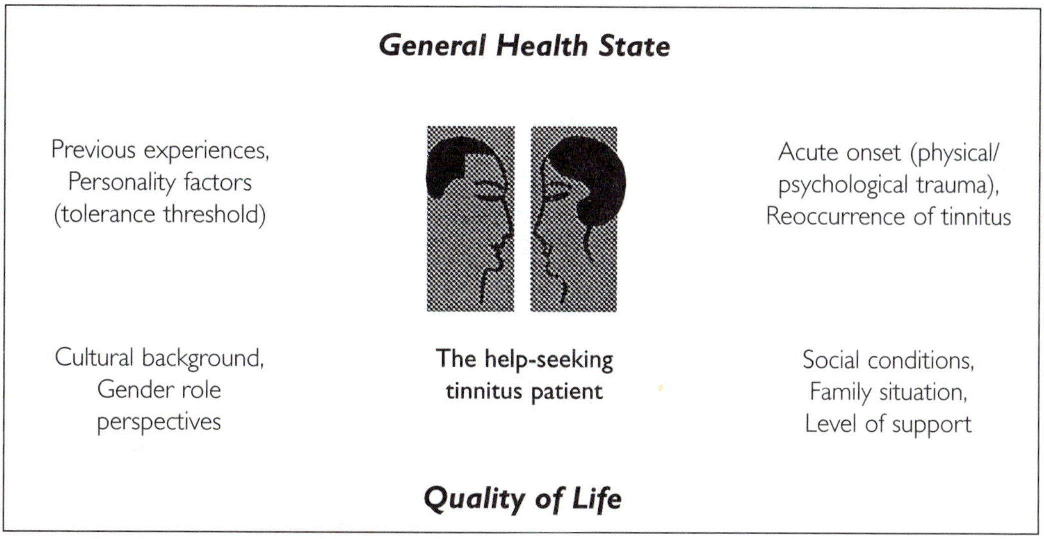

General Health State

Previous experiences,
Personality factors
(tolerance threshold)

Acute onset (physical/
psychological trauma),
Reoccurrence of tinnitus

Cultural background,
Gender role
perspectives

**The help-seeking
tinnitus patient**

Social conditions,
Family situation,
Level of support

Quality of Life

FIGURE 2-1. Interactional causality factors of hypothetical importance for the experience of tinnitus, its onset and reoccurrence.

between the suffering of the patient, the original physical damage (in some cases), previous experiences, gender, the family situation, and cultural background.

There are a number of reports in the older literature attempting to describe and classify signs and symptoms of tinnitus according to a medical regimen with well-defined categories (Jones & Knudsen, 1928; Kafka, 1934; Fowler, 1940; Goodhill, 1952). These models were serious attempts to come to grips with the bothered patients. However, as research and clinical management develop further, new models take form, and more distinctively, it can be of value to bring different research positions together in order to gain a collected view of the difficulties encountered by the tinnitus patients. An obstacle that most often occurs in looking at the fact from more than one frame of reference is that different value systems and schools of thought make it difficult to share and to come to a joint discussion of the problem. The aim of this communication is to approach tinnitus from an eclectic viewpoint and to integrate different lines of thought into a psychological frame of reference.

Getting Beyond the Initial Reaction of Crisis

An individual with tinnitus can spontaneously become totally free from symptoms, but among those who have sought help, this is uncommon. We do not know what the situation is like for individuals who are distressed by tinnitus but who never seek help. Rubinstein (1993) pointed to the limited knowledge of the natural history of tinnitus and to the fact that there exists a great risk for a pessimistic bias concerning the prognosis. Too few studies have focused on the natural course of tinnitus, including the incidence of spontaneous remission of the symptoms. An exaggerated focus on tinnitus as an uncurable disorder seems to be the most common opinion among clinicians. Such a negative bias being forwarded by the professional to his

or her patient may contribute to the patient's view on tinnitus as the worst possible threat that can occur.

Retrospective population studies have pointed to a more favorable developmental course for tinnitus in nonclinical samples. Smith and Coles (1987) argued that the general pattern of severity of tinnitus is likely to decrease gradually soon after the period of onset. Rubinstein, Österberg, Rosenhall, and Johansson (1993) highlighted the importance of studying tinnitus with a longitudinal design of research in order to discover possible fluctuations in tinnitus occurrence and distress. The authors investigated the prevalence of tinnitus in a subsample of a cohort at the age of seventy years and the assessments were repeated when the subjects were seventy-five and seventy-nine years of age. The reports were studied longitudinally at the individual level. There was an increase of tinnitus onset between the ages of seventy and seventy-nine years and remissions seemed to be more frequent than has been assumed in the past.

To suddenly perceive that a persistent sound is located in your ear or in your head can give rise to great concern and worry, which in most cases is a normal reaction. There is, however, a risk that the individual gets stuck in the situation of being overconcerned before tinnitus becomes something that is perceived as more acceptable. When emotional reactions following the event do not seem to be in proportion to the releasing factor, they have to be interpreted from the viewpoint of the individual's earlier experiences in life and his or her personality. A traumatic crisis has been defined by Cullberg (1984; pp. 28) as:

> The individual's mental response and adaptation to an external event of such a sort and degree that the individual experiences his or her physical existence, social identity, security or other goals in life, to be seriously threatened.
>
> (Quotation translated from Swedish by Erlandsson.)

In a qualitative study of tinnitus seen from the process of a traumatic crisis, the participating subjects experienced that they needed to grieve over the loss of silence (Edgren-Sundin, 1993). Instead of silence they had to listen to an annoying, always present tinnitus sound. Several of the participants had been under an increased level of distress before the onset of tinnitus, which was likely to further weaken the mechanisms of defense against anxiety when tinnitus occurred. The situation described is not an unusual chain of events, quite the opposite; it is rather normal to react with regret and sorrow after a sudden onset of tinnitus. However, in those instances in which the traumatic crisis is prolonged and tinnitus becomes chronically distressing, the clinician has to take a stand concerning whether the patient is in need of psychotherapeutic treatment or not.

Gender Aspects of the Subjective Experience of Tinnitus

Gender as an explanatory factor in research of disease, etiology and illness behavior has in the past largely been ignored, however, this state of affairs is rapidly changing. Studies focusing on gender both for descriptions of complaints and reasons for help-seeking are much needed (Unger & Crawford, 1996). The role of gender for the subjective experience of tinnitus remains somewhat untouched as a topic of research. Some research work has, obviously for demanding and/or for practical reasons, mainly focused on the male subject with noise-induced hearing loss. There are some examples in the literature on tinnitus where studies investigating psychological profiles have included male patients only. Using the male as the norm without considering aspects of gender, or even mentioning that a gender difference might exist, limits the conclusions that can be drawn from these data.

In speaking with patients who are distressed by tinnitus, it is essential to try to focus on relevant gender-related factors. The life situation and the gender roles of women are different from those of men, and this affects the divergent ways in which women and men manage an illness. Therefore, it is necessary to obtain a gender perspective in the clinical context. The following examples of possible scenarios are impressions gathered in interviews of female and male sufferers. When a woman seeking help for her tinnitus describes her situation, the listener may detect some of the particular causes of the chronic nature of her problem from her story. The everyday lives of women, in today's society, contain a number of stress factors that tend to be very different from those in men's lives. A female patient suffering from chronic tinnitus may be a woman who has spent her entire life doing things for other people, and who for different reasons no longer can maintain that role. Professional women are often torn between their role as a good spouse and parent and their career (Frankenhaeuser et al., 1989). If such conflicts endure in a woman's life, they may cause her to develop a distance to her deeper feelings and needs which will, however, express themselves sooner or later as covert emotional stress, exhaustion, and unhappiness. Forbidden thoughts and feelings surface, and are repressed at the expense of anxiety and increasing irritation.

Men, in contrast, may find it difficult to face their potential emotional problems directly and constructively, and may have insufficient social networks. They tend to seek help when they have been afflicted with some physical, stress-related illness: high blood pressure, heart disease, or depressed mood manifested in alcohol dependence, and so on. Somehow, they may feel that they are over the hill (a midlife crisis), and the demands on them to renew their outlook on life feel insurmountable. Scicchitano, Lovell, Pearce, Marley, and Pilowsky (1996) showed that male somatizing patients (somatic symptoms for which no organic cause could be established), compared with male nonsomatizing patients (somatic complaints for which an organic cause could be established), were characterized by more signs of affective illness, more acknowledged life stressors and that they were more strongly convinced that they had a physical illness. It was suggested by the authors that although the male somatizer may acknowledge the existence of personal difficulties he does not associate such psychological disturbances with his physical symptoms.

The work situation may be a triggering factor for both men and women; the threat of losing one's job because of a noisy workplace that is a risk factor for a gradual deterioration of hearing and a more intense tinnitus, or of having to do new things at work because of financial cutbacks. But men, in contrast to women, may have difficulties communicating their worries and fears of not being able to compete professionally. Hallberg, Erlandsson, and Carlsson (1992) investigated perceived tinnitus severity and patterns of coping in male patients with noise-induced hearing loss. They found that men with severe tinnitus significantly more often engaged in "escape coping" (for example, wishful thinking, taking drugs and drinking alcohol to make them feel better) than did males with equal hearing status but without tinnitus or with a milder form of tinnitus.

It is a common observation that males tend to ignore their psychological ill-health more than females, and that they are more unlikely to report distress on psychometric scales. However, the frequency of personality disturbances has been found to be higher in male patients than in females (Horwitz & White, 1987). Dineen et al. (1997) demonstrated that female subjects, included in their investigation, reported a higher level of emotional reaction to their tinnitus as measured by the Tinnitus Reaction Questionnaire (Wilson et al., 1991) and by the depression subscale of the Derogatis Stress Profile (Derogatis, 1987). The profile of tinnitus-related distress was somewhat different in the male patients whose stress was more related to personality than emotion related, as was the case with the women. But there were no gender differences in the total scores of the Derogatis Stress Profile,

neither in degree of environmental stress reported nor in problems with neck pain, back pain, jaw pain, and headaches. Female patients in the study by Dineen et al. (1997) also reported more balance problems, an observation that is in accordance with that of Erlandsson et al. (1992).

One reason for studying the quality aspects of tinnitus is that the subjective experience of the sound in the tinnitus sufferer is expected to be colored by emotional factors. A difference in the perceived quality of the tinnitus sound has been observed between men and women. Women more often than men seem to complain about complex tinnitus, that is, a greater variety of the sounds (Meikle & Griest, 1987). The findings were replicated by Dineen et al. (1997) who also observed that females were more likely to report emotional reactions to their tinnitus than males. Hallberg and Erlandsson (1993) noted a contradictory, but nonsignificant difference; that is, complex tinnitus was more prevalent in males than in females. An explanation to the diverse results of the studies mentioned may be that the patients included are different in ways related to tinnitus etiology and mental state.

Summary

Some patients may be able to overcome the crisis on their own, with the help of family and friends, while others are in need of a great deal of professional, psychological support to be able to perceive tinnitus as something natural and acceptable. For those who are accustomed to solving their own problems, it may be an insurmountable task to seek help at all. It is never satisfying when someone seeking help for a sudden onset of tinnitus is left to complete the process of adaptation on his or her own, unless this is the person's request. According to the literature on tinnitus a great number of help-seeking patients have been found to require psychological treatment.

Studies focusing on gender for descriptions of complaints and reasons for help-seeking, will lead to a more precise risk model of vulnerability. There seems to be a gender difference in the frequency of personality disturbances among chronic tinnitus sufferers; the rate is higher in male patients than in females. Men are less likely to report distress on psychometric scales and they tend to ignore their psychological ill-health more than women. It has been reported that women more often than men complain about complex tinnitus, that is, a greater variety of the sounds. If and how the complexity of the sounds is linked to fluctuations of mood and general psychopathology are inquiries considered for further examination.

DIMENSIONAL ASPECTS OF TINNITUS COMPLAINTS

Tinnitus Distress Symptoms in Different Patient Groups Seeking Medical Consultation

The character of the symptomatology of tinnitus can vary between different groups of patients partly due to etiological factors. Tinnitus related to Ménière's disorder seems, for example, to be of a special character; the sound is often of a low pitch (Stouffer & Tyler, 1990). Nodar and Graham (1965) suggested that the type of physiological mechanism that produces the tinnitus associated with Ménière's disease is of another kind than the tinnitus associated with sensory-neural hearing loss. In comparison with nausea and vertigo attacks, tinnitus generally gives rise to less anxiety and worry in this patient group. They soon will learn that tinnitus is a part of the disorder and this may give them a satisfactory explanation and ease their aversive reactions. Ménière-related tinnitus was reported to be fluctuating and at times disturbing by patients participating in focus group interviews (Erlandsson, Eriksson-Mangold, & Wiberg, 1996). Patients with Ménière's disease who felt worried and depressed by the course of their condition, found tinnitus intolerable as it was also a sign of an acute

incidence of vertigo and a reminder of the chronic character of the disorder.

The prevalence of frequent headaches and fatigue/tenderness in jaw muscles was found to be higher in tinnitus patients than in epidemiological samples (Rubinstein, 1993). Approximately one-third of patients with symptoms of craniomandibular disorders had noticed influence on tinnitus of pressure or movements of the temporomandibular joint. Rubinstein (ibid) argued that the relationship between tinnitus complaints and craniomandibular symptoms, including frequent headache, seems to be independent of the degree of hearing loss, occupational noise exposure, general morbidity, medication, and socioeconomic status. Frequent headaches are a common complaint in patients with tinnitus. A prevalence, ranging from 23 percent to 77 percent, has been reported from several studies (Hazell, 1981; Lindberg, Lyttkens, Melin, & Scott, 1984; Rubinstein, Axelsson, & Carlsson, 1990; Erlandsson et al., 1992). In states of anxiety and stress, the tensor tympani muscle reacts with increased activity and contracts reflexively during talking and jaw clenching. The increased activity in the masticatory muscles might increase or even cause the perception of tinnitus (Rubinstein, 1993). Vernon, Griest, and Press (1992) found that 13 percent of patients seen at a tinnitus clinic would be able to alter their tinnitus by jaw movements. A strong relationship between tinnitus complaints and a number of symptoms of craniomandibular disorders including frequent headache has been observed in a community-based sample of elderly (Rubinstein et al., 1993).

Recently there have been attempts to describe whiplash syndrome from a comprehensive and multidisciplinary point of view. Mayou and Radanov (1996) argue that the broader perspective has the advantage of demonstrating similarities between whiplash and other conditions where psychological and social variables interact with the physical symptoms perceived as being a threat to quality of life. The list of different physical symptoms and complaints of the acute whiplash injury includes tinnitus (Chapter 17) and additionally, some of the complaints often reported by patients suffering from tinnitus: neck pain, shoulder pain, arm pain, headache, tinnitus, visual symptoms, dizziness, lower back pain, temporomandibular joint symptoms, parasthesia, memory, and concentration disturbances. According to Mayou and Sharpe (1995) approximately one-fourth of subjects with whiplash syndrome complain of suffering from consequences that seem to be clinically out of proportion. In the United States, the whiplash effect must be considered to be influenced by potential financial gain. Post-traumatic stress disorder has been suggested as a secondary diagnosis for 10 percent of whiplash sufferers describing intrusive thoughts, different symptoms of distress, anxiety, and depression. Sleep disturbances, lack of energy, and poor concentration are also found in subjects with whiplash, but there is a wide variation in outcome.

Mayou and Radanov (1996) report that many subjects with whiplash, not seen by physicians, do not make financial claims of compensation and appear to have an excellent outcome, observations in accordance with tinnitus, where the majority of individuals reporting tinnitus see it as a more or less insignificant problem. Social impairment associated with whiplash symptoms has been found to correlate with psychological outcome. It has also been possible to predict social impairment by baseline mental state and history of previous psychological distress (ibid). The authors emphasize the need for a *well-planned acute care* and assessments of possible effects on mental state and aspects of quality of life in patients with whiplash syndrome. Such clinical considerations would be of no less importance when patients are confronted with a sudden, trauma-induced tinnitus. From yet another viewpoint, the contribution of tinnitus symptoms in the distress profile of the whiplash-injured individual would be interesting to investigate, especially the comparison between tinnitus as a main and as a secondary complaint.

Tinnitus as a symptom can also be found in disorders characterized by disturbances in metabolism, as in the case of hypothyroidism and diabetes mellitus. Little is known about the typical pattern of tinnitus onset and course in these conditions. There is a high risk for women with borderline hypothyroidism to develop a depressive disorder due to their diencephalic system functioning at a lower level of efficiency (Akiskal, 1979). Primary hypothyroidism is an endocrine, rather common disease. The subclinical symptoms can mimic an affective disorder and is therefore sometimes overlooked and diagnosed as depression (Tallis, 1993). Low mood (and tinnitus) can be the only sign of a subclinical hypothyroidism. Between 8 and 14 percent of patients referred to the psychiatric clinic for depression or diagnosed as suffering from an affective disorder were found to have some degree of hypothyrodism. Examples of shared symptoms of primary hypothyroidism and depression are: Dysphoric mood (feeling depressed), loss of interest or pleasure in life, fatigue, concentration disturbances, poor memory. "Deafness" has been defined as one of the exclusive signs of primary hypothyroidism (Tallis, 1993).

Which Dimensions of Complaints are Relevant for the Study of Psychological Profiles of Tinnitus Patients?

Examining the prevalence of psychological and somatic symptoms of distress can be of relevance when considering the psychological profiles of patients with tinnitus. A number of studies using factor analytical solutions for descriptions of complaints have indicated factors such as emotional and cognitive distress, sleep disturbances, auditory perceptual difficulties, social consequences of tinnitus, perceived negative attitudes, and intrusiveness, that is, unpleasantness and loudness of the noises, inability to ignore them and to maintain concentration (Jakes, Hallam, Chambers, & Hinchcliffe,

1985; Hallam, Jakes & Hinchcliffe, 1988; Kuk et al., 1990; Sweetow & Levy, 1990; Wilson et al., 1991; Halford & Anderson, 1991; Hiller & Goebel, 1992; Erlandsson et al., 1992). For a review, see Erlandsson (1992) and Tyler (1993).

By the use of factor analyses, regarding both self-report and audiometric assessments, Jakes et al. (1985) reported two main factors of complaint (emotional distress and intrusiveness) and three specific factors (hearing difficulty, vestibular symptoms, and tinnitus intensity). A further development of the original questionnaire, named the Tinnitus Questionnaire (Hallam et al., 1988), including patients attending the neuro-otology outpatient clinic for tinnitus, resulted in new analyses that revealed a somewhat different set of factors: Mood (depression, anger, irritability, and anxiety), auditory perceptual difficulties, and insomnia. The "intrusiveness" factor was not replicated in its original form in the new study. Hiller and Goebel (1992) investigated the pattern of tinnitus complaints using a German translation of the Tinnitus Questionnaire on adult patients complaining of longstanding and annoying tinnitus seen in a psychosomatic inpatient clinic. The authors used a principal component factor analysis in order to replicate the study by Hallam et al. (1988) and found a similarity between the studies in two factors representing sleep disturbances and auditory perceptual difficulties. Additionally, they were able to define items expressing the intrusive aspects of tinnitus; that is, unpleasantness and loudness of the noises, inability to ignore them and to maintain concentration, in agreement with the previously reported observations by Jakes et al. (1985). The variance explained by the factor structure reported by Hiller and Goebel (1992), was 44.2 percent. The large amount of unexplained variance was suggested to depend on dimensions of tinnitus vulnerability not being included in the analysis.

In a psychometric, evaluative investigation, including a factor-analyzed tinnitus handicap questionnaire, three factors of the patients' responses emerged: Physical, emotional, and social consequences of tinnitus, hearing ability, and patients' view of tinnitus (Kuk et al., 1990). The study sample was heterogenous and included both patients whose primary complaint was tinnitus and patients whose tinnitus was secondary to their hearing loss. Dobie, Sullivan, Katon, Sakai, and Russo (1992) used the same questionnaire in tinnitus patients who were treated with antidepressant medication. It was observed that tinnitus sufferers who were found to be depressed had significantly higher scores on the questionnaire than the nondepressed tinnitus patients. The findings highlighted the importance of tracing both the nature of complaints and the psychological health/illness profile in those seeking help for disturbing tinnitus.

Self-focused attention and awareness of somatic sensations were used as parameters in a cluster analysis by Newman, Wharton, and Jacobson (1997) including fifty-one subjects reporting tinnitus as a primary complaint or as secondary to hearing loss. The subjects rated themselves as low and high on self-attention and somatic-attention measures. A cluster analysis yielded two subgroups of patients; "low self-attenders" and "high self-attenders." The latter group was found, on average, to be more depressed and reported greater emotional distress and greater perceived handicap than the "low self-attenders." Between-group comparisons did not show any statistically significant differences between the two clusters for either tinnitus loudness or pitch. No correlational analysis was reported of the psychometrical tests that were included in the study. The authors observed that the mean level of the Tinnitus Reaction Questionnaire used in their study was very similar to that obtained by Wilson et al. (1991).

So far, there seems to be at least *three different dimensions* of distress that the various studies of tinnitus complaint behavior can agree on. The first are mood and emotional reactions (depression, anger, irritability, and anxiety). Secondly, there is the audiological dimension, including perceptual difficulties or hearing problems giving rise to distress both at an individual level and in demanding social situations. The third dimension is somewhat more blurred. Intrusiveness, that is, the inability to ignore the noises, concentration difficulties, and so on, seems to be a more general factor in which problems with sleep as well as patients' perceived attitudes and view on tinnitus can be included. Underneath the different aspects of intrusiveness, described, we may find a profile of personality characteristics in interaction with critical social circumstances. The three dimensions of tinnitus complaint behavior: emotional, audiological, and intrusiveness, are examplified in the following.

Emotional	Audiological	Intrusiveness
depression, anger, irritability, anxiety	perceptual difficulties (hearing problems in demanding social situations)	continuous focusing on tinnitus, concentration difficulties, insomnia

Summary

The character of the symptomatology of tinnitus can vary between different groups of clients partly due to etiological factors. Sleep disturbances, lack of energy, and poor concentration are symptoms found in patients with whiplash, but as in the case of tinnitus, there is a wide variation in outcome. In comparison with nausea and vertigo attacks, tinnitus in patients with Ménière's disease seems to give rise to less anxiety and worry than in subjects whose primarily complaint is tinnitus. High levels of arousal may cause tension in jaw muscles, tinnitus and insomnia, indicating a psychological profile that is linked to anxiety and high stress reactivity. Another profile would present a symptomatology of tinnitus-related distress more in accordance with depression and emotional fatigue.

It cannot be ruled out that the large amount of unexplained variance in some factorial studies of tinnitus distress depend on dimensions of vulnerability not being included in the analysis. Variability of mood and fluctuations in the way tinnitus distress is perceived is likely to influence the overall level of tinnitus vulnerability. Would such circumstances lead to dishabituation and an intensified cognitive focus on the sound? Dimensions of this kind can only be discovered by a longitudinal approach utilizing repeated daily assessments. Different psychological tests and questionnaires performed in tinnitus research have a high intercorrelation and therefore yield a typical pattern of distress. Is this "distress pattern" of tinnitus patients abnormal or unique, or do patients with other chronic illnesses, such as chronic pain patients, show a similar distress profile? This question is considered in the following sections of this chapter.

DO TINNITUS PATIENTS DIFFER FROM THE GENERAL POPULATION?

Habituation to Tinnitus and Reasons for Dishabituation

Heller and Bergman (1953) showed that normal hearing people in a soundproof room can hear sounds from inside their bodies, heads or ears, sounds that they do not normally perceive. In daily life the environmental noise provides us with a masking effect. The brain has the ability to adapt to sounds (or other stimuli) when they become familiar to the individual, particularly if the sounds are regular and constant. As soon as the stimulus contains some new element, our attentiveness is retriggered: we orient our attention automatically in the direction of the new signal. This process is called habituation. A theoretical model of tinnitus adaptation based on the concept of habituation has been described by Hallam et al. (1984). The authors imply that a gradually increasing tolerance to tinnitus is a normal process, and intolerance or stress accompanies the failure to achieve such tolerance.

Failure to habituate may be caused by a sudden onset of tinnitus, the affective significance of the noises, high levels of tonic arousal, the unpredictability assigned to the noises and/or damage to the neural pathways relating to the habituation process (ibid). The habituation model of tinnitus tolerance has contributed to the understanding of the psychological and psychophysiological aspects of tinnitus, because it offers an explanation to the process of adaptation.

To Konorski (1967), the important factor for habituation was not the repetition of the stimulus, but rather the nature of its relationship to the current adaptive situation. He argued that it is not the change of stimulus characteristics that influences dishabituation most frequently and most powerfully. Halford and Anderson (1991) examined the relationship between a tinnitus variability measure and a number of tinnitus-specific variables and psychological condition. They did not find support for their prediction that greater variability of tinnitus would lead to a heightened cognitive focus making the individual more anxious, depressed, or perceive tinnitus as more severe. Dineen et al. (1997) noted that subjects with constant tinnitus in comparison with subjects reporting intermittent tinnitus found their sounds to be significantly louder and more annoying, however there were no differences between the groups in their level of reaction to the sound or perceived coping ability. The influence of mood and emotions on the perceived tinnitus sound in a particular patient makes the relationship more complicated than what can be studied within a linear causality model.

Two groups of patients with tinnitus, seven complainers and seven noncomplainers, participated in an experiment on short-term habituation to a series of tinnitus-like sound stimuli (Carlsson & Erlandsson, 1991). The skin conductance response and heart rate prior to poststimulus change were chosen as response measures. The only significant difference between the groups was self-reported sleep problems; that is, complaining tinnitus patients reported sig-nificantly more sleep disturbances than non-complainers. Psychophysiological data failed to differentiate between the two groups; however, there was a tendency for complainers to increase their heart rate during the course of exposure to the sound stimulus, which may indicate a greater impact of psychological arousal, in complainers, caused by the experimental situation. The failure to find a short-term orienting response habituation correlate does not necessarily nullify the habituation theory of Hallam et al. (1984), but the processes involved seem to be more complex than those that can be studied within such a paradigm.

A nationwide investigation of tinnitus and the adaptation process including all the hearing centers in Sweden was performed by Scott, Lindberg, Melin, & Lyttkens (1990). A total of 3,372 subjects were asked to take part in a questionnaire study; 9 percent declined participation. Half of the participating subjects reported having tinnitus and the distribution of gender was rather equal (53 percent males/47 percent females). The most pronounced predictor of "current discomfort" was found to be the controllability of the sounds (variance explained was 37 percent). Other predictors were "maskability" (listening to ambvient sounds or to a masker) and "variation in loudness" (would slow the habituation process down). Anxiety, on the other hand, did not seem to belong among the predictor variables explaining discomfort of tinnitus, however concentration difficulties contributed with a minor, significant part. Panic attacks or anxiety in the acute phase is likely to reduce the individual's ability to tolerate the tinnitus, although it might not be responsible for the perceived long-standing discomfort. Tinnitus is not always experienced as a disturbing symptom immediately after its onset, most probably due to the gradual debut in some patients (Stouffer & Tyler, 1990). Someone who had a nondisturbing inner sound for many years, may suddenly find that the condition aggravates, the buzzing may increasingly become a worrying, annoying symptom and the focus of renewed attention.

Around 50 percent of 173 consecutive tinnitus patients attending the Department of Audiology and Otolaryngology at Sahlgrenska University Hospital, Gothenburg, reported a gradual onset. The mean onset of *distressing* tinnitus assessed in this sample was found to take place approximately two years after the tinnitus' first occurrence (Erlandsson et al., 1992).

The actual loudness of the sound may increase, owing to the raised level of alertness in the brain, and to the fact that sounds that normally do not evoke a defensive reaction now do so, because some new, significant meaning has been attached to them. In this way the symptom is reinforced, which, in turn, makes the patient supersensitive to the tinnitus rather than more relaxed about it. Very often, vicious circles arise in which attentiveness to the sounds intensifies as the patient becomes convinced that the problem is there to stay. Another explanation for the increasing intensity of the sound may be that the person's hearing has deteriorated. The masking of environmental sounds can be less efficient and tinnitus become more of a problem for the individual with a gradually deteriorating hearing. A hearing impairment, even a moderate one, often gives rise to psychological distress, owing both to the individual's difficulty in coping with his/her situation, and to the lack of understanding from others (Eriksson-Mangold & Carlsson, 1991). Some reasons for the delayed onset of distress caused by increased tinnitus loudness are summarized as:

- Evoked defensive reactions
- Deterioration of hearing (haircell damage)
- Less efficient masking of ambvient sounds

We know that the tolerance threshold for individuals is influenced by differences in the ways we perceive, select, and process the impressions we receive from both internal and external sources. The subjective experience is personal, and colored by our past as well as by our knowledge of the present situation. Kennedy (1953), a British psychiatrist, viewed tinnitus from a psychoanalytical perspective and in his opinion, the compulsive attentiveness (the factor of preoccupation) to the noise was a very important aspect of understanding the suffering of the patient. What is important with regard to tinnitus, whether or not the individual shows signs of presenting an organic, underlying illness, is the extent to which she or he focuses on the tinnitus. Kennedy (ibid) also suggested that a preexisting sound could come into the awareness of the person during a period of life stress.

Chronic Tinnitus in Comparison with Chronic Pain

Enduring, severe tinnitus is sometimes regarded as a condition comparable to that of chronic pain, such as pain that is not due to a malignant disease. Pain is most often defined as a chronic condition when the duration exceeds six months. As in tinnitus, contradictory evidence of the correlation between pain and pain-related behaviors are reported. Attempts have been made to explain the observed discrepancy between physical findings and the overt behavior of pain (Turk & Floor, 1987). During longstanding pain, the observed clinical picture has usually changed over time and the profile becomes similar to that seen in patients with depressive syndromes (von Knorring, 1975). However, even if an impairment is found, it is difficult to decide whether or not this is an adequate explanation for the presence of the pain behavior. Tinnitus is affected by the same dilemma; that is, there is no clear cutoff point to offer an explanation to the discrepancy found between the medical finding (hearing impairment or tinnitus loudness match) and the complex tinnitus behavior.

Wilson, Henry, and Nicholas (1993) and Chapter 11 have provided an overview of contributions of cognitive theory and therapy to the explanation and management of chronic pain and tinnitus. The authors refer to both aversive pain and tinnitus as giving rise to several stressors besides the pain or tinnitus itself that the individual has to cope with, such as reduced income, marital problems, auditory difficulties or other handicaps associated with the experiences of vulnerability. It was concluded that studies have generally failed to demonstrate an effect of psychological regimens on self-ratings of the severity of pain itself, however, for tinnitus the findings seem to be more contradictory. Wilson et al. (1993) call for more attention to be paid to the development of techniques that will have more long-standing benefits for aversive tinnitus. The identification of a possible subgroup of patients who respond positively to psychological interventions would improve the effectiveness of treatment programs. It was suggested by Axelsson, Coles, Erlandsson, Meikle, and Vernon (1993) that improvement of clinical trials could be obtained through both careful patient selection and the use of standardized and quantitative measures.

How is mood related to tinnitus or to chronic pain? Kirsch, Blanchard, and Parnes (1989) found similarities in psychological profiles and level of depression between patients with chronic pain and patients with severe tinnitus. The authors compared tinnitus patients with patients suffering from chronic headache using a nonheadache and a nontinnitus control group. Tinnitus patients who were classified as a low coping group were very similar to the chronic pain patients in their level of depression and anxiety and the patients defined as a high coping group were similar to the nonclinical group. Assessments of the Mood Adjective Checklist (Sjöberg, Svensson, & Persson, 1979) gave some evidence of the prevalence of low mood in a sample of patients with disabling tinnitus with symptoms of craniomandibular dysfunction, compared to a normative, nonclinical sample and to a sample of patients with rheumatic pain (Erlandsson et al., 1991). In average the tinnitus patients showed mood levels that were significantly lower than those of the chronic pain patients in all three mood dimensions measured (pleasantness/activation/relaxation). The group with the lowest ratings of mood was predominated by male tinnitus subjects with noise-induced hearing loss. The difference in mood levels between the two clinical samples does not have a clear explanation, although Persson and Sjöberg (1987) assumed that painful rheumatoid symptoms are less associated with mood than are diffuse neuroasthenic symptoms. The etiology of tinnitus is also much less clearly defined than that of chronic rheumatism, which can make tinnitus more receptive to images with a frightening and worrying content, influencing mood levels in a negative way.

Almay (1987) investigated the prevalence of depressive symptomatology in two different samples of patients with chronic pain and found that subjects with idiopathic pain syndromes had significantly more inhibition symptoms, such as memory disturbances and concentration difficulties, than subjects with neurogenic pain syndromes. The depressive symptomatology was estimated by means of self-ratings on visual analogue scales and pain drawings. The quality of pain, such as aching, burning, cutting, stabbing, cramping, and numbness, only differed marginally between the two groups of patients. Only pain of an aching type dominated significantly in the idiopathic pain group. The number of different types of pain experienced per subject was 2.47 in the neurogenic pain group and 2.98 in the idiopathic pain group, a nonsignificant difference. The author therefore concluded that detailed analyses of the quality of pain experienced would be of minor importance for the clinical evaluation.

The observation that only a small difference in quality of pain exists between subjects with idiopathic pain syndromes and subjects with neurogenic pain may give rise to questions on the perceived quality of tinnitus and its correlation to etiological aspects, for example noise-induced tinnitus compared to tinnitus in the normal ear.

Meikle, Vernon, and Johnson (1984) reported that tinnitus severity was unrelated to pitch, loudness and symptoms of distress, however the number of sounds noticed seemed to have a positive correlation with severity. Complex tinnitus (several sounds of different character) was also related to the severity of tinnitus in the studies of Hallberg and Erlandsson (1993) and Dineen et al. (1997). There exists a need for more qualitative, descriptive data on the experience of tinnitus and its relation to etiology. Quality aspects of tinnitus may contribute to the understanding of the mechanisms involved at both a neurophysiological and a psychological level.

Personality Patterns Described By the Use of Personality Inventories and Psychiatric Diagnostic Scales

Psychiatric and psychological diagnostic scales utilized in different samples of tinnitus patients are shown in Table 2-1. Assessments of psychopathological disturbances (House, 1981) in patients with tinnitus have indicated the prevalence of neurotic characteristics such as depressive reactions, hysterical conversion reaction, and borderline personality characteristics. Reich and Johnson (1984) found an increase of symptomatic depression and hysterical reactions to stress situations within two groups of tinnitus patients assessed with a shorter form of the Minnesota Multiphasic Personality Inventory (MMPI) at a specialist tinnitus clinic. In a subgroup of seventeen patients with normal hearing, complaining of tinnitus, the assessments indicated paranoid symptoms and elevated scores on a schizophrenia subscale of the MMPI (that is, anxiety, internal conflict, withdrawal, emotional isolation, and nonconformity). It was concluded that for patients whose primary complaint was tinnitus, the elevation in scores was mainly limited to psychotic characteristics and for the patients whose concern primarily was the hearing impairment, the elevation tended to be related to neurotic symptoms. The overall profile on the MMPI was, however, within a normal range.

Collet et al. (1990) applied the short form of the MMPI to one hundred subjects with tinnitus; sixty-three males and thirty-seven females. The group profile was found to be within the normal limits for each scale. A significant positive correlation between elevated scores of the Hysteria subscale and tinnitus duration was observed. The hysteria score was higher in patients reporting bilateral tinnitus. Males showed significantly higher scores on both the depression and the hysteria subscales.

A well-known, psychiatric/psychological scale used for the assessment of somatic distress symptoms in tinnitus research (Harrop-Griffith et al., 1987; Sullivan et al., 1988; Attias et al., 1995) is the Symptom Checklist, SCL-90 (Derogatis & Clearly, 1977) (see Table 2-1). In a study by Harrop-Griffith et al. (1987), the only difference in distress profile between complaining tinnitus patients and noncomplaining patients was the somatization score. In addition, tinnitus patients with current major depression were found to have significantly higher scores on all the scales of the Symptom Checklist compared to the control group. It was concluded that since tinnitus and major depression often coexist, a two-pronged treatment regime may be necessary for effective relief. The study by Attias et al. (1995) comprised males only (active army personnel) divided into two groups having noise-induced hearing losses and tinnitus; help-seeking and nonhelp-seeking subjects, and a control group with males without hearing loss and with no tinnitus. The help-seekers demonstrated significantly more severe symptoms, overall, than the nonhelp-seeking patients. Scores of the obsessive-compulsive and hostility dimensions of the scale were the most severe in help-seekers. Although help-seeking patients were found to have more severe symptoms on the Symptom Checklist, the authors observed that nonhelp-seekers fell into a continuum of symptoms of complaint, disability, and psychopathology making them more vulnerable and at risk for developing serious distress with time.

Table 2-1. General psychiatric and psychological diagnostic scales used in different samples of tinnitus patients.

Author/s (year of publication)	Type of sample	Females / males	(Total N)
Diagnostic and Statistical Manual of Mental Disorders (DSM III)			
Harrop-Griffiths et al. (1987)	Consecutive, tinnitus clinic	24% / 76%	(35)
Simpson et al. (1988)	Selected, not random	52% / 48%	(41)
Erlandsson & Persson (1997)	Selected, tinnitus clinic	30% / 70%	(18)
Hopkins Symptom Checklist (SCL–90)			
Harrop-Griffiths et al. (1987)	Consecutive, tinnitus clinic	24% / 76%	(35)
Sullivan et al. (1988)	Consecutive, tinnitus clinic	24% / 76%	(54)
Hiller et al. (1994)	In–patients, clinical	35% / 65%	(198)
Attias et al. (1995)	Routine, audiologic, check-up	males only	(173)
Newman et al. (1996)	Selected, audiologic, clinic	31% / 69%	(51)
The General Health Questionnaire (GHQ–30)			
Singerman et al. (1980)	Consecutive sample	54% / 46%	(156)
The Derogatis Stress Profile (DSP)			
Dineen et al. (1997)	Community announcements	38% / 62%	(96)
Crisp and Crown Experiential Index (CCEI)			
Stephens & Hallam (1985).	Tinnitus specialist clinic	not specified	(472)
Minnesota Multiphasic Inventory (MMPI)			
House et al. (1977).	Otological/medical, selected	41% / 59%	(41)
Reich & Johnson (1984).	Clinical	not specified	(146)
Gerber et al. (1985).	Sample of NIHL	males only	(45)
Collet et al. (1990).	Referrals to ORL department	37% / 63%	(100)
Beck Depression Inventory (BDI)			
Wood et al. (1983)	Tinnitus sample, selected	62% / 38%	(13)
Wilson et al. (1991)	Referrals from ORL department	33% / 67%	(156)
Newman et al. (1996)	Selected, audiologic, clinic	31% / 69%	(51)
Erlandsson & Persson (1997)	Consecutive, tinnitus clinic	39% / 61%	(106)
State/Trait Anxiety Inventory (STAI)			
Wilson et al. (1991)	Referrals from ORL department	33% / 67%	(156)
Erlandsson et al. (1991)	Consecutive, ORL	36% / 64%	(42)
Halford and Anderson (1991)	Tinnitus self–help group	59% / 41%	(112)
Erlandsson & Persson (1997)	Consecutive, tinnitus clinic	39% / 61%	(106)

The prevalence of symptoms of mental illness in patients referred for audiological examination was measured by the use of the General Health Questionnaire (GHQ-30), a self-administered thirty-item scale (Singerman, Riedner, & Folstein, 1980). The subjects were divided into four groups: patients with normal hearing, unilateral hearing loss, low-tone or high-tone deficit, and with bilateral hearing loss. Patients who had normal hearing, represented nearly 15 percent of the sample. The results showed that symptoms of mental disturbance were, in some way, related to the level of hearing loss; those with bilateral losses showed more such symptoms. However, subjects with no hearing impairment had the highest overall level of symptoms of mental illness. Likewise, Berrios, Ryley, Garvey, and Moffat (1988) investigated the prevalence of psychiatric symptoms in 207 subjects with inner ear disease by the use of the General Health Questionnaire. Within the sample, there was a tendency for tinnitus subjects to score the highest (most symptoms), and presbyacusis patients the lowest on the scale. The two most frequent subtypes of complaints among the cases clustered into a depressive group and an anxiety group. Berrios et al. (1988) suggested that the duration of the symptoms may be of importance; for example, anxiety might be replaced with depression if the annoyance of tinnitus continues for too long. The observations that normal-hearing tinnitus patients suffer from more symptoms of mental illness than other groups of hearing-impaired tinnitus patients are in line with the results of Reich and Johnson (1984).

The occurrence of psychopathology in tinnitus sufferers measured by the *Diagnostic and Statistical Manual of Mental Disorders* (DSM-III-R; APA, 1987) was reported by Harrop-Griffith et al. (1987), Simpson et al. (1988), and Sullivan et al. (1988). Harrop-Griffith et al. (1987) noted that thirteen (62 percent) of twenty-one complaining tinnitus subjects, included in their study of patients attending a newly established tinnitus clinic, had had one or several major depressions in their lifetime compared to three (21 percent) of fourteen control subjects with mild or with no tinnitus. The control group was selected from a general otolaryngology clinic. According to a subsection of somatization disorder of the Diagnostic Interview Schedule, there was a statistically significant difference in the number of somatic symptoms reported between tinnitus complainers and noncomplainers. The authors explained the significant increase of somatic symptoms in complainers as due to the enhanced prevalence of major depression in these patients. Nonsignificant higher than average lifetime

prevalence of alcohol abuse and sexual problems were also found for tinnitus complainers. It needs to be pointed out that the majority of subjects, approximately 75 percent of the participants in the investigation, were males.

The prevalence of personality disorders in the general population has been estimated to reach 10 to 13 percent (Weissman, 1993). Grove and Tellegen (1991) reported that half of the people with personality disorders have more than one disorder. Tinnitus patients under medical examination were investigated in order to define the involvement of anxious and depressed mood in the complaint behavior of the patients (Erlandsson & Persson, submitted). It was hypothesized that some of those who exhibited an average or above average scores of anxious and depressed mood might be afflicted with a more serious disturbance, that is, that of a personality disorder. Of the above average scorers, ten women and twenty-two men (46 percent) were found to be seriously affected by emotional distress. The course of the illness profile was analyzed based on repeated interviews of the Structural Clinical Interview for DSM-III-R, and psychodiagnostic assessments in a subgroup of eighteen subjects who agreed to participate. Eleven patients (85 percent) in the drop-out group reported serious problems due to illness and life stress of a severe character. There were no differences in the initial, psychometric test scores (level of depression and anxiety) between the subjects in the pilot study and the drop-outs.

Of those participating in the pilot study, 50 percent (two women and seven men) were diagnosed as suffering from a personality disorder. Borderline personality disorder was confirmed in three male patients and obsessive compulsive disorder in one female. Comorbidity (two or several disorders in the same individual) was found in the majority of patients. Phobic personality disorder and phobic tendencies were the most common diagnoses. At a follow-up interview, a year and a half later, sixteen subjects were reassessed with the Structural Clinical Interview for DSM-III-R. The agreement between the two different occasions of assessment was approximately 70 percent. One patient, a women, had recovered from her most acute distress. Her social situation and mood had improved significantly and so had her tinnitus. There was a clear trend in the data; patients who initially were diagnosed as suffering from a personality disorder did not change their distress profile (depression and state/trait anxiety) from the first to the third (follow-up) period of assessment. It was therefore suggested that tinnitus might reinforce certain personality traits in an individual who is vulnerable and at the border between psychological health/illness. In such patients a vicious circle is operating in a more serious way due to pronounced intolerance to life stress than in patients who are genuinely, psychologically healthy.

It is often taken for granted that subjects' self-assessments of diverse symptoms of psychological health/vulnerability are unquestionable and show true values. Shedler, Mayman, and Manis (1993) argued that many people who report psychological health on "objective" mental health scales may not be healthy at all due to the scales not being sensitive enough to distinguish between genuine mental health and the illusion of mental health, that is, defensive denial of distress. Psychological distress is often repressed and therefore perceived and expressed only indirectly. We can therefore not rely completely on patients' reports on standard psychometric tests of their mental health status. Defensive denial of psychological health must be taken more seriously and be regarded as crucial within the clinical judgment. The authors found (ibid) that clinical judges could distinguish genuine from illusory mental health, however, "objective" mental health scales could not. These results call for more *qualitative*, clinical methods (interviews) in order to identify tinnitus patients who are at risk for developing a serious condition.

Summary

The brain has the capacity to adapt to stimuli when these become familiar, particularly if they are of a regular and constant type. Although, it was observed that subjects with constant tinnitus in comparison with subjects reporting intermittent tinnitus experienced significantly louder and more annoying sounds. Suggestions have been made that failure to habituate to tinnitus, or dishabituation, might be the result of an overreaction, based on the sound having an implicit noxious meaning. The character of the sound rather than the change in stimulus or variability seems to be of significance for tinnitus complaint behavior and can also secondarily influence the process of habituation.

Joint research and discussions of psychological mechanisms in patients with chronic tinnitus and chronic pain syndrome can give new evidence of value for the understanding of the "cause-effect" dilemma by differentiating coherent factors from specific factors found in the two disorders. The contribution of early experiences and health beliefs as the result of social learning cannot be ignored as explanations for the weak correlations found between the pain of tinnitus and the complaints. A significant increase of somatic symptoms have been observed in tinnitus complainers suffering from major depression. There is some support in the literature that the duration of tinnitus distress might be of importance; for example, anxiety is replaced with depression if the annoyance of tinnitus continues for too long.

It is as essential to use well-defined psychodiagnostic criterias as it is to examine the physiological health of tinnitus patients in order to specialize treatment or to refer patients with severe problems, and/or personality disorders, to professionals in mental health care. Assessments of mental health in patients with annoying tinnitus have indicated the prevalence of different neurotic characteristics (depressive reactions, hysterical conversion reaction, and borderline personality). Several studies on tinnitus have shown that symptoms of mental ill-health are related to the level of hearing loss; subjects with bilateral losses reported more symptoms than those with unilateral losses. Tinnitus patients with no hearing impairment have been found to suffer from the highest overall level of disturbance. In conclusion, a number of results point in the same direction, namely that a profile of vulnerability (personality factors, general anxiety, crucial life stress) is responsible for the duration of severe tinnitus symptoms.

TOLERANCE OR THREAT: THE IMPLICIT MEANING ATTACHED TO THE TINNITUS SOUND

Perceived Character and Quality Aspects of the Tinnitus Sound

It has not been possible to establish a clear, convincing relationship between the loudness of tinnitus measured by a matched stimulus sound and the degree of severity (Meikle et al., 1984; Kuk et al., 1990; Chapter 6). Kuk et al. (1990) reported low correlations between tinnitus handicap and the matched tinnitus sound as well as between the perceived (rated) loudness of tinnitus and the matched sound. The observed relationship between the loudness and the severity of tinnitus has been suggested to largely depend on evaluations that are not sensitive and broad enough to capture the many different ways in which tinnitus can be a problem for the individual (Hallam et al., 1988). But a faint sound may be just as psychologically disturbing as a louder one. Sokolov (1963) reported that weak stimuli, near the threshold, evoke an orienting reflex that is larger and more resistant to habituation than the orienting reflex evoked by stronger stimuli. Psychoacoustical analyses of tinnitus loudness demonstrate that the sensation level normally lies around 5 to 15 decibels above the hearing threshold (Goodwin & Johnson, 1980; Tyler

& Conrad-Armes, 1983). Coles and Baskill (1996) observed somewhat higher mean sensation levels of tinnitus loudness (17.6 decibels) in 103 patients consulting the tinnitus clinic, however, the higher value could be explained by the difference in assessment methods used. These authors reported that instead of focusing on the loudness of tinnitus they are studying tinnitus "dysphony," that is, the unpleasantness of the character of the tinnitus.

Meikle et al. (1984) noted in a study of 1,800 tinnitus patients that self-rated severity of tinnitus was unrelated to most aspects of tinnitus characteristics (pitch, loudness) and symptoms of distress, with the exception of the number of sounds reported and sleep disturbances. Hallberg and Erlandsson (1993) analyzed characteristics of tinnitus sounds that were reported in two samples of patients; "complainers" consulting a tinnitus specialist clinic and "noncomplainers" consulting an otology clinic for problems with hearing. The authors found a difference between the two groups in the type of sounds that was perceived; "complainers" described significantly more often a combination of different sounds (tonal and buzzing) while "noncomplainers" more often reported tonal tinnitus only. Dineen et al. (1997) showed results in agreement with Hallberg and Erlandsson (1993) and with Meikle et al (1984); that is, complex tinnitus sounds give rise to more distress (or highly distressed patients perceive their tinnitus to be more complex in nature). Subjects with multiple tinnitus sounds reported their tinnitus to be louder, more annoying, more difficult to cope with, and they reacted more aversive towards them (Dineen et al., 1997).

The complexity of sounds that seems to be present, particularly, in patients with severe problems, might confirm Kennedy's (1953) suggestion that individuals who are preoccupied by their tinnitus project contents of their own imaginations into the tinnitus sounds, just as the inkblots of the Rorschach test might be interpreted in terms of issues of intrapersonal concerns (see Figure 2-2). In short, the Rorschach test

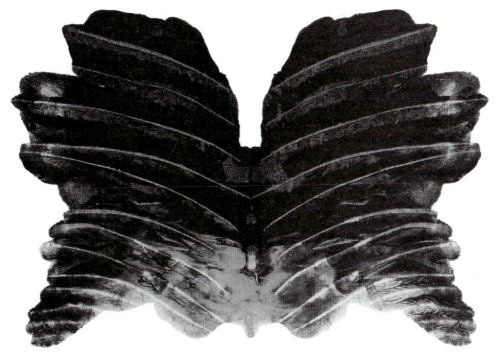

FIGURE 2-2. Illustration (O. Mangold, 1997), resembling a plate of Rorschach's psychodiagnostic test.

is a test of human cognitions and has been assimilated into the psychometric tradition, where it has proven to be useful in clinical settings. Interpretation of the results of the Rorschach test must be based on the context of theoretical expectations about the functions of the mind, the origins of psychopathology, and the psychotherapeutic implications of such factors (Burstein & Loucks, 1989). A great deal of attention is given to observing the ways in which an individual deals with the cognitive problems posed by the nonrepresentational stimuli presented.

The imaginative literature or fiction can give us lively and authentic descriptions of most of what humans can experience in life. Wilhelm Moberg (1898–1973), the well-known Swedish writer, wrote in his book *The Emigrants* about Robert (Moberg, 1949), who was beaten up by his employee, an event which resulted in a middle-ear infection with subsequent cochlear damage and tinnitus in his left ear. Robert's tinnitus sounded like the roaring of the ocean, and

he could listen to it day and night. He attempted to see himself as being privileged in that he could hear the ocean in his ear. Somehow he felt that the ocean called out to him. Robert's interpretation of tinnitus as being something with an implicit positive meaning, helped him to handle the distress. His "inner ocean" became a real experience when he realized his dream to emigrate from the barren Swedish farmland to the United States. However, personal hardships and illness intensified the tinnitus and may have contributed to his premature and tragic death in the New World.

Is Anxiety an Underestimated Factor in Tinnitus Annoyance?

The relationship between anxiety and tinnitus is one of the key factors in the psychological model of tinnitus tolerance or threat (Erlandsson & Archer, 1994). Since anxiety often is being regarded as a consequence of the distress, and not the cause for the patient's increased attention to the tinnitus sound, the anxiety dimension of personality characteristics is too seldom a part of the diagnostic aspects of tinnitus. Reasons for the exaggerated focus on the tinnitus may also be found at the psychophysiological level. Broadbent and Broadbent (1988) showed experimentally that high anxiety increases attention to threat-related stimuli. Anxiety-aggravating causative factors include the obsessive-compulsive syndrome which is characterized by ritual behavior and by certain repetitive thought content, leading to active avoidance; for example, the rituals or thoughts are followed by a decrease of anxiety. Beech and Vaughan (1979) defined the primary difficulty of the obsessional patient as an enhanced potential for becoming aroused and also exhibit strong, defensive reactions to minimal stimulation. An implication of cognitive deficiencies in obsessive-compulsive disorder is the failure to inhibit processing of nonrelevant information.

Examples of obsessive-compulsive behavior in a hearing-impaired population were described by Eriksson-Mangold and Carlsson (1991). Psychological and somatic distress symptoms, experienced disability, and handicap in relation to acquired hearing loss were investigated. Three items in the obsessive-compulsive dimension of the Symptom Checklist (SCL-90) correlated with "tinnitus"; section No. VI included in the Hearing Measurement Scale. These items were: "having to doublecheck what you do," "difficulties in concentration," and "having to repeat your actions." Further, tinnitus correlated significantly with six items in the anxiety dimension of the Symptom Checklist: nervousness/shakiness, trembling, pounding heart, tension, panic spells, and restlessness. It seems to be a somewhat consistent finding that obsessive-compulsive disorder is part of a psychiatric symptomatology related to severe tinnitus complaints in some individuals. So far, studies have demonstrated the prevalence of obsessive compulsive behavior in help-seeking tinnitus patients (Attias et al., 1995; Stephens & Hallam, 1985). In other studies it has been suggested that the compulsive attentiveness

to the tinnitus sound is important for the understanding of the suffering of the patient (Hallam et al., 1984). If a patient with an obsessional-compulsive disorder has an enhanced potential for becoming aroused as suggested by Beech and Vaughan (1979), then even a minimal stimulation, for example, a very faint tinnitus sound, can give rise to a strong defensive reaction in such a person.

More general aspects of anxiety reactions in different tinnitus samples, measured with the State/Trait Anxiety Inventory (Spielberger, 1983) have been reported (see Table 2-1). Level of anxiety, in complaining tinnitus patients, showed levels similar to that of a sample of general medical and surgical patients in the United States (Erlandsson et al., 1991). Ireland, Wilson, Tonkin, and Platt-Hepworth (1985) described similar findings of their assessments of anxiety in patients with tinnitus who participated in a study in which the effects of psychological treatment (relaxation training) was evaluated. A significant but low correlation between overall tinnitus severity and trait anxiety was observed by Halford and Anderson (1991). Self-rated anxiety did not correlate with the intensity and the severity of tinnitus in the study by Erlandsson et al. (1991). These findings are consistent with the experience of pain and anxiety, where state and trait anxiety have been only weakly related to measures of pain intensity. Garron and Leavitt (1983) demonstrated that trait (but not state) anxiety was associated with a chronic character of pain.

Stephens and Hallam (1985) compared subgroups of patients with tinnitus by the use of Crown and Crisp Experiential Index on the basis of gender and whether or not dizziness was complained of. They observed that males with tinnitus alone reported more obsessionality and women with tinnitus alone more somatic complaints. The patients who complained of both dizziness and tinnitus reported more somatic and generalized anxiety problems. It was clearly shown by these results that a different pattern of emotional disturbance appears when dizziness is combined with tinnitus.

Increased arousal and hyperventilation can enhance the sensitivity of the vestibular system. Vestibular dysfunction has been found in a subgroup of patients with panic disorder, but the causal direction of the relationship between panic disorder and vestibular dysfunction is not clear (Jacob & Lilienfeld, 1991). Epidemiological studies show that the occurrence rate of panic disorders in adults has a lifetime prevalence of 2 percent (Wittchen & Essau, 1991) and the consistency rate between different studies seems to be high. Comorbidity was found to be high among patients having either agoraphobia or panic disorder and generalized anxiety (Breier, Charney, & Heninger, 1986).

Anxiety that has an explicit, comprehensible reason, for example anxiety as a reaction to a critical event or injury, is easier to understand and accept than an ill-specified, fluctuating anxiety where the cause remains ambiguous and unknown. High anxiety is likely to negatively influence the patient's perceived level of control of tinnitus, and also generally influence their ability to concentrate. An increase of tension is known to have a negative effect on adaptation to stress and stress-related situations, therefore management of the anxiety in the individual tinnitus patient should be part of any rehabilitation program. Psychological, therapy methods (for example, relaxation training, biofeedback) for handling of the patients' tension and anxiety have been demonstrated in several treatment effect studies (see Chapter 11 for an overview). Lindberg, Scott, Melin, and Lyttkens (1988) reported the use of an Anxiety Management Technique for tinnitus patients in a controlled trial, and showed positive treatment effects, particularly in tinnitus annoyance.

When Things Go Wrong—A Prolonged Reaction Phase Leading to Depression, Despair and Possibly Suicide

Cognitive distortions and emotional distress, found in subjects with severe tinnitus, imply that there are similarities between cognitive, emotional aspects of depression and tinnitus; for example, experienced threats towards self-esteem, negative views of the future and how to manage emotional experiences, helplessness and suicidal idea–tions or connotations. Cognitive disturbances of individuals who are depressed are described and identified as problems in concentration, attention, sleep, learning and implicit memory (Eysenck & Mogg, 1992), complaints that tinnitus patients also report. Patients, with low levels of mood, measured by the Mood Adjective Checklist (Sjöberg et al., 1979), were found to experience significantly more disturbances in concentration compared to tinnitus patients with a more normal pattern of mood (Erlandsson et al., 1991). Difficulties in attention and impaired information processing might lead to an unproportionally intensified attention to tinnitus, which in severe cases can be compared to a form of sensory deprivation. Intense focusing on tinnitus has an impact on the level of awareness and can influence hearing ability in a negative way in patients who are depressed. Low mood can also influence motor reactivity and auditory sensitivity, questioning the reliability of audiological assessments performed on patients who are depressed. Malone and Hemsley (1977) observed that depressed subjects, assessed on an auditory signal detection task, showed lower motor responsiveness and their auditory sensitivity was lowered in comparison with results obtained when they were clinically improved after antidepressant medication.

Vulnerable patients seek help for annoying tinnitus that they neither can meaningfully comprehend nor, deal with. They are often closed off to any other solution than becoming completely free from the sounds. There are several ways in which the first appointment with the general practitioner can go wrong and be a negative experience for this kind of patient. The professional might find the patient's problems difficult to discuss due to the emotional aspects of the condition and therefore leaves him or her without much hope. Statements made over a very short period of time, as often is the rule, can not possibly be based on any extensive knowledge of the individual seeking consultation (Erlandsson, 1998). Some obstacles seen in the interaction between the professional and the client are summarized as follows:

- Tinnitus is regarded by the professional as a physical condition with no effective cure
- The consultation does not give the patient any hope; on the contrary the crisis deepens and the patient withdraws
- The patient becomes depressed when no therapy is available and the distress reaction is therefore prolonged

When grief or conflicts cannot be articulated at the emotional level, they can manifest themselves in the body in the form of tension and psychosomatic symptoms, a phenomenon sometimes referred to as somatization. In this way, tinnitus may turn the identity of the patient into that of a chronic sufferer, because he or she is unable to acknowledge that the perceived distress can arise from covert emotional pain. It has been reported that depressed tinnitus patients are more responsive to medical treatment (lidocain injected intravenously in 30 s, Wood et al., 1983) than less depressed and less neurotic patients. The results should be interpreted with caution due to the small number of cases included and to the lack of a placebo control group. However, if these observations are not only a matter of chance, there are several factors to be discussed. Suffering that is overt, that is, expressed directly through emotional pain, is in a way accessible to the person and therefore easier to communicate, find words for and to compensate for. Patients who have illusionary control over their emotions, with rational explanations and intellectualizing as part of their manic defense, often feel as if they are victimized and persecuted by their tinnitus. In general terms, the latter group would be more resistant to change.

Patients with severe tinnitus have not been helped by treatment, as a rule, even if examples of therapeutic success in some treatment effect studies of psychological interventions exist, like those reported by Jakes, Hallam, Rachman and Hinchcliffe (1986), Lindberg et al. (1988), and Attias, Shemesh, Shoham, Shahar, and Shomer (1990). There is no explicit information of the level of psychopathology of patients included in studies evaluating the effectiveness of treatment. It cannot be ruled out that often the most distressed patients, who are the minority, are excluded due to the study design being a short-term therapy.

Patients who consider themselves to have been misunderstood with regard to their illness and the treatment they are receiving are in the risk zone and may develop a deeper form of depression. In those cases the risk for suicide must also be taken into consideration. The highest suicide rate in the United States has been found among white males and a third of all suicides are committed by persons who are over sixty years of age. Johnston and Walker (1996) highlighted the importance of tracing signs and symptoms of depression and suicidality in the geriatric population. General risk factors reported by Johnston and Walker are sex (male) and marital status (suicide is three times more likely to occur in divorced, widowed, and single elderly males). Psychosocial risk factors include isolation, urban living, retirement, relocation, inadequate social support, disease, personal loss, and change in social roles. The geriatric suicides are related to depression in approximately one-third of the cases. Among risk factors (ibid) identified in one patient who had a history of depression and alcohol abuse were impaired ability to communicate, intractable tinnitus and feelings of helplessness. A review of follow-up studies showed that the lifetime incidence of suicide among depressed patients is 15 percent (Guze & Robins, 1970). Personality disorder has been found in up to 50 percent of the people who later commit suicide (Lewis, Stephens, & Huws, 1992).

Lewis et al. (1992) described six cases of tinnitus sufferers of whom five committed suicide and one was killed by his son. Demographic data showed that four of the individuals were males and five of them had a working-class background. Five lived isolated and two had recently lost their spouses. All of the suicide victims had related psychological disturbances and five of them had consulted a psychiatrist prior to the appointment at the tinnitus clinic. The psychological symptom reported by all six was depression; four were diagnosed as having a major depressive illness and one had schizophrenia. Problems with alcohol could be found in at least two of the subjects. A risk factor mentioned by the authors was *pulsatile tinnitus* which they observed in five of the six cases.

A questionnaire with enquires about demographic factors, psychiatric history and audiological symptoms was distributed worldwide in order to collect data on suicide in association with tinnitus suffering (Lewis, Stephens, & McKenna, 1994). A total of twenty-eight cases were included in the study. It was found that psychiatric symptoms were present in more than 95 percent of the patients at the time of their death. Suicide in the males was more than twice as common as in the women sufferers, which reflect the gender distribution in the general population. Half of the individuals who committed suicide did so within two years of the onset of tinnitus. More than 40 percent of them had been afflicted with tinnitus for less than a year, which again accentuates the importance of early interventions.

Summary

Individuals with long-standing severe tinnitus are often resistant to therapeutic trials and a number of them fall victim to a socially unacceptable situation following long periods of sick leave or early retirement. Reasons for such a negative ending may partly be explained by the prevalence of mental ill health; that is, generalized anxiety problems and obsessive compulsive disorder. It has been suggested that the compulsive attentiveness to the tinnitus

sound is important for the understanding of the suffering of the patient. A patient with an obsessional-compulsive disorder with an enhanced potential for becoming aroused may show a strong defensive reaction to even a minimal stimulation, for example, a very faint tinnitus sound.

Patients suffering from tinnitus who have subsequently committed suicide have previously shown quite clear signs of low mood and severe psychological disturbance, such as depression, schizophrenia and/or alcohol abuse. A demographical description of the suicide victims revealed that being male, elderly and socially isolated were risk factors. Suicide in the males was more than twice as common as in the women sufferers. So far, research indicates that a critical period— soon after the onset of tinnitus— exists.

THE INFLUENCE OF TINNITUS ON PATIENTS' PERCEPTION OF QUALITY OF LIFE

How Does Tinnitus Affect a Patient's Lifestyle and Personal Relationships?

When something we cannot understand on the basis of our previous experience happens to us, we almost always react with worry and uncertainty. Tinnitus is precisely that kind of a phenomenon. Few people are familiar with tinnitus, although they may have a recollection of, say, a grandparent who heard buzzing sounds in his or her old age. To most people, the occurrence of a hearing impairment accompanied by sounds inside one's head or ears, is a sign of aging, and not something that afflicts a young person or someone in the prime of life. Although, tinnitus as a symptom following a rock concert is a rapidly increasing problem that young people now are beginning to become aware of. According to clinical experiences, the amount of young people asking for advice after the onset of acute tinnitus is increasing. Some of them are in acute need of psychological counseling. Tinnitus that occurs during a sensitive period of the young adult's life can bring about a conflict of identity and cause serious interruptions in the social life of the young person.

We tend to fantasize about something that is difficult to pin down and comprehend, and sometimes even experience it as unreal. We might speak of a person losing his or her sense of reality, when the description of tinnitus, for example, takes on disproportionately dramatic dimensions. Such experiences and fantasies may be enriching and useful to a creative artist. Art may also be, and often is, used to process underlying conflicts. One very relevant example of the relationship between creativity and suffering can be found in the work of Fransisco Goya, the Spanish painter and graphic artist who lived between 1746 and 1828. At the age of forty-seven, Goya developed a serious illness which resulted in deafness and tinnitus. His illness is reflected in his art from that period, when his paintings, sketches and etchings took a completely new turn, expressing suffering, dreams of vulnerability, cruelty, and destructiveness: Goya's black period. His work demonstrates how his extraordinary imagination continued until the age of almost eighty.

Some patients may feel that they lose contact with sides of their personality, since they have to give up things that interest them, such as reading, listening to music, going to lectures or the theater, and so on. This, of course, leads to their feeling extremely restricted and handicapped. Reasons for such restrictions cannot be a matter of tinnitus alone; also difficulties related to hearing ability ought to play a part. Kuk et al. (1990) drew the conclusion from results from an evaluative study of tinnitus distress that high scores on both factor 1 (hearing ability) and factor 2 (the patients view on tinnitus) suggest that the patient's perceived handicap may be affected by hearing sensitivity. The relationship between hearing impairment and tinnitus needs to be described and analyzed with inductive methods. Within a psychological perspective we must know if and how emotions, in the individual patient, participate to the perceived tinnitus sound in the process of the deterioration of hearing. The patient with a hearing impairment may experience a general feeling of failure and a loss of control over the situation and become socially insecure (Hetû, 1996). Due to difficulties in communication she or he withdraws from social interactions and the focusing on internal events, such as tinnitus, may be more intense than before. Tinnitus in this case can be seen as a reaction to, and a constant reminder of, the loss of hearing that is perceived to be a lifelong strain and a hindrance to leading a normal life. In such an outcome, depressive reactions from experienced hearing disability may be difficult to differentiate from the negative mood influence of tinnitus. According to clinical experience, patients often emphasize the fact that they are unable to separate the tinnitus distress from the daily strain they perceive as a result of their hearing impairment.

The Nottingham Health Profile is a generic instrument, designed for the assessment of health-related quality of life in different medical conditions. Erlandsson and Holgers (submitted) described the use of the Nottingham Health Profile in a sample of 186 (57 females and 129 males) consecutive tinnitus patients. Significant predictors for the perceived severity of tinnitus were "Emotion," "Sleep," and "Pain," three of the six dimensions of the Nottingham Health Profile. Patterns of health in the present investigation also seemed to be gender-related. Although gender was not a predictive factor in the regression model, explaining 37.8 percent of the variance, four dimensions of the Nottingham Health Profile; "Mobility," "Pain," "Sleep," and "Energy" had a higher severity rate among the females. The women in age group twenty-five to thirty-four reported significantly more health problems compared to a normal female control group in four aspects, such as lack of energy, pain, emotional reactions, and sleep disturbances. The distress profile of the male with tinnitus deviated somewhat from the distress profile of the female. Younger males with tinnitus reported less difficulties than middleaged males. Few studies describing the general aspects of health-related quality of life in tinnitus populations have been reported. The useful and interesting aspect of a generic instrument is that comparisons of health status among a large variety of different diagnoses can be facilitated.

Does Tinnitus Necessarily Cause Sleep Disturbances?

A true story (from the clinical site) is told of the patient who explained to his physician: "Now that I have tinnitus, there is no need for tranquilizers anymore."

Disturbance of sleep is reported by approximately one-half of individuals complaining of tinnitus (Tyler & Baker, 1983; Jakes et al., 1985; Axelsson & Ringdahl, 1989; Chapter 3). Axelsson and Sand (1985) noted that the main forms of discomfort reported by male patients with noise-induced hearing loss and tinnitus were difficulties with speech discrimination, concentration and insomnia. Subjects with tinnitus in comparison with a nontinnitus, hearing-impaired control group were found by Harrop-Griffith et al. (1987) to report significantly more: difficulties with sleep, more problems in relationships with family and friends, more cognitive difficulties, and illness preoccupation. A number of factor analytical studies investigating the nature of tinnitus complaints have shown that problems with sleep belong to the pattern of suffering experienced by the patients (Hallam et al., 1988; Hiller & Goebel, 1992). Erlandsson et al. (1992) found that sleep disturbances had a larger deviation than other variables included in a tinnitus severity questionnaire, which indicates a tinnitus distress profile that is heterogenous.

Hallam (1996) analyzed sleep disturbances recorded during a one-week period in twenty-six patients complaining of tinnitus. The subjects were split into three groups based on the assessor's rating of the degree of sleep disturbance reported: absent, present, and significantly troublesome. Sleep disturbances were *not* related to standardized assessments of anxiety or depression, self-reported emotional distress, irrational beliefs, or auditory perceptual difficulties. There seemed, however, to be some association between sleep problems and tinnitus annoyance in the eight significantly troubled patients. The author noted that absence of sleep disturbances was related to normal hearing over the range 250 Hz to 2 kHz. The observation that insomnia was unrelated to anxious or depressed mood (ibid) was previously reported by Erlandsson et al. (1991), who found that subjects with low levels of mood defined by the assessment of Mood Adjective Checklist did not have significantly more problems with sleep in comparison with subjects reporting more favorable mood levels.

Which characteristics, in more general terms, are significantly related to insomnia? A number of factors of personality characteristics have been linked to sleep disturbance, such as depression, anxiety, obsessive worry, and fear of losing control (Dineen-Wagner, Lorion & Shipley, 1983). According to Roth et al. (1976), middle-aged individuals with sleep problems experience numerous physical symptoms without any apparent organic ground, which can be interpreted as indicative of anxious preoccupation with bodily functions (somatization). Similar observations are found in tinnitus sufferers, who are anxious and obsessed. The most frequent kind of insomnia (35 percent) found in patients consulting Sleep Disorders Centers is insomnia related to a primary psychiatric condition (Coleman & Roffwarg, 1982). Sleep disturbances have been identified in a number of psychiatric disorders: schizophrenia, mood disorders, anxiety disorders, panic disorders, alcoholism, and dementia (Billiard, Partinen, Roth, & Shapiro, 1994). It has been suggested that there is a risk for individuals with insomnia to develop a psychiatric illness, as sleep disturbances may not only be a consequence of psychiatric ill health but rather play a crucial role in the pathogenesis of psychiatric disorders (ibid).

An unsuccessful resolution of the psychosocial crisis in midlife can result in the preoccupation of the self found in middle-aged individuals with sleep disturbances. Erikson (1959) assumed that stagnation in growth is shown by personal impoverishment, self-indulgence and the use of physical problems as a means of expressing self-concern. Dineen-Wagner et al. (1983) reported a study in which the relevance of Erikson's developmental theory to understanding insomnia was examined in two different samples of individuals; the *elderly* and the adolescent. Sleep problems in the elderly were assumed to be associated with the resolution of the psychosocial crisis of "ego versus despair" and in the *adolescent*, of "identity versus role confusion." Members of community organizations (N=122) for the elderly comprised the sample of the first study in the series. The results were in the expected direction: subjects (the elderly) reporting sleep disturbances were found to have more death anxiety, lower life satisfaction, and more negative attitudes toward aging than subjects reporting no sleep disturbances. There were no significant differences found either in demographic or other background data, or in availability of social support between subjects with and without reported sleep disturbances. Neither did health status, measured with respect to number of treated problems, differ between the two groups. An adolescent population of forty-four females and twenty-two males was included in the second study examining "identity versus role confusion." Subjects with and without reported sleep disturbances differed in the expected direction of the Rasmussen ego identity measure (Rasmussen, 1964) as well as on life satisfaction. No significant differences of death anxiety and locus of control were found between the two groups of adolescent subjects.

An interesting finding in the study by Dineen-Wagner et al. (1983) is that quality of sleep was relatively independent of situational factors, such as social class, gender, education, marital status, living arrangements, religion, and number of deaths of children. Social support did not seem to be of any relevance for the occurrence of sleep disturbances. The hypothesis that ineffective resolution of the psychosocial crisis of old age (the absence of "ego integrity" reflected in "despair") is related to sleep disturbances in the elderly was strongly verified by the investigation. Insomnia is linked to old age *per se*, and in some individuals it is also linked to tinnitus because the prevalence of tinnitus increases with age. There are reasons to believe that middle-aged individuals with sleep disturbances show similarities in their profile of distress with a subgroup of tinnitus patients suffering from insomnia in the way they experience physical symptoms as a means of expressing self-concern, indicating an unresolved psychosocial crisis in midlife.

Summary

Difficulties related to hearing ability ought to play some part in tinnitus annoyance. The patient may experience a feeling of failure and a loss of control over the situation and become socially withdrawn due to difficulties in communication. In this way the focusing on internal events, such as tinnitus, may be more intense than before. Depressive reactions from experienced hearing disability may be difficult to differentiate from the negative mood influence of tinnitus and the patients may have difficulties separating the tinnitus distress from the strain they perceive as a result of their hearing impairment. Results have shown a non-significant relationship between insomnia and a number of self-reported factors of emotional distress and auditory perceptual difficulties in tinnitus patients. These results can be viewed in a more general context. Middle-aged individuals with sleep problems have been found to experience numerous physical symptoms without any apparent organic ground. Compared to subjects with no sleep problems, subjects reporting sleep disturbances had more death anxiety, lower life satisfaction, and more negative attitudes toward aging; findings that support the Erikson's developmental theory. Erikson assumed that stagnation in growth is shown by personal impoverishment, self-indulgence and the use of physical problems as a means of expressing self-concern.

WHICH COMES FIRST: PSYCHOLOGICAL VULNERABILITY OR SUFFERING FROM TINNITUS?

Causal Explanations of Tinnitus Distress in Relation to Mental Illness

The difficulties in distinguishing the cause-effect relationships between tinnitus and psychological pathology have been elucidated in some studies assessing mental health and functional disability. The core of the problem seems to be more complicated than research so far has been able to describe. It was suggested that the chronic nature of tinnitus, in large, may be explained by a lifetime of major depression, or that major depression is the primary illness in patients with disabling tinnitus (Harrop-Griffith et al., 1987; Sullivan et al., 1988). Evidence for such interpretations is based on the fact that patients with tinnitus and major depression seem to have significantly more somatic symptoms than nondepressed tinnitus patients. The likelihood that anxiety disorders are accompanied by depressed mood in some tinnitus patients cannot be ruled out. But a complication is that the gender perspective is missing in the majority of studies. Males, for example, are in general more prone to develop an obsessive compulsive disorder than females, among other problems, making them more focused on somatic symptoms. A male patient who already is encumbered with an obsessive disorder may have difficulties adjusting to tinnitus, being unable to control it, and depression develops secondarily. Depression can be secondary to the illness, whether the illness is physical or psychiatric in nature.

The hypothesis that somatopsychic effects would increase with tinnitus duration was examined by Stephens, Erlandsson, Sanchez, and Huws (1992). Anxious and depressive, self-rated complaints as a function of tinnitus duration were examined in 436 subjects. Results showed that there was evidence for sustained tinnitus leading to an increase of depressive but not anxiety-related symptoms. The anxiety-related symptoms; irritability, inability to relax, and stress/tension, did not change significantly as a function of tinnitus duration, which points at the role of anxiety as being a causal factor in tinnitus complaint behavior rather than an effect. Collet et al. (1990) assumed that bilateral tinnitus of long duration can be expected to lead to greater psychological disturbance than shorter unilateral tinnitus. Their assumptions were based on the finding that the hysteria score on the MMPI was higher in patients complaining of bilateral tinnitus. According to clinical observations a subgroup of patients reports that tinnitus appears bilaterally some time after the initial onset in one ear. This might indicate that individuals with tinnitus who demonstrate genuinely high scores on hysteria are intensely occupied by their sound and this is likely to influence their perception of tinnitus as escalating to the other ear (classical, psychoanalytical theory would label this a hysterical conversion reaction).

The subjective nature of tinnitus implies a re-orientation towards system-oriented multicausality models in order to understand the complicated bio-psycho-social processes involved in the pathogenesis of the disorder. According to Carlsson and Jern (1982) the multifactorial views are typically formulated concerning disorders of unknown etiology, that is, hypertension, coronary artery disease, and asthma. Tinnitus belongs to this group of disorders. An illness, regarded as a long-standing condition, will always lead to changes at the bio-psycho-social level. Carlsson and Jern (1982) questioned the linear causality model often used in medical sciences, that is, a "disease is conceived of as the result of the pathogenetic effects of a single noxious factor" (p. 153). The question that guides the researcher in such a paradigm is: "What is the cause of the disorder?" In the multicausality model the different factors are assumed to be in constant interaction with each other, and the researcher using this paradigm asks the question: "Under what conditions may a disease develop?" (ibid).

Conclusions and Implications of What Has Been Discussed

What is the psychological cause of an individual's compulsive preoccupation with tinnitus? Can we apply a psychophysiological and/or a psychodynamic explanatory model to such an obsession? Even if this is possible, we need to understand the interaction that takes place in the neural pathways of the brain and mechanisms involved when tinnitus through preoccupation becomes permanently disabling. Our knowledge of tinnitus related activity at the subcortical level in humans is still limited (See Chapter 4 and Chapter 5). In cases where no clear physical explanation to the tinnitus sound can be found, we would like to have an answer to the question why the particular patient ends up with problematic tinnitus rather than some other form of somatic affliction (although somatic distress symptoms are frequently found in tinnitus sufferers). This is a classical dilemma for those who believe that there must be a logical reason underneath all symptoms. There may be explanations but they rest on assumptions that are too complicated for us to describe with our present knowledge. It seems likely that patients who have not been able to adjust by lowering their responsiveness to the sound, remain stuck in the reaction phase of the crisis following tinnitus onset. A careful investigation into the reasons behind the incidence of major depression might reveal, in some patients, that the mood disorder has occurred during a difficult time in life. Experienced threats

towards life fulfillment by the presence of physical illness, separation anxiety, and the loss of something, or someone, precious in life are examples of this. Low mood following a midlife crisis, a serious illness, or unemployment is a rather common condition in the normal life of an individual.

To comprehend tinnitus distress from a deeper psychological perspective it can be a necessity to interact with patients who have chronic painful symptoms. It should be possible to obtain some guidance from clinical observations and longitudinal research on the psychophysiological and psychodynamic aspects of personality of the tinnitus patient and the interplay between these aspects and the environment. What applies to all patients when they consult a professional with specialist knowledge of tinnitus is that the professional must acknowledge and help them understand that tinnitus has to be viewed in a wider perspective. Too narrow an approach will neither help us move the patient in the direction of insight into his or her general state of mind and health, nor forward insight into the interplay between this state and tinnitus suffering. This is not unique for tinnitus management; early recognition of suffering due to psychological problems can lead to a more favorable outcome in other disorders that encompass a heterogenous accumulation of symptoms with or without a known organic cause.

The patients may have previous experiences of sound (noise) with which they can compare their tinnitus, and they may wish to analyze their subjective experiences. If the individual does not have the desire or ability to be analytical, it will be very difficult if not impossible to find a solution to his or her problems by talking about them. Psychological defense mechanisms can be so strong that the person withdraws from all attempts of professionals to discuss the matter from a psychological point of view. One might say that preoccupation with the somatic symptom, the tinnitus, is an expression of psychological pain, and that not every individual patient is prepared to look into the reasons behind that pain. Psychotherapeutic interventions may ease the symptoms of tinnitus distress by helping the patient begin to process what has happened and in this way gain insight into the constant interplay between the psyche and the soma. When the help-seeking patient leaves the clinic, he or she should have begun to realize what the crisis of having tinnitus may imply; psychologically, emotionally, and socially and should have access to follow-up and further supportive counseling, if necessary.

Tinnitus is often regarded as a chronic condition, but this may be false. Instead we would think of it as a signal of severe distress that interact with crucial circumstances (for example, perceived failure, separation, and loss) in the life of the individual. Such a hypothesis implies that besides adopting a multicausality model, there will be a need for repeated measures in order to describe fluctuations in any part of the bio-psycho-social systems of the individual. Time plays a significant role in the system paradigm. By studying the interrelation between tinnitus and other factors in the model, at different occasions, it is possible to elucidate the causal relation between those factors at a certain developmental state (Carlsson & Jern, 1982).

Even if tinnitus in some cases is likely to disappear altogether, the most common scenario seems to be that after a period of great concern over the symptom, the person manages to weather the crisis, after which his or her attentiveness to the sounds declines. Then, instead of focusing on the tinnitus in any and every context, the individual notices the sounds in times of occasional weakness, when he or she is tired or has a cold. The sound probably does not go away for most people, despite the fact that they stop worrying about whether it is going to get worse. But when their tinnitus no longer arouses so much worry, it takes on less dramatic proportions and is somehow integrated into the individual's personality or identity. Still, there are patients who continue to feel anxious and preoccupied with their symptoms, and in those cases it is a necessity to comprehend tinnitus distress from a deeper psychological perspective. The particular demands on the professional helper are qualities or special skills of sensitivity and keen awareness in the clinical, therapeutic interaction with these patients (Erlandsson, 1998). With a good knowledge base, appropriate clinical skills and some compassion, the professional can help the patient accommodate to their strange, unexpected sounds.

ACKNOWLEDGMENTS

This work was supported by a grant to Professor T. Archer and Dr. S. I. Erlandsson from the Swedish Council for Social Research, C 91-0265:1. The author would like to thank Tonya Pethman for valuable comments on the manuscript.

REFERENCES

Akiskal, H. S. (1979). A biobehavioral approach to depression. In R. S. Depue, (Ed.), *The psychobiology of the depressive disorders. Implications for the effects of stress* (pp. 409–431). New York: Academic Press, Inc.

Almay, B. G. L. (1987). Clinical characteristics of patients with idiopathic pain. *Pain, 29,* 335–346.

Andrade, J. M. P. (1989). Goya, work, life, dreams. Madrid: Siklex Ediciones.

American Psychiatric Association (1987): *Diagnostic and Statistical Manual of Mental Disorders* (3rd ed.). Washington, DC: American Psychiatric Association.

Attias, J., Shemesh, Z., Belich, A., Solomon, Z. B., Alster, J., & Sohmer, H. (1995) Psychological profile of help-seeking and nonhelp-seeking tinnitus patients. *Scandinavian Audiology, 24,* 13–18.

Attias, J., Shemesh, Z., Shoham, C. Shahar, A., & Sohmer, H. (1990). Efficacy of self–hypnosis for tinnitus relief, *Scandinavian Audiology, 19,* 245–249.

Axelsson, A., Coles, R. R. A., Erlandsson, S., Meikle, M., & Vernon, J. (1993). Evaluation of tinnitus treatment: Methodological aspects. *Journal of Audiological Medicine, 2,* 141–150.

Axelsson, A., & Ringdahl, A. (1989). Tinnitus—A study of its prevalence and characteristics. *British Journal of Audiology, 23,* 53–62.

Axelsson, A., & Sand, A. (1985). Tinnitus in noise–induced hearing loss. *British Journal of Audiology, 19,* 271–276.

Beech, H. R., & Vaughan, C. M. (1979). The behavioural treatment of obsessional states. London: Wiley.

Berrios, G. E., Ryley, J. P., Garvey, T. P. N., & Moffat, D. A. (1988). Psychiatric morbidity in subjects with inner ear disease. *Clinical Otolaryngology, 13,* 259–266.

Billiard, M., Partinen, M., Roth, T., & Shapiro, C. (1994). Sleep and psychiatric disorders. *Journal of Psychosomatic Research, 38*(Suppl. 1).

Breier, A., Charney, D. S., & Heninger, G. R. (1986). Agoraphobia with panic attacks: Development, diagnostic stability, and course of illness. *Archives of General Psychiatry, 43,* 1029–1036.

Broadbent, D., & Broadbent, M. (1988). Anxiety and attentional bias: State and trait. *Cognition and Emotion, 2,* 165–183.

Budd, R. J., & Pugh, R. (1996). Tinnitus coping style and its relationship to tinnitus severity and emotional distress. *Journal of Psychosomatic Research, 4,* 327–335.

Burstein, A. G., & Loucks, S. (1989). *Rorschach's test: Scoring and interpretation.* Hemisphere Publishing Corporation.

Carlsson, S. G., & Erlandsson, S. I. (1991). Habituation and tinnitus: An experimental study. *Journal of Psychosomatic Research, 35,* 1–6.

Carlsson, S. G., & Jern, S. (1982). Paradigms in psychosomatic research: A dialectic perspective. *Scandinavian Journal of Psychology,* (Suppl. 1), 151–157.

Coleman, R. M., & Roffwarg, D. B. (1982). Epidemiologic study of sleep disturbances and psychiatric disorders: An opportunity for prevention? *Journal of American Medical Association, 247,* 997–1103.

Coles, R. R. A., & Baskill, J. L. (1996). Absolute loudness of tinnitus: Tinnitus clinic data. In G. E. Reich & J. A. Vernon (Eds.), *Proceedings of the Fifth International Tinnitus Seminar 1995.* Portland, OR: American Tinnitus Association.

Collet, L., Moussu, M. F., Disant, F., Ahamai, T., & Morgan, A. (1990). Minnesota Multiphasic Personality Inventory in tinnitus disorder. *Audiology 29,* 101–106.

Cullberg, J. (1984). Dynamisk psykiatri. (Psychodynamic Psychiatry), Stockholm: Natur och Kultur.

Derogatis, L., & Clearly, P. A. (1977). A confirmation of dimensional structure of the SCL–90: A study in construct validity. *Journal of Clinical Psychology, 33,* 981–989.

Derogatis, L. R. (1987). The Derogatis Stress Profile (DSP): Quantification of psychological stress. *Advances in Psychosomatic Medicine, 17,* 30–54.

Dineen, R., Doyle, J., & Bench, J. (1997). Audiological and psychological characteristics of a group of tinnitus sufferers, prior to tinnitus management training. *British Journal of Audiology, 31,* 27–38.

Dineen Wagner, K., Lorion, R. P., & Shipley, T. E. (1983). Insomnia and psychosocial crisis: Two studies of Erikson's developmental theory. *Journal of Consultant and Clinical Psychiatry, 51,* 595–603.

Dobie, R., Sullivan, M., Katon, W., Sakai, C., & Russo, J. (1992). Antidepressant treatment of tinnitus patients. Interim report of a randomized clinical trial. *Acta Otolaryngologica (Stockholm), 112,* 242–247.

Edgren-Sundin, B. (1993). När tystnaden går förlorad—en pilotstudie om krisprocessen vid tinnitus (When silence is lost—a pilot study of the process of the traumatic experiences in tinnitus). Department of Psychology, Göteborg University, Sweden.

Erikson, E. H. (1959). Identity and the life cycle: Selected papers. New York: International Universities.

Eriksson-Mangold, M., & Carlsson. S. G. (1991). Psychological and somatic distress in relation to perceived hearing disability, hearing handicap, and hearing measurement. *Journal of Psychosomatic Research, 35,* 729–740.

Erlandsson, S. I. (1992). Assessments of tinnitus. A review. In J. M. Aran & R. Dauman (Eds.), *Proceedings of the Fourth International Tinnitus Seminar, Bordeaux, France, 1991* (pp. 545–549). Amsterdam/New York: Kugler Publications.

Erlandsson, S. I. (1998). Psychological counselling in the medical setting—some clinical examples given by patients with tinnitus and Ménière's disease. *International Journal for the Advancement of Counseling, 20,* 265–276.

Erlandsson, S. I., & Archer, T. (1994). Tinnitus, pain and affective disorders. In T. Palomo &

T. Archer (Eds.), *Strategies for studying brain disorders. Vol 1: Depressive, anxiety and drug abuse disorders* (pp. 123–142). London: Farrand Press.

Erlandsson, S. I., Eriksson-Mangold, M., & Wiberg, A. (1996). Ménière's disease: Trauma, distress and adaptation studied through focus interview analyses. In S. I. Erlandsson (Ed.), *Psychological and psychosocial approaches to adult hearing loss* (pp. 45–56). *Scandinavian Audiology, 25*(Suppl 43).

Erlandsson, S. I., Hallberg, L. R. M., & Axelsson, A. (1992). Psychological and audiological correlates of perceived tinnitus severity. *Audiology, 31,* 168–179.

Erlandsson, S. I., & Persson, M. L. Chronic tinnitus suffering: Indications of a personality disorder? Manuscript submitted for publication.

Erlandsson, S. I., & Persson, M. L. (1996). Clinical implications of tinnitus and affective disorders. In G. E. Reich & J. A. Vernon (Eds.), *Proceedings of the Fifth International Tinnitus Seminar 1995* (pp. 557–562). Portland, OR: American Tinnitus Association.

Erlandsson, S. I., Rubinstein, B., Axelsson, A., & Carlsson, S. G. (1991). Psychological dimensions in patients with disabling tinnitus and craniomandibular disorders. *British Journal of Audiology, 25,* 15–24.

Eysenck, M. W., & Mogg, K. (1992). Clinical anxiety, trait anxiety, and memory bias. In S. Å. Christianson (Ed.), *The handbook of emotion and memory: Research and theory* (pp. 429–446). Hillsdale, NJ: Lawrence Erlbaum Associates.

Fowler, E. P. (1940). Head noises—Significance, measurement and importance in diagnosis and treatment. *Archives of Otolaryngology, 39,* 498–503.

Frankenhaeuser, M., Lundberg, U., Fredriksson, M., Melin, B., Tuomisto, M., Myrsten, A. L., Hedman, M., Bergman-Losman, B., & Wallin L. (1989). Stress on and off the job as related to sex and occupational status in white-collar workers. *Journal of Organizational Behaviour, 10,* 321–346.

Garron, D. C., & Leavitt, F. (1983). Chronic low back pain and depression. *Journal of Clinical Psychology, 39,* 487–493.

Goodhill, V. A. (1952). Tinnitus identification test. *Oto-Rhino-Laryngology, 61,* 778–788.

Goodwin, P., & Johnson, R. (1980). The loudness of tinnitus. *Acta Otolaryngologica, 90,* 353–359.

Grove, W. M., & Tellegen, A. (1991). Problems in the classification of personality disorders. *Journal of Personality Disorder, 5,* 31–41.

Guze, S. B., & Robins, C. (1970). Suicide among primary affective disorders. *British Journal of Psychiatry, 117,* 437–438.

Halford, J. B. S., & Anderson, S. D. (1991). Anxiety and depression in tinnitus sufferers. *Journal of Psychosomatic Research, 34,* 1–8.

Hallam, R. S. (1996). Correlates of sleep disturbance in chronic distressing tinnitus. *Scandinavian Audiology, 25,* 263–266.

Hallam, R. S., Jakes, S. C., & Hinchcliffe, R. (1988). Cognitive variables in tinnitus annoyance. *British Journal of Clinical Psychology, 27,* 213–222.

Hallam, R. S., Rachman, S., & Hinchcliffe, R. (1984). Psychological aspects of tinnitus. In S. Rachman (Ed.), *Contributions to medical psychology* (Vol. 3, pp. 31–53). Oxford: Pergamon Press.

Hallberg, L. R. M., & Erlandsson, S. I. (1993). Tinnitus characteristics in tinnitus complainers and noncomplainers. *British Journal of Audiology, 27,* 19–27.

Hallberg, L. R. M., Erlandsson, S. I., & Carlsson, S. G. (1992). Coping strategies used by middle-aged males with noise-induced hearing loss, with and without tinnitus. *Psychology and Health, 7,* 273–288.

Harrop–Griffith, J., Katon, W., Dobie, R., Sakai, C., & Russo, J. (1987). Chronic tinnitus: Association with psychiatric diagnosis. *Journal of Psychosomatic Research, 31,* 613–621.

Hazell, J. W. P. (1981). Patterns of tinnitus: Medical audiological findings. *Journal of Laryngology and Otology* (Suppl. 4), 80–87.

Heller, M. F., & Bergman, M. (1953). Tinnitus Aurium in normally hearing persons. *Annual Otology, 62,* 73–83.

Hétu, R. (1996). The stigma attached to hearing impairment. In S. I. Erlandsson (Ed.), *Psychological and psychosocial approaches to adult hearing loss* (pp. 12–24). *Scandinavian Audiology, 25* (Suppl. 43).

Hiller, W., & Goebel, G. (1992). A psychometric study of complaints in chronic tinnitus. *Journal of Psychosomatic Research, 36,* 337–348.

Horwitz , A. V., & White, H. R. (1987). Gender role orientations and styles of pathology among adolescents. *Journal of Health and Social Behaviour, 28,* 158–170.

House, J. W., Miller, L., & House, P. R. (1977). Severe tinnitus: treatment with biofeedback training (results in 41 cases). *Transactions American Academy of Ophtalmology and Otolaryngology, 4,* 697–703.

House, P. (1981). Personality of the tinnitus patient. In D. Evered & G. Lawrenson (Eds.), *CIBA Foundation Symposium 85. Tinnitus* (pp. 193–198). London: Pitman.

Ireland, C. E., Wilson, P .H., Tonkin, J. P., & Platt-Hepworth, S. (1985). An evaluation of relaxation training in the treatment of tinnitus. *Behaviour Research and Therapy, 33,* 423–430.

Jakes, S. C., Hallam, R. S., Chambers, C., & Hinchcliffe, R. (1985). A factor analytical study of tinnitus complaint behaviour. *Audiology, 24,* 195–206.

Jakes, S. C., Hallam, R. S., Rachman, S., & Hinchcliffe, R. (1986). The effects of reassurance, relaxation training and distraction in chronic tinnitus sufferers. *Behaviour Research and Therapy, 24,* 497–507.

Jacob, R. G., & Lilienfeld, S. O. (1991). Panic disorder: Diagnosis, medical assessment, and psychological assessment. In J. R. Walker, G. R. Norton, & Ross C. A. (Eds.), *Panic disorder and agoraphobia* (pp. 16–102). Pacific Grove, CA: Professional Books.

Johnston, M., & Walker, M. (1996). Suicide in the elderly. Recognizing the signs. *General Hospital Psychiatry, 18,* 257–260.

Jones, I. H., & Knudsen, V. O. (1928). Certain aspects of tinnitus, particularly treatment. *Laryngoscope, 38,* 597–611.

Kafka, M. M. (1934). Tinnitus Aurium, etiology, differential diagnosis, treatment and review of twenty–five cases. *Laryngoscope, 44,* 515–543.

Katon, W., Mark, D., Sullivan, M., Russo, J., Dobie, R., & Sakai, C. (1993). Depressive symptoms and measures of disability: A prospective study. *Journal of Affective Disorder, 27,* 245–254.

Kennedy, A. (1953). Cochlear, neural and subjective factors in tinnitus. *Proceedings of the Royal Society of Medicine, Section of Otology, 46,* 829–832.

Kirsch, C. A., Blanchard, E. B., & Parnes, S. M. (1989). Psychological characteristics of individuals high and low in their ability to cope with tinnitus. *Psychosomatic Medicine, 51,* 209–217.

Konorski, J. E. (1967). *Integrative activity of the brain.* Chicago: University of Chicago Press.

Kuk, F. K., Tyler, R. S., Russel, D., & Jordan, H. (1990). The psychometric properties of a Tinnitus Handicap Questionnaire. *Ear and Hear, 11,* 434–445.

Lewis, J., Stephens, D., & Huws, D. (1992). Suicide in tinnitus sufferers. *Journal of Audiological Medicine, 1,* 30–37.

Lewis, J. E., Stephens, S. D. G., & McKenna, L. (1994). Tinnitus and suicide. *Clinical Otolaryngology, 19,* 50–54.

Lindberg, P., Lyttkens, L., Melin, L., & Scott, B. (1984). Tinnitus—Incidence and handicap. *Scandinavian Audiology, 13,* 287–291.

Lindberg, P., Scott, B., Melin, L., & Lyttkens, L. (1988). Behavioural therapy in the clinical management of tinnitus. *British Journal of Audiology 22,* 265–272.

Malone, J. R. L., & Hemsley, D. R. (1977). Lowered responsiveness and auditory signal detectability during depression. *Psychological Medicine, 7,* 717–722.

Mayou, R., & Radanov, B. P. (1996). Whiplash neck injury. *Journal of Psychosomatic Research 40,* 461–474.

Mayou, R. A., & Sharp, M. (1995). Psychiatric illnesses associated with physical disease. *Balliere's Clinical Psychiatry, 1,* 2.

McKenna, L., Hallam, R. S., & Hinchcliffe, R. (1991). The prevalence of psychological disturbance in neuro-otology outpatients. *Clinical Otolaryngology, 16,* 452–456.

Meikle, M. B., & Griest, S. E. (1987). Gender-based differences in characteristics of tinnitus. *The Hearing Journal, 42,* 68–78.

Meikle, M. B., Vernon, J., & Johnson, R. M. (1984). The perceived severity of tinnitus. *Otolaryngology—Head & Neck Surgery, 92,* 689–696.

Moberg, W. (1949). *Utvandrarna (the Emigrants).* Stockholm: Albert Bonniers Förlag AB.

Newman, C. W., Wharton, J. A., & Jacobson, G. P. (1997). Self-focused and somatic attention in patients with tinnitus. *Journal of American Academy of Audiology, 8,* 143–149.

Nodar, R. H., & Graham, J. T. (1965). An investigation of frequency characteristics of tinnitus associated with Ménière's disease. *Archives of Otolaryngology, 82,* 28–31.

Persson, L. O., & Sjöberg, L. (1987). Mood and positive expectations. *Social Behaviour and Personality, 13,* 171–181.

Rasmussen, J. E. (1964). Relationship of ego identity to psychosocial effectiveness. *Psychological Reports, 15,* 815–825.

Reich, G. E., & Johnson, R. M. (1984). Personality characteristics of tinnitus patients. *Journal of Laryngology and Otology* (Suppl 9.), 228–232.

Roth, T., Kramer, J., & Lutz, T. (1976). The nature of insomnia: A descriptive summary of a sleep clinic population. *Comprehensive Psychiatry, 17,* 217–220.

Rubinstein, B. (1993). Tinnitus and craniomandibular disorders. Is there a link? *Doctoral dissertation, Swedish Dental Journal,* (Suppl. 95).

Rubinstein, B., Axelsson, A., & Carlsson, G. E. (1990). Prevalence of signs and symptoms of craniomandibular disorders in tinnitus patients. *Journal of Craniomandibular Disorder: Facial & Oral Pain, 4,* 186–192.

Rubinstein, B., & Erlandsson, S. I. (1991). A stomatognathic analysis of patients with disabling tinnitus and craniomandibular disorders (CMD). *British Journal of Audiology, 25,* 77–83.

Rubinstein, B., Österberg, T., Rosenhall, U., & Johansson, U. (1993). Tinnitus and craniomandibular disorders in an elderly population. *Journal of Audiological Medicine, 2,* 97–113.

Scicchitano, J., Lovell, P., Pearce, R., Marley, J., & Pilowsky, I. (1996). Illness behaviour and somatization in general practice. *Journal of Psychosomatic Research, 41,* 247–254.

Scott, B., Lindberg, P., Melin, L., & Lyttkens, L. (1990). Predictors of tinnitus discomfort, adaptation and subjective loudness. *British Journal of Audiology, 24,* 51–62.

Shedler, J., Mayman, M., & Manis, M. (1993). The illusion of mental health. *American Psychologist, 48,* 1117–1131.

Simpson, R. B., Nedzelski, J. M., Barber, O. H., & Thomas, M. R. (1988). Psychiatric diagnosis in patients with psychogenic dizziness or severe tinnitus. *Journal of Otolaryngology, 17,* 325–330.

Singerman, B., Riedner, E., & Folstein M. (1980). Emotional disturbance in hearing clinic patients. *British Journal of Psychiatry, 137,* 58–62.

Sjöberg, L., Svensson, E., & Persson, L. O. (1979). The measurement of mood. *Scandinavian Journal of Psychology, 20,* 1–18.

Smith, P., & Coles, R. (1987). Epidemiology of tinnitus: An update. In H. Feldmann (Ed.), *Proceedings of the Third International Tinnitus Seminar, Münster, Germany 1987* (pp. 147–153). Karlsruhe: Harsch Verlag.

Sokolov, E. N. (1963). *Perception and the conditioned reflex.* New York: MacMillan.

Spielberger, C. D. (1983). Manual for the State-Trait Anxiety Inventory (Form Y). Palo Alto, CA: Consulting Psychologists Press.

Stephens, S. D. G., Erlandsson, S. I., Sanchez, L., & Huws, D. (1992). Some psychological aspects of tinnitus. In J. M. Aran & R. Dauman (Eds.), *Proceedings of the Fourth International Tinnitus Seminar, Bordeaux, France 1991* (pp. 433–439). Amsterdam/New York: Kugler Publication.

Stephens, S. D. G., & Hallam, R. S. (1985). The Crown-Crisp Experiential Index in patients complaining of tinnitus. *British Journal of Audiology, 19,* 151–158.

Stouffer, A., & Tyler, R. S. (1990). Characterization of tinnitus by tinnitus patients. *Journal of Speech and Hearing Disorder, 55,* 439–453.

Sullivan, M. D., Katon, W., Dobie, R., Sakai, C., Russo, J., & Harrop-Griffiths J. (1988). Disabling tinnitus. Association with affective disorder. *General Hospital Psychiatry, 10,* 285–291.

Sweetow, R., & Levy, M. (1990). Tinnitus severity scaling for diagnostic and therapeutic usage. *Hearing Instruments, 41,* 20–21, 46.

Tallis, F. (1993). Primary hypothyrodism: A case for vigilance in the psychological treatment of depression. *British Journal of Clinical Psychiatry, 32,* 261–270.

Turk, D. C., & Floor, H. (1987). Pain and pain behaviors: The utility and limitations of the pain behavior construct. *Pain, 31,* 277–289.

Tyler, R. S. (1993). Tinnitus disability and handicap questionnaires. *Sem Hear, 14,* 377–384.

Tyler, R. S., & Baker, L. J. (1983). Difficulties experienced by tinnitus sufferers. *Journal of Speech and Hearing Disorder, 48,* 150–154.

Tyler, R. S., & Conrad-Armes, D. (1983). The determination of tinnitus loudness considering the effects of recruitment. *Journal of Speech and Hearing Research, 26,* 59–72.

Unger, R., & Crawford, M. (1996). *Women and gender. A feminist psychology.* New York: McGraw-Hill.

Vernon, J., Griest, S., & Press, L. (1992). Attributes of tinnitus that may predict temporomandibular joint dysfunction. *Journal of Craniomandibular Practice, 10,* 282–288.

von Knorring, L. (1975). The experience of pain in patients with depressive disorders. *Medical Dissertation,* Umeå University, Sweden.

Weissman, M. (1993). The epidemiology of personality disorders: A 1990 update. *Journal of Personality Disorder* (Suppl.), 44–62.

Wilson, P. A. H., Henry, J., Bowen, M., & Haralambous, G. (1991). Tinnitus reaction questionnaire: Psychometric properties of a measure of distress associated with tinnitus. *Journal of Speech and Hearing Research, 34,* 197–201.

Wilson, P. H., Henry, J. L., & Nicholas, M. K. (1993). Cognitive methods in the management of chronic pain and tinnitus. *Australian Psychologist, 28,* 172–180.

Wittchen, H. U., & Essau, C. A. (1991). The epidemiology of panic attacks, panic disorder, and agoraphobia. In J. R. Walker, G. R. Norton, & C. A. Ross (Eds.), *Panic disorder and agoraphobia* (pp. 103–149). Pacific Grove: CA: Professional Books.

Wood, K. A., Webb, W. L., Orschik, D. J., & Shea J. (1983). Intractable tinnitus: Psychiatric aspects of treatment. *Academy of Psychosomatic Medicine, 24,* 559–561.

CHAPTER 3

Tinnitus and Insomnia

Laurence McKenna, Ph.D.

Almost everyone believes that a good night's sleep is beneficial to health. There is also a widespread belief that poor sleep is somehow harmful and that sleep disturbance needs to be corrected. Sleep disturbance is a frequent complaint of tinnitus sufferers; indeed some patients regarded it as an integral element of the experience of tinnitus. There is an extensive literature on the subject of insomnia and another on tinnitus, but relatively little has been written specifically on tinnitus-related insomnia. This chapter discusses sleep and insomnia and considers tinnitus-related insomnia against this background.

INSOMNIA: PREVALENCE AND DEFINITIONS

Like tinnitus, sleep disorders are extraordinarily prevalent. One in seven Americans has a chronic sleep disorder (Shapiro & Dement, 1993). Bixler, Kales, Soldatos, et al. (1979) reported that 50 percent of adults complain of current or past sleep disorders and 38 percent experience current difficulties with sleep. Although insomnia is one of the most common of all sleep disorders, fig-

ures about its prevalence vary enormously. Liljenberg, Almqvist, Hetta, et al. (1988) reported prevalence rates of less than 2 percent; Bixler et al. (1979) reported that insomnia accounted for 32 percent of the high rate of "current sleep disorders" in their study. The disparity arises from the different definitions and data collection techniques employed by different researchers. The term insomnia covers a range of sleep-related complaints including sleep of insufficient duration, of poor quality or effectiveness. These problems include difficulty falling asleep (initial or early insomnia), waking in the middle of the night and having difficulty returning to sleep (middle insomnia), and waking too early in the morning (terminal or late insomnia). Problems with the quality of sleep usually translate into complaints of sleep being light, broken or restless and not being restorative or refreshing. Espie (1991) suggested a popular definition of insomnia as "not getting enough or a proper sleep." Complaints about associated daytime problems such as tiredness, mood disturbance, and poor performance are also common. Liljenberg et al. (1988) noted that when the complaints about daytime sleepiness were excluded from the definition of insomnia, the prevalence figures for insomnia were three times higher in their study.

Borkovec (1982) lists nine subtypes of insomnia. These include sleep disturbance associated with: respiratory disorders, sleep-related myoclonus and "restless legs," psychiatric disturbance, other medical and environmental conditions, alcohol and drug use, disorders of the sleep wake schedule, and childhood onset insomnia. One of the most prominent subtypes among Borkovec's (1982) list is psychophysiological insomnia. He described this as "insomnia based on chronic, somatized tension-anxiety and negative conditioning" and as "objectively verified insomnia unrelated to medical disease or to serious psychiatric problems" (p. 882). Objective verification relies on psychophysiological measures such as an electroencephalogram (EEG), electromyogram (EMG) and electro-oculogram (EOG). When these types of measures are used collectively, they are referred to as polysomnography. Another important subtype is that of "subjective insomnia" defined by Borkovec (1982) as "a convincing and honest complaint of insomnia made by an individual lacking apparent psychopathology that is not substantiated by polysomnography" (p. 883). In a similar vein, the *Diagnostic and Statistical Manual* (Version IV) of the American Psychiatric Association distinguishes "primary insomnia," that is, "a difficulty in initiating or maintaining sleep that causes clinically significant distress or impairment in daytime functioning," from sleep problems that occur in relation to other medical or psychiatric disorders. Much of the literature on insomnia refers to studies involving subjects suffering from either psychophysiological or subjective insomnia. Many studies do not clearly distinguish between these (or other subtypes) and it is possible that this heterogeneity of samples may account for some inconsistencies in findings.

Most adults report getting 7 to 8½ hours sleep a night; there is, however, considerable variation in "normal" sleep patterns with some people feeling rested and performing well on only three hours sleep, while others apparently require twelve hours sleep (Borkovec 1982). As a consequence the importance of complaints about insomnia often becomes a matter of clinical judgment. Reference needs to be made not only to the total amount of sleep obtained, but to measures of time taken to get to sleep (or initial sleep onset latency), time awake in the middle of the night, and sleep efficiency (time asleep divided by time spent in bed). Some definitions that help to operationalize the term insomnia have been suggested. Morin (1993) proposed that sleep onset problems should refer to a delay of 30 minutes or more, after turning the lights out, before getting to sleep. Similarly, he suggested that middle insomnia be regarded as a delay of 30 minutes or more in getting back to sleep after waking in the night or a total of more than 30 minutes awake in the case of several awakenings. While Espie (1991) concurred that a delay of 30 minutes in getting to sleep must be a minimum criterion for the classification of insomnia, he suggested that 45 minutes as a more appropriate criterion for the classification of sleep disturbance. Morin (1993) proposed that premature awakening in the morning after less than six-and-a-half hours sleep be used to define late insomnia. He also suggested that if the amount of time spent asleep is less than 85 percent of the time spent in bed (namely, sleep efficiency) then the term insomnia can be applied. Morin (1993) suggested that these difficulties should occur at least three nights a week while Espie (1991), again more conservatively, recommended four out of seven nights as a criterion for the classification of insomnia.

THE NATURE AND FUNCTION OF SLEEP

Sleep can be divided (in terms of electrical brain activity) into stages of Rapid Eye Movement (REM) sleep and Non-REM sleep. The latter can be subdivided into four stages that roughly parallel depth of sleep (see Figure 3-1). Stage 1 is a very light or transitional stage between wakefulness and sleep. Sleep then progresses through Stages 2 and 3 to the deepest sleep in Stage 4. After a period of deeper sleep the process reverses with the sleeper passing through lighter stages. There is then a period of REM sleep after which the cycle begins again. This cycle takes about ninety minutes to complete but can vary from seventy to one hundred and twenty minutes. The cycle is repeated four or five times a night in normal young adults. A normal night's sleep also

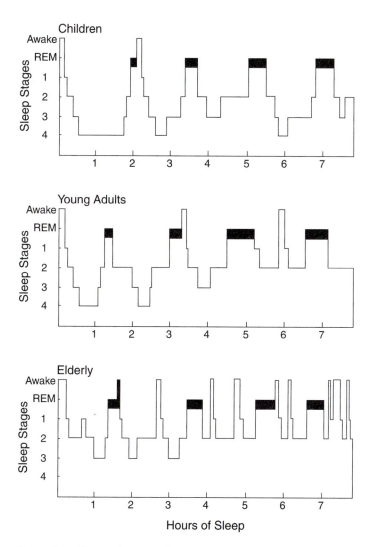

FIGURE 3-1. Sleep cycles across the night in children, young adults and the elderly. REM sleep (darkened areas) occurs cyclically throughout the night at intervals of approximately 90 minutes in all age groups. Stage 4 sleep decreases progressively with age, so little if any is present in the elderly. In addition, the elderly have frequent awakenings and a notable increase in wake time after sleep onset (From *Evaluation and Treatment of Insomnia*, by Anthony Kales and Joyce D. Kales. Copyright (1984 by Anthony Kales and Joyce D. Kales. Used by permission of Oxford University Press, Inc.).

includes several awakenings. These are usually brief and many people are unaware of their occurrence. For many people the first awakening occurs after two or three hours of sleep. Awakenings become more common as the hours of sleep increase. The first awakening often represents a point of change after which the periods of REM sleep become longer and the periods of Non-REM sleep become correspondingly shorter. Clinically, people often described this experience as "little really deep sleep after the first awakening." It is during REM sleep that most dreaming occurs.

Age brings with it changes in the pattern of sleep (see Figure 3-1). Older people experience less deep sleep; Stage 4 sleep may be absent altogether in older people. The number of awakenings also increases with age. Young adults commonly experience two awakenings in a normal night's sleep. An older person may experience as many as nine awakenings in a night. For many elderly people, sleep is experienced as light and fragmented. It is a commonly held belief that older people do not need as much sleep as they did when younger. While older people do tend to get less sleep at night, they also nap more in the daytime. Morin (1993) pointed out that when daytime sleep is added to night time sleep the total sleep achieved remains relatively stable from middle age to later life.

Sleep is thought by most people to be fundamental to their well-being. Many researchers speculate that sleep (in particular slow wave sleep or deep sleep) serves the function of conserving the body's energy or of restoring it in some way. Both the energy conservation and restoration theories have the drop in metabolic rate that occurs during sleep as the focus of their reasoning. It has also been proposed that REM sleep plays a critical role in more psychological functions such as memory and learning (Dean, 1970). There are variations in these theoretical perspectives and no one hypothesis completely explains all of the observations about sleep (Shapiro & Flanigan, 1993). The exact function of sleep remains unknown; nonetheless, there is virtually universal agreement that sleep is necessary for some reason—whatever that might be.

THE CHARACTERISTICS OF INSOMNIA

Poor sleepers commonly define their insomnia by reference to a time when they slept better or by reference to others who sleep well. Considerable variability is seen in the sleep pattern of many insomniacs. Good and bad nights are interspersed and one feature for many sufferers is the unpredictability of sleep rather than simply a lack of it. In fact, Chambers and Keller (1993) concluded from a review of studies comparing good sleepers with insomniacs that the mean total sleep time of the latter was only thirty-five minutes per night less than good sleepers. Although statistically significant, Chambers and Keller (1993) questioned its clinical significance. Some people will habitually take a long time to fall asleep but the predictability of this can lead to acceptance rather than frustration. In any situation in which there is unpredictability there can be a perception of lack of control. This is of fundamental importance in determining distress. An implication of Liljenberg et al.'s (1988) finding that excluding daytime sleepiness from the definition of insomnia tripled the prevalence rate of the problem, is that disturbed sleep does not always result in sleepiness. Daytime sleepiness can be assessed using the Multiple Sleep Latency Test. The patient is offered five twenty-minute naps at two-hour intervals during the day and the time taken to fall asleep is taken as an objective measure of sleepiness. Several studies (for example, Chambers & Keller, 1993; Seidel, Ball, Cohen, et al., 1984) have found no evidence of daytime sleepiness in insomniacs.

There have been many studies comparing insomniacs with good sleepers on measures of psychopathology and personality, most commonly the Minnesota Multiphasic

Personality Inventory (MMPI). Borkovec (1982) briefly reviewed these and concluded that the "insomniac can be characterized as a person who is mildly depressed, anxious, hypochondriacal and overly worrisome." Espie (1991) came to essentially the same conclusion. Borkovec (1982) also pointed out that, apart from the MMPI studies, people experiencing insomnia have been found to score more poorly on other measures of personality and emotional state. These differences were apparent even when studies excluded subjects with gross psychopathology were excluded. Borkovec (1982), however, pointed out that few significant correlations have been found between personality variables and objective sleep parameters (polysomnographic data).

It has been suggested that a loss of sleep has been associated with increased daytime sleepiness and poor performance on a range of psychomotor and cognitive tasks particularly among normal subjects deprived of sleep (Carskadon & Dement, 1982; Dement, Seidel, & Carskadon, 1984; Glenville, Broughton, Wing, & Wilkinson, 1978). While subjective complaints about poorer daytime performance are common among insomniacs, the evidence for impairment of functioning is inconsistent. Williams (1997) cited statistics that suggest that insomniacs have twice as many road traffic accidents as normal sleepers. He also noted that insomniacs are more likely to report that they suffer from poor health and that their work is limited by illness.

Schneider-Helmert (1987) found that general daytime performance of insomniacs was not impaired, but they did more poorly than controls on cognitive tasks performed in the morning. Other studies have found no significant differences in daytime performance between chronic insomniacs and good sleepers (Sugarman, Stern & Walsh, 1985; Seidel, Ball, Cohen, et al., 1984; Mendelson, Garnett & Linnoilal, 1984). Daytime mood disturbance amongst insomniacs has however been reported in a number of studies (Seidel, Ball, Cohen, et al., 1984; Marchini, Coates, Magistad, & Waldum, 1983).

Espie (1991) suggested that sleep and sleep loss should be considered within the twenty-four hour rhythmic cycle. He pointed out that performance decrements in sleep-deprived people occur especially at times when the person would normally be asleep. He also highlighted the importance of the circadian rhythm by reference to the effects of disharmonies such as jet lag and the impact of shift work. Espie (1991) pointed out that "advancing, delaying, extending or reducing established sleep periods has been found to impoverish waking behaviors significantly" (p. 2). It is therefore not clear to what extent the ill effects of a bad night's sleep are the result of the sleep loss per se or to the disruption of the circadian rhythm.

It may be concluded from the literature that complaints about insomnia are not necessarily accompanied by clear sleep deprivation and that the effects of insomnia are variable.

TINNITUS-RELATED INSOMNIA: THE EXTENT OF THE PROBLEM

Sleep disturbance is one of the most common problems associated with tinnitus. Based on data gathered in the United Kingdom National Study of Hearing, Chapter 1 states that 5 percent of the population report sleep-disturbing tinnitus. Tyler and Baker (1983), using an open-ended questionnaire, asked members of a tinnitus self-help group to list the difficulties they had as a result of their tinnitus. Almost fifty-seven percent of respondents listed difficulty in getting to sleep as one of their tinnitus-related problems. As such this was the most commonly listed problem. A large number of respondents in this study also reported emotional problems such as despair, frustration, depression, annoyance, irritation, and an inability to relax. Sanchez and Stephens (1997) administered the same open ended questionnaire in a clinical setting. Their subjects were 473 patients referred to the Tinnitus Clinic at the Welsh Hearing Institute. As in the Tyler and Baker

(1983) study, many respondents listed multiple complaints associated with their tinnitus. Sanchez and Stephens (1997) divided responses into five categories, one of which was sleep-related problems. The complaints listed within this category were "sleep difficulties," problems in "getting to sleep," the use of "sleeping pills" and "early waking." Together these amounted to 14.6 percent of all responses. Twenty-five percent of respondents in this study listed "sleep difficulties" among their tinnitus-related problems. This was the second most commonly listed problem. Problems with "getting to sleep" were listed by 22 percent of respondents while complaints about "sleeping pills" and "early waking" were listed by 4 percent and 3 percent of respondents respectively.

As in the Tyler and Baker (1983) study, many respondents listed psychological problems; such problems amounted to just over thirty percent of all responses. Sleep disturbance is also a significant problem among children complaining of tinnitus. Gabriels (1995) found that 42 percent of her sample of children with tinnitus suffered from sleep disturbance. In a short series of children complaining of tinnitus, Kentish, Crocker and McKenna (in preparation) noted that sleep disturbance was a major problem in over 80 percent of cases.

Axelsson and Sandh (1985) reported that insomnia was one of the most common subjective discomforts associated with tinnitus in patients with noise-induced hearing loss. Axelsson and Ringdahl (1989) assessed the prevalence and characteristics of tinnitus in a Swedish population using a postal questionnaire. They assessed sleep using two questions. One question sought to assess the severity of tinnitus using a four-point descriptive scale. The second highest point on this scale was defined as "tinnitus interferes with my sleep." Twenty-eight percent of their respondents who reported experiencing tinnitus "often or always" rated their tinnitus severity using this category. Axelsson and Ringdahl (1989) described the most severe category as "tinnitus plagues

me all day"; 2.4 percent of their tinnitus sufferers rated their tinnitus using this category. It may be that many of these respondents also suffered from sleep disturbance. The second sleep question examined the severity of sleep disturbance in terms of frequency of difficulty in getting to sleep, or in waking and returning to sleep. They noted that of those who had difficulties in falling asleep only 23 percent to 41 percent rated the severity of their tinnitus as "interferes with my sleep." They suggested that rating the severity of tinnitus in terms of sleep disturbance was not fruitful. Nonetheless, the inclusion of a sleep disturbance variable seems to be an integral part of the assessment of tinnitus.

The importance of sleep disturbance in tinnitus complaint was highlighted by the work of Jakes, Hallam, Chambers, and Hinchcliffe (1985) and Hallam, Jakes and Hinchcliffe (1988). Using questionnaire data these researchers reported three main dimensions to tinnitus complaint: emotional distress, auditory perceptual difficulties, and sleep disturbance. An analysis of their second, refined, questionnaire indicated that sleep disturbance accounted for 43 percent of the variance, that is, the largest single factor (Hallam et al., 1988). The sleep disturbance was expressed in the questionnaire items in terms of all three types of insomnia: delayed sleep onset, middle insomnia, and early morning waking.

Kemp and George (1992) asked tinnitus sufferers who were seeking medical advice to keep diary records of their experience of tinnitus and include in this a rating of difficulty in getting to sleep. All nine of their subjects indicated that tinnitus had some effect on their sleep and three used the upper half of the rating scale to express this difficulty. Jakes et al. (1985) reported that insomnia was considered the main complaint in 50 percent of severe tinnitus sufferers, while Lindberg, Scott, Melin, and Lyttkens (1988) reported that 62 percent of a group of tinnitus patients included in their treatment study listed sleep disturbance among their problems. Slater, Jones, Davis, and Terry (1983) reported that 23 percent of respondents to a tinnitus survey stated that tinnitus woke them at night.

Alster, Shemesh, Ornan and Attias (1993) investigated the prevalence and severity of sleep disturbance in a group of chronic tinnitus patients. Their subjects were military personnel with noise-induced hearing loss. An interview with a psychiatrist excluded formal psychiatric disorder. Subjects were assessed on a range of measures including a Mini Sleep Questionnaire. They compared the tinnitus group's Mini Sleep Questionnaire scores with an existing body of data available for normal controls and a group of thirty military personnel with no history of tinnitus or sleep disorder. Questionnaire scores were found to be higher than for normal controls in 77 percent of the tinnitus subjects. Tinnitus patients with a complaint of sleep disturbance rated Mini Sleep Questionnaire items relating to delayed sleep, morning awakenings, midsleep awakenings, morning fatigue, and chronic fatigue more highly. In contrast, excessive daytime sleep was not rated highly.

Alster et al. (1993) also retrospectively reviewed the records of tinnitus patients seen in a sleep research center. They found that of 1,500 polygraphic studies, only ten patients complained of tinnitus. Most of these ten subjects also complained of other sleep problems such as obstructive sleep apnea, snoring, and periodic leg movements during sleep. Data were available on a number of electrophysiological measures. Sleep latency, REM latency, and sleep efficiency measures were also examined. Alster et al. (1993) concluded that these subjects exhibited severe sleep disturbance including low sleep efficiencies, a high number of sleep awakenings, long sleep onset latencies, early morning awakenings, and short REM latencies which they referred to in terms of "a biological or vulnerability marker for an effective response to stressful life events." Nonetheless, they commented that unless tinnitus subjects have a sleep disorder, in addition to any sleep difficulties related to tinnitus, they are unlikely to seek a sleep

examination. Only two of the ten subjects listed tinnitus as a primary complaint that disturbed their sleep. Four subjects did not connect their tinnitus with their referral for a sleep examination. One subject reported that although his tinnitus had been present for ten years, his sleep had been disturbed for only the last four years; he suffered from obstructive sleep apnea.

Scott, Lindberg, Melin, and Lyttkens (1990) carried out a large-scale questionnaire survey of adaptation processes in tinnitus patients. They measured subjective discomfort, loudness of tinnitus, and psychological complaints among tinnitus patients seen in hearing clinics throughout Sweden. The most important predictors of discomfort from tinnitus and of adaptation to the symptom were "controllability" and the degree to which external sounds masked the tinnitus. The factors that most strongly predicted increased discomfort from and decreased tolerance to tinnitus were depression and insomnia. They also reported that insomnia was a more common problem among tinnitus patients than among control subjects with a hearing loss and no tinnitus. It is not clear how the term insomnia was defined or interpreted by respondents in this study; however, the study included a separate variable referring to difficulty returning to sleep after waking in the night. This latter problem was equally common among tinnitus and hearing impaired subjects.

It is clear from the literature that sleep disturbance is a major problem associated with tinnitus. However, a problem with many of the tinnitus studies mentioned is that insomnia has been only loosely defined, if at all. The very nature of some studies (Sanchez & Stephens, 1997; Tyler & Baker, 1983) has left subjects to make their own definitions. Where criteria have been stated they appear to be less strict than those recommended by insomnia researchers such as Espie (1991) and Morin (1993). For example, Alster, Shemesh, Ornan, and Attias (1993) when examining the sleep records of a group of patients with tinnitus considered sleep latency to be delayed if the time from lights out until the start of Stage 2 exceeded 15 minutes. A delay in sleep onset of twenty minutes has been used to classify tinnitus patients as sleep disturbed in outcome studies carried out by Jakes, Hallam, Rachman, and Hinchcliffe (1986), Davis, McKenna, and Hallam (1995). While in most good sleepers the time until sleep onset is 0 to 15 minutes (Birrell, 1983), the delay can be up to 30 minutes (Espie, 1991). The more conservative figures suggested by Morin (1993) and Espie (1991) therefore seem more appropriate as they are likely to better discriminate normal sleepers from insomniacs. Furthermore, relying on single, or a small number of responses to questionnaires may lead to inaccuracies in the estimation of the prevalence of sleep disorders in tinnitus patients. It is recognized that in a clinical setting patients complaining of insomnia amplify the magnitude of their sleep problems compared with the results of more formal assessment procedures. It is possible therefore that the accounts, to date, of sleep disturbance in tinnitus patients overestimate the extent of the problem. Clearly, tinnitus patients who complain about sleep disorders deserve attention. However, there is a need for a more rigorous assessment of sleep disorders in this population.

ASSESSMENT

The complete assessment of sleep complaints within a sleep clinic includes data from clinical interview, diary records of behavior, questionnaire data and polysomnographic studies. It is also useful to have the benefit of a screening that excludes other sleep disorders such as sleep apnea or periodic limb movements and other medical disorders that might affect sleep, such as hyperthyroidism or anemia. The sleep problem needs to be seen within the context of a formulation of the person's general health and functioning.

Data can be gathered in a number of ways. There are considerable methodological difficulties in obtaining detailed sleep data from an informant other than the complainant. Most assessment procedures therefore rely upon self-report data, of one sort or another, or on objective measures in the form of polysomnography.

Clinical Interview

Once other disorders have been excluded, the central element of the assessment process is obtaining a sleep history. Information needs to be gathered about the nature of the problem, whether it is a difficulty in initiating or in maintaining sleep or both, and about the timing and circumstances of its onset. It is very helpful to obtain an account of the typical 24-hour sleep-wake program, that is, at what time the person goes to bed, how long it takes to go to sleep, how many times and for how long the patient wakes in the night, at what time the patient wakes for the last time and at what time the patient gets up. Information about daytime activity, including naps, should be obtained. This information provides a measure of the severity of insomnia. The number of nights per week that the person experiences poor sleep is yet another expression of the extent of the problem. Information about the effects of the poor sleep on daytime functioning helps to make up a more complete picture; the person can be asked about this in terms of mood changes, fatigue, performance decrements, and changes in social functioning and or relationships.

As in any analysis of behavior, it is important to establish the antecedents and consequences of the insomnia complaint. In this context it is helpful to obtain information about factors such as the person's sleep hygiene, for example, does he or she watch television or do paperwork in bed, are there environmental factors such as light, noise in the background (or possibly the lack of it in the case of some tinnitus patients) contributing to the problem. Information about diet, particularly caffeine and nicotine intake, is sought. Most insomniacs make some attempt to solve their sleep problems through informal means and it is important to question the person about the use of such strategies. In this context, information is sought about the use of "over-the-counter" as well as prescribed medication and also about the use of alcohol. Information is also needed about variations in the typical program, for example changes in routine at weekends or as a result of shift work. It is also important to be alert for possible secondary gains associated with insomnia, such as, providing a justification for other behaviors.

Morin (1993) described an Insomnia Interview Schedule for structuring the data collection during interview. This schedule is intended to obtain a sleep history, to screen for sleep disorders and to gain information about psychological, environmental and medical factors that might be contributing to the sleep problem. The schedule is time consuming to administer but it does provide useful guidelines for assessing insomnia. A person's retrospective account of his or her sleep, however, provides only a rough estimate of the problem. It is common for people to overestimate the severity of their sleep difficulties.

Sleep Diaries

The use of sleep diaries on a nightly basis has been the most favored research and clinical instrument for assessing insomnia. Diaries are used to record most of the information relevant to the person's sleep wake schedule outlined previously. They can also allow sleep efficiency, that is, the amount of time asleep expressed as a percentage of the total time spent in bed, as calculated to provide another measure of the severity of insomnia.

Diary sheets can be provided that allow a summary of a week's sleep pattern at a glance. People are asked to record times as accurately as possible but should be discouraged from "clock watching"; most people are likely to be capable of making estimates to within 5 to 10 minutes. Any error of judgment is likely to be reasonably constant as long as the person completes the diaries in the same way each day. Espie

(1991) concluded that the evidence from the literature indicated that sleep diary data had comparable reliability to electroencephalogram (EEG) assessment. However, it is advisable to ensure that the person has a clear understanding of how to complete the sleep diary, and of the importance of doing so, before starting. An example of a sleep diary for use in a tinnitus clinic setting is provided in Appendix 1. Diaries should be completed within an hour of getting up in the morning. It is standard practice to have the person complete two weeks of sleep diaries as a baseline prior to the commencement of treatment and then throughout the therapy. Compliance with diary-keeping is occasionally a problem. Diaries can be simplified to help improve compliance, but Morin (1993) suggested that estimates of time in bed, sleep time, and wake time represent a minimum data set. The sleep diary is valuable, not only in establishing the extent of the problem, but also in monitoring progress. Morin (1993) pointed out that they represent a practical and economic method of tracking sleep problems over extensive periods of time and as such provide a more representative sample of the person's sleep than one or two nights of polysomnography, particularly given the night-to-night variability in sleep patterns.

While it is relatively straightforward to obtain estimates of time taken to get to sleep and the other similar measures, some ingenuity may be needed to obtain measures of other variables such as quality of sleep or impact on daytime functioning. The use of adjectival, numerical, or visual analogue scales is likely to be the most useful approach to assessing quality of sleep. The sleep diary suggested in the Appendix uses numerical scales for these purposes. These scales are quick and easy to use for most people. Sometimes other methods of assessing the impact of insomnia on daytime functioning suggest themselves, for instance, productivity at work or number of days taken off work.

Careful thought needs to be given to the matter of interpreting data from sleep diaries. Espie, Brooks, and Lindsay (1989) suggested three criteria for the evaluation of clinically significant change in sleep onset latency: (i) absolute (any) reduction in sleep onset latency at posttreatment; (ii) 50 percent reduction in sleep onset latency at post-treatment; (iii) final posttreatment sleep onset latency of 30 minutes or less. Espie (1991) provided a helpful discussion of the interpretation of sleep diary data. He pointed out that the variability in insomniacs' sleep patterns may render an expression of data in terms of mean scores alone uninforma-tive. He suggested that some measure of variance, such as range or standard devia-tion, be used in the consideration of clinical change. He also suggested that therapy goals be agreed in terms that operationalize what is acceptable or functional, and out-come be measured in terms of the achieve-ment of these goals. This approach allows a more clinically meaningful assessment than a reliance on mean scores alone. A goal-planning approach has been used in a range of therapeutic settings, including audiolog-ical rehabilitation (McKenna, 1987).

Assessment of Mood

The importance of assessing mood is high-lighted by the high prevalence of psycho-logical disorder among both insomnia patients (see Borkovec, 1982; Espie, 1993 for reviews) and tinnitus patients (McKenna, Hallam, & Hinchcliffe, 1991; Singerman, Riedner, & Folstein, 1980). Significant mood disorders may need to become the focus of treatment (see Chapter 2 and Chapter 11). Mood may be assessed through the use of standard questionnaires. There are a number of highly suitable instruments available and the choice of questionnaire will inevitably be a matter of familiarity and personal preference. The Beck Depression Inventory (Beck, Steer, & Brown, 1996) and Beck Anxiety Inventory (Beck & Steer, 1990) are quick to administer, provide easily inter-pretable scores, and are widely accepted instruments. The Speilberger State-Trait Anxiety Inventory (Speilberger, Gorsuch, & Lushene, 1970) has the advantage of pro-viding a measure of trait anxiety, or con-stitutional predisposition to anxiety, as well as of current anxiety level but takes slightly longer to complete and score. The General Health Questionnaire (Goldberg, 1978) is intended as a screening device for significant psychological disorder in nonpsychiatric clinic populations. It is quick to complete and score and has the advan-tage that it has been used with tinnitus patients (McKenna et al., 1991; Singerman et al., 1980).

Sleep Questionnaires

A number of sleep questionnaires have been developed, for example, the Pittsburgh Sleep Quality Index (Buysse, Reynolds, Monk, et al., 1989). Sleep questionnaires are of limited clinical value because they pro-vide retrospective estimates that may include significant reporting biases and the value of the average figures that they provide is questionable given the variability in many insomniacs' sleep patterns. Espie (1991) argued against the use of sleep ques-tionnaires but conceded that they are inex-pensive and easy to administer and that they can provide helpful data when there are large numbers of subjects to be surveyed or screened.

Polysomnographic Recordings

Data from sleep diaries also tend to repre-sent an overestimation of the difficulties experienced compared with polysomno-graphic data (Borkovec & Weerts, 1976; Bixler, Kales, Leo, & Slye, 1973). Morin (1993) described nocturnal polysomnography as the "gold standard" for sleep measurement. It involves electrographic monitoring of sleep (in terms of electroencephalogram, electromyogram and electro-oculogram), respiration, cardiac function, oxygen desat-uration, and leg movements. It is helpful in determining the severity of the problem and in highlighting any discrepancy between subjective complaints and actual sleep. It can help to reveal otherwise obscured con-ditions, for example, it may provide the first opportunity for observing periodic leg movements, or for it may reveal REM latencies that suggest depression and therefore provide helpful data in people who strongly deny psychological disorder. Electrophysiological measurement in the form of the Multiple Sleep Latency Test has also been used in the assessment of daytime functioning. The Multiple Sleep Latency Test provides a measure of daytime sleepiness. However, as mentioned above the value of this test has been called into question (Chambers & Keller, 1993; Seidel, Ball, Cohen, et al., 1984). Polysomnography is a relatively expensive process and, outside the United States, sleep laboratories are not a standard facility in even major medical centers. There is also an issue about how representative one or two nights' polysomnography are for most people complaining of insomnia. The variability that characterizes many insomniacs' sleep patterns can make it difficult to generalize from data gathered in the unusual circumstances of a sleep laboratory to the person's home life. It is also the case that polysomnography does not allow any comment to be made about sleep quality—one of the most important of variables in sleep assessment. Most tinnitus sufferers do not request formal sleep assessments and little polysomnograph data are available on tinnitus patients (Alster et al., 1993). This remains an area for further investigation.

Other Behavioral Assessments

A number of other behavioral assessment devices such as a switch-activated clock (Franklin, 1981) or the use of tape recorders that prompt responses from people if they are awake (Lichstein, Nickel, Hoelscher, & Kelley, 1982) have been used to gather sleep data. One of the more popular devices is the wrist actigraph (Hauri & Wisbey, 1992). This device uses an accelerometer to monitor the occurrence and degree of motion. Sleep is scored in the absence of movement according to preset criteria, for example, if no movement is recorded in a given recording epoch and if there is no movement recorded in adjacent epochs. This device permits a profile of the person's sleep geography, including most of the parameters derived from diary records, to be complied in their home environment and in a relatively nonintrusive way. As such it provides a useful supplement to diary data. This approach does require specialized equipment and appropriate computer software for data recovery and processing; however, it is less demanding on resources than polysomnography.

It is worth remembering that insomniacs' complaints are often not corroborated by objective data. A subjective complaint of disturbed sleep or of disturbed daytime functioning is therefore necessary and usually sufficient for the patient's distress to be accepted. *The Diagnostic and Statistical Manual* (IV edition) of the American Psychiatric Association (1994) classification requires only a subjective complaint and does not demand objective evidence of sleep disturbance.

Any or all of the assessment methods described are likely to be relevant and applicable to the patient with tinnitus-related insomnia. In practice, however, the clinical interview and sleep diary are likely to prove the most convenient and useful methods of assessment in most clinical settings. It may also be useful to employ additional tinnitus-related assessment devices. In a clinical setting many patients refer to a vicious circle of tinnitus intrusiveness and annoyance and sleep disturbance. Tinnitus intrusiveness and annoyance are commonly assessed on numerical or visual analogue scales. Hallam's (1996) tinnitus questionnaire includes an insomnia factor and is useful not only as a research tool but also as a means of assessing progress in a clinical setting (see Chapter 11).

MODELS OF INSOMNIA

Most theoretical models of insomnia have the concept of an elevated level of arousal as a central theme; the arousal may be physiological or psychological in nature. It has been suggested that insomniacs may have particularly sensitive nervous systems and that they are very reactive to external stimulation (Coursey, Buchsbaum, & Frankel, 1975). The idea that insomnia may result from heightened levels of autonomic nervous system arousal associated with tension and difficulty in relaxing has not received strong support. Borkovec (1982) noted the inconsistent nature of the evidence about autonomic arousal among people with insomnia. He pointed out that there was no relationship between declines in physiological activity during relaxation treatment and subjective and objective sleep outcomes. This argues against the idea that autonomic hyperactivity is involved in insomnia. However, he concluded that there remains a possibility that insomnia is mediated by autonomic activity. Espie (1991) stated that the use of relaxation techniques in the management of insomnia does not, in itself, lend support to an autonomic arousal model.

An alternative to the idea of heightened physiological arousal is the suggestion that insomnia may be the result of psychological overarousal. This may be due to either high levels of cognitive activity, such as "a busy mind," or to emotional arousal. Insomniacs' reports of "a racing mind" have been recorded by many researchers (Borkovec, 1982) and this phenomenon is frequently noted in clinical practice. Lichstein and Rosenthal (1980) asked insomniacs to attribute their sleep difficulties to a series of somatic and cognitive factors; they found that the majority of subjects (55 percent) identified cognitive factors as more important while many others (35 percent) rated it as of at least equal importance to somatic arousal. The findings of Espie, Brooks, and Lindsay (1989) support this view. They reported on a principal component analysis of a Sleep Disturbance Questionnaire that revealed "mental anxiety" as the first factor accounting for 40 percent of the total variance. In his review of the literature Borkovec (1982) noted the frequent finding that when insomniacs are awakened during Stage 2 sleep they often report having been

awake. Espie (1991) also pointed to this frequent observation and proposed that continuing mental activity even in Stage 2 sleep is interpreted by insomniacs as wakefulness. Both Borkovec (1982) and Espie (1991) concluded from their reviews that there is considerable evidence supporting the idea that insomniacs are highly cognitively aroused. The cause and effect relationship, however, remains unconfirmed.

Other mechanisms apart from heightened arousal may be important in creating or maintaining insomnia. The effect of disrupted circadian rhythms can be profound. The experiences of jet lag and shift work are known by many people. The effects may take place at the time of the disruption or a long time after. Sleep disturbance is more common in former shift workers ten years after stopping shift work than among controls who never did shift work (Shapiro & Dement, 1993). It is possible that the higher incidence of insomnia complaints in middle-aged and elderly women results from disrupted sleep years before, during child-rearing. In a slightly different vein, Chambers and Keller (1992) have suggested that many people complaining of insomnia are in reality short sleepers who erroneously believe that they require more sleep than they are getting. They suggested that the anxiety associated with this may be responsible for daytime fatigue.

TINNITUS-RELATED INSOMNIA: MECHANISMS

Insomnia may be primary in nature, (without any apparent physical disorder or a mental illness etiology), or secondary, (symptomatic of an underlying medical or psychological state). Clearly, the insomnia experienced by tinnitus patients is secondary in nature. Whether it is secondary to the tinnitus *per se* or to emotional or cognitive arousal is less clear. If the former is the case, then tinnitus may be understood as a specific arousal factor that may be similar to other sleep disrupters such as restless legs.

The evidence on this issue is mixed. Axelsson and Ringdahl (1989) reported a relationship between the severity of tinnitus and difficulties in falling asleep. They pointed out, however, that in some patients quite severe tinnitus has no influence on their sleep, while others with a moderate degree of tinnitus find sleep difficult. They also reported that it was unusual for the target population to be awakened by tinnitus. Meikle, Vernon, and Johnson (1984) also reported that tinnitus severity correlated highly with sleep disturbance. Alster et al., (1993) reported that subjects whose sleep scores were more pathological demonstrated more severe tinnitus symptomology than subjects with normal sleep scores. Interestingly, Kemp and George (1992) found that sleep disturbance was only weakly correlated with subjective ratings of tinnitus loudness and annoyance. These authors suggested that this may have been because of the "fairly widespread" use of sleeping medications among their study population.

The factor analytic studies carried out by Hallam et al. (1988) and by Hiller and Goebel (1992) imply that sleep disturbance represents an independent factor in tinnitus complaint, specifically, separate from emotional distress. Hallam et al. (1988) also suggested that the sleep complaint was related to tinnitus rather than to a preexisting sleep disorder. It should be noted, however, that Hallam et al. (1988) carried out two analyses of their questionnaire data, and their initial analysis indicated that sleep disturbance was related to difficulty in ignoring the noises and to difficulty in relaxing and to a depressed mood. Alster et al. (1993) also reported that sleep disturbance in tinnitus subjects was associated with depressed mood. Davies, McKenna, and Hallam (1995) reported that 50 percent of patients entering a study of psychological treatments for tinnitus listed sleep disturbance as a significant problem. The study included a follow-up assessment four months after the completion of therapy. Part of that assessment involved the completion of a one-week diary

record of several sleep variables. Hallam (1996a) reported on this aspect of the assessment. Sleep disturbance was indicated by reports of a sleep onset latency in excess of twenty minutes, waking in the night, taking sleeping tablets and in terms of number of hours sleep. He found that sleep disturbance was related to self-report ratings of tinnitus annoyance made each evening. Sleep disturbance was not related to more general ratings of annoyance and loudness made with reference to the preceding week rather than to individual evenings. Nor was it related to standardized measures of depression or anxiety or to the Emotional Distress Scale of the Tinnitus Questionnaire (Hallam et al, 1988; Hallam, 1996). In this respect Hallam's (1996a) findings contrast with those of Alster et al. (1993) who reported that 37 percent of their tinnitus subjects obtained scores on the Zung depression scale (Zung, 1967) that were indicative of depression and that there was a significant correlation between the Zung scores and the Mini Sleep Questionnaire mean score suggesting a link between emotional state and sleep disorder.

The fact that emotional problems and sleep disturbance often coexist creates the possibility that the two are related and there must be a strong probability that sleep disturbance is symptomatic of the emotional disturbance. This would seem to be a more parsimonious explanation than the postulation that sleep disturbance is a direct result of tinnitus per se. Attributing sleep disturbance to emotional distress rather than tinnitus also provides a more optimistic basis for counseling patients. While it is good scientific practice to accept the most parsimonious explanation that can account for the data, it must be recognized that the body of data on tinnitus-related insomnia is not adequate enough to permit firm conclusions.

A model that formulates tinnitus as a specific sleep irritant must take account of the large number of tinnitus sufferers who do not suffer from sleep disturbance. The division of tinnitus patients into subgroups is not a new idea. Tyler and Baker (1983) noted that some of their respondents avoided noisy situations while others avoided quiet environments. These preferences are frequently observed in clinical settings. Tyler and Baker (1983) speculated that this division might point to two subcategories of tinnitus with different etiologies. They suggested that those who prefer noisy situations might be good candidates for tinnitus maskers. It might also be the case that those who prefer noisy situations are more vulnerable to tinnitus-related sleep disturbance because the quietness that is typical of the bedroom may lead to tinnitus being more intrusive. To the author's knowledge, there has been little basic information on this point. Axelsson and Ringdahl (1989) did report that of those who responded to their questionnaire indicating that tinnitus bothers them in quiet surroundings just under 20 percent reported sleep disturbance; the remaining 80 percent reported that they did not have difficulty falling asleep. This percentage figure does not seem to lend strong support to the idea of a subdivision of tinnitus patients based on preference for noise in the environment and sleep disturbance.

An alternative division of tinnitus patients in this context may be on the basis of hearing loss. Alster et al. (1993) reported that sleep disturbance in tinnitus subjects was associated with greater hearing loss. Hallam (1996) also reported that sleep disturbance was related to hearing loss in as much as those subjects without sleep problems had essentially normal hearing while the mean level of hearing loss among those subjects who were regarded as sleep disturbed was 19.5 dB HL in the left ear and 23 dB HL in the right ear. Hallam (1996) suggested that hearing loss further diminishes the masking effects of already reduced ambient noise levels of the night time. This seems similar to the idea that those who find tinnitus more disturbing in quiet surroundings will be more prone to sleep problems. Whatever the merits and problems of that idea the possible division of tinnitus

patients on the basis of hearing loss remains an interesting one. McKenna (1997, unpublished thesis) assessed the cognitive functioning of tinnitus patients and of patients with hearing loss. He found that some deficits in information processing were apparent in tinnitus patients only when hearing loss was controlled. Lyxell (1994) also reported that hearing loss was associated with deficits in information processing and it may be worth considering whether it is associated with the sort of cognitive arousal that has been linked with insomnia.

Alster et al. (1993) suggested that sleep complaints in tinnitus patients might be the result of a combined effect in which tinnitus disrupts or delays sleep which in turn is further exacerbated by emotional disturbance. There are clearly other possible explanations for tinnitus related insomnia. Tinnitus related sleep problems may be related to the increasing prevalence of tinnitus with age (Coles, 1984). It is possible that tinnitus alerts sufferers to what Espie (1991) referred to as "developmental insomnia" associated with older age. Coles (1984) reported that the prevalence of tinnitus that is sufficiently severe to interfere with sleep was negatively correlated with socioeconomic status. The prevalence of insomnia is also negatively correlated with socioeconomic status (Gallup Organization, 1991). Factors such as socioeconomic status or age may have a causative influence in tinnitus-related insomnia. The idea that age is a mediating factor again offers what seems like a parsimonious explanation. None of the alternatives has been tested.

THE MANAGEMENT OF INSOMNIA

Medication

Most insomniacs have been prescribed medication of one type or another. Borkovec (1982) pointed out that although no sleep medication is effective when taken persistently for months or years, most sleep disorder specialists agree that the occasional use of such medicine may be indicated in severe cases of insomnia. He added that usually sleep medication taken once or twice per week may help to break the vicious cycle of insomnia feeding on itself. He pointed out that care needs to be taken when using sleep medication with patients with other medical problems such as liver or kidney disease and that because of their respiratory depressant effects, they may aggravate sleep apnea. Behavioral interventions are likely to be the treatment of choice in most insomnia cases (Williams, 1997).

Behavioral Treatment

Insomnia that is judged to be primary in nature (not secondary to another medical or psychiatric condition) or that is related to sleep-induced respiratory impairment or to restless legs syndrome, may be managed within a sleep disorders clinic. It is widely accepted that the management of a person suffering from insomnia that is secondary to a medical or psychiatric disorder should focus on the removal of that primary condition. However, if insomnia has been present for more than a few months, then it is highly likely that behavioral factors will be aggravating or at least maintaining it. These behavioral factors will almost certainly need to be a focus for treatment.

Relaxation Therapy

Borkovec (1982) reviewed the literature on behavioral treatments for insomnia. He concluded that the majority of studies examining the efficacy of relaxation treatment indicate that it is superior to placebo or no treatment conditions. He concluded that relaxation therapy achieved an average reduction of 45 percent in reported sleep onset latency and that there is some objective (polysomnographic) evidence of this improvement. Morin (1993) also evaluated the efficacy of cognitive behavioral treatments across a number of published studies. The outcome measures included sleep onset latency,

time awake after sleep onset, number of awakenings, and total sleep time. He concluded that relaxation therapy is associated with an average of 41 percent improvement in sleep onset and 28 percent improvement in time awake after sleep onset.

Stimulus Control Techniques

The use of stimulus control techniques have also been widely investigated. Stimulus control treatments seek to eliminate conditioned associations between sleep incompatible behaviors and stimuli related to sleeping. The essential ingredients of this approach are to encourage the patient to go to bed only when tired, to avoid daytime sleeping, to wake at the same time each day, to avoid activity that is incompatible with sleep (for instance, reading, watching TV, or listening to music) in the bedroom and to leave the bedroom if not asleep after about 20 minutes and to return to bed when sleepy again. Clinically, most stimulus control programs would also advise poor sleepers to limit their caffeine and nicotine intake and to avoid the use of alcohol as a hypnotic; the latter may help induce sleep initially but provokes a more restless night's sleep. Poor sleepers are advised to avoid going to bed hungry. A light snack before bed may help induce sleep however the person should avoid eating while awake in the night in case the body is trained to be hungry in the night. Advice is usually given to avoid using other drugs, including nonprescribed medicines such as antihistamines as hypnotics. Poor sleepers are often advised to take regular exercise. Fit people tend to sleep better than unfit people. Also the increase in body temperature induced by exercise helps to promote sleep onset. Care should be taken, however, to avoid exercise immediately before bed as arousal levels may interfere with sleep onset. It is good practice to introduce one element of a stimulus control program at a time. This avoids the possible adverse effects of a general upheaval of routines and allows a clearer identification of the items that are efficacious in the individual case. Stimulus control studies that focus on the essential ingredients of the approach have been reviewed by Borkovec (1982) and by Balter and Uhlenhuth (1992) and by Morin (1993) all of whom concluded that this treatment approach is superior to placebo and no treatment controls. Borkovec (1982) estimated that stimulus control procedures achieve an average of 70 percent reduction in sleep onset latency while Morin (1993) in his more inclusive analysis found a 48 percent improvement across his outcome measures associated with the procedure.

Paradoxical Intention

This is another commonly used behavioral management technique. In this approach the person with poor sleep is asked to remain awake as long as possible. It is widely presumed that this instruction helps to reduce performance anxiety surrounding the demand to sleep and as a result, the probability of sleep is increased. Borkovec (1982) summarized his review of treatment studies by stating that paradoxical intention produces a 58 percent improvement in sleep onset latency compared with pretreatment levels. Morin (1993) reported that paradoxical intention was associated with a 28 percent improvement in sleep onset latency and with a 54 percent improvement in time awake after sleep onset. He noted, however, that many people are reluctant to comply with this procedure.

Sleep Restriction

More recently, Spielman, Saskin, and Thorpy (1987) proposed a method of insomnia management known as sleep restriction. This approach literally restricts the amount of time that the person spends in bed. It is based on the observation that insomniacs spend excessive amounts of time in bed compared with good sleepers; this is in an attempt to compensate for the poor nature of their sleep. In a sleep restriction program, the person's sleep is monitored over a two-

week period and the average amount of sleep per night is calculated. The person is instructed to spend only that average amount of time in bed each night. A waking time is set for the morning according to the person's daytime needs. Bedtime is calculated by deducting the average amount of sleep time from the set rising time. The poor sleeper is instructed to follow this new schedule for several weeks. It is thought that this procedure reestablishes a more helpful circadian rhythm. In order to maximize compliance it is best to avoid restricting time in bed to less than 4 hours, whatever the results of the sleep log. As sleep becomes more consolidated, so the retiring time is gradually made earlier until an optimal sleep duration is achieved. Adjustments are made to the routine on a weekly basis; generally the bedtime is moved to be made fifteen to thirty minutes earlier as sleep efficiency reaches 85 percent for the previous week. Spielman et al. (1987) reported that sleep restriction led to significant improvements in most sleep measures, particularly in sleep efficiency. They also noted a reduction in night-to-night variation in sleep patterns. However, Spielman et al.'s (1987) treatment program was difficult to follow for many of their subjects; they reported a 16 percent subject attrition rate. Morin (1993) reported an improvement of 62 percent associated with sleep restriction methods.

Both sleep restriction and stimulus control techniques commonly lead to reduced time asleep in the early stages of therapy. In other words, they lead to a slightly greater degree of sleep deprivation than already existed. It is presumed that this, in turn, leads to faster sleep onset, improved continuity and deeper sleep. It has been argued (Lundh, in press) however, that the effects of these behavioral management strategies may be mediated by either restricting the amount of time available for presleep ruminations or by distracting the patient from otherwise intrusive cognitions. Even progressive relaxation, which ostensibly focuses on somatic sensations, involves a degree of mental relaxation and distraction from other cognitive events.

Approaches to the management of intrusive cognitions

Cognitive Therapy

There have been a number of approaches that have attempted to influence the cognitive variables associated with insomnia more directly. A cognitive therapy approach is aimed at helping the patient to reevaluate their thinking about sleeplessness and its consequences. It involves identifying dysfunctional sleep-related cognitions, challenging their accuracy and replacing them with more adaptive beliefs (Morin, 1993). Espie and Lindsay (1987) suggested that poor sleepers try a "worry session" in the early evening during which they attempt to write down their current problems and possible steps that might be taken to resolve them. The person is encouraged to spend about thirty minutes doing this each evening. If disturbed by worries in the night the person is encouraged to remind him or herself that the problem is being dealt with in the worry session and to postpone further consideration of the issue until the next day's session. They reported success with this approach in a case study.

Thought Stopping

This is a behavioral approach used for controlling intrusive cognitions. Levey, Aldaz, Watts, and Coyle (1991) described a thought stopping technique known as articulatory suppression. It is assumed that intrusive thoughts are primarily verbal in nature. It is also assumed that the cognitive systems involved in processing information have a limited capacity, and temporal storage, and that the processing of verbally based information can be disrupted by the introduction of other verbal stimuli. Articulatory suppression involves the poor sleeper repeating a nonsense syllable or nonemotive word (such as "the") subvocally while awaiting

sleep onset. The pace at which the word or syllable is repeated should be as nonregular as possible. The authors suggested that most people will find a comfortable rate themselves; if it is too slow, thoughts will intrude and if it is too fast, the process will be arousing and therefore defeat the object. The essential ingredient of the technique is that the vocal apparatus is engaged (to produce subvocal speech); simply imagining the word will not work. The postulation is that the person is unable to simultaneously entertain intrusive cognitions and carrying out this subvocalization. Levey, Aldaz, Watts, and Coyle (1991) described the successful use of the technique in an informal case series and also in a controlled case study. They suggested that while many behavioral techniques are helpful in reducing sleep onset latency, articulatory suppression may be particularly effective for sleep maintenance insomnia.

THE MANAGEMENT OF TINNITUS-RELATED INSOMNIA

The management of tinnitus-related insomnia with medication requires considerable care. Luxon (1993) pointed out that, while benzodiazepines may benefit some anxious patients, they may make a depressed patient with tinnitus worse. She pointed to the link between tinnitus and depression and noted that treatment with trycyclic antidepressants has been common practice. The newer selective serotonin re-uptake inhibitor antidepressants (for example, Prozac) are also widely used by tinnitus patients. Some of these, however, have sleep antagonist properties and again care is needed in their use. From a clinical perspective, the use of cognitive-behavioral management approaches is likely to be more straightforward. Any (or all) of the cognitive-behavioral approaches described earlier is likely to be relevant and valuable in cases of tinnitus-related insomnia. The choice of which cognitive-behavioral technique will depend on the individual patient's presentation.

There is clearly some common ground between the cognitive-behavioral management of insomnia and that of tinnitus. While only a few studies have incorporated any form of specific intervention for tinnitus-related insomnia, it might be assumed that the cognitive-behavioral techniques used in tinnitus management (see Chapter 13) would result in some relief of associated sleep problems. Unfortunately, many psychological treatment studies in the tinnitus field have not included any measures of sleep (Scott, Lindberg, Lyttkens, & Melin, 1985; Goebel, Hiller, Fruhauf, & Fichter, 1992). However, some have done so. Ireland, Wilson, Tonkin, and Platt-Hepworth (1985) and Haralambous, Wilson, Platt-Hepworth et al. (1987) included sleep measures when assessing the efficacy of relaxation and of biofeedback in the treatment of tinnitus. In the first study, subjects completed detailed sleep diaries while in the second they rated difficulty in sleep onset on a five-point scale. Ireland et al. (1985) described their subjects as suffering from "high levels of sleep difficulties." However, neither study directed any interventions specifically at sleep. Unfortunately, in neither study was there evidence for the efficacy of the interventions on any of the measures taken, although Ireland et al. (1985) did report a nonsignificant decrease in sleep onset latency. Henry and Wilson (1996) went on to report significant treatment effects associated with a cognitive/educational approach to tinnitus management. Unfortunately, they did not report on sleep specifically.

Lindberg, Scott, Melin, and Lyttkens (1988) used individualized behavioral analyses that allowed somatic symptoms associated with tinnitus, such as sleep disorder, to be treated. Their general interventions involved providing information and discussion about tinnitus, relaxation and cognitive strategies. They did not report the details of this behavioral analysis nor the specific ways in which sleep problems were treated. Sleep disturbance was assessed by an interview question. Eighty-two percent of their patients who listed sleep disturbance as a problem in a pretreatment interview reported an improvement at follow-up. Lindberg, Scott, Melin, and Lyttkens (1989) described an experimental evaluation of the use of relaxation combined with behavioral or cognitive coping strategies. They did not make any specific sleep intervention, but as part of their package of measures they administered a questionnaire, at follow-up, that included a sleep-related item. Most subjects reported an improvement in their sleep following therapy but some reported no change and one reported a worsening of sleep.

There was no difference in this respect between the behavioral and cognitive coping strategy conditions. Attias, Shemesh, Shoham et al. (1990) compared the efficacy of self-hypnosis with that of a brief auditory stimulus in the alleviation of tinnitus. Sleep was assessed by a single item on a tinnitus questionnaire and no specific sleep intervention was carried out. They found that self-hypnosis was associated with an improvement in most of the tinnitus-related symptoms assessed, including insomnia but with no corresponding improvement in audiometric parameters. In a subsequent study, Attias, Shemesh, Sohmer, et al. (1993) found that self-hypnosis was again associated with improvements in most tinnitus-related symptoms, but not on this occasion with improvements in sleep. Goebel and Hiller (1996) evaluated the benefits of their inpatient multimodal behavioral treatment (including relaxation, assertiveness training, and body-related therapies) of tinnitus using a German version of Hallam's (Hallam et al, 1988; Hallam, 1996) Tinnitus Effects Questionnaire. They found significant treatment effects for all of the aspects of tinnitus complaint assessed except sleep disturbance. Jakes et al. (1986) assessed the value of reassurance, relaxation and distraction for chronic tinnitus sufferers. They did address sleep specifically but only to the extent of advising subjects to "use relaxation as a general stress reducer and to facilitate sleep." Sleep was assessed by asking subjects to keep daily diary records of whether they had difficulty falling asleep and whether they woke in the night and by reference to sleep-related items on an early version of the Tinnitus Effects Questionnaire (Jakes, Hallam, Chambers, & Hinchcliffe, 1985) and on the Hamilton scale for depression (Hamilton, 1967). The effects of their interventions on sleep were mixed; an improvement was noted on diary records but no significant changes were observed on the questionnaire items. The authors also noted that the improvement in diary records of sleep was evident after the provision of information about tinnitus but before the start of relaxation training, suggesting that cognitive variables, rather than just behavioral ones, were important in bringing about the observed changes.

In a later study, in which no specific sleep intervention was made, Jakes, McKenna, and Hinchcliffe (1992) reported that cognitive therapy resulted in a reduction in emotional distress scores on a tinnitus complaint questionnaire but not in a corresponding significant improvement on insomnia scores. Davis, McKenna, and Hallam (1995) carried out a comparison of the effects of relaxation and cognitive therapy in tinnitus management. They noted that about half of their subjects suffered from sleep disturbance. They included behavioral techniques (mainly stimulus control) for the management of insomnia, alongside the principal mode of intervention. Sleep was assessed through the use of the tinnitus effects questionnaire completed pre- and posttherapy and at follow-up. Subjects also completed sleep diaries in a post hoc fashion one week prior to follow-up; for each night they recorded whether they had taken longer than 20 minutes to fall asleep, whether they had woken in the night, and an estimate of how many hours they slept. Insomnia scores on the questionnaire improved from pre- to posttherapy, but deteriorated to pretreatment levels again at follow-up. The diary records

indicated that sleep remained a significant problem for many subjects.

The pattern of results from these studies makes it difficult to draw conclusions about the benefits of cognitive-behavioral for tinnitus related insomnia, not least because most of the sleep assessments were very crude and some post hoc in nature. They do point to the need for a more careful assessment of tinnitus-related insomnia in outcome studies. Furthermore, these studies have either not addressed their interventions specifically at sleep or have done so only minimally. It is clear that there is a need to systematically investigate the benefits of cognitive-behavioral interventions with tinnitus-related insomnia as a primary and specific target. In this context it is worth mentioning a number of commonly encountered issues concerned with tinnitus-related insomnia that are likely to be important in the management of patients through psychological techniques.

Many people believe that tinnitus prevents sleep or wakes the individual from sleep. Such beliefs are clearly going to make the experience of tinnitus all the more distressing. The approach to this issue taken by the tinnitus therapist will depend on whether it is accepted that tinnitus is a specific arouser. If it is not accepted that tinnitus acts in this way, then challenging this belief, through the use of basic education about the nature of sleep, may be helpful. In a similar vein, many people may be alerted to essentially normal sleep processes for the first time and may interpret these as pathological. Espie (1991) refers to the age-related changes in sleep as a form of "developmental insomnia" that may be best regarded as a "nonpathological sleep disturbance." In some cases education about the normality of such changes may be all that is necessary to relieve the distress of some people with tinnitus and concerns about their sleep.

Related to this issue the author has encountered a few people, in a clinical setting, who have expressed a fear that their tinnitus might get to a point where it would intrude into their sleep. In the author's experience this has always been expressed as a fear of potential intrusion rather than tinnitus actually intruding into sleep. Again, there is no clear research evidence about whether or not tinnitus does intrude into people's sleep; this has not been a feature of people's tinnitus complaints in studies such as Tyler and Baker (1983) or Sanchez and Stephens (1997). Nonetheless, the possibility that insomniacs may mistake cognitive activity in Stage 2 sleep for wakefulness and the fact that some processing of external information continues when people are asleep must make it a possibility that tinnitus intrudes into some people's sleep. For many people, this possibility is likely to be alarming and could represent quite a challenge for the cognitive therapy approach. It may be that some benefit could be had from attributing the difficulty to a high level of cognitive arousal rather than tinnitus per se. Such patients may benefit from techniques designed to reduce arousal such as early evening worry sessions, relaxation, and articulatory suppression. It should be remembered, however, that most people who are concerned that tinnitus might intrude into their sleep can be reassured that this is not likely to happen.

Beliefs about an inability to control sleep are widely held among insomniacs. This results not only from the deterioration in sleep but also from the unpredictability of their sleep. Not knowing whether the night ahead will be one of good or bad sleep leads many insomniacs to believe that they are personally ineffective in controlling the process. In this context, the attribution of a deterioration in sleep to the onset of or change in tinnitus has face validity. It is easy to see how beliefs about the uncontrollability of tinnitus interacting with those about the uncontrollability of sleep help to create the familiar vicious circle of tinnitus intrusiveness, distress, and autonomic arousal and poor sleep. However, as already mentioned, the idea that insomnia can be directly attributed to tinnitus per se may yet prove to be erroneous. It is possible that

developmental changes in sleep patterns may be misinterpreted as a loss of control over sleep. Beliefs about the importance of sleep loss may add to the patient's emotional distress and heighten arousal so making sleep more elusive and tinnitus more intrusive.

SUMMARY AND CONCLUSIONS

Sleep and insomnia, like tinnitus, are complex matters. There is a range in the amount of sleep, and in other sleep parameters, that can be regarded as normal or acceptable. The exact functions of sleep remain uncertain but there is an acceptance that it is important. Insomnia is one of the most prevalent of complaints, but there is still a debate about its nature and consequences and, perhaps surprisingly, complaints about insomnia do not necessarily reflect sleep deprivation. It does seem clear that insomnia has many behavioral and cognitive, rather than anaepathic, antecedents. There are guidelines for the assessment of insomnia and there is evidence that it can be managed effectively through cognitive-behavioral strategies. In these ways it is not unlike tinnitus.

Insomnia is perhaps the most prevalent of problems associated with tinnitus. It is therefore surprising so few studies have made tinnitus-related insomnia a central focus. The nature of the problem has to be gleaned from a consideration of studies that have addressed it as part of a more general concern about tinnitus. The vast majority of tinnitus studies have not made reference to, nor been enlightened by, the insomnia literature. As a result, the definitions, guidelines, and assessment procedures employed have, for the most part, not been as rigorous as those to be found in the insomnia literatures. It is therefore difficult to arrive at firm conclusions about tinnitus-related insomnia, other than to repeat that it is a major problem. For example, whether insomnia is secondary to tinnitus per se, as many patients believe, or is secondary to a poor emotional state, remains uncertain. This is an important question, the answer to which could have implications for management. The evidence on the matter is somewhat inconsistent, but more importantly, the data are not of an adequate nature to properly address this issue.

There appear to be some similarities in the presentation of tinnitus sufferers and that of insomniacs, for example, both groups are characterized by psychological distress involving worry, anxiety, and depression. It is possible to speculate on other similarities. For example, insomnia is thought to be mediated by high levels of arousal and it might be expected that insomniacs would have difficulty in achieving reduced levels of arousal and in habituating to external stimuli. It may be that there is a commonality in terms of central nervous system arousal between those people who have difficulty in habituating to tinnitus and those who suffer from insomnia. Another similarity between tinnitus and insomnia is the preeminence given to the patient's self-report of distress or dissatisfaction in the assessment process. Further, tinnitus, like insomnia, can be managed through cognitive-behavioral therapy. To date, however, the evidence is that the impact of these psychological therapies on tinnitus-related insomnia is no more than modest. However, few studies have made specific sleep-related interventions and where such interventions have been made they have been of a very superficial nature. Again, the standard of data concerning sleep that has been collected has been poorer than recommended in the insomnia literature. There is a clear need for an outcome study in which tinnitus-related insomnia is the central target and which does not rely on isolated and ad hoc measures.

It was suggested by Shapiro and Flannigan (1993) that poor sleep is the thing that leads people to complain that their medical condition is more pernicious, and their quality of life poorer, than those whose sleep is not disrupted. This is clearly a view that many tinnitus sufferers would agree with. As insomnia is one of the most important problems seen in a tinnitus clinic, it seems extraordinary that we have invested so little of our energies in it to date. The community of researchers and clinicians in the tinnitus field have a responsibility to investigate tinnitus-related insomnia more carefully and to seek solutions to the problem.

REFERENCES

Alster, J., Shemesh, Z., Ornan, M., & Attias, J. (1993). Sleep disturbance associated with chronic tinnitus. *Biological Psychiatry, 34,* 84–90.

American Psychiatric Association. (1994). *Diagnostic and statistical manual of mental disorders* (4th ed.). Washington, DC: Author.

Attias, J., Shemesh, Z., Shoham, C., Shahar, A., & Sohmer, H. (1990). Efficacy of self-hypnosis for tinnitus relief. *Scandinavian Audiology, 19,* 245–249.

Attias, J., Shemesh, Z., Sohmer, H., Gold, S., Shoham, C., & Faraggi, D. (1993). Comparison between self-hypnosis, masking and attentiveness for alleviation of chronic tinnitus. *Audiology, 32,* 205–212.

Axelsson, A., & Ringdahl, A. (1989). Tinnitus: A study of its prevalence and characteristics. *British Journal of Audiology, 23,* 53–62.

Axelsson, A., & Sandh, A. (1985). Tinnitus in noise induced hearing loss. *British Journal of Audiology, 19,* 271–276.

Balter, M., & Uhlenhuth, E. (1992). New epidemiological findings about insomnia and its treatment. *Journal of Clinical Psychiatry, 53* (Suppl. 12), 34–39.

Beck, A., & Steer, R. (1990). *Beck Anxiety Inventory.* The Psychology Corporation. San Antonio, TX: Harcourt Brace Jovanovich.

Beck, A., Steer, R., & Brown, G. (1996). *Beck Depression Inventory* (2nd ed.). The Psychology Corporation. San Antonio, TX: Harcourt Brace & Company.

Birrell, P. (1983). Behavioral, subjective and electroencephalographic indices of sleep onset latency and sleep duration. *Journal of Behavioural Assessment, 5,* 179–190.

Bixler, E., Kales, A., Soldatos, C., Kales, J., & Healey, S. (1979). Prevalence of sleep disorders in the Los Angeles Metropolitan Area. *American Journal of Psychiatry, 136,* 1257–1262.

Borkovec, T. (1982). Insomnia. *Journal of Consulting and Clinical Psychology, 50,* 880–895.

Borkovec, T., & Weerts, T. (1976). Effects of progressive relaxation on sleep disturbance: An electroencephalographic evaluation. *Psychosomatic Medicine, 38,* 173–180.

Buysse, D., Reynolds, C., Monk, T., Berman, S., & Kupfer, D. (1989). The Pittsburgh Sleep Quality Index: A new instrument for psychiatric practice and research. *Psychiatry Research, 28,* 193–213.

Chambers, M., & Keller, B. (1993). Alert insomniacs: Are they really sleep deprived? *Clinical Psychology Review, 13,* 649–665.

Coles, R. (1984). Epidemiology of tinnitus: (2) Demographic and clinical features. *Journal of Laryngology and Otology, 9*(Suppl.), 195–202.

Coursey, R., Buchsbaum, M., & Frankel, B. (1975). Personality measures and evoked responses in chronic insomniacs. *Journal of Abnormal Psychology, 84,* 239–249.

Davis, S., McKenna, L., & Hallam, R. (1995). Relaxation and cognitive therapy: A controlled trial in chronic tinnitus. *Psychology & Health, 10,* 129–143.

Dean, E. (1970). The programming "p" hypothesis for REM sleep. In E. Hartmann (Ed.), Sleep and dreaming. *International Psychiatry Clinic Series* (Vol. 7). Boston: Little Brown.

Espie, C. (1991). *The psychological treatment of insomnia.* Chichester: Wiley.

Espie, C., Brooks, D., & Lindsay, W. (1989). An evaluation of tailored psychological treatment of insomnia. *Journal of Behaviour Therapy and Experimental Psychiatry, 20,* 143–153.

Espie, C., & Lindsey, W. (1987). Cognitive strategies for the management of severe sleep maintenance insomnia: A preliminary investigation. *Behavioural Research and Therapy, 15,* 388–395.

Espie, C., Lindsay, W., & Brooks, D. (1988). Substituting behavioural treatment for drugs in the treatment of insomnia: An exploratory study. *Journal of Behaviour Therapy and Experimental Psychiatry, 19,* 51–56.

Franklin, J. (1981). The measurement of sleep onset latency in insomnia. *Behavioural Research and Therapy, 19,* 547–549.

Gabriels, P. (1995). Children with tinnitus. In G. Reich & J. Vernon (Eds.), *Proceedings of the Fifth International Tinnitus Seminar.* Portland, OR: The American Tinnitus Association.

Gallup Organization. (1991). *Sleep in America.* Princeton, NJ: Author.

Glenville, M., Broughton, R., Wing, A., & Wilkinson, R. (1978). Effects of sleep deprivation on short duration performance measures compared to the Wilkenson Vigilance Task. *Sleep, 1,* 169–176.

Goebel, G., & Hiller, W. (1996). Effects and predictors of a therapeutic inpatient treatment for chronic tinnitus. In G. Reich & J. Vernon (Eds.), *Proceedings of the Fifth International Tinnitus Seminar.* Portland, OR: American Tinnitus Association.

Goebel, G., Hiller, W., Fruhauf, K., & Fichter, M. (1992). Effects of inpatient multimodal behavioral treatment on complex chronic tinnitus. In J. Aran & R. Dauman (Eds.), *Tinnitus 91. Proceedings of the Fourth International Tinnitus Seminar* (pp. 465–470). Amsterdam: Kugler Publications.

Goldberg, D. (1978). *Manual of the General Health Questionnaire.* National Foundation for Educational Rsearch. Slough, United Kingdom.

Hallam, R. (1996). *Manual of the tinnitus questionnaire.* The Psychology Corporation. London: Harcourt Brace & Company.

Hallam, R. (1996a). Correlates of sleep disturbance in chronic distressing tinnitus. *Scandinavian Audiology, 25,* 263–266.

Hallam, R., Jakes, S., & Hinchcliffe, R. (1988). Cognitive variables in tinnitus annoyance. *British Journal of Clinical Psychology, 27,* 213–222.

Hamilton, M. (1967). Development of a rating scale for primary depressive illness. *British Journal of Social and Clinical Psychology, 6,* 278–299.

Haralambous, G., Wilson, P., Platt-Hepworth, S., Tonkin, J., Hensley, R., & Kavanagh, D. (1987). EMG biofeedback in the treatment of tinnitus: An experimental evaluation. *Behaviour Research and Therapy, 25*(1), 49–55.

Hauri, P., & Wisbey, J. (1992). Wrist actigraphy in insomnia. *Sleep, 15,* 293–301.

Henry, J., & Wilson, P. (1992). Psychological management of tinnitus: An evaluation of cognitive interventions. In J. Aran & R. Dauman (Eds.), *Tinnitus 91. Proceedings of the Fourth International Tinnitus Seminar* (pp. 447–480). Kugler Publications.

Hiller, W., & Goebel, G. (1992). A psychometric study of complaints in chronic tinnitus. *Journal of Psychosomatic Research, 36,* 337–348.

Ireland, C., Wilson, P., Tonkin, J., & Platt-Hepworth, S. (1985). An evaluation of relaxation training in the treatment of tinnitus. *Behaviour Research and Therapy, 23*(4), 423–430.

Jakes, S., Hallam, R., Chambers, C., & Hinchcliffe, R. (1985). A factor analytical study of tinnitus complaint behaviour. *Audiology, 24,* 195–206.

Jakes, S., Hallam, R., McKenna, L., & Hinchcliffe, R. (1992). Group cognitive therapy for medical patients: An application to tinnitus. *Cognitive Therapy and Research, 16*(1), 67–82.

Jakes, S., Hallam, R., Rachman, S., & Hinchcliffe, R. (1986). The effects of reassurance, relaxation training and distraction on chronic tinnitus sufferers. *Behaviour Research and Therapy, 24*(5), 497–507.

Kemp, S., & George, R. (1992). Diaries of tinnitus sufferers. *British Journal of Audiology, 26,* 381–386.

Levey, A., Aldaz, J., Watts, F., & Coyle, K. (1991). Articulatory suppression and the treatment of insomnia. *Behaviour Research and Therapy, 29,* 85–89.

Lichstein, K., Nickel, R., Hoelscher, T., & Kelley, J. (1982). Clinical evaluation of a sleep assessment device. *Behavioural Research and Therapy, 20,* 292–297.

Lichstein, K., & Rosenthal, T. (1980). Insomniacs' perceptions of cognitive versus somatic determinants of sleep disturbance. *Journal of Abnormal Psychology, 89,* 105–107.

Liljenberg, B., Almqvist, M., Hetta, J., Roos, B., & Agren, H. (1988). The prevalence of insomnia: The importance of operationally defined criteria. *Annals of Clinical Research, 20,* 393–398.

Lindberg, P., Scott, B., Melin, L., & Lyttkens, L. (1988). Behavioural therapy in the clinical management of tinnitus. *British Journal of Audiology, 22,* 265–272.

Lindberg, P., Scott, B., Melin, L., & Lyttkens, L. (1989). The psychological treatment of tinnitus: An experimental evaluation. *Behaviour Research and Therapy, 27*(6), 593–603.

Luxon, L. (1993). Tinnitus: Its causes, diagnosis and treatment. *British Medical Journal, 306,* 1491–1492.

Lyxell, B., Ronnberg, J., & Samuelsson, S. (1994). Internal speech functioning and speech reading in deafened and normal hearing adults. *Scandinavian Audiology, 23,* 179–185.

Marchini, E., Coates, T., Magistad, J., & Waldum, S. (1983). What do insomniacs do, think and feel during the day? *Sleep, 6,* 147–155.

McKenna, L. (1987). Goal planning in audiological rehabilitation. *British Journal of Audiology, 21,* 5–11.

McKenna, L. (1997). *Psychological aspects of auditory disorders: Cognitive functioning and psychological state.* Unpublished Ph.D. thesis, The City University, London.

McKenna, L., Hallam, R., & Hinchcliffe, R. (1991). The prevalence of psychological disturbance in neuro-otology outpatients. *Clinical Otolaryngology, 16,* 452–456.

Meikle, M., Vernon, J., & Johnson, R. (1984). The perceived severity of tinnitus. Some observations concerning a large population of tinnitus clinic patients. *Otolaryngology, Head & Neck Surgery, 92,* 689.

Mendelson, W., Garnett, D., & Linnoila, M. (1984). Do insomniacs have impaired daytime functioning? *Biological Psychiatry, 19,* 1261–1264.

Morin, C. (1993). *Insomnia: Psychological assessment and management.* New York: Guilford Press.

Sanchez, L., & Stephens, D. (1997). A tinnitus problem questionnaire in a clinic population. *Ear and Hearing, 18*(3), 210–217.

Schneider-Helmert, D. (1987). Twenty-four hour sleep-wake function and personality patterns in chronic insomniacs and healthy controls. *Sleep, 10,* 452–462.

Scott, B., Lindberg, P., Lennart, M., & Lyttkens, L. (1990). Predictors of tinnitus discomfort, adaptation and subjective loudness. *British Journal of Audiology, 24,* 51–62.

Scott, B., Lindberg, P., Lyttkens, L., & Melin, L. (1985). Psychological treatment of tinnitus. *Scandinavian Audiology, 14,* 223–230.

Seidel, W., Ball, S., Cohen, S., Patterson, N., Yost, O., & Dement, W. (1984). Daytime alertness in relation to mood, performance and nocturnal sleep in chronic insomniacs and noncomplaining sleepers. *Sleep, 7,* 230–238.

Shapiro, C., & Dement, W. (1993). Impact and epidemiology of sleep disorders. In C. Shapiro (Ed.), *ABC of Sleep Disorders.* BMJ Publishing.

Shapiro, C., & Flanigan, M. (1993). Function of sleep. In C. Shapiro (Ed.), *ABC of Sleep Disorders.* BMJ Publishing.

Singerman, B., Riedner, E., & Folstein, M. (1980). Emotional disturbance in hearing clinic patients. *British Journal of Psychiatry, 137,* 58–62.

Slater, R., Jones, D., Davis, B., & Terry, M. (1982). *Project into psychological aspects of adjustment to subjective tinnitus and the effectiveness of tailored masking.* Report to Department of Health & Social Security.

Speilberger, C., Gorsuch, R., & Lushene, R. (1970). *Manual of the State-Trait Anxiety Inventory.* Palo Alto, CA: Consulting Psychologist Press.

Spielman, A., Saskin, P., & Thorpy, M. (1987). Treatment of chronic insomnia by restriction of time in bed. *Sleep, 10,* 45–56.

Sugarman, J., Stern, J., & Walsh, J. (1985). Daytime alertness in subjective and objective insomnia: Some preliminary findings. *Biological Psychiatry. 20,* 741–750.

Tyler, R., & Baker, L. (1983). Difficulties experienced by tinnitus sufferers. *Journal of Speech and Hearing Disorders, 48,* 150–154.

Williams, A. (1997). An effective strategy for sleep. *The Practitioner, 241,* 606–610.

Zung, W. (1967). A self-rating depression scale. *Archives of General Psychiatry, 12,* 63–70.

Appendix

SLEEP DIARY

Name_____ Date/Week beginning _____

	Example	Mon.	Tues.	Wed.	Thurs.	Fri.	Sat.	Sun.
Time spent napping in the day	30 mins.							
Amount of medication or alcohol	7.5 mg sleepwell							
Bed time & Lights out time	10:45 11:30							
Time taken to fall asleep	55 mins.							
Number of times you woke in the night	4							
Amount of time awake in the night	60 mins.							
Final wake up time & time you get up.	6:00 7:30							
Quality of sleep 0 = very poor sleep 10 = very good sleep	3							
Tinnitus annoyance 0 = no annoyance 10 = extremely annoying	7							

Time in bed (TIB)	8 hours 45 mins.							
Total sleep time (TST)	4 hours 35 mins.							
Sleep efficiency TST/TIB × 100	52%							

Daytime functioning 0 = very poor 10 = no problems	7							

SLEEP DIARY INSTRUCTIONS

In order to be able to help you with your sleep problems it is important to get information about what is happening to your sleep. Please fill in the sleep diary each day within an hour of getting up so that you can still remember what happened during the night. Each day you fill in the column for the previous day. For example on Sunday morning you fill in the column for Saturday —you are referring to Saturday night's sleep, even if you went to bed after midnight. Please estimate the times in each case. Do not watch the clock in order to get accurate times. Instead guess the times involved; it should be possible to guess to within five or ten minutes. Daytime functioning should be estimated at the end of the day. See the following.

Napping: Add up all the times that you napped in the previous day and write the total time down. Napping means sleeping when you are not in bed, whether or not you meant to fall asleep.

Medication/Alcohol: Please write down the names and dose of any medication you take at night time. Also write down the amount of alcohol you take to help you sleep.

Bedtime and lights out time: Write down what time you got in to bed and also what time you turned the lights off and settled down to sleep. These times may be different and you should write both down.

Time taken to fall asleep: Write down how long it took you to fall asleep. Remember this is an estimate.

Number of times you woke in the night: Write down how many times you woke up in the night.

Amount of time awake in the night: Add up all of the times that you are awake in the middle of the night. Estimate the time; do not watch the clock.

Wake up time and get up time: Write down when you woke up for the final time. Also write down what time you got out of bed. For many people this will be different from when they woke up.

Quality of sleep: Estimate the quality of your sleep by choosing a number between 0 and 10 where 10 is very good quality sleep. The quality of sleep refers to how well you slept, and whether it was the sort of sleep you feel you need, for example, was it refreshing and/or natural sleep. If you feel you slept well you will pick a high number, if it was poor quality or restless sleep you should pick a low number.

Tinnitus annoyance: State how annoying your tinnitus was during the night by choosing a number between 0 and 10 where ten is extremely annoying.

Time in bed (TIB), Total Sleep Time (TST) and Sleep Efficiency (SE): TIB is the time between getting into bed and getting up in the morning. TST is TIB less all of the time you were not asleep. SE is TST divided by TIB times 100 percent.

Daytime functioning: State how well you believe you did during the day by choosing a number between 0 and 10 where ten is extremely good performance without any problems. This is a statement about how well you carried out the things that you needed to do in the day. Remember, estimate this at the end of the day, so at the end of Sunday fill in how well you did that day in the Saturday column.

CHAPTER 4

Physiological Mechanisms and Neural Models

Jos J. Eggermont, Ph.D.

INTRODUCTION

This review considerably extends previous ones (Jastreboff, 1990; Eggermont, 1990) in the light of many new experimental findings and ideas. I start with a review of normal spontaneous activity in the auditory system, followed by electrophysiological results obtained from animals and humans with sensorineural hearing loss and tinnitus. The second part of this review presents a comprehensive survey of models proposed to explain tinnitus together with experimental evidence. The third part, labeled "where in the brain is tinnitus," interprets these facts and models about the action of tinnitus-inducing agents within a "levels of description" approach: from the systems level down to the molecular level. Finally, a short natural history of tinnitus as emerging from this review is proposed.

FACTS

Spontaneous Activity in the Auditory System

Spontaneous Activity: Noise or Information Carrier?

Spontaneous activity in the nervous system is cursorily defined as neural activity that occurs in the absence of an external stimulus. Spontaneous activity is reflected, for instance, in fluctuations from the resting membrane potential level in an inner hair cell, in the number of action potentials per second fired by an auditory nerve fiber, or in the spontaneous electroencephalographic (EEG) activity. Spontaneous activity is by some considered as neuronal noise which adds to the stimulus-induced activity (Siebert, 1965). The presence of this internal noise results in variable stimulus-related activity and thereby sets a limit to the detection capabilities of the central nervous system and makes perceptual decisions probabilistic. Another viewpoint is that spontaneous activity reflects the main process in the nervous system and that stimulation merely perturbs or modulates this activity (Rodieck et al., 1962). In this view, spontaneous activity acts as an information carrier. The first point of view likely applies more to the sensory periphery, whereas the second conforms more to the situation in the central nervous system. Auditory nerve fibers can be grouped in two or three categories (depending on the animal species) with low, (middle) and high spontaneous firing rates (Dallos & Harris, 1978; Liberman, 1978). Auditory nerve fibers with spontaneous firing rates below 0.5 spikes/s (that is, they tend to fire on average once per two seconds) have approximately 20 dB higher thresholds for tone stimulation than nerve fibers with higher spontaneous firing rates. (Liberman, 1978), suggesting that there are benefits derived from high spontaneous activity (or that high spontaneous activity accompanies higher sensitivity) and that the modulation theory may also apply to the high spontaneous group of nerve fibers in the auditory nerve. If we do not take either of these two extreme points of view, but consider the action of a stimulus to add neural activity as well as to modulate the existing spontaneous activity, then the emphasis on what an external stimulus does shifts from mostly adding spikes at the peripheral level to mostly modulating the spontaneous firing rate at the central level.

The two distinct views of spontaneous activity, either as unwanted noise or as information carrier, may determine the proposed mechanism for tinnitus (Table 4-1). If one considers spontaneous activity as unwanted noise in the auditory system, the favored concept about tinnitus is likely that it results from too much neural noise. The suggested functional substrate of tinnitus will then be increased spontaneous firing rates in the auditory nervous system. In that case, the stimulus-evoked or added activity, also called the driven activity, should not change after experimentally induced tinnitus for low intensity stimuli. The saturation value, that is, the upper boundary of the neuron's firing rate, however, may be reached at lower stimulus levels. This suggests that, according to this model, the driven rate might actually decrease for higher intensities after experimentally induced tinnitus. On the other hand, spontaneous activity may be considered as the information carrier of the auditory nervous system, the rate of which is modulated by sound. Tinnitus might then arise from a pathological modulation of the spontaneous activity of peripheral or central neurons. In this case, the driven firing rate will change after induced tinnitus, because it will also be modulated by the tinnitus causing pathology. An interference, not unlike that produced by presenting two tones simultaneously, might also occur and *could* cause suppression of the tinnitus by an external stimulus.

When the spontaneous activity in a substantial fraction of auditory nerve fibers is depressed as a result of deafferentation by inner hair cell loss, sprouting, or synapse

Table 4-1. Views of spontaneous activity and Tinnitus

Spontaneous activity	Tinnitus model
Considered as noise	Too much noise: tinnitus results from increase in firing rate
Considered as information carrier	Pathological modulation of spontaneous activity: tinnitus results from increased neural synchrony

reorganization at higher neural levels may create large arrays of neurons previously responsive to the deafferented peripheral neurons that have "retuned" and are responding to the "edge" of the remaining healthy parts of the cochlear array (Rajan et al., 1993). Hence, these edge-tuned neurons might fire very similarly and more or less synchronously even in the absence of sound (Salvi et al., 1996a; and Chapter 5). This synchrony would be analogous to that caused by stimulation with edge-frequency tones or narrow-band noise. Hence, tinnitus with a pitch resembling that of such a stimulus will result.

Spontaneous Otoacoustic Emissions

Spontaneous otoacoustic emissions are low level sounds emitted by the healthy normal ear that are recordable with sensitive microphones inserted in the ear canal (Zurek, 1981). In about 6 to 12 percent (or at least 4 percent according to a recent review by Penner and Jastreboff, 1996) of normal hearing persons spontaneous otoacoustic emissions are considered at least partially responsible for the tinnitus (Kemp, 1981; Norton et al., 1990; Chapter 8). Plinkert et al. (1990), elaborating on a proposal by Kemp (1981), speculate that the pathological long-term movements of a small local group of not more than sixty affected outer hair cells may account for tonal tinnitus. Similar ideas were presented also by O-Uchi and Tanaka (1988). In most cases, however, spontaneous otoacoustic emissions and tinnitus are independent phenomena (Wilson & Sutton,

1981; Penner & Burns, 1987; Penner, 1992). Although spontaneous emissions likely produce increased "spontaneous firing" in neurons innervating the basilar membrane at the emission site, central nervous system adaptation may preclude their audibility. Occasionally, some subjects hear intermittent spontaneous otoacoustic emissions as intermittent tinnitus (Burns & Keefe, 1992). It appears to me that relatively fast changes in spontaneous emission frequencies or levels will avoid this adaptation and thus might be audible.

Normal Spontaneous Auditory Neural Activity

In general, spontaneous neural activity in the peripheral auditory system is attributed to spontaneous transmitter release from the inner hair cells. Destruction of the inner hair cells destroys spontaneous activity in all auditory nerve fibers innervating these hair cells (Dallos & Harris, 1978; Liberman & Kiang, 1978) whereas destruction of the outer hair cells does not have this effect. Auditory nerve fibers with spontaneous firing rates of more than 1 spike/s appear to innervate the inner hair cells at the side facing the outer hair cells, whereas low spontaneous activity neurons innervate the inner hair cells on the other side. Each inner hair cell is contacted by about twenty auditory nerve fibers representing the full range of spontaneous firing rates (Liberman & Oliver, 1984).

As we have seen, auditory nerve fibers can be distinguished on the basis of their spontaneous firing rates (Table 4-2). These

Table 4-2. Auditory nerve fibers with low, medium and high spontaneous activity

Property	Low spontaneous	Medium spontaneous	High spontaneous
Firing rate	< 1 spikes/s	1 < rate < 20 spikes/s	> 20 spikes/s
Threshold for tones	highest thresholds > 30 dB SPL	sensitivity in between	most sensitive: threshold < 10 dB SPL
Dynamic range	large (> 30 dB)	in between	small (< 20 dB)

firing rates correlate well with the size of the dendritic terminals of the nerve fibers as well as with their threshold for tonal stimulation. The larger the size of the synaptic terminal, the higher the spontaneous firing rate. High-spontaneous rate fibers have lower thresholds than low-spontaneous rate fibers. Small, medium, and large terminals are found on all inner hair cells. These findings support the idea that the major determinant of the spontaneous rate is the effect of the transmitter spontaneously arriving at the auditory nerve fiber, which is roughly proportional to its synaptic terminal size. Although there appears to be a topographic mapping onto the cochlear nucleus reflecting the dorsoventral arrangement in the spiral ganglion in addition to the fine-grained tonotopic mapping, there is no evidence that fibers with different spontaneous firing rates project differentially (Leake & Snyder, 1989). The dynamic range, the difference between the threshold, just above the spontaneous activity, and the stimulus level above which no further increase in firing rate occurs, is generally less than 20 dB for the high spontaneous fibers and more than 30 dB for the low spontaneous fibers.

Spontaneous firing rates of up to 150 spikes per second are not unusual in the cat's auditory nerve (Kiang et al., 1965), but can also be found in the cat's cochlear nucleus (Pfeiffer & Kiang, 1965; Koerber et al., 1966) and in the superior olivary complex (Goldberg et al., 1964). Spontaneous firing rates are considerably lower in more central nuclei, for example, in inferior colliculus the average rate is about 5 spikes per second (Chen & Jastreboff, 1995; Manabe et al., 1997). In the auditory cortex about 50 percent of the cells discharge with less than one spike per second. However, the remainder discharge at rates of 1 to 35 spikes per second even in the unanesthetized preparation (Goldstein et al., 1967). Despite these neurons with high spontaneous firing rates, the mean spontaneous firing rate in the primary auditory cortex of the ketamine anesthetized cat is only about one spike per second (Eggermont, 1992b; Ochi &

Eggermont, 1996). In awake animals, spontaneous firing rates in auditory cortex tend to be substantially higher than in anesthetized animals.

It is assumed that, even in the absence of sound, the inner hair cell is partially depolarized as a result of a leaking potassium current flowing through the transduction channels at the top of the hair cells (Hudspeth, 1989). This steady depolarization opens calcium channels at the base of the hair cell. The entry of calcium ions results in spontaneous transmitter release. Blocking the calcium channels reduces the spontaneous firing rate in proportion to the extracellular concentration of the blocking agent (for example, cobalt or manganese ions; Sewell, 1990). In contrast, a reduction of the extracellular calcium concentration to very low levels increases the spontaneous activity with additional burst firing in *Xenopus* lateral line afferents (Russell, 1971), likely due to an outward calcium flow that reduces the intracellular concentration. Reducing the intracellular free calcium concentration in cortical neurons with chelating agents also results in bursting behavior (Friedman & Gutnick, 1989).

In the auditory nerve of the cat or guinea pig, nearly all fibers show spontaneous activity with interspike-intervals that are exponentially distributed and are independent of each other (Kiang et al., 1965). This means that the duration of the interval between two action potentials is independent of the length of the previous interval. The exponential nature of the interspike-interval distribution indicates that there are many short intervals and very few long ones. Because of the auditory nerve fiber's refractory period of 0.8 to 1.6 ms, there is a decreasing number of intervals below 1.6 ms (Manley & Robertson, 1976). It has been suggested that fibers with the same characteristic frequency, and thus possibly innervating the same inner hair cell, have uncorrelated spontaneous firing patterns (Johnson & Kiang, 1976).

In the auditory cortex, the spontaneous firing patterns are not that simple; unimodal, bimodal and multimodal interspike-interval distributions can be found. The dominant modes (most frequent intervals) are between 1 and 10 ms and between 75 to 150 ms (Eggermont, 1992). This can be interpreted as cells firing in bursting fashion (3 to 10 spikes with inter-spike intervals in the 1 to 10 ms range) that repeat every 75 to 150 ms (Smith & Smith, 1965; Pernier & Gerin, 1975). The inter-burst repetition rate is likely determined by the EEG-spindle frequency (Kenmochi & Eggermont, 1997). If no spindling occurs, then more unimodal firing patterns will be found since the bursts would follow each other with random intervals. Burst firing, while absent in auditory nerve fibers, is a common feature in many cortical neurons (Legendy & Salcman, 1985; Eggermont et al., 1993). In cortical layer V, burst-firing is an intrinsic property of the pyramidal cells (McCormick et al., 1985), whereas in other layers it may be determined by the way the cortical neurons are interconnected.

Why is Spontaneous Neural Activity Inaudible?

From this summary we conclude that spontaneous activity is a prominent property of the normal auditory nervous system. The question that thus should arise is: "Why don't we perceive this spontaneous activity as sound?". The short answer is "because we are used to it and have adapted to it" just as one adapts to a constant tactile stimulus; one is not constantly aware of sitting in a chair or wearing a ring. This adaptation view may assume that our auditory nerve fibers are fast adapting like the somatosensory fibers innervating the Pacinian corpuscles responsible for tactile sensations. However, auditory nerve fiber firings adapt only partially. This receptor adaptation occurs during 30 to 100 ms after stimulus onset after which an adapted steady-state firing rate is reached (Eggermont, 1985). A steady state sound generally produces no change in firing rate in auditory cortex, except for an onset transient increase, com-pared to spontaneous activity (deCharms and Merzenich, 1996; Eggermont, 1997), whereas changes in sound amplitude generally produce changes in firing rate. So constant spontaneous activity may be like continuous stimulation as to its effect on the cortex. However, continuous stimulation produces a sound sensation whereas spontaneous activity does not.

It is more likely that we do not hear spontaneous activity because sound sensation relies on synchronized firings of neighboring neurons (Eggermont, 1984, 1990). Synchronization of firing means that action potentials from different neurons tend to fire at nearly the same time (say within less than 5 ms). Under normal spontaneous firing conditions such interneuron synchrony is presumed to be largely or completely absent in the auditory nerve (Johnson & Kiang, 1976). Thus auditory nerve fibers tend to fire independently in silence. In auditory cortex, some neuronal synchrony is present during spontaneous activity (Eggermont, 1992b) but continuous stimulation produces an increase in that synchrony (deCharms and Merzenich, 1996; Eggermont, 1997).

In auditory nerve fibers with characteristic frequencies below 5 kHz, low-level stimulation with continuous tones or noise evokes a change in the interval distribution of the firings and, at higher intensities, also in the mean firing rate. The change in interval distribution, that is detectable below behavioral threshold levels, is caused by the tendency of the firings to become phase-locked to the period of the tone or to the band-pass filtered (by the basilar membrane-outer hair cell filter) noise (Eggermont et al., 1983; Javel et al., 1988; Nuttall et al., 1997). The phase-locking will introduce preferred intervals equal to those of the stimulating waveform. Thus, the spontaneous exponential interspike-interval distributions tend to be replaced by more symmetric ones during pure tone stimulation with frequencies below about 4 kHz. For auditory nerve fibers with characteristic-frequency above about 4 kHz, which do not show phase-locking to the stimulus, an increase in steady-state firing rate of is the most obvious response to the continuous presence of a low-level sound. The firing rate of auditory nerve fibers also tends to follow the amplitude modulation of complex or high frequency pure tone sounds up to modulation rates of 1 to 3 kHz (Møller, 1976; Javel, 1981; Joris & Yin, 1992). This modulation-following pattern also causes deviations in the exponential interspike-interval distribution of the nerve fiber discharges. On this basis, one could argue that both the mean firing rate (a zero-order statistic) and the interval histogram (a first-order statistic) carry information about the presence or absence of sound in single auditory nerve fibers. Higher order statistics, such as serial dependencies between interspike-intervals as in burst firing (Chen & Jastreboff, 1995), may also be important for sound detection.

The emergence of synchronized firing activity in neighboring auditory nerve fibers as a result of increased stimulus levels may lead to stronger activation of certain anteroventral cochlear nucleus cells, such as the bushy cells, whose activation partially depends on coincident input from different auditory nerve fibers (Oertel et al., 1988). Coincidence detection mechanism in anterior ventral cochlear nucleus cells, therefore, can not only signal the presence of an external signal but also can enhance stimulus detection in noisy backgrounds. As a result, they enhance neural synchronization to the stimulus in cochlear nucleus (Joris et al., 1994). The strength of the resulting neural synchrony may reflect the relative strength of the stimulus (Voigt & Young, 1980). Thus, the cooperative effort of several neurons enhances the speed and accuracy of representing sound levels, and extends the dynamic range of the output neuron if the input neurons represent a certain range of threshold values.

A correlation mechanism combined with a spike count mechanism that transmits only sufficiently coincident spikes to higher order nuclei will cause a reduction in the spontaneous firing rates in higher auditory nuclei and simultaneously extend the dynamic range of these neurons as well as their range of threshold values. This transformation of firing synchrony into firing rate, postulated to appear at or below the level of the inferior colliculus (Langner, 1997), may diminish the role of firing synchrony relative to the role of firing rate when advancing up the neuraxis. In this view, a sound sensation must be related to a "sufficiently strong" activation of the higher centers of the auditory nervous system. This "combination theory" requires a threshold mechanism that determines what "sufficiently strong" activation is in order to allow the decision that spontaneous activity does not represent sound.

In cortex, the size of the postsynaptic potential produced by a single synapse is so small (Abeles, 1991) that at least 30 or so coincident inputs have to occur before an output spike can be elicited. Under asynchronous conditions, that is, those during spontaneous activity, the number of active excitatory inputs required is estimated at about 300. Because at most only 10 percent of inputs to pyramidal cells in layer IV or deep layer III of cortex are from the specific auditory thalamus, the main determinant of spontaneous activity in the auditory cortex will be the input from other cortical sources.

Increasing sound intensity causes a monotonic increase in the firing rate for monotonic cortical neurons and, an initial increase followed by a decrease in the activity for nonmonotonic units. Strong post-activation suppression effects, reflecting the absence of firings for up to 100 ms after the onset response, are found especially in drowsy or anesthetized animals. Thus, under these conditions, most cortical neurons respond only in an onset fashion to continuous stimulation. When transient stimuli of moderate length (such as with a duration of about 100 to 200 ms) are used, the average (over the stimulus duration) firing rate of neurons with high spontaneous activity is only modestly above the spontaneous rate (Eggermont, 1997). This relative mean firing rate constancy is due to a pronounced reorganization of the firing times into an onset response followed by a relatively long postactivation suppression.

Correlations between the spontaneous firings of neuron pairs in primary auditory cortex are found in at least 60 percent of the pairs recorded from within primary auditory cortex (Dickson & Gerstein, 1974; Eggermont, 1992b) and between different cortical fields (Eggermont, 1997). These correlations may result from direct synaptic interactions between the neurons (although very few have actually been demonstrated in correlation studies; Toyama et al., 1981; Eggermont, 1992b). Other sources are common input due to the divergence of specific thalamic afferents as well as from pyramidal cell axon collaterals (Wallace et al., 1991). Thus, the phenomenon of correlated neural activity in primary auditory cortex in itself will not be sufficient to signal whether a stimulus is present or not. Changes in correlation strength must also be involved. This returns to the problem of how much change is required to decide on the presence or absence of a stimulus. A potential additional function of stimulus-induced synchrony may be "binding" of the particular stimulus features analyzed in parallel by the various cortical areas (Eggermont, 1977; for related ideas in the visual system but based on synchrony accompanying gamma band oscillations in cell membrane potentials, see Gray & Singer, 1988).

Summary

1. Spontaneous activity in the auditory nerve increases the sensitivity of sound detection. Part of this may result from spontaneous basilar membrane motion.
2. Spontaneous firing rates decrease from auditory nerve to auditory cortex, especially from the inferior colliculus onward, and become less and less dependent on the spontaneous transmitter release from the inner hair cells.
3. Spontaneous activity of neighboring neurons is uncorrelated in the auditory

periphery, whereas there is a small but consistent correlation between the spontaneous firings of both neighboring and distant neurons in auditory cortex.

The Role of Calcium in the Auditory System

Hair Cells

Sound increases basilar membrane motion above its spontaneous activity (Nuttall et al., 1997). The resulting movement of inner and outer hair cells results in displacement of their stereocilia from their resting position. This causes ion-conducting channels in these stereocilia to open. The resulting potassium influx from the endolymph depolarizes the hair cells which in turn, causes an opening of voltage-gated calcium channels in the basal part of the hair cell. An influx of calcium ions results because the concentration of calcium in the hair cell is much lower than in the surrounding perilymph. The increase of the calcium concentration in the hair cells is responsible for the slow motility response in outer hair cells and for transmitter release in inner hair cells. Antagonists of calmodulin, a secondary messenger for the metabotropic calcium channel, block the slow motility (Wangemann & Schacht, 1996). Repolarization of the hair cell is partially accomplished by an outward calcium-activated potassium current. Much of the calcium entering the cell diffuses away from the membrane and will be buffered to proteins within a few milliseconds. This is an intermediate step to sequestering the calcium in the endoplasmic reticulum which happens in a time span of about 10 ms. Subsequently any excess free calcium as well as most of the sequestered calcium will slowly exit the cell through an adenosinetriphosphate (ATP)-driven pump modulated by calmodulin (Blaustein, 1988).

Calcium is the dominant factor that links membrane activity to cellular metabolism. Calcium is also critical for mechanosensory adaptation because it regulates a myosin-type adaptation motor in the outer hair cells (Lenzi & Roberts, 1994). If the intracellular concentration of calcium becomes too high, the cell may die. Intense mechanical stimulation of isolated outer hair cells results in increased intracellular calcium levels (Fridberger & Ulfendahl, 1996). Nimodipine, an L-type calcium channel blocker abolishes the negative summating potential suggesting the involvement of these channels in the functioning of hair cells (Bobbin et al., 1990; 1991) although this drug in higher concentrations also blocks voltage-dependent potassium channels in outer hair cells (Lin et al., 1995).

Calcium is involved in both spontaneous and evoked transmitter release from inner hair cells. Spontaneous activity appears to be mostly dependent on the entry of extracellular calcium through basal hair cell membrane ion channels whereas evoked release also requires the liberation of calcium from intracellular calcium stores (Guth et al., 1991). An influx of calcium from the endolymph compartment has been postulated as the trigger for this liberation of intracellular calcium (Ohmori, 1989; Yamamoto & Karaide, 1990).

Nervous System

In the nervous system, both a decrease in extracellular calcium concentration (Russell, 1971; Dietzel & Heinemann, 1986) or a reduction in the intracellular calcium concentration (Friedman & Gutnick, 1989) results in burst-firing behavior. Caffeine, which in sensitive subjects induces tinnitus,

increases the tendency of the intracellular calcium release channels in the endoplasmic reticulum to open, by activation of the ryanodine receptors, and thus increases intracellular free calcium (Shirokova & Ríos, 1996a,b; Berridge, 1997). Salicylates and quinine also appear to increase intracellular free calcium (reviewed in Ochi & Eggermont, 1997, Table 4-3) and this would thus likely prevent burst firing. This suggests that bursting in itself may not be a causal factor in tinnitus, but that an increased intracellular free calcium concentration may be. Such increase may potentially result in higher spontaneous transmitter release and thus potentially increased spontaneous firing rates in the activated neurons.

Summary

1. Abnormal neural activity can arise from both enhanced and strongly reduced extracellular calcium concentrations.
2. Most tinnitus-inducing agents appear to affect the intracellular free calcium concentration in hair cells as well as in neurons.

Neural Activity Correlates of Cochlear Hearing Loss and Tinnitus

Do Animals Have Tinnitus?

Because all information presented here is based on animal research, the crucial element for its interpretation is whether animals experience tinnitus. A behavioral model that validates this assumption is thus needed.

Table 4-3. Effects of salicylates and quinine on cell K^+ and Ca^{2+}

Salicylate	Quinine
Increases K^+ channel conductances	Blocks voltage-dependent K^+ channels
Increases Ca^{2+} channel conductance	Increases Ca^{2+} channel conductance
Increases intracellular free Ca^{2+} concentration	Increases intracellular free Ca2+ concentration
Activates Ca^{2+}-dependent K^+-conductance	Blocks Ca^{2+}-dependent K^+-conductance

To establish a salicylate- and quinine-based animal model of tinnitus (Jastreboff et al., 1988; 1991), male pigmented rats were conditioned to suppress licking during presentation of noise. Subsequently, after injection of salicylate or quinine, the animals showed this suppression of licking. This may be interpreted as being caused by a sensation, analogous to that of the conditioning noise, that was induced by the application of the drug. Thus, it is reasonable to assume that rats may experience tinnitus, and that this can be extended to other mammals.

The following overview details the summary presented in Table 4-4, where shaded entries show clear effects attributable to tinnitus-inducing agents, specifically noise and drugs such as salicylates and quinine. Whereas Table 4-4 puts the cortex on top and the cochlea at the bottom, in the following description we will start with the cochlea.

Cochlea

Application of acetylsalicylic acid has no detectable effect on outer hair cell membrane potential fluctuations, suggesting that the mechanoelectrical potassium transduction current under spontaneous conditions is not affected (Preyer et al., 1997). Under conditions where the whole cochlear partition is stimulated by a transverse electric current, resulting in a polarized outer hair cell basolateral membrane, the outer hair cells produce sufficient forces to distort the basilar membrane position. These forces are reversibly reduced by superfusion with 10 mM sodium salicylate. It is thus likely that salicylates directly inhibit the outer hair cell motor (Mammano & Ashmore, 1993). Many of the effects of salicylate on hearing loss may arise from this effect, likely caused by the partitioning of the salicylate molecule into the membrane of the outer hair cell (Tunstall et al., 1995; Kakehata & Santos-Sacchi, 1996).

A daily dosage of 3.9 grams of aspirin reduces the level of otoacoustic emission in humans (McFadden & Plattsmier, 1984;

Long & Tubis, 1988) and moderate doses of quinine sulfate (325 mg) eliminate spontaneous acoustic emissions in humans within 7 hours. (McFadden & Pasanen, 1994). These findings suggest a specific involvement of the outer hair cells in the generation of otoacoustic emissions. In contrast to normal hearing subjects or subjects with mild noise-induced hearing loss, click-evoked otoacoustic emissions in tinnitus sufferers with either noise-induced hearing loss or normal hearing, show increased emission amplitudes during contralateral masking (Attias et al., 1996). This suggests that a reduction of efferent activity, responsible for the contralateral masking, could account for tinnitus in some patients (see also Graham et al., 1996).

The sharpness of the mechanical tuning in the cochlea depends on the patency of the outer hair cells. Tinnitus-inducing agents cause changes in the outer hair cells and are thus likely to affect the motion of the basilar membrane. Frequency tuning of basilar membrane displacements in the 15 kHz region of the guinea-pig cochlea, as measured by laser Doppler interferometry, is affected during perfusion of the scala tympani with 2.5 or 5 mM salicylate solutions. The tips of frequency-tuning curves become up to 45 dB less sensitive, the characteristic frequency shifts 2 kHz to lower frequencies and the tail of the frequency-tuning curve becomes sensitized by about 10 dB. This change can be explained by a reduction in outer hair cell amplifier action, and by an increased compliance of the basilar membrane as a result of reduced turgidity of the outer hair cells. The time it takes to produce a change in basilar membrane mechanics, cochlear microphonics and compound action potential from the onset of salicylate perfusion is about 6 minutes, similar to the time course of the salicylate-induced reduction in motility, turgor pressure and axial stiffness of outer hair cells *in vitro*. However, the duration of the salicylate-induced changes in the cochlear microphonics and compound action potential outlasts those in the basilar membrane. This can partly be

Table 4-4. Effects of tinnitus inducing agents (salicylates, quinine, and noise)

Measure Brain Area	Amplitude (stim. induced) or spont. activity	Spontaneous Firing Rate	Spontaneous inter-spike intervals	Spontaneous Bursting	Synchrony
Cortex	2-DG activity up Effect on EEG	No change in primary areas. Up in secondary	Rebound response later	No change	Increased in cortex and between areas
Medial Geniculate Body	2-DG activity up				
Other inferior colliculus nuclei	C-fos increased in pericentral nucleus	Up for all agents		Number of bursts with > 4 spikes up	
Central nucleus of the inferior colliculus		Up for all agents	More regular		
Inferior colliculus	2-DG activity shows banded pattern. Evoked potentials up				
Dorsal cochlear nucleus	C-fos no change after salicylate	Strongly up after noise trauma			
Ventral cochlear nucleus	C-fos no change after salicylate	Same or down after noise trauma			
Auditory nerve	Compound action potential amplitude down. Tuning broader. Thresholds up	Up for high dose of salicylate, same for lower dose	Mostly normal	Number of spike doublets up in neurons with high thresholds	
Summating potential	Salicylate no effect. Quinine down				
Cochlear micophonics	Salicylate no effect. Quinine down				
Endolymphatic potential	Salicylate and quinine no effect				
Outer hair cells	Motility and turgidity down (all for salicylate)				

explained by the independent, longer lasting, action of salicylates on transmitter release at the inner hair cell synapse compared to those on the outer hair cell motility (Murugasu & Russell, 1995).

Perfusion of the perilymphatic space of the guinea pig cochlea with salicylate (Puel et al., 1990) results, for high-frequency tone burst stimulation, in a reduction in the cochlear microphonics but has no effect on the summating potential. The perfusion reduces the compound action potential amplitude at low stimulus levels but has no effect at high stimulus levels (suggesting a recruitment type of hearing loss). In the cat, similar findings for summating potential and compound action potential but accompanied by an increase in cochlear microphonics amplitude were reported by Stypulkowski (1990). This suggests that salicylate does not antagonize the hair cell transmitter in the cochlea and that altered prostaglandin levels following salicylate application may not be the cause of the compound action potential changes. Quinine reduced the compound action potential amplitude at all levels (resulting in a parallel shift of the amplitude-intensity curves) and reduced the cochlear microphonics as well as the summating potential. Quinine toxicity may be caused by the inhibition of an ATP-sensitive K^+ channel or a Ca^{2+}-activated K^+ channel. Neither salicylate or quinine affects the endolymphatic potential, thus eliminating involvement of the stria vascularis (Puel et al., 1990) despite the fact that systemically applied salicylate (Didier et al., 1993) and quinine (Jung et al., 1993) may cause a decreased blood flow, potentially affecting the stria vascularis, that may contribute to the ototoxicity of these drugs.

Auditory Nerve

After several hours of noise exposure and long survival times, cat auditory nerve fibers in characteristic frequency regions with normal thresholds still have normal spontaneous activity and normal interspike-interval statistics. Units that no longer respond to sound have significantly decreased spontaneous firing rates and also have a tendency to fire in spike bursts separated by long periods of silence. These abnormally-firing, bursty, fibers might innervate partially damaged inner hair cells (Liberman & Kiang, 1978), whereas units without spontaneous activity likely originate from regions where all inner hair cells are completely damaged.

In the frog, salicylate affects the ion channels involved in action potential generation. When applied intracellularly or to the bathing solution, salicylate slows the falling phase of the action potential at the node of Ranvier, with little effect on the amplitude. This may be due to salicylate crossing the membrane and binding preferentially to a receptor at the external surface, thus changing the surface potential, or might be the result of a rise in intracellular calcium concentration (by releasing calcium ions from mitochondria) following inhibition of oxidative phosphorylation (Attwell et al., 1979; Ricciopo Neto, 1980). Similar effects on the shape of the action potential have been noted after application of quinine sulfate to auditory nerve fibers (Lin, 1997).

Cats given 400 mg/kg sodium salicylate intravenously showed threshold increases of 30 to 40 dB (the maximum was reached 5 to 10 hours after application) with broadened frequency-tuning curves. The drug produced a significant increase of 10 to 20 spikes/second (sp/s) in the spontaneous discharge of medium-spontaneous (20 to 59 sp/s) fibers, in stark contrast with the effects of other, for example, aminoglycoside, ototoxic agents that typically reduce the spontaneous firing rate. A tendency for double spiking occurred analogous to that found with sound stimulation (Evans et al., 1981; Evans & Borerwe, 1982). Salicylate administration in cats at a lower dose (200 mg/kg) produced no significant change in the mean spontaneous rates in the low- and high-spontaneous firing rate populations of nerve fibers following drug administration. In some individual cells, however, significant increases in firing rate were seen (Stypulkowski, 1990). Salicylate applied into scala media (or scala tympani) of the pigeon elevates auditory nerve fiber tip threshold by 5 to 35 dB. The mean spontaneous discharge rate either increases slightly or remains unchanged in the majority of fibers (Shehate-Dieler et al., 1994).

For the diagnosis of Ménière's disease, tinnitus is a prerequisite symptom (see Chapter 9). Surgical obliteration of the endolymphatic sac in guinea pigs is an accepted animal model of Ménière's disease. After development of endolymphatic hydrops and low-frequency hearing loss, spontaneous firing rates in auditory nerve fibers are unchanged. However, on occasion fibers without spontaneous discharge are found. Some fibers show abnormal bursting activity (intermittent groups of spikes having very short intervals often less than 1 ms (smaller than their relative refractory period), both in the spontaneous and in the driven discharge (Harrison & Prijs, 1984). Atrophy of outer hair cell stereocilia is found in such hydroptic guinea pig cochleas. Comparison of the morphopathology with the compound action potential audiograms indicates a close association between the low-frequency hearing loss and this atrophy of stereocilia (Rydmarker & Horner, 1991).

Auditory nerve fiber activity is zero in the absence of inner hair cells (Dallos & Harris, 1978). Thus, the origin of changes in spontaneous activity must be the inner hair cells. Modulation of the spontaneous activity of auditory nerve fibers can of course also be produced by changes in ionic content inside and outside the auditory nerve fibers. Decreases in extracellular calcium produce increased spontaneous activity with bursting behavior in lateral line afferent nerve fibers (Russell, 1971). Zenner and Ernst (1995) propose several features in the action of outer hair cells and inner hair cells that may result in altered spontaneous activity. First among these are changes in the motility of the outer hair cells, which may be accompanied by changes in spontaneous

otoacoustic emissions. Second there are changes in both outer and inner hair cell transduction channels, caused by pathological deflections of stereocilia (LePage, 1995) or ion channel malfunctioning. Third there are changes in the biochemistry surrounding the release of the transmitter substance by inner hair cells. All these changes may involve calcium conductance alterations affecting the calcium-activated potassium channels responsible for repolarization of the hair cell. If these channels are blocked or not activated, likely the result of a reduction in extracellular calcium concentration, then the hair cell stays polarized and may release transmitter continuously and at an elevated rate. If there is too much extracellular calcium, then calcium spikes may result producing a burstlike release of transmitter. Thus, a delicate homeostasis of the extracellular, most likely that in the perilymph, calcium concentration is required to prevent abnormal hair cell functioning. Nimodipine, an L-type calcium channel blocker, appears to abolish quinine-induced tinnitus in rats in a dose-dependent manner (Jastreboff et al., 1991), suggesting that excess extracellular calcium may be involved. Strangely, dietary calcium supplements were also effective in partly abolishing the conditioned reduction of the licking response. This suggests that it would rather be a leaking of intracellular calcium down the concentration gradient that is prohibited by Nimodipine.

Auditory Brain Stem

Chinchillas exposed to an 86 dB SPL, 4 kHz noise band for about four days show at 2 to 12 hours postexposure strongly decreased spontaneous firing rates for cochlear nucleus neurons with characteristic frequencies in the region with elevated thresholds (Salvi et al., 1978). Adult hamsters exposed for 4 hours to a 10 kHz tone at levels between 125 and 130 dB SPL, showed after thirty to fifty-eight days of survival a major increase in spontaneous multi-unit activity (from 4 to 42 spikes/s) in the characteristic frequency regions with increased neural thresholds in the dorsal cochlear nucleus (Kaltenbach & McCaslin, 1996; Kaltenbach et al., 1996a,b). In another study, neurons in dorsal cochlear nucleus were recorded from before and after exposure to an intense tone with a frequency above the neuron's characteristic frequency. The exposure had no effect on thresholds at characteristic frequency but improved "tail" thresholds by as much as 40 dB, in addition spontaneous and driven firing rates increased (Salvi et al., 1996a,b). In contrast to the ventral cochlear nucleus, spontaneous activity in the dorsal cochlear nucleus is not abolished after sectioning of the auditory nerve (Koerber et al., 1966). These old and new findings thus suggest that the increased spontaneous activity in the dorsal cochlear nucleus may result from a shift in the balance of excitation and inhibition due to loss of normal input to inhibitory units.

Auditory Midbrain

Exposure of chinchillas to a 2 kHz pure tone of 105 dB SPL produces 20 to 30 dB of permanent threshold shift in the region from 2 to 8 kHz. Generally, less than 60 percent of outer hair cells are missing. Evoked potential amplitude level functions at 4 and 8 kHz in the inferior colliculus are of the recruitment type. At 2 kHz the functions show mostly over-recruitment whereas at 500 Hz, where no hearing loss was induced, the curve is also steeper than normal and reaches substantially larger amplitudes than normal (Salvi et al., 1990). Single units with characteristic frequency below the region of damage show a hypersensitive tail (Salvi et al., 1996a,b). For the rat, tone exposure (4 kHz tone, 104 dB SPL, 30 minutes) the evoked potential amplitude in the inferior colliculus is also increased. Baclofen, a GABA$_B$ agonist, reverses the increased amplitude induced by this tone exposure in a dose-dependent manner (Szczepaniak & Møller, 1995; 1996). This suggests that noise trauma causes a loss of GABA$_B$ mediated lateral inhibition.

Evaluation of the discharge patterns of 40 neurons in the central nucleus of the inferior colliculus before and after acute cochlear trauma induced by a 15 to 25 minutes high intensity (95 to 115 dB) pure tone at a frequency above the unit's characteristic frequency shows (Wang et al., 1996): (1) a significant increase in the suprathreshold discharge rates in 70 percent of all neurons studied (93 percent of neurons with non-monotonic discharge rate level functions), (2) almost no effect on post-stimulus-time histograms of onset or sustained responders, (3) in 75 percent of pauser-neurons (neurons that respond with a sharp onset, followed by a suppression period, the pause, after which the firing rate gradually increases) a decreased pause duration and increased sustained discharge rate. This suggests that the response properties of neurons with extreme narrow frequency-tuning curves and nonmonotonic rate-intensity functions are shaped by an inhibitory circuit acting above the high-frequency flank of the frequency tuning curve. These neurons show much broader tuning curves after noise exposure, suggesting a reduction in lateral inhibition. This inhibition is obviously reduced by frequency-selective damage to the hair cells in the cochlea.

Diffuse inner hair cell loss does not give rise to abnormally broad tuning or hypersensitivity. Following nearly total inner hair cell damage induced by carboplatin, frequency selectivity remains normal for those few neurons in inferior colliculus that were still responding to sound, suggesting that frequency selectivity in the auditory system may remain present with small numbers of surviving inner hair cells, provided the outer hair cells remain normal (Wake et al., 1996).

In the inferior colliculus of guinea pigs, 200 mg/kg sodium salicylate increases mean spontaneous firing rates from about 5 sp/s to about 19 sp/s at 100 minutes after application, firing rates then declined to baseline after 10 hours. In control animals (saline infusion) the firing rate did not change significantly (Manabe et al., 1997).

Administration of 450 mg/kg of sodium salicylate to guinea pigs caused in inferior colliculus neurons a decrease in the inter-spike-interval histogram mode from about 3 to 1.2 ms. A significant proportion of the cells also show activity with a much higher regularity of discharges than before drug application (Jastreboff & Sasaki, 1986). Recordings from 471 units in the external nucleus of the inferior colliculus in the rat revealed that salicylate (233 mg/kg) increased spontaneous activity from about 6 sp/s to about 9 sp/s. The probability of bursts consisting of fewer than 5 spikes was identical before and after salicylate application. However, after salicylate, bursts with up to 13 spikes were noted in a small percentage (about 0.1 percent). The effect was dominant for units with characteristic frequencies from the 10 to 16 kHz range (Chen & Jastreboff, 1995).

Using indicators of neural metabolism (radioactive labeled 2-deoxyglucose) and gene expression (c-fos) also suggests specific changes in the auditory midbrain after application of salicylates. The inferior colliculus of rats normally shows a uniform and diffuse deoxyglucose uptake in silence, but after salicylate administration a heterogeneous banded pattern of alternating reduced and increased uptake was seen (Jastreboff & Jastreboff, 1996a; Wallhäusser-Franke et al., 1996). After application of salicylate in gerbils (Wallhäusser-Franke, 1997) a c-fos study showed some increase in the pericentral nucleus of the inferior colliculus, but no change in other auditory brain stem nuclei. Jastreboff and Jastreboff (1996b) also found increased expression of c-fos in the inferior colliculus after salicylate administration. However, the locus coeruleus, the midbrain peri-aquaductal grey and the lateral parabrachial nucleus (regions also activated by stress or pain, which affect arousal and anxiety) show increased expression (Wallhäusser-Franke, 1997). This suggests that brain areas related to stress and pain may be involved in tinnitus (Hallam et al., 1984; Levine, 1994).

Auditory Thalamus and Cortex

Because tinnitus is a perceptual phenomenon, one expects the auditory cortex, or at least some of its many areas, to show effects after application of tinnitus-inducing agents. Following four days of salicylate treatment (200 to 350 mg/kg i.p. daily) auditory cortex of gerbils showed a reduced uptake of deoxyglucose along some isofrequency contours (always 2 to 3 bands). The medial geniculate body showed increased uptake after treatment but without an apparent systematic frequency dependent effect (Wallhäusser-Franke et al., 1996).

Ochi and Eggermont (1996; 1997) investigated single-unit firing activity in primary auditory cortex of cats following systemically applied salicylate and quinine. Sodium salicylate (200 mg/kg) was administered intraperitoneally, while quinine hydrochloride (100 mg/kg or 200 mg/kg) was administered intramuscularly. Recordings from the same units were performed prior to application and continuously up to six hours after administration. For salicylate, all animals showed 20 to 30 dB threshold shift about 2 hours after administration, without recovery during the following 4 hours. Input-output curves were invariably of the recruitment type. For quinine, all animals showed 10 to 40 dB threshold shift about one-half hour after administration.

Both salicylate and quinine produce small but significant changes in spontaneous firing rates. Low-spontaneous rate units (initial firing rate < 1spike/s) become more active while the activity of high-spontaneous rate units (initial firing rate > 1 spike/s) decreased. However, averaged across all units, no change in spontaneous firing rate occurred.

Peak cross-correlation coefficients for the firing patterns of simultaneously recorded cells increased significantly for quinine, whereas for salicylate the correlogram's central peak became significantly narrower after application. This reflection of increased synchronization of the spontaneous firings across different neurons observed after application of both drugs may be related to tinnitus (Eggermont and Ochi, 1996; Ochi and Eggermont, 1997).

The best modulation frequency in response to stimulation with periodic click trains decreases after administration. Recently, we showed that salicylate and quinine both decrease the EEG-spindle frequency and that EEG-spindle frequency accounts for more than half of the variance in the best modulation frequency (Kenmochi & Eggermont, 1997 a,b). The concurrent changes in the EEG-spindle-frequency and in the temporal modulation transfer function also suggest that salicylates and quinine affect both the auditory periphery and the auditory cortex or thalamus.

In more recent studies, involving simultaneous recording from three auditory cortical areas (primary auditory cortex, anterior auditory field, and secondary auditory cortex) in cat (Eggermont & Kenmochi, 1998) it was shown that after both salicylate and quinine application, spontaneous firing rates increased in secondary auditory cortex whereas they decreased slightly in primary auditory cortex and in the anterior auditory field.

Behavioral Studies in Animals

As a consequence of mild hearing loss, certain groups of central auditory neurons become more sensitive to electrical stimulation of the auditory system (Gerken et al., 1984). Behaviorally measured thresholds for the detection of brief trains of electrical pulses applied to the cochlear nucleus and inferior colliculus of the cat were determined before and after 48 hours exposure to a 1 kHz 110 dB SPL tone. Although the average permanent threshold shift across cats and frequencies for acoustic stimulation was 19 dB, the mean shift in electrical stimulation threshold was only 10.4 dB. This suggests that those neurons became hypersensitive to electrical stimulation. Temporal integration for this electrical stimulation

was also reduced after noise exposure (Gerken et al., 1991). This points to central changes in neural properties as a result of only modest changes in hearing loss. Such changes may also occur in certain forms of tinnitus.

Physiological Measurements in Humans

Tinnitus, considered as a positive symptom disorder characterized by "neuronal hyperactivity due to loss of afferent inhibition" (Jeanmonod et al., 1996), has been linked to bursting neural activity in the medial thalamus, recorded prior to medial thalamotomy, in humans. In one study, over 2,000 single units were recorded in 104 patients, six of which had tinnitus. About 99 percent of the 2,000 single units, were unresponsive to sensory stimulation or motor activation, while 41 percent of the total showed rhythmic (at about 4 Hz) or random burst-firing typical for low-threshold calcium spike bursts (Jeanmonod et al., 1996). This suggests a linkage between some forms of tinnitus and EEG spindling which is initiated by rhythmic bursting in the thalamus.

In assessing candidate subjects for a cochlear implant, it has been observed that negative currents applied to the round window are more effective for inducing hearing sensations than positive currents. Positive currents, however, suppressed tinnitus possibly by hyperpolarization of the nerve fibers which might inhibit some pathological activity (Cazals et al., 1978; Aran, 1981; Aran & Cazals, 1981; and Chapter 16 of this text). *In vitro* studies in the hippocampus have shown that electrical stimulation with currents, similar to those used to stimulate nerves in the CNS, can inhibit penicillin- or picrotoxin-induced synchronized epileptic burstlike neuronal activity (Durand, 1986).

Functional magnetic resonance imaging has been used to study gaze-induced tinnitus (Cacace et al., 1996) or oral facial movements (Lockwood et al., 1998). In patients in which certain directions of gaze are accompanied by, foci of activity in the tinnitus patient were localized in the superior colliculus and frontal eye fields in cortex. Presently it is not clear whether this reflects activity related to the motor act (gaze) that induces tinnitus or to the percept of tinnitus itself. In patients able to modulate the loudness of their tinnitus by oral facial movements, the loci of activity were in the auditory cortex contralateral to the ear in which the tinnitus was perceived as well as in limbic structures.

Summary

Table 4-4 presents a summary of this section:

1. Noise trauma or application of salicylate and quinine slightly reduces or does not alter spontaneous activity in auditory nerve fibers, in cells of the ventral cochlear nucleus and likely also in some parts of the inferior colliculus. Activity in both primary auditory cortex and anterior auditory field is reduced. Thus, the tonotopically organized lemniscal auditory pathway shows mainly a reduction in spontaneous activity.
2. Noise trauma greatly increases spontaneous activity in the dorsal cochlear nucleus, salicylate results in elevated spontaneous activity in the external nucleus of the inferior colliculus, and both quinine and salicylate cause increased spontaneous firing in secondary auditory cortex. This suggests that the multimodal, extralemniscal pathway may be selectively involved by tinnitus-inducing agents.
3. Increases in spontaneous activity are generally accompanied by changes in the temporal properties of neuronal firing. These changes may reflect loss of post-activation suppression, occasionally leading to prolonged duration bursting such as in the external nucleus of the inferior colliculus. Other changes may reflect a loss of off-characteristic frequency (or lateral) inhibition resulting in broadening of the frequency response area and hypersensitivity.

4. Changes in interneuronal firing synchrony, reflected in increased strength and narrowed central peaks in cross-correlograms, are observed in primary auditory cortex.

Hearing Loss and Biochemical Changes

Salicylate and Quinine

The mechanisms of salicylate and quinine ototoxicity appear to be multifaceted. Morphological studies indicate no permanent cochlear damage after salicylate- or quinine-induced ototoxicity. Electrophysiologic and morphologic data conclusively demonstrate that salicylates and quinine reversibly affect outer hair cells. In addition, both drugs appear to decrease cochlear blood flow (Jung et al., 1993). Salicylates inhibit prostaglandin-forming cyclooxygenase, and recent studies suggest that abnormal levels of arachidonic acid metabolites consisting of decreased prostaglandins and increased leukotrines may mediate salicylate ototoxicity (Jung et al., 1997). The action of salicylates is considerably weaker than that of acetyl salicylic acid (Packham, 1982). Unlike with salicylate, however, the role of prostaglandins in quinine ototoxicity has not been clearly demonstrated. One of quinine's principal actions, blocking of calcium-dependent potassium channels, has yet to be investigated for its potential role in ototoxicity (Jung et al., 1993). Some of the similarities and differences in the ion channel action of salicylates and quinine are shown in Table 4-3 (from Ochi & Eggermont, 1997). Neither salicylate nor quinine affect the endolymphatic potential thus eliminating involvement of the stria vascularis (Puel et al., 1990).

Acoustic Trauma

In the guinea pig, a slight but significant elevation of the endolymphatic potential and an alkalization of the endolymph has been induced by acoustic overstimulation (2,000 Hz at 120 dB SPL for 309 minutes), with little change in the K^+, Na^+, Cl^- and HCO_3^- concentrations. The Ca^{2+} concentration in endolymph increased abruptly to 48 times the pre-exposure value, whereas no significant change in the Ca^{2+} concentration was observed in the perilymph (Ikeda et al., 1988).

Experimental Endolymphatic Hydrops

An increased endolymphatic calcium concentration may explain the occurrence of an endolymphatic hydrops (Meyer zum Gottesberge-Orsulakova & Kaufmann, 1986). During the development of experimental endolymphatic hydrops, disturbed Ca^{2+} homeostasis occurs, reflected in the elevation of the endolymphatic calcium concentration and in the concentration of intracellular calcium in the light cells and the melanocytes of the vestibular organ. A striking correlation exists between the rising endolymphatic calcium concentration and the decreasing endolymphatic potential. Accumulation of calcium may be the result of an increase in Ca^{2+} influx into the cells and/or an insufficient outward pumping mechanism and/or dysfunction of the internal Ca^{2+} storage. An enhanced free systolic calcium concentration may increase the osmotic pressure, which may cause an influx of water and an increase in cell volume (Meyer zum Gottesberge, 1988).

Summary

1. A reduction in the endolymphatic potential is found in experimental endolymphatic hydrops, a slight increase occurs after noise trauma, whereas salicylates and quinine have no effect on the endolymphatic potential.
2. Endolymphatic calcium concentrations are elevated after noise trauma and in experimental endolymphatic hydrops but not after application of salicylate and quinine.
3. Changes in endolymph and endolymphatic potential are thus not likely primary factors in the causation of tinnitus.

Hearing Loss and Changes in CNS Organization

Slow Changes

Analysis of the cortical effects of unilateral cochlear lesions suggests that the adult auditory cortical frequency map undergoes a slow reorganization in cases of partial deafness (Robertson & Irvine, 1989; and Chapter 5). The effect thirty-five to eighty-one days after such damage is that the area of contralateral auditory cortex in which the lesioned frequency range would normally be represented becomes partially occupied by an expanded representation of frequencies adjacent to the range damaged by the lesion, with normal thresholds for these frequencies. This reflects a gradual reorganization since the responses of neuron clusters examined within hours of making similar cochlear lesions showed only small shifts in characteristic frequency towards frequencies spared by the lesion, with greatly elevated thresholds (about 32 dB) compared to normal.

Similar changes are observed two to eleven months after a unilateral cochlear lesion in adult cats. Along the tonotopic axis of the primary auditory cortex the total representation of cochlear lesion-edge frequencies may extend up to 2.6 mm rostral to the area of normal frequency representation. In contrast, the map of the unlesioned ipsilateral cochlea does not differ from those in normal animals. Thus, in the lesioned animals ipsilateral and contralateral tonotopic maps in the same primary auditory cortex differ in the region of the lesion only, in contrast to the normal very good matching of ipsilateral and contralateral primary auditory cortex maps. This suggests that the cortical reorganization also reflects subcortical changes in the representation of the contralateral cochlea (Rajan et al., 1993).

After three months of recovery, newborn kittens with aminoglycoside induced hearing loss show an extensively reorganized primary auditory cortex with almost all units in the region of initial hearing loss tuned to a border frequency between normal and damaged hair cell regions (Harrison et al., 1991). Substantial reorganization of tonotopic maps in the central nucleus of the inferior colliculus occurs, following sustained neonatal high-frequency sensorineural hearing loss, indicating an overrepresentation of input arising from the high-frequency border of the damaged cochlea. It appears that cortical frequency map reorganization is more extensive following neonatal lesions compared with those in the adult, suggesting an additional set of mechanisms that may operate only during early postnatal development (Harrison et al., 1996).

Major alterations occur in the tonotopic map of the dorsal cochlear nucleus following damage to a portion of the cochlea. These changes, however, are typically characterized by some combination of threshold shifts and characteristic frequency gaps in the region representing the cochlear lesion. In the edge-frequency regions, expanded areas characterized by more or less constant characteristic frequencies are found, largely confined to the low-frequency side of the characteristic frequency gaps but these regions always have abnormal characteristic frequency thresholds. All of the characteristics of tuning found in the expanded map areas of the dorsal cochlear nucleus are features that have been found in auditory nerve fibers following restricted cochlear lesions (Kaltenbach et al., 1996a,b).

In genetic (C57) mouse, sensorineural hearing loss begins during adulthood with principal involvement of the basal cochlea and progresses to include lower frequencies as well, thus featuring an animal model for studying the effects of presbycusis on central nervous system changes. An overrepresentation of middle frequencies exists in inferior colliculus, indicating that plastic reorganization is also present subcortically and is likely caused by a *diminished inhibition with age* (Willott, 1996).

Transient Changes

Deoxyglucose studies in adult guinea pigs showed that 2 hours after unilateral cochlea removal, the ipsilateral cochlear nucleus activity was reduced, combined with a reduction in the contralateral medial superior olive and the inferior colliculus and some reduced uptake in the contralateral medial geniculate body. In contrast, ten to forty-eight days after cochlea removal, the only reduction observed was in the contralateral medial superior olive, all other structures were normal. Studies in which both cochlea were ablated also resulted in increased uptake in all auditory structures after twelve days of survival time (Sasaki et al., 1980). This suggests that there is increased neuronal activity in central auditory structures after deafferentation. Because deoxyglucose uptake reflects largely metabolic demands in the generation of excitatory as well as inhibitory postsynaptic potentials, increased uptake does not necessarily imply increased spontaneous firing rates.

The fact that the tonotopic map of the auditory cortex is altered does not mean that the primary locus of reorganization resides in the cortex. Further evidence comes from a study using traumatizing tones above the excitatory response area of neurons in inferior colliculus. This can acutely and dramatically alter the firing pattern of inferior colliculus neurons that have nonmonotonic discharge rate-level functions and inhibitory response areas above characteristic frequency. The excitatory response area expands dramatically along the low-frequency side of the tuning curve, and the maximum driven discharge rate increases significantly. The broadening of the frequency tuning curve appears to be due to the reduction in off-characteristic frequency inhibition, which is normally mediated by GABAergic inputs. The magnitude of the effect appeared to be much less in dorsal cochlear nucleus than in inferior colliculus (Salvi et al., 1996a,b) suggesting at least two different mechanisms.

Summary

1. Peripheral lesions produce some instantaneous changes in neural response properties and also pronounced long

lasting changes in the representation of the cochlea in structures such as dorsal cochlear nucleus, central nucleus of the inferior colliculus and primary auditory cortex.

2. The changes in neural organization appear more pronounced for more central locations and include a vastly expanded number of neurons in the central structure that were previously tuned to the damaged cochlear area and are now tuned to the frequencies representing the low-frequency edges of the cochlear lesions. This edge frequency likely determines the pitch of the tinnitus.

3. Organizational changes in the brain stem may be the result of changed tuning properties of the neurons in these structures, rather than changed synaptic strengths.

THEORIES

Introduction

The general belief, expressed in the literature, is that most tinnitus results from altered spontaneous activity in the auditory nerve. Opinions then diverge as to which changes in auditory nerve fiber activity are causing the effect. Changes can occur at the individual neuron level, such as changes in spontaneous firing rate or in the temporal properties of single-neuron spike trains.

Changes in population activity are also proposed, specifically in the synchrony of firings of subsets of neurons or in the changed activity patterns across characteristic frequency. I will review the rate, temporal and synchronization aspects of neural firing as they relate to proposed models for tinnitus (Table 4-5). The format I will use is that of a brief statement and some argumentation that captures the essence of the theory followed by experimental evidence for that statement. Thus theories are not considered as opposite to facts, the contents of the previous section, but rather as proposals for mechanisms of tinnitus for which, at present, there is likely not sufficient experimental evidence to completely support or refute them.

Firing Rates

Theory: Tinnitus is the Result of Increased Neural Activity

The most straightforward theory is that tinnitus results from an increased firing rate in auditory nerve fibers (Tyler, 1984), generating an overall enhancement of activity in the central nervous system. This idea is likely based on studies by Evans et al. (1981) who found a considerable increase in spontaneous activity after application of high doses (400 mg/kg) of salicylate in cat. In general, however, insults to the human auditory system that are accompanied by

Table 4-5. Tinnitus Theories

Theory (Tinnitus results from:)	Experimental Evidence
Increased firing rates	Demonstrated in extralemniscal pathway: In the dorsal cochlear nucleus, in the pericentral and external nuclei of the inferior colliculus and in the secondary auditory cortex
Increased burst firing	Demonstrated in auditory nerve and inferior colliculus
Pathological neural firing synchrony	Demonstrated in primary auditory cortex
Hypersensitivity due to loss of inhibition	Demonstrated in inferior colliculus
Reorganization of cortical maps (long-standing tinnitus)	Demonstrated after induced hearing loss

tinnitus decrease spontaneous firing rates in animal auditory nerve fibers (Table 4-6; Kiang et al., 1976; Liberman & Kiang, 1978; Stypulkowski, 1990). Thus, increased firing rates in the auditory nerve are not likely to be causal to tinnitus.

It remains somewhat of a problem that the observed changes in spontaneous firing rates in primary auditory cortex after application of quinine or salicylates are also very small (Ochi & Eggermont, 1996; 1997) even after salicylate doses as high as 400 mg/kg (Eggermont, 1992). One could propose that the intricate balance of excitation and inhibition that generally exists in auditory cortex is not sufficiently disturbed and that there are no secondary effects at the single cell level accompanying the tinnitus. In other words, the manifestation of tinnitus may involve central auditory structures that are not necessarily impaired (Lenarz et al., 1995).

Tinnitus as a result of increased spontaneous activity conforms to the idea that spontaneous activity in the auditory system is unwanted noise, as well as to the idea that

Table 4-6. Tinnitus: Level of Description and Type of Treatment

---

Systems Level

Tinnitus, triggered by peripheral lesions, affects the entire auditory nervous system.
Initial effects: hypersensitivity, increased spontaneous activity and increased synchronization.
Long-standing tinnitus also involves a reorganization of the auditory cortex and inferior colliculus. This may affect peripheral parts of the auditory system by the action of localized interconnected feedback loops.

Interference by desynchronization or inducing reorganizational changes through electrical stimulation or noise masking.

Network Level

Tinnitus may result from a specific activation of the extralemniscal system resulting in increased spontaneous firing rate.
In addition, increased synchronization of activity in auditory cortical fields is found.

Interference by specific interaction with the extralemniscal system through tactile or electric stimulation.

Neuron Level

Tinnitus may result from neurons that show dramatically altered temporal firing properties such as increased burst-firing, caused by decreased intracellular calcium.

Interference by increasing intracellular calcium, potentially through an extracellular calcium supplement.

Synapse Level

Tinnitus may result from decreased GABA levels and increased NMDA activity in the auditory system.

Interference by supplying GABA agonists such as backlofen and benzodiazepines.

Molecular Level

Tinnitus may result from changes in calcium channel conductance. Increased intracellular calicum may give rise to increased transmitter release and higher firing rates. Reduced intracellular calcium concentration, potentially resulting from low extracellular calcium, may increase burst-firing.

Interference by applying Nimodipine, an L-type calcium channel blocker.

---

firing rates code for all aspects of a sound. The latter idea has been given some impetus by the success of artificial neural networks that learn by adjusting their connection strengths solely based on firing rates propagating through the network. If a rate code for sound applies, then the pitch of a sound could be determined by the location of strong activity peaks across the array of auditory nerve fibers. Timbre, in turn, might be determined by the overall distribution of firing rates across characteristic frequency. Such activity profiles may be faithfully represented along the lemniscal pathway up to the auditory cortex. The emergence of non-monotonic units in cortex, however, results in an intensity dependent spatial representation of activity in primary auditory cortex (Phillips et al., 1994). Thus, simple rate models of timbre have to be modified to remain intensity independent (but see Schulze & Langner, 1997).

Evidence: Increased Firing Rates in Extralemniscal Pathway

Evidence is now abundant for enhanced spontaneous activity after noise trauma in the dorsal cochlear nucleus (Kaltenbach & McCaslin, 1996; Kaltenbach et al., 1996a,b; Salvi et al., 1996a,b) which directly inputs to the inferior colliculus, where increased spontaneous activity has also been demonstrated (Jastreboff & Sasaki, 1986; Chen & Jastreboff, 1995; Manabe et al., 1997). In order to reconcile this with the commonly found reduced spontaneous activity in the auditory nerve, Eggermont (1984) suggests that increased spontaneous activity at higher levels may result from a decreased inhibition in the type II cells of the dorsal cochlear nucleus giving rise to increased activity of the type IV output cells. Møller (1995) suggests an additional disinhibition in the inferior colliculus. This reduction could reflect diminished GABA activity (Brummett, 1995; Møller, 1995; Salvi et al., 1996a,b) that is partially restored by application of benzodiazepines or baclofen, which often depress tinnitus (Table 4-7; Brummett, 1995; Szczepaniak & Møller, 1995). Thus, decreased spontaneous activity in the auditory nerve appears to be compatible with increased spontaneous activity in the inferior colliculus.

Møller et al. (1992b) proposed that tinnitus might be a special manifestation of increased spontaneous activity in the extralemniscal pathways because of interaction effects between the perception of tinnitus and somatosensory stimuli. In particular, the dorsal cochlear nucleus and external nucleus of the inferior colliculus receive substantial somatosensory input. Chen and

Table 4-7. Action of some potential tinnitus suppressing drugs

Drug	Na+ channels	K+ channels	Cl− channels	Ca²⁺ channels
Lidocaine	use dependent block in central nervous system			
Benzodiazepine			modulates GABA_A release	
Baclofen		GABA_B agonist, prolongs after-hyperpolarization		
Nimodipine		blocks voltage-dependent currents in outer hair cells		blocks L-channels in hair cells and in neurons

Jastreboff (1995) and Manabe et al. (1997) have demonstrated increased spontaneous activity in the external nucleus of the inferior colliculus which is the proposed branching off point of the extralemniscal pathway. If this is the case, then a more likely cortical area for the detection of changes in spontaneous activity is the secondary auditory cortex which receives a strong direct input from the extralamniscal pathway. Recently, Eggermont and Kenmochi (1997) demonstrated that increased spontaneous activity was indeed present in the secondary auditory cortex, but not in the primary auditory cortex and anterior auditory field, after salicylate and quinine application.

The extralemniscal pathway has also been implicated in auditory plasticity and in classical conditioning based learning, whereas the lemniscal pathway is far less sensitive (Weinberger, 1995). It may thus be that the extralemniscal pathway is selectively involved in transient changes produced by noise trauma or the application of ototoxic drugs. The lemniscal pathway reacts transiently by a reduction of activity to changes in auditory nerve spontaneous activity. However, in addition a vast reorganization in the tonotopic maps in the central nucleus of the inferior colliculus and primary auditory cortex slowly occurs as a result of changes in the spatial activity pattern across the auditory nerve.

Temporal Structure of Spike Trains

Theory: Tinnitus Results from Increased Burst-firing

One of the effects of low level sound stimulation is that the temporal properties of spike trains are changed. Neurons may start firing in phase-locked fashion to the stimulus and the percentage of spikes in bursts increases. Thus, a complete reorganization of the temporal structure of the spike trains results. It is conceivable that tinnitus is caused by a pathological reorganization of spontaneous firing patterns resembling that

found during sound stimulation. Normal spontaneous activity in individual high-spontaneous auditory-nerve fibers can be described as resulting from a Poisson process, that is, the firings are independent and the interspike intervals have an exponential probability distribution. Because low-level sound stimulation alters these properties, Eggermont (1984) suggested that changes in the temporal structure of spike trains, likely resulting in increased interneural synchronization, are sufficient to produce auditory sensations.

Increased extracellular calcium concentrations produce calcium spikes in saccular hair cells (Hudspeth & Corey, 1977). This in turn may produce enhanced transmitter release from these hair cells and may give rise to burst-firing in auditory nerve fibers (Eggermont, 1990).

Burst-firing in the central nervous system has commonly been attributed to activation of NMDA-type glutamate receptors (Sherman, 1996). Pujol (1992) reports the presence of NMDA as well as non-NMDA glutamate receptors on Type I afferent fibers (that innervate the inner hair cells) in the auditory nerve. Normally, these NMDA receptors are only affected by high intensity sound, but abnormal activity of NMDA receptors may result in spontaneous epileptic-like spike bursts. This was proposed as a likely cause of tinnitus. Activation of NMDA receptors in the spinal cord also appears to be critical in the production of chronic pain (Dickenson, 1996) a condition often likened to tinnitus (Tonndorf, 1987).

Bursts of action potentials are an efficient way to ensure synaptic transmission by allowing temporal integration of the resulting postsynaptic potentials. Although burst-firing does not appear to increase the amount of information transmitted, it appears to lower the detection threshold even when the overall firing rate has decreased (Bair et al., 1994; Sherman, 1996). Bursting may in fact enhance the overall firing rate of the recipient neurons, by up to a factor 20 (Dickenson, 1996). If spontaneous bursting manifests itself throughout the auditory system, it may be one of the substrates for tinnitus.

Jeanmonod et al. (1996) postulated that the causal event of a positive symptom (such as some forms of tinnitus) is low-threshold calcium spike bursting in the medial thalamus. The bursting output converges on the reticular thalamic nucleus reinforcing its rhythmic low-threshold calcium spike-bursting pattern. The effect on the cortex of rhythmic bursting activity in reticular thalamic nucleus in general is drowsiness and a slow wave sleeplike state with 7 to 14 Hz spindles modulated by delta waves (1 to 4 Hz, in sleep) or theta waves (2 to 6 Hz, in the awake subjects). Recently, we showed that salicylate and quinine both decrease the EEG-spindle frequency and that EEG-spindle frequency accounts for more than half of the variance in the best modulation frequency (Kenmochi & Eggermont, 1997 a,b).

Evidence: The Probability of Burst-firing Increases

In most studies involving damage to the cochlea, either after noise-induced hearing loss (Liberman & Kiang, 1978), application of ototoxic drugs (Kiang, Moxon & Levine, 1970), or after the introduction of an endolymphatic hydrops (Harrison and Prijs, 1984), an increase in the number of spike pairs and short bursts over and above that expected from a Poisson process is observed in those fibers with reduced spontaneous activity. Increased burst-firing also occurs after salicylate application in the external nucleus of the inferior colliculus (Chen & Jastreboff, 1995). Whereas cortical neurons tend to burst in synchrony with EEG-spindles (Eggermont, 1992; Eggermont & Smith, 1995), the amount of bursting observed in cortex after salicylate or quinine application does not change (Ochi & Eggermont, 1996; 1997).

An apparent inconsistency arises when one considers the excess activity in the extralemniscal pathway after noise trauma or salicylate and quinine application. This pathway converges on the dorsal region of the specific thalamus and should largely offset the reduced input to the medial thalamus from the lemniscal pathway which supposedly causes rhythmic bursting. One possible explanation may be that the long-standing tinnitus due to bursting activity in the medial thalamus has a different origin than that following acute hearing loss.

Synchrony of Firing

Theory: Tinnitus Results from a Pathological Synchronization of Neural Activity

Møller (1984) proposed pathological neural synchrony, thought to result from disruptions in the myelin sheath of auditory nerve fibers, to explain tinnitus in acoustic neuroma patients. At the same time, Eggermont (1984) introduced interneural synchronization as a more general phenomenon underlying any sound sensation, stimulus-induced or pathological, as follows:

> This [reorganization of firings] actually means that there are instantaneous rate changes in the individual nerve fiber firing patterns, but above all it means that activity patterns of small groups of nerve fibers become synchronized. This is a cooperative effect and it is now postulated that such cooperative effects in the central nervous system or auditory periphery may give rise to spontaneous sensations of sound, to tinnitus.

This idea was specifically elaborated to include both the myelin disruption mechanism and a mechanism for the induction of synchrony among the twenty or so nerve fibers innervating the same hair cell (Eggermont, 1990). The proposal was based on the observed calcium spikes in saccular hair cells for increased extracellular calcium concentrations. Detailed modeling showed that increased calcium concentration in the inner hair cells could produce temporal changes in individual neuron spike trains as well as synchrony between the firings of neighboring nerve fibers.

The effect of increased interneuronal synchrony is generally to provide a more efficient excitation of cells, especially at the cortical level. About 30 coincident inputs suffice to fire a cortical pyramidal cell in contrast to the 300 needed when their firings are random (Abeles, 1991). Besides that, synchronized firings between distant auditory cortex neurons appear to code the presence of sound in the absence of any change in firing rate (deCharms & Merzenich, 1996; Eggermont, 1997) and provide a greater salience for sounds in the presence of background noise as well as more selectivity in the coding of sound in inferior colliculus (Epping & Eggermont, 1987; Eggermont & Epping, 1987).

Evidence: Increased Synchronization of Firings Found in Cortex

Experimental findings relevant for the neural synchrony model of tinnitus were reported by Schreiner & Snyder (1987) and Martin et al. (1993), who recorded ensemble activity from the surface of the exposed cat cochlear nerve, and from the exposed auditory nerve in human subjects during intraoperative monitoring (Martin, 1995). After salicylate application, the normally present 1 kHz peak in spectrum of the spontaneous activity disappears and a clear peak emerges around 200 Hz. This was interpreted as a sign of changed synchronized rhythmic ensemble activity (Lenarz et al., 1995). Cazals and Huang (1996) also found a strong 1 kHz peak in the average activity spectrum recorded from the round window or from the auditory nerve surface of guinea pigs, which was decreased by contralateral masking. They suggest that "some kind of synchrony on a short time basis, of about 1 ms, should exist among a group of fibers innervating a limited cochlear area centered around 16 kHz." In this reviewer's opinion, the emerging 200 Hz peak could also represent the increased appearance of neural components with a typical duration of 5 ms such as calcium-spikes accompanied by

stereotypical fast-spike bursts of that duration. Because periodic 200 Hz activity, nor periodic 1,000 Hz activity, has never been observed in individual auditory nerve fibers, it is difficult to account for synchronized activity with that signature. Lenarz et al. (1996) recently stated that this 200 Hz component does not originate in the auditory nerve.

Increased interneuronal synchrony has in fact been established in the primary auditory cortex of the cat after application of both sodium salicylate and quinine hydrochloride (Ochi & Eggermont, 1996; 1997), drugs that induce tinnitus in humans and presumably in rats (Jastreboff, 1990). It is not clear if this increased synchrony in cortex is the result of an upward propagated synchrony from the level of the auditory nerve or if it reflects an additional central effect of these drugs.

Activity Patterns Across Characteristic Frequency

Theory: Tinnitus Results from Hypersensitivity and Reorganization

After finding decreased behavioral thresholds and reduced temporal integration for electrical stimulation in cochlear nucleus or inferior colliculus (Gerken et al., 1984; 1991) after noise trauma, lateral inhibition (or rather absence thereof) models generating profound edge effects in evoked activity in the inferior colliculus have been proposed as the cause of tinnitus (Gerken, 1996 a,b; Kral & Majernik, 1996).

Salvi et al. (1996a) suggest in their "tuned-cluster" model of tinnitus that

> large clusters of cortical neurons tuned to a narrow frequency range could give rise to phantom auditory sensations, particularly if the neural activity in these clusters were to become synchronized, as often happens in cases of epilepsy. This type of population coding does not require an increase in discharge rate of individual neurons.

Harrison et al. (1996) suggest that this overrepresentation could also be the basis for increased susceptibility to audiogenic seizures. It is feasible that the large isofrequency representations that develop in the central nucleus of the inferior colliculus consist of a population of neurons of similar response properties that could fire synchronously to optimal seizure-inducing sound frequencies. This exaggerated response to sound, which could be more important in determining loudness recruitment than peripheral changes, might further trigger additional neural activity, leading to seizure-like motor responses or, more likely, tinnitus.

The pitch of tinnitus resulting from noise trauma is frequently similar to the characteristic frequencies on the edge of the damaged area. Meikle (1995) proposed that the combination of a cortical reorganization with hypersensitivity of neurons near the edge of the damaged area provides the substrate for tinnitus (see also Chapter 6). It may also alter the severity of tinnitus by modulating the sympathetic nervous system, which may affect the hypersensitivity of partially deafferented neurons. Involvement of nonauditory nuclei in "affect" regions of the brain in the percept of tinnitus has also been suggested by the c-fos studies of Wallhäusser-Franke (1997) and positron emission tomography scans in humans by Lockwood et al. (1998).

Evidence: Cortical Reorganization Occurs After Trauma

Restricted high-frequency cochlear damage results in a profound reorganization of the auditory cortex. Cortical neurons that had characteristic frequencies corresponding to those in the damaged parts of the cochlea show a characteristic frequency equal to the edge-frequency of the damaged area (Harrison et al., 1991; 1996; Rajan et al., 1993; Robertson & Irvine, 1989). This has two implications. First, there is an excess of cortical cells representing a very restricted area of the cochlea. Second, the spontaneous

and stimulated activity of those cells is likely more synchronized than it was before the damage.

Increased incidence of tinnitus with age may also be the result of changes in neural organization (Willott, 1996).

Tinnitus in Neural Space and Time

Peripheral Versus Central Tinnitus

Spontaneous local field potential spindle frequencies in cat primary auditory cortex estimated from the local field potential trigger autocorrelogram before and after application of sodium salicylate and quinine sulfate decrease significantly (from 8.7 Hz to 7.6 Hz). The best modulation frequencies for 251 single units recorded in primary auditory cortex in response to periodic click train stimulation also decreased (from 10 Hz to 8.6 Hz) after application of these tinnitus-inducing drugs. The results strongly suggest a central effect of salicylates and quinine in addition to their peripheral ototoxic effects (Kenmochi & Eggermont, 1997). The single-unit recordings from the medial thalamus by Jeanmonod et al. (1996), in patients with positive symptom tinnitus, suggest a change in the firing patterns of the medial thalamus resulting from reduced specific afferent input. The gradual reorganization of the central nervous system after peripheral lesions also suggests that the distinction of peripheral versus central tinnitus is likely not very relevant.

Transient Versus Long-standing Tinnitus

The mechanisms that cause transient and long-standing tinnitus may be quite different. Consider the action of loud music provided by a local rock group. This may induce in the admiring audience a temporary threshold shift accompanied by transient tinnitus or in more sensitive persons a permanent high-frequency hearing loss and also permanent tinnitus. In the latter case, a complete reorganization of the auditory cortex will slowly occur so that the long-lasting tinnitus effects may be related to an overrepresentation of the audiometric edge-frequencies. In the first case, such reorganization has not yet occurred, but increased firing rates in dorsal cochlear nucleus, external nucleus of the inferior colliculus and secondary auditory cortex, combined with increased synchronization of firings within individual cortical areas may be related to the tinnitus sensation. These changes could be brought about by any combination of reduced off-characteristic frequency inhibition, synaptic potentiation or involvement of NMDA glutamate receptors, and enhancement of spontaneous or weak activity by increased release of neuromodulators, likely through involvement of the "affect" systems of the brain including the amygdala. The latter is directly innervated by the magnocellular part of the medial geniculate body which is part of the extralemniscal pathway (Weinberger, 1995).

WHERE IN THE BRAIN IS TINNITUS?

There are many correlates of tinnitus, from the molecular level to the systems level. Because tinnitus is a perceptual phenomenon (Jastreboff & Hazell, 1993; Levine, 1994), the path to understanding it has to proceed from the top down. We will follow this path (Table 4-6) as we recapitulate experimental findings with reflection to the levels of description of the central nervous system (Churchland & Sejnowski, 1992).

Systems Level

The auditory system is a massively parallel system although it is presently not clear what sound features each of the many possible paths processes. The most peripheral sign of parallel processing is in the multi-fold innervation of the inner-hair cells by a set of auditory nerve fibers with different sensitivities. This allows stimulus levels to be coded locally in an activity pattern

across the twenty or so fibers innervating a single inner hair cell. In addition, stimulus levels are coded globally across an array of inner hair cells. The second level of parallelism is found at the cochlear nucleus where each auditory nerve fiber trifurcates to project tonotopically to each of the three cochlear nucleus divisions. Activity from the anterioventral cochlear nucleus passes through the medial and lateral superior olivary complex nuclei where comparisons are made with activity from the contra-lateral ear for the purpose of sound localization. Activity from the posterioventral cochlear nucleus and dorsal cochlear nucleus also feed directly into the inferior colliculus together with directional information from the superior olivary complex. Within each of these brain stem nuclei there are also different cell types that likely have different roles in extracting, integrating, and passing information to the auditory midbrain.

The inferior colliculus is the nexus between the lower auditory system and the thalamocortical system and is also considered the branching point for the lemniscal and extralemniscal pathways to the cortex. The lemniscal pathway is defined as strictly auditory, narrowly tuned to frequency, starting in the ventral cochlear nucleus and projecting in strict topographic fashion to the primary auditory cortex and the anterior auditory field. The extralemniscal pathway is more broadly tuned, more diffusely organized and is considered more plastic and context dependent (Weinberger & Diamond, 1987), and also receives input from the somatosensory system. Given these properties, the extralemniscal pathway could well be extended to include the dorsal cochlear nucleus. While the dorsal cochlear nucleus is characterized by sharp tuning and strict tonotopic organization (Young et al., 1992), it also has a demonstrated sensitivity to somatosensory stimuli (Young et al., 1995). The somatosensory input to the dorsal cochlear nucleus occurs through the granule cell horizontal fiber system that runs perpendicular to the isofrequency sheets and likely provides information about pinna position, which is integrated with information about auditory sound localization cues. Thus, in this tentative model the branching point between lemniscal and extralemniscal pathways could be in the lower brain stem, specifically in the cochlear nucleus. The two lemniscal sections of the medial geniculate body feed dominantly into primary auditory cortex and anterior auditory field respectively, whereas the extralemniscal sections project to layers III/IV of secondary auditory cortex areas and also diffusely to layer I of all cortical areas.

The auditory system is also a reentrant system characterized by multiple, loosely interconnected, regional feedback loops (Spangler & Warr, 1991). At the lowest level, a loop between cochlea and the superior olivary complex exists, this comprises the olivocochlear bundle. A second loop is found between the lower brain stem nuclei and the inferior colliculus. A third loop is formed between the inferior colliculus and the thalamocortical system which, in itself, consists of a feedback loop between thalamus and cortex. More specifically, the auditory cortex projects back to the medial geniculate body with ten times as many fibers than the number of afferents from the medial geniculate body to auditory cortex. The auditory cortex also connects with the inferior colliculus, but with exclusion of the central nucleus (Winer, 1992). The central and external inferior colliculus subnuclei both project back to the dorsal cochlear nucleus. The dorsal cochlear nucleus in turn feeds back to the ventral cochlear nuclei. The olivocochlear bundle projects to both outer hair cells (medial olivocochlear neurons), thus regulating both the slow motility of the outer hair cells and thus the stiffness of the basilar membrane, and (lateral olivocochlear neurons) to especially low spontaneously active auditory nerve fibers synapsing with the inner hair cells (Spangler & Warr, 1991). It seems that the strongest contiguous projections from cortex to the periphery involve the nuclei of the extra-

lemniscal pathway, including the dorsal cochlear nucleus.

Thus, as recognized before (Jastreboff & Hazell, 1993; Feldman, 1995), the whole brain must somehow be involved in the sensation of tinnitus, specifically through the closed loop type interaction between the periphery and the CNS, potentially amplified by the action of the sympathetic nervous system (Hallam et al., 1984; Meikle, 1995). Permanent changes in cortical organization will alter the descending activity from the auditory cortex to the periphery (Zhang et al., 1997), especially through the components of the extralemniscal pathway in the thalamus and midbrain to the dorsal cochlear nucleus.

Network Level

Several spatially restricted neural networks can be identified that are potentially involved in tinnitus. These are: (1) the auditory cortex and, to a lesser extent, the inferior colliculus as the main loci of reorganization following peripheral hearing loss, and (2) the extralemniscal system that seems to be a network within the auditory system where peripheral lesions transiently result in increased spontaneous firing rates and hypersensitivity.

A neural network implicated in certain forms of tinnitus, and in the case of neurogenic pain, is the thalamocortical spindle loop (Jeanmonod et al., 1996). When hyperpolarized by permanent or temporary reduction of sensory activity to the specific thalamus, this loop goes into a rhythmic burst-firing mode. This mode forms the natural correlate of drowsiness or initial stages of slow-wave sleep. It has been observed that in positive-symptom patients, including subjects suffering from tinnitus, single units in the medial thalamus showed excessive rhythmic burst-firing. A cortical correlate of this burst-firing mode of the thalamus is pronounced spindling activity. Application of salicylate or quinine lowers the "natural" EEG-spindle frequency present under light ketamine anesthesia. This suggests a potential involvement of these tinnitus-inducing drugs with the thalamo-cortical spindle system. Tinnitus has also been likened to pain (Tonndorf, 1987; Møller, 1996), and some forms of neurogenic pain appear to fit the same physiological substrate of thalamic bursting, thus the pain hypothesis may be covered under this framework. The known involvement of the NMDA glutamate receptor in chronic pain and the link of NMDA activation with burst-firing is one extra aspect of a similarity between different pain states (Dickenson, 1996) and various forms of tinnitus.

As hypothesized by Meikle (1995), the sympathetic nervous system may be involved in modulating the amount of hypersensitivity of partially denervated neurons. Thus, other networks besides specific sensory ones may be involved in tinnitus. The definition of "pain as an unpleasant sensory and emotional experience associated with actual or potential tissue damage, or described in terms of such damage" (Merskey, 1979) may apply to tinnitus as well. Recent positron emission tomography (Lockwood et al., 1998) and c-fos studies (Walhaüsser-Franke, 1997) point to involvement of the anxiety areas of the brain in tinnitus. Because c-fos is expressed by novel stimuli, and not by stress (Hillman et al., 1997), the induction of tinnitus or other sensations by salicylate may be sufficiently different from that of an external sound to activate these anxiety areas. The involvement of this network offers a plausible explanation for the effect of stress on the severity of tinnitus (through the sympathetic system) as well as the fact that tinnitus may cause anxiety.

We have already discussed the dominant involvement of the extralemniscal system in tinnitus: it may be the only part of the auditory system that responds to tinnitus-inducing agents by increasing spontaneous firing rates. Møller et al. (1993) suggests its potential involvement based on studies showing that tactile stimuli can interfere with the sensation of tinnitus. One of the main characteristics of the extralemniscal system is its bimodality; most of its neurons are sensitive to both somatosensory and auditory stimuli. In bimodally sensitive neurons, stimulation with both sensory modalities simultaneously often shows enhanced responses that far exceed the sum of the response to each modality alone (Stein & Meredith, 1993). Our finding that the driven response rate is also enhanced in AII after salicylate or quinine suggests potentially that these neurons respond as if a bimodal stimulus was present. This idea is corroborated by findings of Møller et al. (1992) who showed that in about half of twenty-six tinnitus patients stimulation of the median nerve increased the tinnitus noticeably, whereas in the other half no noticeable change was noted.

Neuron Level

Some neurons in parts of the extralemniscal system such as dorsal cochlear nucleus, external nucleus of the inferior colliculus and secondary auditory cortex, increase their spontaneous firing rates in response to tinnitus-causing agents. This altered spontaneous firing is invariably accompanied by changes in temporal response properties that result in bursting. Rhythmic bursting in thalamic geniculate relay cells is generally considered to be the hallmark of slow-wave sleep, whereas random bursting occurs when the subject is awake but not paying attention (Sherman, 1996). Bursting in visual cortex has been related to the presence of local field potential activity in the 20 to 60 Hz band (Bair et al., 1994) which usually signals an attentive state, and is considered to be an intrinsic cell property because of the independence of burst length and stimulus level. A link to learning is present through the ability of these cells to accumulate calcium at their presynaptic terminals during a burst; this is thought to be responsible for various forms of synaptic facilitation and augmentation. Bursting may greatly increase detectability at low signal levels (Eggermont & Smith, 1996), at the expense of detailed timing information.

Disinhibition in the external nucleus of the inferior colliculus has been credited as the major cause of prolonged burst-firing (Chen & Jastreboff, 1995). In order to show disinhibition, the neurons in the external nucleus of the inferior colliculus should have inhibitory input similar to that of the principal cells (fusiform and giant cells) in the dorsal cochlear nucleus which receive such input from the vertical interneurons (Young et al., 1992). Candidate neurons in the central nucleus of the inferior colliculus and external nucleus of the inferior colliculus must abound, since the nucleus shows high GABA levels resulting from both intrinsic and extrinsic (dorsal nucleus of the lateral lemniscus) inhibitory neurons (Faingold et al., 1991). It could also be that a reduced postactivation suppression, resulting from an interference with the strength and duration of the after-hyperpolarization mediated by a calcium-activated potassium current, is the main factor in determining the strength of bursting. During stimulation with short tone bursts, spike-burst length in primary auditory cortex is longest at stimulus levels just above threshold, and the number of spikes in a burst decreased for higher stimulus levels (Eggermont & Smith, 1996). Prolonged burst-firing could thus be the result of a reduction in the calcium-activated potassium current which could occur for a decrease in intracellular calcium. Recent evidence from the dentate gyrus (Pan & Stringer, 1997) suggests that both an increased extracellular potassium concentration and a decreased extracellular calcium concentration have to be present, both within rather narrow limits to induce bursting. In behavioral studies, dietary calcium supplements appear to eliminate or reduce the response to salicylate and quinine. This could be understood as a result of alleviating decreased calcium levels. On the other hand, L-type calcium channel blockers also reduce the suppressed licking response, likely by reducing the spontaneous activity in auditory nerve fibers. It is interesting to note that both salicylate and quinine appear to increase intracellular calcium, albeit that this obviously does not fit into the theory of tinnitus resulting from excessive "burst-firing."

Synapse Level

The intracellular free calcium concentration combined with the L-type calcium channel conductance determines the amount of transmitter release from the inner hair cells and afferent neurons in the auditory system. A lack of excitatory input to the dorsal cochlear nucleus and inferior colliculus appears to reduce the activation of $GABA_A$ receptors resulting in hyperactivity and hypersensitivity. Systemic application of the GABA-agonists, benzodiazepines and baclofen, appears to reverse this. Activation of $GABA_A$ receptors results in conformational changes in the receptor, thereby allowing the conduction of Cl^- across the membrane and resulting in fast inhibitory postsynaptic potentials, the inhibitory counterpart of rapid excitatory postsynaptic potentials in cortex. The intricate balance between these two postsynaptic potentials is required for normal cortical activity, reduction of $GABA_A$-receptor mediated inhibition may result in out of bound excitation of the cortical network. Activation of $GABA_B$ receptors (for example, by baclofen) results in a slower inhibitory postsynaptic potentials through the activation of a slower K^+ conductances mediated by G-proteins (McCormick et al., 1993). In cortex, inhibition and excitation are usually well-balanced; the sources are manifold and under control of the thalamus. Any change in the polarization level of cortical pyramidal cells as a result of changes in neuromodulator activity by serotonin, dopamine, or acetylcholine transmitting neurons causes pronounced alterations in spontaneous firing rates and in the temporal structure of the firings (McCormick et al., 1993). For instance the depolarization of cortical layer V burst-firing neurons through application of acetylcholine results in a switch of firing mode from rhythmic bursting to single-spike activity. This occurs because of a reduction of at least four specialized K^+ currents. Quinine, one of the common tinnitus-inducing drugs exerts a blocking action on these K^+ channels, and might potentially produce the same effect. This again could link burst-firing to tinnitus.

Molecular Level

Membrane-ion channels are crucial for living cells in allowing ions to pass from the outside to the inside of the cell and vice versa. Ion channels can be gated by voltage gradients across the membrane, by ligands such as neurotransmitters and, indirectly, by metabotropic channels that use calcium ions as second messengers. The activation of the second messenger system is mediated by specialized G-proteins that may also directly modulate calcium channel conductivity. Thus, calcium is an important determinant of channel conductance. Calcium-activated potassium channels open in response to an increase in cytoplasmic calcium concentration as well as to membrane depolarization. L-type calcium channels are voltage-gated. These channels are found, for instance, at the base of the hair cells and are involved in spontaneous and stimulated transmitter release and indirectly affect outer hair cell motility. Salicylates and quinine increase the L-type channel conductance. The blocking action of Nimodipine combined with its apparent relief of quinine-induced tinnitus in rats (Jastreboff et al., 1991) suggests that these calcium channels may be involved in spontaneous activity changes that cause tinnitus. Blocking L-type channels likely eliminates or reduces spontaneous transmitter release across the hair cell array. The effect would be larger on healthy inner hair cells than on damaged ones, thereby reducing the spontaneous activity gradient in the auditory nerve. This could lead to a smaller edge-effect and less differential activation of higher order nuclei. Caution has to be expressed because Nimodipine in concentrations larger than 1µM also inhibits potassium currents in outer hair cells (Lin et al., 1995).

The specialized potassium channels that are activated by $GABA_B$ receptors play a role in postactivation suppression. The resulting hyperpolarization may be deep enough to activate the low-threshold calcium currents that give rise to rebound bursting activity. We have demonstrated (Ochi & Eggermont, 1996) that salicylate increases this time to rebound, suggesting an involvement with the duration of the postactivation suppression and thus with at least one of the potassium currents.

SUMMARY: A NATURAL HISTORY OF TINNITUS

A perceived sound that cannot be attributed to an external source is called tinnitus. The initiator is likely a prolonged discontinuity in the spatial activity pattern across fibers in the auditory nerve, caused by functional loss of outer hair cells in those regions where inner hair cells are preserved. This may result in a reduction of inhibition at more central levels that induces hypersensitivity and hyperactivity specifically in auditory nuclei that are part of the extralemniscal pathway. This multimodal pathway comprises the dorsal cochlear nucleus, the external nucleus of the inferior colliculus, the magnocellular nucleus of the medial geniculate body and the secondary auditory cortex. The neural activity in the parallel, strictly auditory and tonotopically organized, lemniscal pathway is typically reduced but exhibits increased neuronal synchrony thus mimicking one aspect of normal sound stimulation. Persisting changes in the normal cochlear output pattern across characteristic frequency result in a slow reorganization of the lemniscal cortical areas with increased numbers of neurons tuned to a limited range of frequencies at the edge of the cochlear lesion. These edge-frequency neurons are likely to exhibit enhanced synchrony in their firings and, by their sheer number, enhanced sensitivity to peripheral activity changes. The involvement of affect centers of the brain could plausibly account for the often high emotional state of many individuals affected by tinnitus.

ACKNOWLEDGMENTS

Research supported by the Alberta Heritage Foundation for Medical Research, the Natural Sciences and Engineering Research Council of Canada, the Campbell McLaurin Foundation and the American Tinnitus Association. Manny Don commented and Curtis Ponton provided detailed critical and editorial feedback upon several previous versions of this manuscript.

REFERENCES

Abeles, M. (1991). *Corticonics. Neural circuits of the cerebral cortex.* Cambridge: Cambridge University Press.

Aran, J. M. (1981). Electrical stimulation of the auditory system and tinnitus control. *British Journal Laryngol. Otol. 95*(Suppl 4), 153–162.

Aran, J. M., & Cazals, Y. (1981). Electrical suppression of tinnitus. In *Tinnitus, Ciba Foundation Symposium, 85* (pp. 217–231).

Attias, J., Bresloff, I., & Furman, V. (1996). The influence of the efferent auditory system on otoacoustic emissions in noise induced tinnitus: clinical relevance. *Acta Otolaryngologica (Stockholm) 116*, 534–539.

Attwell, D., Bergman, C., & Ojeda, C. (1979). The action of salicylate ions on the frog node of Ranvier. *Journal of Physiology 175*, 69–81.

Bair, W., Koch, C., Newsome, W., & Britten, K. (1994) Power spectrum analysis of bursting cells in area MT in the behaving monkey. *Journal of Neuroscience 14*, 2870–2892.

Berridge, M. J. (1997). Elementary and global aspects of calcium signalling. *Journal of Physiology 499.2*, 291–306.

Blaustein, M. P. (1988). Cellular calcium: nervous system. In B. E. C. Nordin (Ed.), *Calcium in human biology* (pp. 339–366). London: Springer Verlag.

Bobbin, R. P., Fallon, M., & Kujawa, S. G. (1991). Magnitude of the negative summating potential varies with perilymph calcium levels. *Hearing Research 56*, 101–110.

Bobbin, R. P., Jastreboff, P. J., Fallon, M., & Littman, T. (1990). Nimodipine, an L-channel Ca^{2+} antagonist, reverses the negative summating potential recorded from the guinea pig cochlea. *Hearing Research, 46*, 277–288.

Brummett, R. E. (1995). A mechanism for tinnitus? In J. E. Vernon & A. R. Møller (Eds.) *Mechanisms of Tinnitus* (pp. 7–10). Boston: Allyn & Bacon.

Burns, E. M., & Keefe, D. H. (1992). Intermittent tinnitus resulting from unstable otoacoustic emissions. In J. M. Aran & R. Dauman (Eds.), *Tinnitus 91* (pp. 89–94). Amsterdam: Kugler Publications.

Cacace, A. T., Cousins, J. P., Moonen, C. T. W., van Gelderen, P., Miller, D., Parnes, S. M., & Lovely, T. J. (1996). In-vivo localization of phantom auditory perceptions during functional magnetic resonance imaging of the human brain. In G. E. Reich & J. E. Vernon (Eds.), *Proceedings of the Fifth International Tinnitus Seminar 1995* (pp. 397–401). Portland, OR: American Tinnitus Association.

Cazals, Y., & Huang, Z. W. (1996). Average spectrum of cochlear activity: A possible synchronized firing, its olivocochlear feedback and alterations under anesthesia. *Hearing Research, 101*, 81–92.

Cazals, Y., Negrevergne, M., & Aran, J. M. (1978). Electrical stimulation of the cochlea in man: Hearing induction and tinnitus suppression. *Journal of American Audiological Society, 3*, 209–213.

Chen, G., & Jastreboff, P. J. (1995). Salicylate-induced abnormal activity in the inferior colliculus of rats. *Hearing Research, 82*, 158–178.

Churchland, P. S., & Sejnowski, T. J. (1992). *The computational brain.* Cambridge, MA: The MIT Press.

Dallos, P., & Harris, D. (1978). Properties of auditory nerve responses in absence of outer hair cells. *Journal of Neurophysiology, 41*, 365–383.

deCharms, R. C., & Merzenich, M. M. (1996). Primary cortical representation of sounds by the coordination of action-potential timing. *Nature 381*, 610–613.

Dickenson, A. H. (1996). Balances between excitatory and inhibitory events in the spinal cord and chronic pain. *Progress in Brain Research 110*, 225–231.

Dickson, J. W. and Gerstein, G. L. (1974). Interaction between neurons in auditory cortex of the cat. *Journal of Neurophysiology, 37*, 1239–1261.

Didier, A., Miller, J. M., & Nuttall, A. L. (1993). The vascular component of sodium salicylate ototoxicity in the guinea pig. *Hearing Research, 69*, 199–206.

Dietzel, I., & Heinemann, U. (1986). Dynamic variations of the brain cell micro-environment in relation to neuronal hyperactivity. *Ann. N.Y. Acad. Sci. 481*, 72–83.

Durand, D. (1986). Electrical stimulation can inhibit synchronized neuronal activity. *Brain Research, 382*, 139–144.

Eggermont, J. J. (1984). Tinnitus: Some thought about its origin. *Journal of Laryngology and Otology* (Suppl. 9), 31–37.

Eggermont, J. J. (1985). Peripheral auditory adaptation and fatigue: A model oriented review. *Hearing Research, 18*, 57–71.

Eggermont, J. J. (1990). On the pathophysiology of tinnitus: A review and a peripheral model. *Hearing Research, 48*, 111–124.

Eggermont, J. J. (1991). Rate and synchrony measures of periodicity coding in cat primary auditory cortex. *Hearing Research, 56*, 153–167.

Eggermont, J. J. (1992). Salicyl-induced changes in the spontaneous activity. In J. M. Aran & R. Dauman (Eds.), *Tinnitus, 91* (pp. 293–298). Amsterdam: Kugler Publications.

Eggermont, J. J. (1992a). Neural interaction in cat primary auditory cortex. Dependence on recording depth, electrode separation and age. *Journal of Neurophysiology, 68*, 1216–1228.

Eggermont, J. J. (1992b). Stimulus induced and spontaneous rhythmic firing of single units in cat primary auditory cortex. *Hearing Research, 61*, 1–11.

Eggermont, J. J. (1997). Firing rate and firing synchrony distinguish dynamic from steady state sound. *NeuroReport, 8*, 2709–2713.

Eggermont, J. J., & Epping, W. J. M. (1987). Coincidence detection in auditory neurons: A possible mechanism to enhance stimulus specificity in the grassfrog. *Hearing Research, 30*, 219–230.

Eggermont, J. J., Johannesma, P. I. M., & Aertsen, A. M. H. J. (1983). Reverse correlation methods in auditory research. *Quarterly Review of Biophysics, 16*, 341–414.

Eggermont, J. J., & Kenmochi, M. (1998). Salicylate and quinine selectively enhance spontaneous firing rates in secondary auditory cortex. *Hearing Research, 117*, 149–160.

Eggermont, J. J., & Ochi, K. (1996). The effect of salicylate and quinine on temporal coding in cat auditory cortex. In G. E. Reich & J. E. Vernon (Eds.), *Proceedings of the Fifth International Tinnitus Seminar 1995* (pp. 402–403). Portland, OR: American Tinnitus Association.

Eggermont, J. J., & Sininger, Y. (1995). Correlated neural activity and tinnitus. In J. E. Vernon & A. R. Møller (Eds.), *Mechanisms of Tinnitus* (pp. 21–34). Boston: Allyn & Bacon.

Eggermont, J. J., & Smith, G. M. (1996). Burst-firing sharpens frequency-tuning in primary auditory cortex. *NeuroReport, 7*, 753–757.

Eggermont, J. J., Smith, G. M., & Bowman, D. (1993). Spontaneous burst-firing in cat primary auditory cortex. Age and depth dependence and its effect on neural interaction measures. *Journal of Neurophysiology, 69*, 1292–1313.

Epping, W. J. M., & Eggermont, J. J. (1987). Coherent neural activity in the auditory midbrain of the grassfrog. *Journal of Neurophysiology, 57*, 1464–1483.

Evans, E. F., & Borerwe, T. A. (1982). Ototoxic effects of salicylates on the responses of single cochlear nerve fibres and on cochlear potentials. *British Journal of Audiology, 16*, 101–108.

Evans, E. F., Wilson, J. P., & Borerwe, T. A. (1981). Animal models of tinnitus. In *Tinnitus, Ciba Foundation Symposium 85* (pp. 108–138).

Faingold, C. L., Gehlbach, G., & Caspary, D. M. (1991). Functional pharmacology of inferior colliculus neurons. In R. A. Altschuler, R. P. Bobbin, B. M. Clopton, & D. W. Hoffman (Eds.), *Neurobiology of hearing: The central auditory system* (pp. 223–251). New York: Raven Press.

Feldman, H. (1995). Mechanisms of tinnitus. In J. E. Vernon & A. R. Møller (Eds.), *Mechanisms of Tinnitus* (pp. 35–49). Boston: Allyn & Bacon.

Fridberger, A., & Ulfendahl, M. (1996). Acute mechanical overstimulation of isolated outer hair cells causes changes in intracellular calcium levels without shape changes. *Acta Otolaryngologica (Stockholm), 116*, 17–24.

Friedman, A., & Gutnick, M. J. (1989). Intracellular Calcium and control of burst generation in neurons of guinea-pig neocortex in vitro. *European Journal of Neuroscience, 1*, 374–381.

Gerken, G. M. (1996a). Central tinnitus and lateral inhibition: An auditory brainstem model. *Hearing Research, 97*, 75–83.

Gerken, G. M. (1996b). Central auditory mechanisms and the generation of tinnitus. In G. E. Reich & J. E. Vernon (Eds.), *Proceedings of the Fifth International Tinnitus Seminar 1995* (pp. 410–417). Portland, OR: American Tinnitus Association.

Gerken, G. M., Saunders, S. S., & Paul, R. E. (1984). Hypersensitivity to electrical stimulation of auditory nuclei follows hearing loss in cats. *Hearing Research, 13,* 249–259.

Gerken, G. M., Solecki, J. M., & Boettcher, F. A. (1991). Temporal integration of electrical stimulation of auditory nuclei in normal-hearing and hearing-impaired cat. *Hearing Research, 53,* 101–112.

Goldberg, J. M., Adrian, H. O., & Smith, F. D. (1964). Response of neurons of the superior olivary complex of the cat to acoustic stimuli of long duration. *Journal of Neurophysiology, 27,* 706–749.

Goldstein, M. H., Hall, J. L., & Butterfield, B. O. (1967). Single unit activity in the primary auditory cortex of unanesthetized cats. *Journal of Acoustical Society of America, 43,* 444–455.

Graham, R. L., Jastreboff, P. J., & Hazell, J. W. P. (1996). Contralateral suppression of transient evoked otoacoustic emissions: Is there a tinnitus effect?. In G. E. Reich & J. E. Vernon (Eds.), *Proceedings of the Fifth International Tinnitus Seminar 1995* (pp. 418–419). Portland, OR: American Tinnitus Association.

Gray, C. M., & Singer, W. (1988). Stimulus-specific neuronal oscillations in orientation columns of cat visual cortex. *Proc. Natl. Acad. Sci. USA, 86,* 1698–1702.

Guth, P. S., Aubert, A., Ricci, A. J., & Norris, C. H. (1991). Differential modulation of spontaneous and evoked neurotransmitter release from hair cells: Some novel hypotheses. *Hearing Research, 56,* 69–78.

Hallam, R. S., Rachman, S., & Hinchcliffe, R. (1984). Psychological aspects of tinnitus. In S. Rachman (Ed.), *Contributions to Medical Psychology* (pp. 31–34). Oxford: Pergamon Press.

Harrison, R. V., Ibrahim, D., Stanton, S. G., & Mount, R. J. (1996). Reorganization of frequency maps in chinchilla auditory midbrain after long-term basal cochlear lesions induced at birth. In R. J. Salvi, D. Henderson, F. Fiorino, & V. Colletti (Eds.), *Auditory system plasticity and regeneration* (pp. 238–255). New York: Thieme Medical Publ. Inc.

Harrison, R. V., Nagasawa, A., Smith, D. W., Stanton, S., & Mount, R. J. (1991). Reorganization of auditory cortex after neonatal high frequency cochlear hearing loss. *Hearing Research, 54,* 11–19.

Harrison, R. V. & Prijs, V. F. (1984). Single cochlear fibre responses in guinea pigs with long-term endolymphatic hydrops. *Hearing Research, 14,* 79–84.

Hillman, D. E., Gordon, C. E., Troublefield, Y., Stone, E., Giacchia, R. J., & Chen, S. (1997). Effect of unilateral tympanotomy on auditory induced c-fos expression in cochlear nuclei. *Brain Research, 748,* 77–84.

Hudspeth, A. J. (1989). How the ear's works work. *Nature, 341,* 397–404.

Hudspeth, A. J., & Corey, D. P. (1977). Sensitivity, polarity and conductance change in the response of vertebrate hair cells to controlled mechanical stimuli. *Proc. Natl. Acad. Sci. USA, 74,* 2407–2411.

Ikeda, K., Kusakari, J. & Takasaka, T. (1988). Ionic changes in cochlear endolymph of the guinea pig induced by acoustic injury. *Hearing Research, 32,* 103–110.

Jastreboff, M. M., & Jastreboff, P. J. (1996a). Modification of metabolic activity in the inferior colliculus related to salicylate-induced tinnitus. In G. E. Reich & J. E. Vernon (Eds.), *Proceedings of the Fifth International Tinnitus Seminar 1995* (pp. 423–425). Portland, OR: American Tinnitus Association.

Jastreboff, M. M., & Jastreboff, P. J. (1996b). Tinnitus-related modulation of c-fos expression. In G. E. Reich & J. E. Vernon (Eds.), *Proceedings of the Fifth International Tinnitus Seminar 1995* (pp. 426–428). Portland, OR: American Tinnitus Association.

Jastreboff, P. J. (1990). Phantom auditory perception (tinnitus): Mechanism of generation and perception. *Neuroscience Research, 8,* 221–254.

Jastreboff, P. J., Brennan, J. F., & Sasaki, C. T. (1988). Phantom auditory sensation in rats: An animal model for tinnitus. *Behav. Neuroscience, 102,* 811–822.

Jastreboff, P. J., Brennan, J. F., & Sasaki, C. T. (1991). Quinine-induced tinnitus in rats. *Arch. Otolaryngol Head and Neck Surgery, 117,* 1162–1166.

Jastreboff, P. J., & Hazell, J. W. P. (1993). A neurophysiological approach to tinnitus: Clinical implications. *British Journal of Audiology, 27,* 7–17.

Jastreboff, P. J., & Sasaki, C. T. (1986). Salicylate-induced changes in spontaneous activity of single units in the inferior colliculus of the guinea pig. *Journal of Acoustical Society of America, 80,* 1384–1391.

Javel, E. (1981). Suppression of auditory nerve responses. I. Temporal analysis, intensity effects and suppression contours. *Journal of Acoustical Society of America, 69,* 1735–1745.

Javel, E., McGee, J. A., Horst, J. W., & Farley, G. R. (1988). Temporal mechanisms in auditory stimulus coding. In G. M. Edelman, W. E. Gall & W. M. Cowan (Eds.), *Auditory function. Neurobiological basis of hearing* (pp. 515–558). New York: J. Wiley.

Jeanmonod, D., Magnin, M., & Morel, A. (1996). Low-threshold calcium spike bursts in the human thalamus. Common physiopathology for sensory, motor and limbic positive symptoms. *Brain, 119*, 363–375.

Johnson, D. H., & Kiang, N. Y. S. (1976). Analysis of discharges recorded simultaneously from pairs of auditory nerve fibers. *Biophysical Journal, 16*, 719–734.

Joris, P. X., Carney, L. H., Smith, P. H., & Yin, T. C. T. (1994). Enhancement of neural synchronization in the anteroventral cochlear nucleus. I. Responses to tones at the characteristic frequency. *Journal of Neurophysiology, 71*, 1022–1036.

Joris, P. X., & Yin, T. C. T. (1992). Responses to amplitude-modulated tones in the auditory nerve of the cat. *Journal of Acoustical Society of America, 91*, 215–232.

Jung, T. T. K., Kim, J. P. S., Bumme, J., Davamony, D., Duncan, J., & Fletcher, W. H. (1997). Effect of leukotrine inhibitor on salicylate induced morphological changes of isolated cochlear outer hair cells. *Acta Otolaryngologica (Stockholm), 117*, 258–264.

Jung, T. T. K., Rhee, C. K., Lee, C. S., Park, Y. S., & Choi, D. C. (1993). Ototoxicity of salicylate, nonsteroidal anti-inflammatory drugs, and quinine. *Otolaryng Clin. North Am., 26*, 791–810.

Kakehata, S., & Santos-Sacchi, J. (1996). Effects of salicylate and Lanthanides on outer hair cell motility and associated gating charge. *Journal of Neuroscience, 16*, 4881–4889.

Kaltenbach, J. A., Godfrey, D. A., McCaslin, D. L., & Squire, A. B. (1996a). Changes in spontaneous activity and chemistry of the cochlear nucleus following intense sound exposure. In G. E. Reich & J. E. Vernon (Eds.), *Proceedings of the Fifth International Tinnitus Seminar 1995* (pp. 429–440), Portland, OR: American Tinnitus Association.

Kaltenbach, J. A., & McCaslin, D. L. (1996). Increases in spontaneous activity in the dorsal cochlear nucleus following exposure to high intensity sound: A possible neural correlate of tinnitus. *Auditory Neuroscience, 3*, 57–78.

Kaltenbach, J. A., Meleca, R. J., & Falzarano, P. R. (1996b). Alterations in the tonotopic map of the cochlear nucleus following cochlear damage. In R. J. Salvi, D. Henderson, F. Fiorino & V. Colletti (Eds.), *Auditory system plasticity and regeneration* (pp. 317–332). New York: Thieme Medical Publishers, Inc.

Kemp, D. T. (1981). Physiologically active cochlear micromechanics—one source of tinnitus. In *Tinnitus, Ciba Foundation Symposium 85* (pp. 54–81).

Kenmochi, M. & Eggermont, J. J. (1997). Salicylate and quinine affect the central nervous system. *Hearing Research, 113*, 110–116.

Kiang, N. Y. S., Liberman, M. C., & Levine, R. A. (1976). Auditory-nerve activity in cats exposed to ototoxic drugs and high intensity sounds. *Ann. Otol. Rhinol. Laryngol., 85*, 752–768.

Kiang, N. Y. S, Moxon, E. C., & Levine, R. A. (1970). Auditory-nerve activity in cats with normal and abnormal cochleas. In G. E. W. Wolstenholm & J. Knight (Eds.), *Sensorineural hearing loss* (pp. 241–276). London: J. A. Churchill.

Kiang, N. Y. S., Watanabe, T., Thomas, E. C., & Clark, L. F. (1965). *Discharge patterns of single fibers in the cat's auditory nerve.* Cambridge, MA: MIT Press.

Kitahara, M., Kitano, H., Suzuki, M., & Kitajima, K. (1995). Tinnitus and spontaneous activity in the auditory system. In J. E. Vernon & A. R. Møller (Eds.), *Mechanisms of Tinnitus* (pp. 95–100). Boston: Allyn & Bacon.

Koerber, K. C., Pfeiffer, R. R., Warr, W. B., & Kiang, N. Y. S. (1966). Spontaneous spike discharges from single units in the cochlear nucleus after destruction of the cochlea. *Exp. Neurology, 16*, 119–130.

Konishi, T., Teas, D. C., & Wernick, J. S. (1970). Effects of electrical current applied to cochlear partition on discharges in individual auditory-nerve fibers. I. Prolonged direct-current polarization. *Journal of Acoustical Society of America, 47*, 1519–1526.

Kral, A. & Majernik, V. (1996). On lateral inhibition in the auditory system. *Gen. Physiol. Biophys., 15*, 109–127.

Langner, G. (1997). Neural processing and representation of periodicity pitch. *Acta Otolaryngologica (Stockholm)* Suppl. 532, 68–76.

Leake, P. A., & Snyder, R. L. (1989). Topographic organization of the central projections of the spiral ganglion in cats. *Journal of Comparative Neurology, 281,* 612–629.

Legendy, C. R., & Salcman, M. (1985). Bursts and recurrences of bursts in the spike trains of spontaneously active striate cortex neurons. *Journal of Neurophysiology, 53,* 926–939.

Lenarz, T., Schreiner, C., Snyder, R. L., & Ernst, A. (1995). Neural mechanisms of tinnitus. The pathological ensemble spontaneous activity of the auditory system. In J. E. Vernon & A. R. Møller (Eds.), *Mechanisms of Tinnitus* (pp. 101–113). Boston: Allyn & Bacon.

Lenarz, T., Schreiner, C., Snyder, R. L., & Ernst, A. (1996). Neural mechanisms of tinnitus. In G. E. Reich & J. E. Vernon (Eds.), *Proceedings of the Fifth International Tinnitus Seminar 1995* (pp. 441–448), Portland, OR: American Tinnitus Association.

Lenzi, D., & Rogers, W. M. (1994). Calcium signalling in hair cells: Multiple roles in a compact cell. *Current Opinion in Neurobiology, 4,* 496–502.

LePage, E. (1995). A model for cochlear origin of subjective tinnitus: excitatory drift in the operating point of the inner hair cells. In J. E. Vernon & A. R. Moller (Eds), *Mechanisms of Tinnitus,* 115–147. Boston: Allyn & Bacon.

Levine, R. A. (1994). Tinnitus. *Current Opinion in Otolaryngology & Head and Neck Surgery, 2,* 171–176.

Liberman, M. C. (1978). Auditory-nerve responses from cats raised in a low-noise chamber. *Journal of Acoustical Society of America, 63,* 442–455.

Liberman, M. C., & Kiang, N. Y. S. (1978). Acoustic Trauma in cats. Cochlear pathology and auditory-nerve activity. *Acta Otolaryngologica,* (Suppl 358), 1–63.

Liberman, M. C., & Oliver, M. E. (1984). Morphometry of intracellularly labeled neurons of the auditory nerve: Correlations with functional properties. *Journal Comparative Neurology, 223,* 163–176.

Lin, X. (1997). Action potentials and underlying voltage-dependent currents in cultured spiral ganglion neurons in the postnatal gerbil. *Hearing Research, 108,* 157–179.

Lin, X., Hume, R. I., & Nuttal, A. L. (1995). Dihydropyridines and verapamil inhibit voltage-dependent K^+ current in isolated outer hair cells of the guinea pig. *Hearing Research, 88,* 36–46.

Lockwood, A. H., Salvi, R. J., Coad, M. L., Towsley, M. L., Wack, D. S., & Murphy, B. W. (1998). The functional neuroanatomy of tinnitus. Evidence for limbic system links and neural plasticity. *Neurology, 50,* 114–120.

Long, G. R., & Tubis, A. (1988). Modification of spontaneous and evoked otoacoustic emissions and associated psychoacoustic microstructure by aspirin consumption. *Journal of Acoustical Society of America, 84,* 1343–1353.

Mammano, F. & Ashmore, J. F. (1993). Reverse transduction measured in the isolated cochlea by laser Michelson interferometry. *Nature, 365,* 838–841.

Manabe, Y., Yoshida, S., Saito, H., & Oka, H. (1997). Effects of lidocaine on saliylate-induced discharge of neurons in the inferior colliculus of the guinea pig. *Hearing Research, 103,* 192–198.

Manley, G. A., & Robertson, D. (1976). Analysis of spontaneous activity of auditory neurons in the spiral ganglion of the guinea pig cochlea. *Journal of Physiology, 258,* 323–336.

Martin, W. H. (1995). Spectral analysis of brain activity in the study of tinnitus. In J. E. Vernon & A.R. Møller (Eds.), *Mechanisms of Tinnitus* (pp. 163–180). Boston: Allyn & Bacon.

Martin, W. H., Schwegler, J. W., Scheibelhoffer, J., & Ronis, M. (1993). Salicylate-induced changes in cat auditory nerve activity. *Laryngoscope, 103,* 600–604.

McCormick, D. A., Connors, B. W., Lighthall, J. W., & Prince, D. A. (1985). Comparative electrophysiology of pyramidal and sparsely spiny stellate neurons of the neocortex. *Journal of Neurophysiology, 54,* 782–806.

McCormick, D. A., Wang, Z., & Huguenard, J. (1993). Neurotransmitter control of neocortical activity and excitability. *Cerebral Cortex, 3,* 387–398.

McFadden, D., & Pasanen, E. G. (1994). Otoacoustic emissions and quinine sulfate. *Journal of Acoustical Society of America, 95,* 3460–3474.

McFadden, D., & Plattsmier, H. S. (1984). Aspirin abolishes spontaneous otoacoustic emissions. *Journal of Acoustical Society of America, 76,* 443–448.

Meikle, M. B. (1995). The interaction of central and peripheral mechanisms in tinnitus. In J. E. Vernon & A. R. Møller (Eds.), *Mechanisms of Tinnitus* (pp. 181–206). Boston: Allyn & Bacon.

Merskey, H. (1979). Pain terms: A list with definitions and a note of usage. Recommended by the International Association for the Study of Pain (IASP) Subcommittee on Taxonomy. *Pain, 6,* 249–252.

Meyer zum Gottesberge, A. M. (1988). Imbalanced calcium homeostasis and endolymphatic hydrops. *Acta Otolaryngologica (Stockholm), 460*(Suppl.), 18–27.

Meyer zum Gottesberge-Orsulakova, A. M., & Kaufmann, R. (1986). Is an imbalanced calcium-homeostasis responsible for the experimentally induced endolymphatic hydrops? *Acta Otolaryngologica (Stockholm), 102,* 93–98.

Møller, A. R. (1976). Dynamic properties of primary auditory fibers compared with cells in the cochlear nucleus. *Acta Physiol. Scand., 98,* 157–167.

Møller, A. R. (1984). Pathophysiology of tinnitus. *Ann. Otol. Rhinol. Laryngol., 93,* 39–44.

Møller, A. R. (1995). Pathophysiology of tinnitus. In J. E. Vernon & A. R. Møller (Eds.), *Mechanisms of Tinnitus* (pp. 207–217). Boston: Allyn & Bacon.

Møller, A. R. (1996). Similarities between tinnitus and pain. In G. E. Reich & J. E. Vernon (Eds.), *Proceedings of the Fifth International Tinnitus Seminar 1995* (pp. 449–454), Portland, OR: American Tinnitus Association.

Møller, A. R., Møller, M. B., & Yokota, M. (1992). Some forms of tinnitus may involve the extralemniscal pathway. *Laryngoscope, 102,* 1165–1171.

Murugasu, E., & Russell, I. J. (1995). Salicylate ototoxicity: The effects on basilar membrane displacement, cochlear microphonics, and neural responses in the basal turn of the guinea-pig cochlea. *Auditory Neuroscience, 1,* 139–150.

Norton, S. J., Schmidt, A. R. & Stover, L. J. (1990). Tinnitus and otoacoustic emissions: Is there a link? *Ear and Hearing, 11,* 159–166.

Nuttall, A. L., Guo, M., Ren, T., & Dolan, D. F. (1997). Basilar membrane velocity noise. *Hearing Research, 114,* 35–42.

Ochi, K., & Eggermont, J. J. (1996). Effects of salicylate on neural activity in cat primary auditory cortex. *Hearing Research, 95,* 63–76.

Ochi, K., & Eggermont, J. J. (1997). Effects of quinine on neural activity in cat primary auditory cortex. *Hearing Research, 105,* 105–118.

Oertel, D., Wu, S. H., & Hirsch, J. A. (1988). Electrical characteristics of cells and neuronal circuitry in the cochlear nucleus studied with intracellular recordings from brain slices. In G. M. Edelman, W. E. Gall & W. M. Cowan (Eds.), *Auditory function. Neurobiological basis of hearing* (pp. 313–336). New York: J. Wiley.

Ohmori, H. (1989). Mechano-electrical transduction of the hair cell. *Jap. J. Physiology, 39,* 643–657.

O-Uchi, T., & Tanaka, Y. (1988). Study of so-called cochlear mechanical tinnitus. *Acta Otolaryngologica (Stockholm)* Suppl., 447, 94–99.

Packham, M. A. (1982). Mode of action of acetylsalicylic acid. In H. J. M. Banett, J. Hirsh, & J. F. Mustard (Eds.), *Acetylsalicylic acid: New uses for an old drug* (pp. 63–86). New York: Raven Press.

Pan, E., & Stringer, J. L. (1997). Role of potassium and calcium in the generation of cellular bursts in the dentate gyrus. *Journal of Neurophysiology, 77,* 2293–2299.

Penner, M. J. (1992). Audible and annoying spontaneous otoacoustic emissions. In J. M. Aran & R. Dauman (Eds.), *Tinnitus 91* (pp. 85–87). Amsterdam: Kugler Publications.

Penner, M. J., & Burns, E. M. (1987). The dissociation of SOAEs and Tinnitus. *Journal of Speech Hearing Research, 30,* 396–403.

Penner, M. J., & Jastreboff, P. J. (1996). Tinnitus: psychophysical observations in humans and an animal model. In T. R. Van De Water, A. N. Popper, & R. R. Fay (Eds.), *Clinical aspects of hearing,* (pp. 258–304). New York: Springer Verlag.

Pernier, J., & Gerin, P. (1975). Temporal pattern analysis of spontaneous unit activity in the neocortex. *Biol. Cybernetics, 18,* 123–136.

Pfeiffer, R. R., & Kiang, N. Y. .S. (1965). Spike discharge patterns of spontaneous and continuously stimulated activity in the cochlear nucleus of anaesthetized cats. *Biophysical Journal, 5,* 301–316.

Phillips, D. F., Semple, M. N., Calford, M. B., & Kitzes, L. M. (1994). Level-dependent representation of stimulus frequency in cat primary auditory cortex. *Exp. Brain Res., 102,* 210–226.

Plinkert, P. K., Gitter, A. H., & Zenner, H. P. (1990). Tinnitus associated spontaneous otoacoustic emissions. *Acta Otolaryngologica (Stockholm), 110,* 342–347.

Preyer, S., Meyer, J., Zenner, H. P., & Gummer, A. W. (1997). Acetylcalicylic acid and spontaneous mechanoelectrical transduction current of outer hair cells. *ARO Abstract,* 293.

Puel, J. L., Bobbin, R. P. & Fallon, M. (1990). Salicylate, mefenamate, meclofemamate, and quinine on cochlear potentials. *Otolaryngology-Head and Neck Surgery, 1,* 66–73.

Pujol, R. (1992). Neuropharmacology of the cochlea and tinnitus. In J. M. Aran & R. Dauman (Eds.), *Tinnitus 91* (pp. 103–107). Amsterdam: Kugler Publications.

Rajan, R., Irvine, D. R. F., Wise, L. Z., & Heil, P. (1993). Effect of unilateral partial cochlear lesions in adult cats on the representation of lesioned and unlesioned cochleas in primary auditory cortex. *Journal of Comparative Neurology, 338,* 17–49.

Riccioppo, Neto, F. (1980). Further studies on the actions of salicylates on nerve membranes. *European Journal of Pharmacology, 68,* 155–162.

Robertson, D., & Irvine, D. R. F. (1989). Plasticity of frequency organization in auditory cortex of guinea pigs with partial unilateral deafness. *Journal of Comparative Neurology, 282,* 456–471.

Rodieck, R. W., Kiang, N. Y. S., & Gerstein, G. L. (1962). Some quantitative methods for the study of spontaneous activity of single cells. *Biophysical Journal, 2,* 351–368.

Russell, I. J. (1971). The pharmacology of efferent synapses in the lateral line system of Xenopus laevis. *J. Exp. Biology, 54,* 643–658.

Rydmarker, S., & Horner, K. C. (1991). Atrophy of outer hair cell stereocilia and hearing loss in hydroptic cochlea. *Hearing Research, 53,* 113–122.

Salvi, R. J., Hamernik, R. P., & Henderson, D. (1978). Discharge patterns in the cochlear nucleus of the chinchilla following noise induced asymptotic threshold shift. *Exp. Brain. Research, 32,* 301–320.

Salvi, R. J., Saunders, S. S., Gratton, M. A., Arehole, S., & Powers, N. (1990). Enhanced evoked response amplitudes in the inferior colliculus of the chinchilla following acoustic trauma. *Hearing Research, 50,* 245–258.

Salvi, R. J., Wang, J., & Powers, N. L. (1996a). Plasticity and reorganization in the auditory brainstem: Implications for tinnitus. In G. E. Reich & J. E. Vernon (Eds.), *Proceedings of the Fifth International Tinnitus Seminar 1995* (pp. 457–466), Portland, OR: American Tinnitus Association.

Salvi, R. J., Wang, J., & Powers, N. L. (1996b). Rapid functional reorganization in the inferior colliculus and cochlear nucleus after acute cochlear damage. In R. J. Salvi, D.

Henderson, F. Fiorino, & V. Colletti (Eds.), *Auditory system plasticity and regeneration* (pp. 275–296). New York: Thieme Medical Publishers, Inc.

Sasaki, C. T., Kauer, J. S., & Babitz, L. (1980). Differential [^{14}C]2-deoxyglucose uptake after deafferentation of the mammalian auditory pathway—a model for examining tinnitus. *Brain Research, 194,* 511–516.

Schreiner, C. E., & Snyder, R. L. (1987). A physiological animal model of peripheral tinnitus. In H. Feldman (Ed.), *Proceedings of the Third International Tinnitus Seminar* (pp. 100–106). Karlsruhe: Harsch Verlag.

Schulze, H., & Langner, G. (1997). Representation of periodicity pitch in the primary auditory cortex of the mongolian gerbil. *Acta Otolaryngologica (Stockholm)* Suppl. 532, 89–95.

Sewell, W. F. (1990). Synaptic potentials in afferent fibers innervating hair cells of the lateral line organ in Xenopus laevis. *Hearing Research, 44,* 71–82.

Shehata-Dieler, W. E., Richter, C. P., Dieler, R., & Klinke, R. (1994). Effects of endolymphatic and perilymphatic application of salicylate in the pigeon. I: Single fiber activity and cochlear potentials. *Hearing Research, 74,* 77–84.

Sherman, S. M. (1996). Dual response modes in lateral geniculate neurons: Mechanisms and functions. *Visual Neuroscience, 13,* 205–213.

Shirokova, N., & Ríos, E. (1996a). Activation of Ca^{2+} release by caffeine and voltage in frog skeletal muscle. *Journal of Physiology, 493.2,* 317–339.

Shirokova, N., & Ríos, E. (1996b). Caffeine enhances intramembranous charge movement in frog skeletal muscle by increasing cytoplasmic Ca^{2+} concentration. *Journal of Physiology, 493.2,* 341–356.

Siebert, W. M. (1965). Some implications of the stochastic behavior of primary auditory neurons. *Kybernetik, 2,* 206–215.

Smith, D. R., & Smith, G. K. (1965). A statistical analysis of the continual activity of single cortical neurones in the cat unanaesthetized isolated forebrain. *Biophysical Journal, 5,* 47–74.

Spangler, K. M., & Warr, W. B. (1991). The descending auditory system. In R. A. Altschuler, R. P. Bobbin, B. M. Clopton, & D. W. Hoffman (Eds.), *Neurobiology of hearing: The central auditory system* (pp. 27–45). New York: Raven Press.

Stein, B. E., & Meredith, M. A. (1993). *The merging of the senses.* Cambridge, MA: The MIT Press.

Stypulkowski, P. H. (1990). Mechanisms of salicylate ototoxicity. *Hearing Research, 46,* 113–146.

Szczepaniak, W. S. & Møller, A. R. (1995). Effects of (-)-baclofen, clonazepam, and diazepam on tone exposure-induced hyperexcitability of the inferior colliculus in the rat: Possible therapeutic implications for the pharmacological management of tinnitus and hyperacusis. *Hearing Research, 97,* 46–53.

Szczepaniak, W. S., & Møller, A. R. (1995). Evidence of decreased GABAergic influence on temporal integration in the inferior colliculus following acute noise exposure: A study of evoked potentials in the rat. *Neuroscience Letters, 196,* 77–80.

Tonndorf, J. (1987). The analogy between tinnitus and pain: A suggestion for a physiological basis of chronic tinnitus. *Hearing Research, 28,* 271–275.

Toyama, K., Kimura, M., & Tanaka, K. (1981). Cross-correlation analysis of interneuronal connectivity in cat visual cortex. *Journal of Neurophysiology, 46,* 191–201.

Tunstall, M. J., Gale, J. E., & Ashmore, J. F. (1995). Action of salicylate on membrane capacitance of outer hair cells from guinea-pig cochlea. *Journal of Physiology, 485,* 739–752.

Tyler, R. S. (1984). Does tinnitus originate from hyperactive nerve fibers in the cochlea? *Journal Laryngol. Otol. Suppl., 9,* 38–44.

Voigt, H. F., & Young, E. D. (1980). Evidence of inhibitory interactions between neurons in dorsal cochlear nucleus. *Journal of Neurophysiology, 44,* 76–96.

Wake, M., Takeno, S., Mount, R. J., & Harrison, R. V. (1996). Recording from the inferior colliculus following cochlear inner hair cell damage. *Acta Otolaryngol (Stockholm), 116,* 714–720.

Wallace, M. N., Kitzes, L. M., & Jones, E. G. (1991). Intrinsic inter- and intralaminar connections and their relationship to the tonotopic map in cat primary auditory cortex. *Exp. Brain Res., 86,* 527–544.

Wallhäusser-Franke, E. (1997). Salicylate evokes c-fos expression in the brain stem: Implications for tinnitus. *NeuroReport, 8,* 725–728.

Wallhäusser-Franke E., Braun, S., & Langner, G. (1996). Salicylate alters 2-DG uptake in the auditory system: A model for tinnitus? *NeuroReport, 7,* 1585–1588.

Wang, J., Salvi, R. J., & Powers, N. (1996). Plasticity of response properties of inferior colliculus neurons following acute cochlear damage. *Journal of Neurophysiology, 75,* 171–183.

Wangemann, P., & Schacht, J. (1996). Homeostatic mechanisms in the cochlea. In P. Dallos, A. N. Popper, & R. R. Fay (Eds.), *The cochlea* (pp. 130–185). New York: Springer Verlag.

Weinberger, N. M. (1995). Retuning the brain by fear conditioning. In M. S. Gazzaniga (Ed.), *The cognitive neurosciences* (pp. 1071–1089) Cambridge, MA: The MIT Press.

Weinberger, N. M., & Diamond, D. M. (1987). Physiological plasticity in auditory cortex: Rapid induction by learning. *Progr. Neurobiology, 29,* 1–55.

Willot, J. F. (1996). Auditory system plasticity in the adult C57BL/6J mouse. In R. J. Salvi, D. Henderson, F. Fiorino, & V. Colletti (Eds.), *Auditory system plasticity and regeneration* (pp. 297–316). New York: Thieme Medical Publishers, Inc.

Wilson, J. P., & Sutton, G. J. (1981). Acoustic correlates of tonal tinnitus. In *Tinnitus, Ciba Foundation Symposium 85* (pp. 82–107).

Winer, J. A. (1992). The functional architecture of the medial geniculate body and the primary auditory cortex. In D. B. Webster, A. N. Popper & R. R. Fay (Eds.), *The mammalian auditory pathway: Neuroanatomy* (pp. 222–409). New York: Springer Verlag.

Yamamoto, H., & Karaide, H. (1990). Release of intracellularly stored Ca^{2+} by inositol 1,4,5 triphosphate—An overview. *General Pharmacology, 21,* 387–393.

Young, E. D., Nelken, I., & Conley, R. A. (1995). Somatosensory effects on neurons in dorsal cochlear nucleus. *Journal of Neurophysiology, 73,* 743–765.

Young, E. D., Spirou, G. A., Rice, J. J., & Voigt, H. F. (1992). Neural organization and responses to complex stimuli in the dorsal cochlear nucleus. *Phil. Trans. R. Soc. Lond. B, 336,* 407–413.

Zenner, H. P., & Ernst, A. (1995). Cochlear motor tinnitus, transduction tinnitus, and signal transfer tinnitus: Three models of cochlear tinnitus. In J. E. Vernon & A. R. Møller (Eds.), *Mechanisms of tinnitus* (pp. 237–254). Boston: Allyn & Bacon.

Zhang, Y., Suga, N., & Yan, J. (1997). Corticofugal modulation of frequency processing in bat auditory system. *Nature, 387,* 900–903.

Zurek, P. M. (1981). Narrow-band acoustic signals emitted by human ears. *Journal of Acoustical Society of America, 62,* 514–523.

CHAPTER 5

Neural Plasticity and Tinnitus

Richard J. Salvi, Ph.D.
Alan H. Lockwood, M.D.
Robert Burkard, Ph.D.

INTRODUCTION

Tinnitus often develops soon after the auditory system is damaged. This suggests that important clues about the biological mechanisms of tinnitus might be gained by understanding how the auditory system responds to various types of ototraumatic insults. Over the past four to five decades, considerable progress has been made in elucidating the functional changes that occur in the peripheral auditory system after the cochlea is damaged (Salvi, Henderson, & Hemernik, 1983). However, the physiological changes observed in the periphery cannot account for several different aspects of tinnitus. A clear-cut example of this is the tinnitus that develops after the auditory nerve is sectioned (House & Brackman, 1981). The fact that tinnitus develops after the neural output of the cochlea is eliminated indicates that tinnitus may have its origins in the central auditory pathway (Risey, Guth, & Amedee, 1995; Tyler, 1981); however, the mechanisms by which this occurs remain obscure. The general thesis put forward in this chapter is that central auditory system reorganization is an impor-tant, and in some cases, unwanted, by-product of cochlear damage. If the reorganization is extensive and uncontrolled, it may result in tinnitus.

While much of the information presented here has been derived from physiological studies in animals, the basic findings are likely to have parallels in the human central nervous system. The basic science results provide an empirical foundation and conceptual framework from which one can begin to formulate testable hypotheses regarding the neural basis of tinnitus. A few decades ago it would have been difficult, if not impossible, to study the neural substrate of tinnitus in the living human brain. However, in the past few decades, rapid advances in brain imaging technology have provided clinicians and researchers with powerful new tools to view some of the functional properties of the human brain and to relate the results to more fundamental data obtained from animals.

The central auditory system has traditionally been thought of as a hardwired system that receives inputs from a series of cochlear bandpass filters. When a segment of the cochlea is damaged or destroyed, the inputs to a specific frequency region within the central auditory system are reduced or eliminated (Koerber Pfeiffer, Warr, & Kiang, 1966). How does the central auditory system respond to the loss of some of its peripheral input? Clinical insights into the underlying nature of the problem can be gleaned from patients with sensorineural hearing loss and tinnitus. In regions of hearing loss, where the neural input to the central auditory system is greatly reduced, patients show an abnormally rapid growth of loudness (Zheng & Turner, 1991), and in some cases, an inability to tolerate the loudness of sounds presented at suprathreshold levels (Goldstein & Shulman, 1996). The abnormally rapid growth of loudness that occurs in cases of sensorineural hearing loss suggests that the central auditory system can compensate for the loss of peripheral inputs, perhaps by increasing the gain of the system. These compensatory changes could give rise to aberrant patterns of spontaneous neural activity that may result in subjective tinnitus. Chapter 4 describes some of the neural mechanisms that may contribute to tinnitus. In addition, Chapter 7 and Chapter 8 discuss some of the abnormal psychophysical and physiological measures that have been observed in humans with tinnitus. In this chapter, we provide a brief overview of some of the results obtained in other sensory systems. These results have provided scientists and clinicians with important clues about the reorganization of the central nervous system and these results may help us understand peripheral damage may contribute to phantom sensations.

REORGANIZATION OF SOMATOSENSORY SYSTEM AND PHANTOM LIMB PAIN

Amputation of a finger, hand, or arm eliminates the somatosensory inputs from a restricted region of the receptor surface (Figure 5-1). Despite the loss of peripheral sensory inputs from the amputated region, patients often experience phantom limb sensations and phantom limb pain. Recent electrophysiological studies suggest that phantom limb pain may be linked to the reorganization of the central nervous system (Dostrovsky, Millar, & Wall, 1976; Jenkins & Merzenich, 1987). In adult mammals, removal of peripheral afferent inputs by transection of a peripheral nerve or amputation of a finger causes the deprived area of the somatosensory cortex to respond to regions of the body bordering the lesion (Jenkins & Merzenich, 1987; Merzenich & Kaas, 1982; Pons et al., 1991; Rasmusson, 1982). Similarly, removal of select vibrissae causes the deprived cortical barrels in the somatosensory cortex to become more sensitive to stimulation of vibrissae adjacent to the vibrissae-deprived area (Welker et al., 1996). Thus, if a finger is amputated (Figure 5-1), the "finger cortex" may be activated by stimulation of the thumb and adjacent region of the hand bordering the amputated region, resulting in the misperception of the phantom finger.

To appreciate how the reorganization occurs, it is useful to review some of the fundamental characteristics of neurons in the somatosensory cortex. Each neuron in the somatosensory cortex is excited by stimulation to a specific region of the body surface (Figure 5-2). The width and strength of the excitatory and inhibitory response area vary with location on the surface of the body. This excitatory region (+ + + +) occurs in the area where excitation is stronger than inhibition; this defines the center of the neuron's receptive field. The central excitatory region is surrounded by an inhibitory area (– – – – – –) where inhibition is stronger than excitation. Because the inhibitory and excitatory regions overlap, stimulation delivered to the inhibitory surround can suppress the activity elicited by stimulation of the central excitatory region, depending on the strength of the inhibitory signal. The response properties of each cortical neuron arise from the delicate interplay between its excitatory and inhibitory inputs. Thus, the inhibitory surround serves to restrict and sharpen the excitatory response area or receptive field.

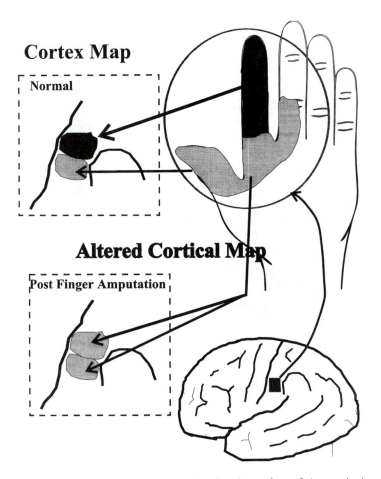

FIGURE 5-1. Lower right: Schematic showing the surface of the cerebral cortex. Shaded area shows approximate location of somatosensory cortex. Upper right: Schematic of hand with somatotopic map of the index finger (black area) and thumb (shaded area). Upper left: Schematic showing a portion of the map of the normal somatosensory cortex. Black area represents approximate region of somatosensory cortex activated by stimulation of index finger. Shaded area represents areas of somatosensory cortex activated by thumb and adjacent region of hand. Lower right: Altered map of somatosensory cortex following amputation of index finger. Note expanded area of the somatosensory cortex that is activated by stimulation of thumb and adjacent region of hand following amputation of index finger.

Damage to a segment of the surface of the body can perturb the balance between the excitatory and inhibitory inputs to the receptive field. As illustrated in Figure 5-3, when a small segment of the body surface (digit) is amputated or anesthetized on the wing of the flying fox bat, the excitatory receptive field shifts to an adjacent region of the body surface and/or expands in size (Calford & Tweedale, 1988). Because the excitatory receptive field is shaped by surround inhibition, the rapid reorganization of the excitatory receptive field is thought to arise from disinhibition or unmasking of preexisting excitatory inputs. Some of the preexisting excitatory inputs are normally

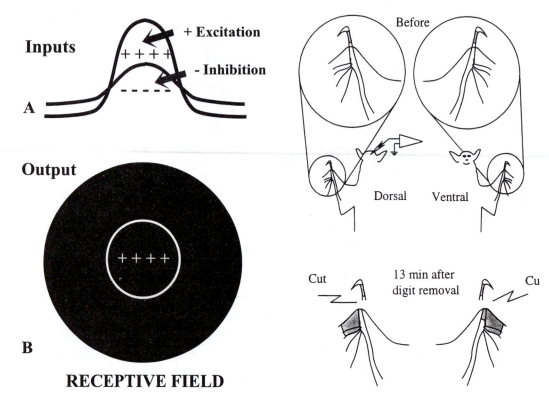

RECEPTIVE FIELD

FIGURE 5-2. (**A**) Schematic showing the hypothetical location and strength of the excitatory (+) and inhibitory (–) inputs of the receptive field of a neuron in the somatosensory cortex. Response to stimulation is excitatory if the strength of the excitatory input exceeds the inhibitory input. (**B**) Schematic showing the resulting output of the receptive field.

FIGURE 5-3. Schematic showing the excitatory receptive field of a neuron in the somatosensory cortex of the flying fox bat. Top and middle panel. Neuron normally responds to tactile stimulation of the digit on the wings. Bottom panel. Amputation (cut) of the digit causes a rapid shift in neuron's receptive field to adjacent regions of the wing that surround the amputated region.

inhibited by inputs from regions of the body adjacent to the amputated or denervated area (Calford & Tweedale, 1988; Calford & Tweedale, 1990). The full extent of the excitatory receptive field can be demonstrated by blocking the inhibitory inputs with various drugs. Blocking the GABAergic inputs in the somatosensory cortex results in a large, rapid expansion of the neuron's excitatory receptive field (Hicks & Dykes, 1983). These results indicate that each cortical neuron receives low-threshold excitatory inputs from a relatively large expanse of the body surface, but these inputs are partially covered up or masked by lateral inhibition. When these inhibitory inputs are inactivated as a result of amputating the appro-

priate receptor inputs, a new excitatory region will be expressed.

Obviously, there must be some limits to the degree of cortical reorganization. Complete reorganization or filling-in of a portion of the somatosensory cortex occurs if sensory inputs are removed from a small part of the hand, but if inputs are removed from more than half the hand, some regions of the cortex will remain unresponsive to stimulation (Wall & Kass, 1986). The upper limit for complete reorganization was thought to extend approximately 1 to 2 mm in the somatosensory cortex. However, after prolonged deafferentation, massive reorganization, extending up to 10 to 14 mm, has been observed in adult monkeys (Pons et al.,

1991). These results suggest that the duration of deafferentation influences the degree of reorganization.

Experience and practice are important factors that can shape the somatotopic maps. Trained musicians who play string instruments show an increased cortical representation of the fingers of the left hand compared to normals (Elbert, Pantev, Wienbruch, Rockstroh, & Taub, 1995). Anomalous cross-sensory activation of visual cortex has been observed in blind patients. Braille reading by blind subjects results in activation of primary visual cortex (Sadato et al., 1996). These results suggest that the visual cortex can be activated by inputs from the somatosensory system when the normal inputs to the visual cortex have been eliminated.

Patients who lose a limb often experience phantom limb sensations and phantom limb pain. Recent brain imaging studies have shown that the region of the body surface surrounding the amputated limb is expanded in the human somatosensory cortex. Interestingly, the amount of reorganization in the somatosensory cortex is strongly correlated with the degree of phantom limb pain. These results suggest that the degree of functional reorganization may be an important factor mediating phantom limb pain (Flor et al., 1995) as well as other phantom sensations such as tinnitus.

Reorganization in Visual Cortex

Like the somatosensory system, the visual system of adult mammals is capable of reorganizing if the retina is damaged. If one eye is removed and a 5 to 10° lesion is made in the other eye, then the retinotopic maps in the primary and secondary visual cortex are immediately altered. Cortical neurons that normally respond to light presented to the destroyed area of the retina now respond to light that is delivered to regions of the retina surrounding the lesions (Kaas et al., 1990). If the retinal lesions are large (10 to 15°), the cortical neurons associated with the center of the lesion become unresponsive to light

stimulation whereas neurons located just inside the boundaries of the retinal lesion now respond to light presented just outside the lesioned retinal area.

The visual cortex receives numerous inputs from the lateral geniculate nucleus. Lesions of the retina initially cause complete inactivation of the neurons in the lateral geniculate nucleus whose visual receptive fields lie within the lesion (Eysel, Gonzalez-Aguilar, & Mayer, 1981). However, after a thirty-day recovery period, light-excitable cells can be found within the region of the lateral geniculate nucleus that was initially unresponsive to light. These neurons now respond to light presented just outside the lesioned area of the retina. These results suggest that some of the reorganization observed in the cortex may originate at more peripheral sites within the visual pathway.

Mechanisms of Reorganization

A variety of mechanisms have been implicated in the functional reorganization seen in the visual and somatosensory system. The functional changes observed immediately after lesioning the periphery have been attributed to disinhibition or the unmasking of intrinsic neural circuits. In contrast, the functional changes observed weeks or months following the lesion are thought to have a structural basis (Eysel, Gonzalez-Aguilar, & Mayer, 1980; Eysel et al., 1981). The structural changes that have been implicated in long-term reorganization include axonal sprouting and the formation of additional synaptic contacts (Darian-Smith & Gilbert, 1994; Liu & Chambers, 1958; Rubel, Smith, & Steward, 1981), translocation of synapses (Lynch, Deadwyler, & Cotman, 1973a; Lynch, Stanfield, & Cotman, 1973b) and increased efficiency of existing synapses (denervation hypersensitivity) (Sharpless, 1975). Sprouting and developing axons can be labeled with antibodies to GAP-43 (Kalil & Skene, 1986; Meiri, Pfenninger, & Willard, 1986; Skene & Willard, 1981). GAP-43 is expressed in the somatosensory cortex in arrays representing the pattern of vibrissae on the snout (Erzurlumlu, Jhaveri, & Benowitz, 1990). When whiskers are removed, there is a rapid alteration in the pattern of GAP-43 immunostaining, suggesting that there is a reorganization of the afferent inputs. GAP-43 immunostaining also reappears in the dorsal root ganglion and sciatic nerve during regenerative sprouting (Van der Zee et al., 1989). These results provide a structural basis for some of the long-term functional changes observed in the central nervous system.

CENTRAL AUDITORY SYSTEM REORGANIZATION

Reorganization of Tonotopic Maps

One of the hallmarks of the normal auditory system is its precise tonotopic organization. The tonotopic organization originates in the mechanical response of the cochlea and is recapitulated at each subsequent level of the auditory pathway up to the cortex. When all of the hair cells are destroyed within a narrow segment of the cochlea, neural activity ceases (silent neurons) within a discrete frequency band within the cochlea and in each subdivision of the cochlear nucleus where the auditory nerve projects (Koerber et al., 1966). If the central auditory system were completely hardwired, then these silent neurons should also be present at higher levels of the auditory pathway. This is in fact what is observed in the auditory cortex immediately after damaging a segment of the cochlea (Robertson & Irvine, 1989). The portion of auditory cortex that is tuned to the lesioned area of the cochlea becomes silent and unresponsive to sound. However, if measurements are made several months later, the previously silent region of the cortex now contains neurons that have nearly normal thresholds and tuning. However, the tonotopic organization of the cortex is dramatically altered such that many more neurons are tuned to frequencies just outside the region corresponding to the cochlear lesion. One consequence of this reorganization is that the cortical tonotopic map contains an overabundance of neurons that are tuned to frequencies at the edges of the hearing loss (Harrison, Nagasawa, Smith, Stanton, & Mount, 1991; Harrison, Smith, Nagasawa, & Mount, 1992; Robertson & Irvine, 1989; Willott, Aitkin, & McFadden, 1993). Consequently, an abnormally large segment of the auditory cortex will be activated by a narrow range of frequencies on the low and high frequency borders of the hearing loss. The overrepresentation of these border frequencies could conceivably lead to an increase in the perceptual salience of these frequencies, and the endogenous spontaneous neural activity in these regions could give rise to the phantom sensation of tinnitus.

Although the tonotopic map can be reorganized in the cortex, this does not necessarily mean that the cortex is the only site within the auditory pathway where this type of reorganization can take place. As shown in Figure 5-4, the tonotopic map of the inferior colliculus shows signs of remodeling in adult mammals following a cochlear lesion. However, the degree of reorganization is less pronounced and occurs less frequently than in the auditory cortex (Harrison, Stanton, Ibrahim, Nagasawa, & Mount, 1993; Irvine & Rajan, 1994; Salvi, Wang, & Powers, 1996b). On the other hand, the dorsal cochlear nucleus shows little evidence of tonotopic reorganization following cochlear damage (Kaltenbach, Czaja, & Kaplan, 1992).

It is well known that experience and practice can result in an improvement in one's ability to detect or discriminate a stimulus. A similar type of training effect can be demonstrated electrophysiologically in cortical and certain subcortical regions of the auditory pathway (Weinberger, Javid, & Lepan, 1993; Weinberger, 1995). Presenting a sound (the conditioned stimulus, CS) prior to an electric shock (the unconditioned stimulus, UCS), can modify a neuron's response properties. For example, a neuron

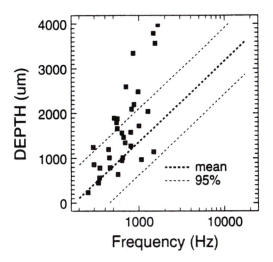

IC TONOTOPIC MAP

FIGURE 5-4. Tonotopic organization of the inferior colliculus of the chinchilla. Characteristic frequency of neurons increases from low-to-high frequencies (abscissa) as the electrode depth increases along the dorsal-ventral axis of the inferior colliculus. Thick dashed line and thin dashed lines show the mean and 95 percent confidence interval of tonotopic map in normal-hearing chinchillas. Filled squares show the tonotopic organization of chinchillas with a severe high frequency hearing loss above 1,000 Hz. Tonotopic map is normal for neurons with characteristic frequencies below 1,000 Hz, but near the boundary of the hearing loss (1,000 Hz), the characteristic frequencies remain nearly constant as the electrode penetration increases from 1,500 to 4,000 m.

in the auditory cortex that normally responds robustly to a 4 kHz tone, but weakly to a 2 kHz tone, can be conditioned to produce its maximum response to the 2 kHz tone by presenting the CS (2 kHz tone) followed by the UCS (electric shock). Classical and operant conditioning paradigms can modify the tuning, characteristic frequency and discharge rate of a neuron. Results such as this provide a scientific rationale for clinical intervention strategies that attempt to train the auditory brain to ignore a phantom sound (Jastreboff & Hazell, 1993). This retraining therapy approach is more fully described in Chapter 15. Conversely, one can also imagine how tinnitus might take on

its negative emotional characteristics if it were repeatedly paired with a stressful event.

Enhancement of Neural Activity

When the cochlea is damaged by ototoxic drugs or acoustic overstimulation, the neural activity flowing into the central nervous system is reduced, particularly when there is significant damage to the IHCs and auditory nerve (Salvi, Hamernik, & Henderson, 1978; Trautwein, Hofstetter, Wang, Salvi, & Nostrant, 1996; Wang et al., 1997). The reduced neural activity flowing out of the cochlea would presumably cause a corresponding reduction in the neural activity in more central regions of the auditory pathway. Surprisingly, the activity in the central auditory pathway sometimes increases after the cochlea is damaged. Noise-induced damage to the cochlea can lead to an enhancement of evoked potential amplitude in the auditory cortex even though response thresholds are elevated (Syka, Rybalko, & Popelar, 1994). Cortical evoked potentials are enhanced for hours or days even though responses from the inferior colliculus and auditory nerve are reduced (Popelar, Syka, & Berndt, 1987; Syka et al., 1994).

In normal animals, evoked potentials recorded from the ipsilateral auditory cortex have higher thresholds and smaller amplitudes than those recorded from the contralateral auditory cortex. Surprisingly, when one cochlea is destroyed with aminoglycoside antibiotics, the evoked potentials from the ipsilateral auditory cortex show an improvement in threshold within two to six days (Popelar, Erre, Aran, & Cazals, 1994). In addition, the amplitude of the evoked response from the ipsilateral auditory cortex increases during the first two to three weeks following the exposure.

The enhancement of evoked potential amplitude has also been observed in the auditory midbrain. The deafness mouse (dn/dn) shows progressive degeneration of spiral ganglion neurons with age. Although the neural output of the cochlea decreased with age, the evoked potential amplitudes from the inferior colliculus of the deafness mouse were larger than in normal mice; however, no changes in threshold or latency of the evoked response were noted (Steel & Bock, 1984). Evoked potential amplitudes from mice with 50 percent loss of ganglion cells were approximately twice as large as normal. Hair cell degeneration and hearing loss are also seen in certain strains of mice that develop audiogenic seizures following a brief exposure to intense sounds. As expected, the thresholds of mice primed for audiogenic seizures are higher than the thresholds of unprimed mice. However, at high stimulus levels, the evoked potentials of primed mice are considerably larger in amplitude than those of unprimed animals (Henry & Saleh, 1973; Saunders, Bock, James, & Chen, 1972). Genetically normal animals can also develop enhanced evoked potentials in the inferior colliculus after acoustic overstimulation (Gerken, Simhadri-Sumithra, & Bhat, 1986; Salvi, Powers, Saunders, Boettcher, & Clock, 1992; Salvi, Saunders, Gratton, Arehole, & Powers, 1990). In the region of greatest hearing loss, the amplitude of the evoked response increased at an abnormally rapid rate once threshold was exceeded; however, the maximum response amplitude was normal. Surprisingly, the maximum evoked response amplitude was sometimes two-to-three times larger than normal at frequencies located just outside the region of hearing loss (Salvi et al., 1992; Salvi et al., 1990).

Most evoked potential studies have failed to find enhanced response amplitudes at the level of the cochlear nucleus. In fact, the responses from the cochlear nucleus are generally depressed after acoustic stimulation (Salvi et al., 1992; Salvi et al., 1990). The most convincing evidence that the enhancement phenomenon originates in the central auditory pathway comes from electrical stimulation studies of animals with hearing loss. Behavioral thresholds elicited by electrical pulses delivered to different regions of the auditory brain show substantial improvement after the cochlea is damaged.

(Gerken et al., 1986; Gerken, 1979; Gerken, Saunders, & Paul, 1984; Gerken, Saunders, Simhadri-Sumithra, & Bhat, 1985). These results indicate that neurons in the central auditory pathway become more sensitive to electrical stimulation when the cochlea is damaged (inactivated). The increased sensitivity is similar to the denervation hypersensitivity seen in other sensory systems. This hypersensitivity may involve the upregulation of ion channels or receptors for excitatory neurotransmitters. Other potential mechanisms include the loss of inhibition due to the down regulation of inhibitory neurotransmitters or their receptors (Caspary, Blomquist, Wilson, Salvi, & Milbrandt, 1996) or the rapid inactivation of lateral inhibitory circuits resulting from partial destruction of the cochlea (Wang, Salvi, & Powers, 1996).

Lateral Inhibition and Rapid Reorganization

Evoked potential amplitude enhancement is generally most pronounced along the low frequency border of the hearing loss. This suggests that enhancement could result from the loss of lateral inhibition (disinhibition). Figure 5-5 is a model that illustrates how damage to the auditory periphery could lead to a loss of lateral inhibition and cause an increase in the amplitude of the evoked response. Low, medium and high-frequency tones selectively excite hair cells and auditory nerve fibers in the apical, middle and basal regions of the cochlea, respectively (Panel A). Each auditory nerve fiber has a V-shaped frequency-threshold tuning curve with a low-threshold, narrowly tuned tip. The frequency with the lowest threshold on the tuning curve is referred to as the characteristic frequency. Neurons with low characteristic frequencies contact IHCs in the apex of the cochlea and those with high characteristic frequencies contact hair cells in the base of the cochlea. Each auditory nerve fiber projects into the cochlear nucleus where it branches to contact neurons in anteroventral cochlear nucleus (AVCN), posteroventral cochlear

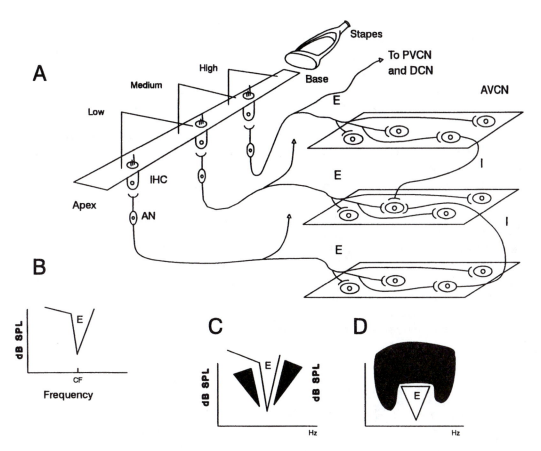

FIGURE 5-5. (**A**) Schematic showing the organization of the cochlea, auditory nerve and cochlear nucleus. High frequency sounds produce maximum excitation in base of cochlea, medium and low frequency sounds produce maximum vibration at progressively more apical region along the cochlea. Neurons from the auditory nerve (AN) contact inner hair cells (IHCs) and the axon of each AN fiber projects to the anteroventral cochlear nucleus (AVCN), posteroventral cochlear nucleus (PVCN) and dorsal cochlear nucleus (DCN). Schematic shows AN fibers making excitatory (E) contacts with neurons in isofrequency lamina in the AVCN. Neurons in each isofrequency sheet send inhibitory (I) inputs to isofrequency sheets tuned to higher or lower frequencies. (**B**) Schematic showing frequency-threshold response area of a cochlear nucleus neuron that has an excitatory (E) response area with a low-threshold, narrowly tuned tip near its characteristic frequency and a high-threshold, broadly tuned, low-frequency tail. (**C**) Response area map of cochlear nucleus neuron that has an excitatory response area (E) that is surrounded by an inhibitory response (black) area above characteristic frequency and below characteristic frequency. (**D**) Response area map of a cochlear nucleus neuron that has an enclosed excitatory response area near characteristic frequency that is completely surrounded by an inhibitory response area (black).

nucleus (PVCN) and dorsal cochlear nucleus (DCN). The cochlear nucleus is tonotopically organized into isofrequency laminae (sheets) in which all of the neurons are excited (E) by the same characteristic frequency.

Neurons in the AVCN with high characteristic frequencies are located near the dor-sal surface of the cochlear nucleus and those with low characteristic frequencies are located near the ventral surface. Neurons within the isofrequency sheet receive inhibitory (I) inputs that presumably originate from neurons in isofrequency laminae tuned to higher and lower characteristic frequencies. Thus, the response properties of neurons in the cochlear nucleus, as well as those in higher auditory centers, reflect the combination of both excitatory and inhibitory inputs. Because neurons in the central auditory pathway receive numerous excitatory and inhibitory inputs, their frequency response areas can be extremely complex as illustrated by the schematic in Figure 5-5. Some neurons (panel A) have excitatory response areas that are flanked by inhibitory areas while others have excitatory response areas that are surrounded by inhibitory areas (Ryan & Miller, 1978; Young, 1984). The darkly shaded areas in panels C and D show the frequency-intensity combinations that inhibit (I) a neuron. The solid lines show the frequency-intensity combinations that excite (E) the neuron. Since high intensity sounds produce a relatively broad vibration pattern that spreads towards the

high frequencies, a stimulus presented at or below characteristic frequency will activate both the excitatory inputs and inhibitory inputs at high stimulus levels. This in turn should reduce the neuron's discharge rate at suprathreshold levels. If the inhibitory inputs are eliminated by destroying the region of the cochlea that turns on the inhibition, then neurons in the central auditory system should be disinhibited. This should theoretically result in an increase in the maximum discharge rate and a broadening of the excitatory response area. A logical place to test this model is in the inferior colliculus where the enhancement effect has been seen after acoustic trauma.

The tuning curves of some neurons in the inferior colliculus, such as the one shown in Figure 5-6A, are extremely narrow (Wang, et al., 1996). This neuron was excited by a

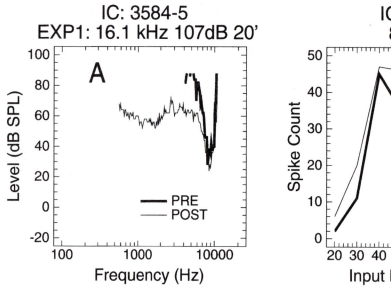
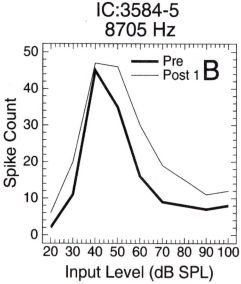

FIGURE 5-6. (**A**) Frequency-threshold tuning curve of narrowly tuned neuron in the inferior colliculus. Tuning curve measured preexposure (thick line) and postexposure (thin line). Neuron's preexposure characteristic frequency approximately 8 kHz at 28 dB SPL. Traumatizing tone presented at 16.1 kHz at 107 dB SPL for 20 minutes. Note that characteristic frequency-threshold is unchanged after the exposure. Neuron develops a low-frequency tail after the exposure and threshold in the low-frequency tail of the tuning curve improves after the exposure. (**B**) Discharge-rate versus SPL near the neuron's characteristic frequency preexposure and postexposure. Note the increase in discharge rate after the exposure, particularly at near-threshold levels (20 to 30 dB SPL) and at suprathreshold levels (40 to 100 dB SPL). Neuron's discharge rate-level function is strongly nonmonotonic.

small range of frequencies near characteristic frequency and was inhibited by a broad range of frequencies above and below characteristic frequency (data not shown). To damage the inputs to the inhibitory region above the characteristic frequency, an intense tone was presented for 15 minutes in the inhibitory response area above the characteristic frequency. When the traumatizing tone was turned on, it initially suppressed the spontaneous discharge rate, but as the exposure continued the discharge gradually increased. This increase in spontaneous rate suggests that the inhibition was reduced by the traumatizing tone. At the end of the traumatizing exposure, the neuron's response properties were remeasured. The neuron's postexposure spontaneous discharge rate increased approximately 50 percent. In addition, the neuron's excitatory tuning curve showed a dramatic expansion along the low frequency side of the tuning curve (Figure 5-6A) and thresholds in the 4 to 5 kHz region improved by as much as 25 dB.

Figure 5-6B shows the number of spike discharges that the neuron produced in response to tone bursts of increasing intensity (input/output function). The preexposure input/output function near the neuron's characteristic frequency (Figure 5-6B) was strongly nonmonotonic. The number of spike discharges initially increased, reached a maximum around 40 dB SPL and then dropped precipitously at higher intensities. This decline in the discharge rate is presumably due to the activation of inhibitory inputs to the cell.

After the traumatizing exposure, the spike count increased significantly in the nonmonotonic region of the input/output function suggesting that the inhibitory inputs to the cell were reduced. However, the rate decreased at higher intensities suggesting that the inhibition was still present. The neuron was generally unresponsive to sounds below characteristic frequency and therefore the input/output function was nearly flat at the low frequencies (data not

shown). However, after the traumatizing exposure, the neuron responded vigorously to low-frequency sounds greater than 50 dB SPL. Several aspects of these results are significant. First, intense sounds that damage a segment of the inner ear may actually cause the spontaneous activity and sound-evoked activity to increase in inferior colliculus neurons with characteristic frequencies located below the region of hearing loss. Second, traumatizing sounds presented above the excitatory response area can cause a dramatic expansion of the excitatory response area and significant improvement in threshold below characteristic frequency. The increase in discharge rate and the expansion of the excitatory response area are likely to contribute to the evoked response amplitude enhancement seen in the inferior colliculus. Approximately 40% of the neurons in the inferior colliculus showed an expansion of their excitatory response areas and an increase in discharge rate after the traumatizing tone was presented above the neuron's characteristic frequency. Neurons exhibiting increased responsiveness tended to have very narrow excitatory response areas and nonmonotonic input/output functions. These results indicate that a subset of neurons in the central auditory system become hyperactive after a segment of the cochlea is damaged.

Reflex Modulation

The preceding results indicate that cochlear damage can modify the functional properties of neurons in the central auditory pathway. However, it is important to determine if these neurophysiological changes have any effect on hearing or behaviors that rely on hearing. One technique that can be used to address this question is the acoustic startle modification paradigm (Willott, 1996; Willott, Carlson, & Chen, 1994). This paradigm uses a high intensity noise burst (S2) to evoke a standard behavioral startle response that can be quantified by the degree of movement of the animal. The magnitude of the startle response can be reduced by a low intensity stimulus (S1) that precedes S2. The reduction of the startle response by S1 is referred to as prepulse inhibition. If the S1 stimulus is a salient cue for the animal, it will significantly reduce the startle response. Conversely, if the S1 stimulus has little effect on the magnitude of the startle reflex, then S1 presumably has little behavioral relevance. In mice that develop age-related hearing loss, prepulse inhibition is greatly reduced in the region of high frequency hearing loss suggesting that information in this region may be less relevant than normal. On the other hand, prepulse inhibition is significantly enhanced at the low frequency edge of the hearing loss where hearing is fairly well preserved. Frequencies that manifest enhanced prepulse inhibition correspond well to regions where the greatest evoked response enhancement and greatest expansion of the tonotopic map occur.

Reorganization Reflected in Aberrant Cross Modality Interactions

Although the pathophysiology that underlies the development of tinnitus is unknown, the observation that sensorineural hearing loss can result in significant reorganization of the central auditory pathway provides a scientific basis for understanding several unusual forms of tinnitus. Interestingly, a substantial number of patients are able to alter the loudness and/or pitch of their tinnitus by voluntarily activating motor centers or nonauditory sensory systems. It has been hypothesized that cochlear damage may, in some severe cases, result in cross-modality interactions due to the rewiring of nonauditory centers with nuclei in the classical auditory pathway (Cacace, Lovely, McFarland, Parnes, & Winter, 1994; Lockwood et al., 1996).

In the early 1980s, a series of brief papers described an usual group of patients who developed an unusual form of tinnitus fol-lowing surgical removal of a tumor that resulted in the destruction of the auditory nerve (House, 1982; Whittaker, 1982; Whittaker, 1983). Approximately one month following surgery, the patients reported that they could control the loudness and/or pitch of their tinnitus by moving their eyes. Wall subsequently reported more detailed observations made on two such patients and concluded that this symptom was best explained by an abnormal interaction between the cochlear nucleus and the brain stem neural integrator controlling eye movements (Wall, Rosenberg, & Richardson, 1987a; Wall, Rosenberg, & Richardson, 1987b). Both of these patients also reported brief phantom visual sensations that were evoked by eye movements. Cacace and colleagues have identified additional cases and also concluded that this rare phenomenon is the result of aberrant connections between the auditory and eye-control systems (Cacace et al., 1994; Cacace, Lovely, Parnes, Winter, & McFaland, 1996b).

An association between temporomandibular joint dysfunction and tinnitus has also been noted (for review, see Chan & Reade, 1994). Many explanations for this association have been advanced, including mechanical effects of jaw movement on the Eustachian tube, co-contraction of muscles innervated by the facial nerve, and common embryological origins of many affected structures from the first pharyngeal arch. During the course of evaluations designed to probe links between tinnitus and temporal mandibular joint dysfunction (Rubinstein, Axelsson, & Carlsson, 1990; Vernon, Griest, & Press, 1992) researchers noted that exaggerated jaw movements changed the perceptual characteristics of the tinnitus. The Rubinstein study was derived from consecutive patients that visited an audiological clinic, whereas the Vernon study was composed of patients with and without temporal mandibular joint dysfunction. They found that among the patients with temporal mandibular joint dysfunction, 36 percent reported changes in the perception of their tinnitus with jaw movement, whereas only 11 percent of the comparison group reported such changes.

Cacace and colleagues (Cacace et al., 1995; 1996) have reported a subject in which tinnitus could be evoked by cutaneous stimulation to the back of the hand. This subject developed gaze-evoked tinnitus several weeks following complete resection of the seventh and eighth nerve to remove a glomus jugulare tumor. Her gaze-evoked tinnitus was evoked whenever the eyes deviated to the left, or vertically. When the subject's eyes were straight ahead, the gaze-evoked tinnitus disabled, stimulation of the left upper anterior hand near the wrist evoked a tonal tinnitus. Moller et al. (1992b) evaluated the interaction of the somatosensory and auditory systems by investigating the effects of electrical stimulation of the median nerve located near the wrist of subjects with tinnitus. In twenty-six subjects evaluated, median nerve stimulation resulted in a noticeable increase in the magnitude of the tinnitus in four subjects, and six subjects noticed a decrease in the magnitude of the tinnitus. The reports of Cacace et al. (1995; 1996) and Moller et al. (1992b) are instructive, because they tell us that stimulation of the somatosensory system other than that mediated by the trigeminal nerve can modulate tinnitus. In the case of gaze-evoked tinnitus or tinnitus modulation by oral-facial movements, one can look at the distribution of the trigeminal nerve and its central projections, or the vestibulo-ocular system, and suggest that these apparently aberrant cross-modality interactions require close approximation of the peripheral sensory receptors or central projections of the two systems. This makes the collateral sprouting hypothesis attractive. The patient with cutaneous-evoked tinnitus reported by Cacace et al. (1995; 1996) suggests that this proximity is not requisite. Cacace et al. (1994a) interpret gaze-evoked tinnitus to be a maladaptive consequence of nervous sys-

tem plasticity. Cacace uses the term plasticity in the functional sense, rather than pointing to any specific mechanism. The time course of development of both gaze-evoked and cutaneous tinnitus is on the order of four to six weeks (Cacace et al., 1994b), which might support an anatomical mechanism such as collateral sprouting, where one would predict a comparatively long time course to rewire. An alternative hypothesis would be that the tinnitus is a consequence of changes in the synaptic input to multimodal neurons. For example, there are neurons in the external and paracentral nuclei of the inferior colliculus that respond to both auditory and somatosensory stimulation (Aitkin et al., 1975; 1978; 1981). If the auditory input to these neurons is disrupted by eighth-nerve section, these inactivated auditory inputs over time may degenerate, or be replaced (either anatomically or functionally) by the somatosensory input. The results of such changes may lead to the aberrant auditory perception of tinnitus. The interaction of tinnitus and oral-facial movements may be the result of changes in multimodal neurons meant to suppress the perception of self-generated sounds during chewing and related behaviors. The value of this circuit for survival is obvious. That about one-third of subjects with temporomandibular joint problems can modulate their tinnitus by oral-facial movements (Rubinstein et al, 1990) supports this hypothesis. The interaction between the auditory and oculomotor system could similarly be the result of a reduction of auditory input during activities requiring visual pursuit, where attentional resources must be allocated to the visual system. However, it is harder to rationalize the interaction of the cutaneous receptors on the hand and the auditory system. Cacace and colleague's subject with cutaneous modulation of tinnitus makes the "normal function laid bare" concept of tinnitus as the result of inactivation of the auditory inputs to multimodal neurons tenuous.

PHYSIOLOGIC/METABOLIC MANIFESTATIONS OF TINNITUS IN HUMAN SUBJECTS

Auditory-Evoked Potentials

Moller et al. (1992a) have recorded the compound action potential from the exposed eighth nerve of nineteen patients suffering from tinnitus. In general, the latencies of N_1 and N_2 were highly similar in the tinnitus subjects and in patients with similar audiograms but no tinnitus. In only one subject were distinct compound action potential abnormalities found that were unattributable to hearing loss. These data would appear to suggest that any physiologic manifestations of tinnitus are not observed in the compound action potential.

As we are promoting the theory that tinnitus is a perceptual manifestation of auditory plasticity, it is instructive to review the studies that have investigated auditory evoked potentials known to emanate from the central auditory nervous system. Reports on auditory brain stem response abnormalities and tinnitus have been inconsistent. Schulman and Seitz (Shulman & Seitz, 1981) reported a variety of auditory brain stem response abnormalities in tinnitus patients, including latency and interwave interval increases and abnormal amplitude ratios. However, interpretation of their data is hampered by the absence of a control group. Moller et al. (1992a), in addition to recording the compound action potential from the exposed eighth nerve, recorded the auditory brain stem response. Wave III latencies in tinnitus patients were not significantly different than the control group with similar audiograms. However, wave V latency was significantly *shorter* in the tinnitus subjects than the control subjects. Ikner and Hassen (1990) compared the latencies and inter-peak intervals of the auditory brain stem response in tinnitus patients and in a control group matched for gender and audiometric thresholds (1 to 4 kHz). With the exception of a prolonged wave I latency

in the female tinnitus patients, there were no significant differences in auditory brain stem response peak latencies and interwave intervals in tinnitus and control groups. Barnea et al. (1990) investigated the auditory brain stem response to 120 dB SPL clicks in tinnitus sufferers with normal hearing, comparing responses with a control group matched for gender and age. The two groups were not significantly different in terms of high-frequency (9 to 20 kHz) thresholds, and there were no significant differences across groups in terms of the latency or amplitudes of waves I, III or V, or the I-V interval. Taken as a whole, the auditory brain stem response in tinnitus patients appears to be minimally different than in a control group matched for age, gender and hearing loss.

Several studies have investigated event-related potentials in tinnitus patients. Shiraishi et al. (1991) found that the contingent negative variation (CNV) amplitude was enhanced in tinnitus patients, as compared to age-matched controls. However, the latency and amplitude of the N100 (N1) and P300 (P3) waves did not differ between tinnitus and control groups. Attias et al. (1993) evaluated event-related potentials to repetitive 1 kHz tone bursts and to stimuli presented by the oddball paradigm, using 1 kHz "target" tones and 2 kHz "nontarget" tones. Experimental groups included a tinnitus group and an age- and hearing-matched control group. Although no latency differences were seen across groups, the amplitudes of N1, P2, and P3 were significantly smaller in the tinnitus group. There were no differences in the latencies, interwave intervals or amplitudes of the various auditory brain stem response peaks across subject groups. Attias et al. compared auditory and visual event-related potentials in tinnitus patients with an age- and hearing-matched control group. P3 latencies were prolonged in tinnitus patients for both auditory and visual stimuli. While P3 amplitudes were reduced in tinnitus patients for auditory stimulation, they were not significantly different from those of the control group for visual stimulation. Attias et al. (1993) also found that N1 and N2 to nontarget auditory stimuli were prolonged in the tinnitus group. Although the effects seem to vary across study, it appears that event-related potentials differ in tinnitus patients when a control group is used that matches for age and hearing loss.

Magnetic-Evoked Potentials

A serious shortcoming of obtaining auditory-evoked potentials by recording the electrical activity from the scalp is the inability to unambiguously identify the specific site of the neural generators within the auditory pathway. One technique that partially overcomes the problem of localizing the neural generators involves the use of sensitive and extremely sophisticated instrumentation to record the magnetic fields that are produced by a current source within the brain. Unlike electrical potentials, the magnetic fields are minimally distorted by the brain, dura, skull or scalp, at least for magnetic-field frequencies below 1,000 Hz (Kaufman & Williamson, 1982). This facilitates the localization of a current dipole source within the brain. The recording of magnetic evoked potentials requires a device that can convert magnetic fields to voltages. This device is called a superconducting, quantum interference device (SQUID). At the heart of the SQUID is a second-order gradiometer, which facilitates the detection of small-magnitude (on the order of tens to hundreds of femtoteslas), nearby magnetic fields produced by groups of neurons in the brain. A unique feature of the gradiometer is its ability to separate the weak, but nearby magnetic fields in the brain from the very large (on the order of 70 microteslas), but more distant, magnetic field generated by the earth (Kaufman & Williamson, 1982; Williamson & Kaufman, 1988). The gradiometer is placed in a Dewar flask containing liquid helium maintained at a temperature of −269° C. This puts the device into a superconducting state, which makes it possible for the device to detect extraordinarily small magnetic fields. Once the magnetic field is converted to an electrical voltage, the voltage is amplified and time-domain signal averaging is used to extract the magnetic evoked potential from the background magnetic "noise." The current dipole can be viewed as having a tangential and radial component at right angles to each other, with the total current the vector sum of the two components. In magnetic-evoked potentials, one can only measure the magnetic fields that are generated by a current dipole flowing tangentially to the surface of the head (Kaufman & Williamson, 1982). This means that the magnetic field measured with the magnetic evoked potentials is not only dependent on the magnitude of the current dipole (basically the number of neurons responding) and the distance of this current dipole from the surface of the head, but also the orientation of the equivalent dipole. It is worth keeping this latter point in mind when interpreting magnetic-evoked potential data.

Magnetic-Evoked Potentials and Tinnitus

Several studies have investigated auditory magnetic-evoked potentials in tinnitus patients. Hoke et al. (1989) reported that patients suffering from tinnitus showed differing magnetic-evoked potential amplitudes than a control group of normal hearing young adults. Specifically, the amplitude of the M100 wave (the magnetic homologue of N1 of the late components of the auditory-evoked potentials) was augmented in the tinnitus patients (as compared to controls), while wave M200 (corresponding to AEP wave P2) was poorly developed in tinnitus subjects. They reported a M200/M100 amplitude ratio of less than 0.5 in all patients suffering from tinnitus, while a ratio of greater that 0.5 was found in control subjects who were less than fifty years of age. The M200/M100 amplitude ratio decreased with age, and hence the tinnitus and control group M200/M100 amplitude ratios overlapped for ages greater than fifty years.

Both groups had normal hearing at the test frequency of 1,000 Hz, but no attempt was made to control for hearing loss at higher frequencies across groups. Pantev and colleagues (Pantev, Hoke, Lutkenhoner, Lehnertz, & Kumpf, 1989) followed a patient who reported the onset of tinnitus following mild noise-induced hearing loss (<25 dB HL at 3 to 4 kHz). This patient showed a M200/M100 amplitude ratio of substantially less than 0.5 up to 69 days posttrauma. During this time, the tinnitus reportedly changed from continuous to intermittent. By 100 days posttrauma, the tinnitus only reappeared for a few hours when the patient was exposed to loud music. By 256 days posttrauma, the patient was completely free of tinnitus. At this time, their M200/M100 ratio was 1.1 and it was suggested (Pantev et al., 1989) that these findings supported those of Hoke et al. (1989); that is, that a M200/M100 ratio of less than 0.5 is correlated with the perception of tinnitus. Jacobson et al. (1991) compared auditory magnetic-evoked potentials in normal hearing young adults with those of subjects with monaural tinnitus and hearing loss. They found no significant difference in the M200/M100 amplitude ratios between the normal-hearing group and the tinnitus/hearing-impaired group. Furthermore, there were no differences in the M200/M100 ratio when comparing magnetic-evoked potentials obtained by stimulating the normal ear with those elicited by stimulating the hearing-loss/tinnitus ear in the unilateral tinnitus/hearing-loss group. Colding-Jorgensen and colleagues (Colding-Jorgensen, Lauritzen, Johnsen, Mikkelsen, & Saermark, 1992) compared magnetic-evoked potentials in a group of tinnitus subjects and an age- and gender-matched control group. Although audiograms were not matched across groups, all subjects had thresholds of 20 dB HL or better at 1,000 Hz, the frequency of tone bursts used to elicit the magnetic evoked potentials. In agreement with Jacobson et al., Colding-Jorgensen et al. found no differences in the two subject groups in the latency or amplitude of the N100 or

P200 magnetic-evoked potential peaks. Available magnetic-evoked potential data do not consistently demonstrate differences in auditory magnetic-evoked potentials between nontinnitus and tinnitus subjects. Future studies should consider matching tinnitus and nontinnitus groups for hearing loss.

Brain Imaging Techniques

During the past two decades, enormous advances in functional brain imaging technology have provided clinicians and researchers with powerful new tools to investigate the neural substrates of tinnitus. While techniques such as positron emission tomography, single photon emission computerized tomography and functional magnetic resonance imaging represent giant technological steps forward in terms of studying brain pathologies, each method has certain advantages as well as technological limitations.

Functional brain imaging is based on techniques that have emerged from more conventional clinical imaging strategies such as x-ray-computed tomography, magnetic resonance imaging, and positron emission tomography. Instead of showing an image of brain structure, as with x-ray-computed tomography or magnetic resonance imaging, functional images portray biochemical or physiological processes such as blood flow. The development of statistical methods to compare these images has made it possible to create maps of the brain that quantitatively depict the functional differences between two states (for example, different experimental conditions, groups of subjects, and so on). The functional changes can be quantified and assigned to specific anatomical sites. These images identify specific brain regions where neural activity differs between two states or conditions. The images are usually presented in a standard stereotaxic frame of reference or as a statistical image superimposed on an anatomical scan of the brain such as a T_1-weighted magnetic resonance imaging scan. Since the nature of the tasks to be studied is not usually a limiting factor, these methods have been used to investigate a variety of functions ranging. For example, one can map brain regions activated by simple formless visual stimuli (Phelps, Mazziotta, & Huang, 1982), or map brain regions activated by very complex tasks such as those that differentiate the formation of past tenses of regular versus irregular English verbs. (Jaeger et al.). Initial functional imaging techniques were based on the use of positron emission tomography. More recently, magnetic resonance imaging technology has been adapted to produce functional images, functional magnetic resonance imaging, in addition to more standard anatomical images.

Positron emission tomography and functional magnetic resonance imaging techniques depend on the fact that the brain has virtually no reserves of energy, in spite of the fact that 15 to 20 percent of the resting cardiac output is required to supply glucose and oxygen to meet cerebral energy demands. As a result, as the amount of brain work and the rate of energy consumption change, there must be parallel and proportional increments (or decrements) in the delivery and consumption of metabolic substrates. Since the normal brain uses aerobic glucose metabolism as its only source of energy, measurements of glucose or oxygen metabolic rates, or measurements of cerebral blood flow, reflect brain activity. Thus, in a steady state, changes in metabolism or cerebral blood flow mirror the changes in neural activity that are associated with changes in brain function. In practice, measurements of glucose metabolism and cerebral blood flow form the basis for positron emission tomography techniques, while changes in oxygenation of blood underlie magnetic resonance imaging-based techniques.

Glucose metabolism and cerebral blood flow are both measured with relative ease using positron emission tomography. Glucose metabolism is measured by quantifying the cerebral uptake of 2-fluoro-2-deoxy-D-glucose labeled with ^{18}F (FDG). This glucose analog is transported across the blood-brain barrier and is phosphorylated by the same systems that transport and catalyze the metabolism of glucose. Unlike glucose, the metabolism of FDG stops after phosphorylation and FDG-6-phosphate remains trapped in the brain at the site of uptake and metabolism. Thus the amount of ^{18}F in the brain 40 minutes after the injection of FDG is proportional to the rate of glucose metabolism (40 minutes is required for complete uptake and phosphorylation to occur). The FDG technique is limited by the 40-minute uptake period and the 110-minute half-life of ^{18}F. Although most FDG is taken up in the first 15 minutes after the injection of the tracer, it is difficult to maintain a steady state uptake for this length of time. This occurs because of subject fatigue and the high probability that task familiarity and learning lead to alterations in the amount of energy the neural systems require to perform the task. The isotopic half-life also makes it impractical to conduct sequential studies in a given subject. For these reasons, FDG studies are usually restricted to comparisons of resting states where no specific task is being performed.

An alternative method of assessing brain activity, which overcomes some of the limitations of glucose metabolism, is to assess cerebral blood flow. Since typical tracers of cerebral blood flow have short half-lives, repeated measurements requiring short imaging times (and hence short behavioral steady-state times) are practical. This overcomes some of the limitations imposed by glucose metabolism. Since ^{15}O has a 123-second half-life and labeled water diffuses in and out of the brain rapidly, its biological half-life in the brain is very short, and serial studies of the same subject in the same experimental session are feasible. Typically, 1-minute data acquisition times are employed for each brain scan sequence. In some studies, more than a dozen different scans may be obtained. Statistical power is gained if tasks are repeated. For example, in a six-scan sequence there may be two repetitions of each of three tasks. Although single-subject studies are possible, functional positron emission tomography studies usually require multiple subjects, even with task repetition, to gain sufficient statistical power to yield reliable results. Positron emission tomography cameras typically image all or most of the brain, an advantage over functional magnetic resonance imaging techniques that are usually restricted to the acquisition of data from a single tomographic plane.

Since the changes in glucose metabolism and cerebral blood flow that are associated with changes in neural activity are relatively small in comparison to either resting glucose metabolism or cerebral blood flow, most functional neuroimaging studies are based on relative rather than absolute measurements of these variables. This reality simplifies substantially the experimental measurements, since absolute quantification requires arterial blood sampling in addition to the acquisition of brain images.

In contrast to positron emission tomography, functional magnetic resonance imaging techniques rely on changes in the paramagnetic properties of hemoglobin as it gains or loses oxygen (Hunter, 1996; Kwong, 1995). The blood oxygen level dependent (BOLD) technique is the most widely used of the magnetic resonance imaging techniques. As neural activity increases in a brain region, there are local increases in cerebral blood flow and cerebral blood volume. Since the blood volume increase outstrips the increase in oxygen metabolism, cerebral venous blood in the brain region that is activated is more highly oxygenated than at rest. This difference in oxygenation can be detected using suitably designed magnetic resonance imaging pulse sequences and magnetic resonance imaging systems equipped with magnets of 1.5 Teslas or more. The time interval required to acquire enough data to produce a reliable image using this technique is shorter than with positron emission tomography. Typically, multiple brief stimuli are presented (for instance, a checkerboard pattern in which the squares alternately

change from black to white to stimulate the visual system) and data from the two states are acquired in a sequence. The data from these two states forms the image after statistical treatment. The functional study is usually preceded by a conventional imaging session that is used to select the regions of interest for the functional study and to provide an anatomical framework on which to superimpose the functional data. The final result is a high-resolution, between-state statistical image superimposed on an anatomical image of a single subject.

Both positron emission tomography and magnetic resonance imaging functional imaging techniques can be applied to the study of single subjects or groups of subjects. Each technique has advantages and disadvantages (Nadeau & Crosson, 1995; Sergent, 1994). For studies of the auditory system, functional magnetic resonance imaging protocols are hampered by the high levels of background acoustic noise produced by magnetic resonance imaging systems. Typically, magnetic resonance imaging units produce background sounds that are in excess of 75 dB SPL, and thus relatively high stimulus levels may be required. The high levels of background noise may drive some neurons in the auditory pathway into saturation and prevent them from responding to the test stimulus. Since certain equipment containing wires or magnets (for example, speakers, microphones) will not function properly in the strong magnetic fields of functional magnetic resonance imaging unit, many technical obstacles must be overcome to solve these and other problems.

Application of Brain Imaging Techniques to Tinnitus

Single Photon Emission Computerized Tomography

The earliest radioisotope technique applied to the study of tinnitus involved single photon emission computerized tomography. Shulman and his associates (Shulman, 1995;

Sulman et al., 1995) used single photon emission computerized tomography to measure cerebral blood flow in several patients with severe tinnitus. They reported perfusion abnormalities in a number of brain regions including mesial temporal lobe structures such as the hippocampus and amygdala, and asymmetry of flow in frontal, temporal, and parietal cortical regions. They conclude that tinnitus is due to an organic dysfunction of the brain that involves mesial temporal structures. While single photon emission computerized tomography imaging can provide a qualitative picture of differences in regional CFB; the interpretation of the results are limited by the nonquantitative nature of the imaging methods.

Positron Emission Tomography

We have recently identified several patients who are able to exert voluntary control over the loudness of their tinnitus by performing oral-facial movements (Lockwood, Salvi, Coad, Wack, & Murphy, 1997; Salvi et al., 1996a). Two of these subjects experienced an increase in tinnitus loudness while two experienced a decrease in loudness.

The ability of patients to modulate the loudness of their tinnitus provides us with a unique opportunity to compare the pattern of brain activity under two different tinnitus states, the normal tinnitus condition and the condition where the oral-facial movements makes the tinnitus louder or quieter. We used positron emission tomography to measure the changes in cerebral blood flow during the oral-facial movements. A control group of subjects had normal hearing and no tinnitus. In normal subjects, we predicted that the oral-facial movements would only cause a change in cerebral blood flow (activation) in the region of the somatosensory and motor cortices associated with the jaw and lower face. However, in the tinnitus patients, we predicted that the oral-facial movements would not only activate the somatosensory and motor cortex, but also the auditory cortex, since the change in cerebral blood flow

in this region would presumably correspond to the change in tinnitus loudness. In the control subjects, the oral-facial movements produced the expected increase in activation in the somatosensory and motor cortices and the supplementary motor areas of the brain without affecting auditory centers. However, in tinnitus patients, the oral-facial movements produced striking changes in cerebral blood flow in auditory cortical areas as well as somatosensory and motor areas of the brain. Figure 5-7 shows the results in three patients who all report a change in the loudness of right ear tinnitus while performing the oral-facial movements. A prominent region of activation was observed in the left primary auditory cortex. The data from these patients provide convincing evidence for aberrant neural links between the somatosensory and motor systems and the auditory system.

In additional studies performed in this group of subjects, we examined the effects of stimulating the auditory system with low-frequency tones (0.5 and 2 kHz), as both subject groups had normal low-frequency hearing. When we compared brain regions activated by the 2.0 kHz tones in normal hearing subjects versus the regions activated in our tinnitus patients with high frequency sensorineural hearing loss, we found more extensive activation in the temporal lobe of the experimental group compared to controls. Since the 2.0 kHz stimulus was in a region of normal hearing at the edge of the hearing loss, the expanded area of activation is consistent with animal studies showing an expanded cortical representation at frequencies adjacent to the cochlear lesion (Recanzone, Schreiner, & Merzenich, 1993; Willott, Aitkin, & McFadden, 1993). In addition to excess activation of auditory cortex, we also found that sound stimulation activated portions of the limbic system of experimental (tinnitus) subjects, but not controls. These data indicate that abnormal neural links have developed between the limbic system, an important emotional center, and the auditory system. These abnormal links may help explain why

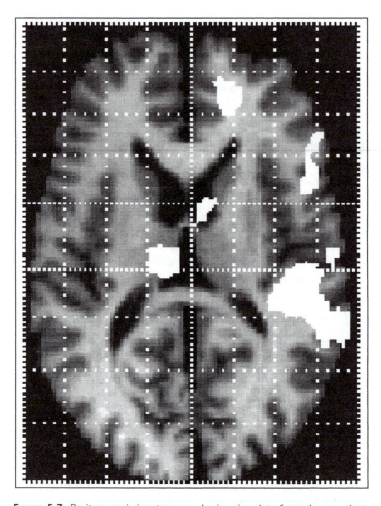

FIGURE 5-7. Positron emission tomography imaging data from three patients able to change tinnitus loudness by performing an oral-facial movement had cerebral blood flow measured at rest and during oral-facial movements. Regions where cerebral blood flow changed significantly are shown in white and are superimposed on a T_1-weighted composite magnetic resonance imaging image. A prominent area of altered cerebral blood flow is seen in the left temporal lobe including primary auditory cortex. The data link changes in the loudness of tinnitus and suggest that the phantom sounds of tinnitus affect this part of the brain.

tinnitus can be so emotionally disabling in some tinnitus patients.

The data from this study provide evidence for substantial reorganization of neural pathways related to auditory function. The loudness modulation induced by oral-facial movements appears to be associated with aberrant connections between sensory-motor and auditory pathways. In addition, there is an expansion of the auditory cortical response area to pure tones, an indication that the auditory system itself has developed a modified tonotopic map in these patients. Finally, we have found links between the auditory and limbic systems that may be related to the development of the powerful psychological symptoms that often accompany tinnitus. These tantalizing brain-imaging data pose more questions than they answer. What is the relative importance of tinnitus and hearing loss in these subjects? How representative of the general tinnitus population are these subjects who can modulate their tinnitus? The answers to these and other questions await additional studies.

Functional Magnetic Resonance Imaging

At about the same time that the positron emission tomography imaging studies were being performed, Cacace and his associates used functional magnetic resonance imaging techniques to study two patients who could modulate the loudness and pitch of their tinnitus with eye movements or cutaneous stimulation (Cacace et al., 1996a; Cacace et al., 1996b). In their gaze-evoked tinnitus patients, but not in normal subjects, eye movements evoked abnormal foci of activity in the upper brain stem and frontal cortex. They suggested that functional magnetic resonance imaging might be a powerful tool for evaluating the neural structures involved with gaze-evoked tinnitus. As the background noise in the scanners is reduced, the value of functional magnetic resonance imaging for localizing pathological activity in the auditory brain is likely to increase.

SUMMARY AND CONCLUSION

It is clear from recent relevant experimental studies in hearing, vision and taction that the central nervous system is capable of substantial functional reorganization following insult to the peripheral receptor surface in all three sensory systems. While the mechanisms underlying functional reorganization are currently unknown, it appears that auditory cortical regions rendered quiescent by cochlear damage are taken over by adjacent frequency regions, resulting in an expanded cortical representation of frequency regions adjacent to the damaged region. A review of experimental findings in

tinnitus patients demonstrates the presence of aberrant cross-modality interactions in some individuals. It has been known for some time that a small subgroup of patients can modulate the loudness and pitch of their tinnitus by moving and/or touching the lower jaw or face. This cross-modality interaction is extremely difficult to explain if one adopts the classical, hardwired view of the nervous system, particularly since these motor and somatosensory activities normally do not produce or modulate our auditory experiences. However, our recent positron emission tomography imaging studies show that movement of the jaw and lower face, which normally activate only the somatosensory and motor cortex in normal subjects, also activate regions of the auditory brain in patients with severe tinnitus. We suggest that tinnitus may be a maladaptive manifestation of the functional reorganization of the auditory system that occurs after cochlear damage. This same hypothesis has been offered as an explanation for phantom limb pain. Patients with the most severe limb pain exhibited the greatest amount of reorganization of the somatosensory cortex. It is important to recognize that not all patients with cochlear damage develop tinnitus. It may be that the degree of auditory system reorganization in some individuals is insufficient to produce these phantom auditory sensations. Conversely, some individuals have tinnitus, but appear to have normal hearing and presumably a normal cochlea. Cases such as this appear to be inconsistent with a tinnitus model based on cochlear damage and central nervous system reorganization. There could be several reasons for this. First, patients with so-called normal hearing may in fact have discrete cochlear lesions that are undetected by conventional audiometry, particularly damage that corresponds to regions of the cochlea that are associated with frequencies above 8 kHz. Second, focal lesions to lower brain stem regions are unlikely to be detected with conventional audiometry, but such damage could nevertheless give rise to cortical reorganization.

ACKNOWLEDGEMENTS

Work supported in part by a grant from the American Tinnitus Association and grants from NIDCD (NIH grant R01 DC00166, R01 DC03306).

REFERENCES

Aitkin, L. M., Dickhaus, H., Schult, W., & Zimmermann, M. (1978). External nucleus of inferior colliculus: Auditory and spinal somatosensory afferents and their interactions. *Journal of Neurophysiology, 41,* 837–847.

Aitkin, L. M., Kenyon, C. E., & Philpott, P. (1981). The representation of the auditory and somatosensory systems in the external nucleus of the cat inferior colliculus. *Journal of Comparative Neurology, 196,* 25–40.

Aitkin, L. M., Webster, W. R., Veal, J. L., & Crosby, D. C. (1975). Inferior colliculus. I. Comparison of response properties of neurons in central, pericentral and external nuclei of adult cat. *Journal of Neurophysiology, 38,* 1196–1207.

Attias, J., Furman, V., Shemesh, Z., & Bresloff, I. (1996). Impaired brain processing in noise-induced tinnitus patients as measured by auditory and visual event-related potentials. *Ear & Hearing, 17*(4), 327–333.

Attias, J., Urbach, D., Gold, S., & Shemesh, Z. (1993). Auditory event related potentials in chronic tinnitus patients with noise induced hearing loss. *Hearing Research, 71*(1–2), 106–113.

Barnea, G., Attias, J., Gold, S., & Shahar, A. (1990). Tinnitus with normal hearing sensitivity: Extended high-frequency audiometry and auditory-nerve brain-stem-evoked responses. *Audiology, 29*(1), 36–45.

Cacace, A. T., Cousins, J. P., Moonen, C. T. W., van Geldren, P., Miller, D., Parnes, S. M., & Lovely, T. J. (1996a). In-vivo localization of phantom auditory perceptions during functional magnetic imaging. In G. E. Reich & J. A. Vernon (Eds.), *Proceedings of the Fifth International Tinnitus Seminar* (pp. 397–401). Portland, OR: American Tinnitus Association.

Cacace, A. T., Lovely, T. J., McFarland, D. J., Parnes, S. M., & Winter, D. F. (1994). Anomalous cross-modal plasticity following posterior fossa surgery: some speculations on gaze-evoked tinnitus. *Hearing Research, 81*(1–2), 22–32.

Cacace, A. T., Lovely, T. J., Parnes, S. M., Winter, D. F., & McFarland, D. J. (1996b). Gaze-evoked tinnitus following unilateral peripheral auditory deafferentation: A case for anomolous cross modality plasticity. In R. J. Salvi, D. Henderon, F. Fiorino, & V. Colletti (Eds.), *Auditory System Plasticity and Regeneration* (pp. 1354–1358). New York: Thieme Medical Publishers.

Calford, M. B., & Tweedale, R. (1988). Immediate and chronic changes in responses of somatosensory cortex in adult flying-fox after digit amputation. *Nature, 332,* 446–448.

Calford, M. B., & Tweedale, R. (1990). Interhemispheric transfer of plasticity in the cerebral cortex. *Science, 249,* 805–807.

Caspary, D. M., Blomquist, T. S., Wilson, M. C., Salvi, R., & Milbrandt, J. C. (1996). GAD immunoreactivity in the inferior colliculus following acute sound exposure: Loss of inhibition? *Abstract of Association for Research in Otolaryngology.*

Chan, S. W. Y., & Read, P. C. (1994). Tinnitus and temporomandibular pain-dysfunction disorder. *Clinical Otolaryngology, 19,* 370–380.

Colding-Jorgensen, E., Lauritzen, M., Johnsen, N. J., Mikkelsen, K. B., & Saermark, K. (1992). On the evidence of auditory evoked magnetic fields as an objective measure of tinnitus. *Electroencephalography Clinical Neurophysiology, 83,* 322–327.

Darian-Smith, C., & Gilbert, C. D. (1994). Axonal sprouting accompanies functional reorganization in adult cat striate cortex. *Nature, 368,* 737–740.

Dostrovsky, J. O., Millar, J., & Wall, P. D. (1976). The immediate shift of afferent drive of dorsal column nucleus cells following deafferentation: A comparison of acute and chronic deafferentation in gracile nucleus and spinal cord. *Experimental Neurology, 52,* 480–495.

Elbert, T., Pantev, C., Wienbruch, C., Rockstroh, B., & Taub, E. (1995). Increased cortical representation of the fingers of the left hand in string players. *Science, 270,* 305–307.

Erzurlumlu, R. S., Jhaveri, S., & Benowitz, L. I. (1990). Transient patterns of GAP-43 expression during the formation of barrels in the rat somatosensory cortex. *Journal of Comparative Neurology, 292,* 443–456.

Eysel, U. T., Gonzalez-Aguilar, F., & Mayer, U. (1980). A functional sign of reorganization in the visual system of adult cats: Lateral geniculate neurons with displaced receptive fields after lesions of the nasal retina. *Brain Research, 191,* 285–300.

Eysel, U. T., Gonzalez-Aguilar, F., & Mayer, U. (1981). Time-dependent decrease in the extent of visual deafferentation in the lateral geniculate nucleus of adult cats with small retinal lesions. *Experimental Brain Research, 41,* 256–263.

Flor, H., Elbert, T., Knecht, S., Wienbruch, C., Pantev, C., Birbaumer, B., Larbig, W., & Taub, E. (1995). Phantom-limb pain as a perceptual correlate of cortical reorganization following arm amputation. *Nature, 375,* 482–484.

Gerken, G., Simhadri-Sumithra, R., & Bhat, H. H. V. (1986). Increase in central auditory responsiveness during continuous tone stimulation or following hearing loss. In R. J. Salvi, R. P. Hamernik, D. Henderson, & V. Colletti (Eds.), *Basic and applied aspects of noise induced hearing loss* (pp. 195–212). New York: Plenum Press.

Gerken, G. M. (1979). Central denervation hypersensitivity in the auditory system of the cat. *Journal of the Acoustical Society of America, 66*(3), 721–727.

Gerken, G. M., Saunders, S. S., & Paul, R. E. (1984). Hypersensitivity to electrical stimulation of auditory nuclei following hearing loss in cats. *Hearing Research, 13,* 249–259.

Gerken, G. M., Saunders, S. S., Simhadri-Sumithra. R., & Bhat, K. H. (1985). Behavioral thresholds for electrical stimulation applied to auditory brain stem nuclei in cat are altered by injurious and noninjurious sound. *Hearing Research, 20*(3), 221–231.

Goldstein, B., & Shulman, A. (1996). Tinnitus-Hyperacusis and the loudness discomfort level test: A preliminary report. *The International Tinnitus Journal, 2,* 83–89.

Harrison, R. V., Nagasawa, A., Smith, D. W., Stanton, S., & Mount, R. J. (1991). Reorganization of auditory cortex after neonatal high frequency cochlear hearing loss. *Hearing Research, 54,* 11–19.

Harrison, R. V., Smith, D. W., Nagasawa, A., & Mount, R. J. (1992). Developmental plasticity of auditory cortex in cochlear hearing loss: Physiological and psychophysical findings. *Advances in Biosciences, 83,* 625–633.

Harrison, R. V., Stanton, S. G., Ibrahim, D., Nagasawa, A., & Mount, R. J. (1993). Neonatal cochlear hearing loss results in developmental abnormalities of the central auditory pathways. *Acta Oto-laryngologica, 113,* 296–302.

Henry, K. R., & Saleh, M. (1973). Recruitment deafness: functional effect of priming-induced audiogenic seizures in mice. *Journal of Comparative & Physiological Psychology, 84*(2), 430–435.

Hicks, T. P., & Dykes, R. W. (1983). Receptive field size for certain neurons in the primary somatosensory cortex is determined by BAS-mediated intracortical inhibition. *Brain Research, 274,* 160–164.

Hoke, M., Feldmann, H., Pantev, C., Lutkenhoner, B., & Lehnertz, K. (1989). Objective evidence of tinitus in auditory evoked magnetic fields. *Hearing Research, 37,* 281–286.

House, J. W., & Brackman, D. E. (1981). Tinnitus: Surgical treatment. In D. Evered & G. Lawrenson (Eds.), *CIBA Foundation Symposium 85: Tinnitus* (pp. 204–212). London: Pitman.

House, W. F. (1982). Letter to the editor. *American Journal of Otology, 4,* 188.

Hunter, J. V. (1996). Functional neuroimaging radiology: Radiology. *Current Opinion in Neurology, 9,* 37–41.

Ikner, C. L., & Hassen, A. H. (1990). The effect of tinnitus on ABR latencies. *Ear & Hearing, 11*(1), 16–20.

Irvine, D. R. F., & Rajan, R. (1994). Plasticity of frequency organization in inferior colliculus of adult cats with restricted cochlear lesions. *Abstract of Association for Research in Otolaryngology, 17,* 21.

Jaeger, J. J., Lockwood, A. H., VanValin, R. D., Kemmerer, D. X., Murphy, B. W., & Khalak, H. G. (1996). A positron emission tomographic study of regular and irregular verb morphology in English. *Language, in press.*

Jastreboff, P. J., & Hazell, J. W. P. (1993). A neurophysiological approach to tinnitus: Clinical implications. *British Journal of Audiology, 27,* 7–17.

Jenkins, W. M., & Merzenich, M. M. (1987). Reorganization of neocortical representations after brain injury: A neurophysiological model of the bases of recovery from stroke. *Progress in Brain Research, 71,* 249–266.

Kaas, J. H., Krubitzer, L. A., China, Y. M., Langston, A. L., Polley, E. H., & Blair, N. (1990). Reorganization of retinotopic maps in adult mammals after lesions of the retina. *Science, 248,* 229–231.

Kalil, K., & Skene, J. H. P. (1986). Elevated synthesis of an axonally transported protein correlates with axon outgrowth in normal and injured pyramidal tracts. *Journal of Neuroscience, 6,* 2563–2570.

Kaltenbach, J. A., Czaja, J. M., & Kaplan, C. R. (1992). Changes in the tonotopic map of the dorsal cochlear nucleus following induction of cochlear lesions. *Hearing Research, 59,* 213–223.

Kaufman, L., & Williamson, S. (1982). Magnetic location of cortical activity. In I. Bodis-Wollner (Ed.), *Evoked potentials* (Vol. 88, pp. 197–213). New York: Annal New York Academy of Sciences.

Koerber, K. C., Pfeiffer, R. R., Warr, W. B., & Kiang, N. Y. S. (1966). Spontaneous spike discharges from single units in the cochlear nucleus after destruction of the cochlea. *Experimental Neurology, 16,* 119–130.

Kwong, K. K. (1995). Functional magnetic resonance imaging with echo planar imaging. *Magnetic Resonance Quarterly, 11,* 1–20.

Liu, C. N., & Chambers, W. W. (1958). Intraspinal sprouting of dorsal root axons. *Archives of Neurology and Psychiatry, 79,* 46–61.

Lockwood, A. H., Salvi, R. J., Coad, M. L., Sakowitz, A., Towsley, M., Murphy, B. W., & Khalak, H. (1996). Neural correlates of subjective tinnitus identified by positron emission tomography (PET) of cerebral blood flow. *Abstract of Association for Research in Otolaryngology.*

Lockwood, A. H., Salvi, R. J., Coad, M. L., Wack, D. S., & Murphy, B. W. (1997). Neural plasticity in patients with tinnitus and sensorineural hearing loss. In J. Syka (Ed.), *Auditory Signal Processing in the Central Auditory System.* Plenum Publishing Corp.

Lynch, G., Deadwyler, S., & Cotman, C. (1973a). Postlesion axonal growth produces permanent functional connections. *Science, 180,* 1364–1367.

Lynch, G., Stanfield, B., & Cotman, C. (1973b). Developmental differences in post-lesion axonal growth in the hippocampus. *Brain Research, 59,* 155–168.

Meiri, K. F., Pfenninger, K. H., & Willard, J. B. (1986). Growth-associated protein, GAP-43, a polypeptide that is induced when neurons extend axons, is a component of growth cones and corresponds to pp46, a major polypeptide of a subcellular fraction enriched in growth cones. *Proceedings of the National Academic Science of the United States, 83,* 3537–3541.

Merzenich, M. M., & Kaas, J. H. (1982). Organization of Mammalian somatosensory cortex following peripheral nerve injury. *Trends in Neuroscience, 5,* 4428–4436.

Moller, A. R., Moller, M. B., Jannetta, P. J., & Jho, H. D. (1992a). Compound action potentials recorded from the exposed eighth nerve in patients with intractable tinnitus. *Laryngoscope, 102,* 187–197.

Moller, A. R., Moller, M. B., & Yokota, M. (1992b). Some forms of tinnitus may involve the extralemniscal auditory pathway. *Laryngoscope, 102,* 1165–1171.

Nadeau, S. E., & Crosson, B. (1995). A guide to the functional imaging of cognitive processes. *Neuropsychiatry, Neuropsychology and Behavioral Neurology, 8,* 143–162.

Pantev, C., Hoke, M., Lutkenhoner, B., Lehnertz, K., & Kumpf, W. (1989). Tinnitus remission objectified by neuromagnetic measurements. *Hearing Research, 40,* 261–264.

Phelps, M. E., Mazziotta, J. C., & Huang, S. C. (1982). Study of cerebral function with positron computed tomography. *Journal of Cerebral Blood Flow Metabolism, 2,* 113–162.

Pons, T., Garraghty, P. E., Ommaya, A. K., Kaas, J. H., Taub, E., & Mishkin, M. (1991). Massive cortical reorganization after sensory deafferentation in adult macaques. *Science, 252,* 1857–1860.

Popelar, J., Erre, J. P., Aran, J. M., & Cazals, Y. (1994). Plastic changes in ipsi-contralateral differences of auditory cortex and inferior colliculus after injury to one ear in the guinea pig. *Hearing Research, 72,* 125–134.

Popelar, J., Syka, J., & Berndt, H. (1987). Effect of noise on auditory evoked responses in awake guinea pigs. *Hearing Research, 26,* 239–247.

Rasmusson, D. D. (1982). Reorganization of raccoon somatosensory cortex following removal of the fifth digit. *Journal of Comparative Neurology, 205,* 313–326.

Recanzone, G. H., Schreiner, C. E., & Merzenich, M. M. (1993). Plasticity in the frequency representation of primary auditory cortex following discrimination training in adult owl monkeys. *Journal of Neuroscience, 13,* 87–103.

Reivich, M., Kuhl, D., Wolf, A., Greenberg, J., Phelps, M., Ido, T., Casella, V., Fowler, J., Hoffman, E., Alavi, A., Som, P., & Sokoloff, L. (1979). The [18F] fluorodeoxyglucose method for the measurement of local cerebral glucose utilization in man. *Circ. Res., 44,* 127–137.

Risey, J. A., Guth, P. S., & Amedee, R. G. (1995). Furosemide distinguishes central and peripheral tinnitus. *The International Tinnitus Journal, 1,* 99–103.

Robertson, D., & Irvine, D. R. F. (1989). Plasticity of frequency organization in auditory cortex of guinea pigs with partial unilateral deafness. *Journal of Comparative Neurology, 282,* 456–471.

Rubel, E. W., Smith, Z. D., & Steward, O. (1981). Sprouting in the avian brain stem auditory pathway: Dependence on dendritic integrity. *Journal of Comparative Neurology, 202,* 397–414.

Rubinstein, B., Axelsson, A., & Carlsson, G. (1990). Prevalence of signs and symptoms of craniomandibular disorders in tinnitus patients. *Journal of Craniomandibular Disorders: Facial and Oral Pain, 4,* 186–192.

Ryan, A., & Miller, J. (1978). Single unit responses in the inferior colliculus of the awake and performing monkey. *Experimental Brain Research, 32,* 389–407.

Sadato, N., Pascual-Leone, A., Grafman, J., Ibanez, V., Deiber, M.-P., Dold, G., & Hallett, M. (1996). Activation of the primary visual cortex by Braille reading in blind subjects. *Nature, 380,* 526–528.

Salvi, R. J., Hamernik, R. P., & Henderson, D. (1978). Discharge patterns in the cochlear nucleus of the chinchilla following noise induced asymptotic threshold shift. *Experimental Brain Research, 32,* 301–320.

Salvi, R. J., Henderson, D., & Hamernik, R. P. (1983). Physiological basis of sensorineural hearing loss. In J. Tobias & E. Schubert (Eds.), *Hearing Research and Theory* (2nd ed., pp. 173–231). New York: Academic Press.

Salvi, R. J., Lockwood, A. H., Sakowitz, A., Coad, M. L., Towsley, M., Khalak, H., & Murphy, B. W. (1996a). Identification of cerebral sites mediating tinnitus. *Neurology, 46,* A219.

Salvi, R. J., Powers, N. L., Saunders, S. S., Boettcher, F. A., & Clock, A. E. (1992). Enhancement of evoked response amplitude and single unit activity after noise exposure. In A. Dancer, D. Henderson, R. J. Salvi, & R. Hamernik (Eds.), *Noise-induced hearing loss* (pp. 156–171). St. Louis: Mosby Year Book.

Salvi, R. J., Saunders, S. S., Gratton, M. A., Arehole, S., & Powers, N. (1990). Enhanced evoked response amplitudes in the inferior colliculus of the chinchilla following acoustic trauma. *Hearing Research, 50,* 245–258.

Salvi, R. J., Wang, J., & Powers, N. L. (1996b). Plasticity and reorganization in the auditory brain stem: Implications for tinnitus. In G. E. Reich & J. A. Vernon (Eds.), *Proceedings of the Fifth International Tinnitus Seminar* (pp. 457–466). Portland, OR: American Tinnitus Association.

Saunders, J. C., Bock, G. R., James, R., & Chen, C. S. (1972). Effects of priming for audiogenic seizure on auditory evoked responses in the cochlear nucleus and inferior colliculus of BALB-c mice. *Experimental Neurology, 37*(2), 388–394.

Sergent, J. (1994). Brain-imaging studies of cognitive function. *Trends in Neuroscience, 17,* 221–227.

Sharpless, S. K. (1975). Disuse supersensitivity. In A. H. Riesen (Ed.), *The Developmental Neuropsychology of Sensory Deprivation* (pp. 125–152). New York: Academic Press.

Shiraishi, T., Sugimoto, K., Kubo, T., Matsunaga, T., Nageishi, Y., & Simokochi, M. (1991). Contingent negative variation enhancement in tinnitus patients. *American Journal of Otolaryngology, 12,* 267–271.

Shulman, A. (1995). A final common pathway for tinnitus: The medial temporal lobe system. *The International Tinnitus Journal, 1,* 115–126.

Shulman, A., & Seitz, M. R. (1981). Central tinnitus—diagnosis and treatment. Observations simultaneous binaural auditory brain responses with monaural stimulation in the tinnitus patient. *Laryngoscope, 91*(12), 2025–2035.

Shulman, A., Strashun, A. M., Afriyie, M., Aronson, F., Abel, W., & Goldstein, B. (1995). SPECT imaging of brain and tinnitus—neurotologic/neurologic implications. *International Tinnitus Journal, 1,* 13–29.

Skene, J. H. P., & Willard, M. (1981). Changes in axonally transported proteins during axon regeneration in toad retinal ganglion cells. *Journal of Cell Biology, 89,* 86–95.

Steel, K. P., & Bock, G. R. (1984). Electrically-evoked responses in animals with progressive spiral ganglion degeneration. *Hearing Research, 15,* (1), 59–67.

Syka, J., Rybalko, N., & Popelar, J. (1994). Enhancement of the auditory cortex evoked responses in awake guinea pigs after noise exposure. *Hearing Research, 78,* 158–168.

Trautwein, P., Hofstetter, P., Wang, J., Salvi, R., & Nostrant, A. (1996). Selective inner hair cell loss does not alter distortion product otoacoustic emissions. *Hearing Research, 96*(1–2), 71–82.

Tyler, R. S. (1981). Comment on Animal models of tinnitus. In D. Evered & G. Lawrenson (Eds.), *Tinnitus* (p. 136): Pitman Books, Ltd.

Van der Zee, C. E. E. M., Nielander, H. B., Vos. J. P., Lopes da Silva, S., Verhaagen, J., Oestreicher, A. B., Schrama, L. H., Schotman, P., & Gispen, W. H. (1989). Expression of growth-associated protein B-50 (GAP-43) in dorsal root ganglia and saciatic nerve during regenerative sprouting. *Journal of Neuroscience, 9,* 3505–3512.

Vernon, J., Griest, S., & Press, L. (1992). Attributes of tinnitus that may predict temporomandibular joint dysfunction. *Craniology, 10,* 282–288.

Wall, J. T., & Kaas, J. H. (1986). Long-term cortical consequences of reinnervation errors after nerve regeneration in monkeys. *Brain Research, 372,* 400–404.

Wall, M., Rosenberg, M., & Richardson, D. (1987a). Gaze-evoked tinnitus. *Neurology, 37*(6), 1034–1036.

Wall, M., Rosenberg, M., & Richardson, D. (1987b). Gaze-evoked tinnitus. *Neurology, 37,* 1034–1037.

Wang, J., Powers, N. L., Hofstetter, P., Trautwein, P., Ding, D., & Salvi, R. J. (1997). Effect of selective IHC loss on auditory nerve fiber threshold, tuning, spontaneous and driven discharge rate. *Hearing Research, 107,* 67–82.

Wang, J., Salvi, R. J., & Powers, N. (1996). Rapid functional reorganization in inferior colliculus neurons following acute cochlear damage. *Journal of Neurophysiology, 75,* 171–183.

Weinberger, N., Javid, R., & Lepan, B. (1993). Long term retention of learning-induced receptive field plasticity in the auditory cortex. *Proceedings of the National Academic Science of the United States, 90,* 2394–2398.

Weinberger, N. M. (1995). Dynamic regulation of receptive fields and maps in the adult sensory cortex. *Annual Review of Neuroscience, 18,* 129–158.

Welker, E., Armstrong-James, M., Bronchti, G., Ourednik, F., Gheorghita-Baechler, F., Dubois, R., Guernsey, D. L., Van der Loos, H., & Neumann, P. E. (1996). Altered sensory processing in the somatosensory cortex of the mouse mutant barrelless. *Science, 271,* 1864–1867.

Whittaker, C. K. (1982). Letter to the editor. *American Journal of Otology, 4,* 188.

Whittaker, C. K. (1983). Letter to the editor. *American Journal of Otology, 4,* 273.

Williamson, S., & Kaufman, L. (1988). Auditory evoked magnetic fields. In F. Jahn & J. Santos-Sacchi (Eds.), *Physiology of the Ear* (pp. 497–505). New York: Raven Press.

Willott, J. F. (1996). Auditory system plasticity in the adult C57BL/6J mouse. In R. J. Salvi, D. Henderson, F. Fiorino, & V. Colleti (Eds.), *Auditory plasticity and regeneration: Basic science and clinical implications* (pp. 297–316). New York: Thieme Medical Publishers.

Willott, J. F., Aitkin, L. M., & McFadden, S. L. (1993). Plasticity of auditory cortex associated with sensorineural hearing loss in adult C57BL/6J mice. *Journal of Comparative Neurology, 329,* 402–411.

Willott, J. F., Carlson, S., & Chen, H. (1994). Pre-pulse inhibition of the startle response in mice: Relationship to hearing loss and auditory system plasticity. *Behavioral Neuroscience, 108,* 703–713.

Young, E. (1984). Response characteristics of neurons of the cochlear nucleus. In C. Berlin (Ed.), *Hearing Science* (pp. 423–460). San Diego: College-Hill.

Zheng, F. G., & Turner, C. W. (1991). Binaural loudness matches in unilaterally impaired listeners. *The Quarterly Journal of Experimental Psychology, 43A,* 565–583.

CHAPTER 6

The Psychoacoustical Measurement of Tinnitus

Richard S. Tyler, Ph. D.

INTRODUCTION

The quantification of a symptom is fundamental to understanding its mechanisms and treatments. If we cannot measure it, we cannot study it. In this chapter, I focus on psychoacoustical measurements of tinnitus, both experimental and clinical. Physiological measurements of tinnitus are discussed in Chapters 4, 7, and 8. Several questionnaires are available to measure tinnitus handicap. These are discussed in Chapter 11 and by Tyler (1993).

WHY MEASURE TINNITUS?

There are several reasons why it might be desirable to measure tinnitus (Tyler, 1992a). These include:

1. To provide reassurance to the patient that their tinnitus is real.
2. To be able to reproduce a similar sound to demonstrate to family and significant others some of the characteristics of the tinnitus experienced by the patient.

3. To provide information that might assist in the determination of site in the auditory system where the tinnitus originates.
4. To distinguish different subcategories of tinnitus.
5. To determine whether the tinnitus has changed.
6. To determine if a treatment has had an effect.
7. To provide treatment guidelines.
8. To determine which patients are likely to benefit from some types of treatment.
9. To assist in legal issues.

Providing Reassurance

Many patients feel insecure that they perceive a sound that others cannot hear. The ability to measure tinnitus reassures them that tinnitus is real.

Producing a Tinnitus Simulation

Often, a parent, partner, sibling, or child cannot appreciate the devastating nature of tinnitus. Once tinnitus has been measured, a pure tone can be presented at the pitch-match frequency and at the tinnitus loudness so that the other person can get some indication of what the tinnitus patient is going through. It is also possible to simulate other detailed aspects of the tinnitus quality. While it might not be possible to reproduce exactly what a patient hears, the complexity and annoyance can be conveyed (Hazell, 1981; Penner, 1993).

Determination of the Site of Tinnitus

Tinnitus has many sources throughout the auditory system (see Chapters 4 and 5). It could be helpful to identify specific sources that contribute to the perception of tinnitus. For example, some measurements are more consistent with tinnitus originating in the cochlea, auditory nerve, brain stem, or central nervous system (see "Central versus Peripheral" on page 171). It is also possible that tinnitus in an individual may have multiple sources. Psychoacoustical measurements can provide insights into the source of tinnitus and the neural systems involved.

Distinguish Different Subcategories of Tinnitus

One of the more remarkable things about the measurement of tinnitus is the wide range of responses across patients. Some, for example, can have their tinnitus masked at low levels, whereas in others, the tinnitus cannot be masked at all. Even though patients often describe their tinnitus similarly, their responses to psychoacoustical measurements often result in clear subcategories. This observation could have many important implications. For example, it could indicate which neural pathways are involved, or which treatments could be more effective.

Determining Whether the Tinnitus has Changed

In many patients, tinnitus is not stable; it changes its perceptual characteristics in its normal course. It could be helpful to substantiate a patient's claim that their tinnitus has improved, gotten worse, or remained stable. For example, the tinnitus itself might have remained stable, but their reaction to it might have improved substantially.

Measure Treatment Effectiveness

Measurements are essential to determine whether a treatment has had an effect. Measurements made before, during, and after treatment are critical to evaluating the effectiveness of a treatment. Multiple baseline measures are needed to establish whether any changes are the result of normal fluctuations or of treatment.

Provide Treatment Guidelines

Some measurements could be helpful in the application of treatments. For example, the level at which a broadband noise can mask tinnitus or the tinnitus pitch-match frequency could provide guidelines for the level and spectrum to be used in tinnitus maskers (see Chapter 14).

Determine Which Patients are Likely to Benefit from Some Types of Treatment

Tinnitus has many causes and possibly many mechanisms are involved. It is likely that one treatment might not be effective for all. Many patients react very different when listening to the same acoustical stimulus. For example, tinnitus can be masked with low-level stimuli in some patients, whereas in others it cannot be masked at all. Furthermore, some patients have a pronounced enhancement in their tinnitus following a masker. These observations can be utilized to determine which treatment might be suitable for which patients.

Legal Issues of Tinnitus

In legal cases it is often necessary to validate the presence of tinnitus, and determine the degree of impairment, disability and/or handicap. Measurements can be used to show that tinnitus does exist, and measurements of loudness and "maskability" can address its severity (see "Legal Issues," on page 173 and Chapter 17).

VARIABILITY OF TINNITUS MEASUREMENTS

Like all measures, there is variability associated with the measurement of tinnitus. In addition, tinnitus measurement has sources of variations, which are not present in the measurement of acoustic tones. The sources of variability include:

- Test-retest variability.
- The normal fluctuation of the tinnitus present in some patients.
- Changes in the tinnitus produced by the measurement stimulus in some patients.

Errors in judgment as to what constitutes an equal pitch or loudness, and what has been masked, is observed in normal hearing individuals and should be expected in tinnitus patients. Burns (1984) for example, noted that patients' demonstrating tinnitus pitch matching that was at least an order of magnitude greater than pitch matching of acoustic tones.

Tinnitus fluctuates daily in some patients (Penner, 1983b; Stouffer & Tyler, 1990a). In these patients, the tinnitus is inherently variable. It is possible to measure tinnitus on successive days to distinguish test-retest variability from day-to-day fluctuations.

Finally, in some patients, the test stimulus itself could alter the tinnitus (Tyler & Conrad-Armes, 1983b). For example, the test stimulus could alter the tinnitus pitch or loudness. Presenting a matching stimulus to the opposite ear might reduce such effects, but because of central interactions, might not eliminate them entirely.

Tinnitus measurement is inherently variable. This means it is essential to perform repeated measures of the characteristic under investigation, and to report the variability along with the mean value of the measurement.

THE INTERPRETATION OF THE PATIENT'S DESCRIPTION OF QUALITY

Patients' descriptions of tinnitus include many sounds; such as buzzing, rushing, ringing, roaring, and whistling. Stouffer and Tyler (1990a) reported that 38 percent of their subjects described their tinnitus as ringing and 11 percent as buzzing (see Table 6-1). Since these descriptions depend on the patient's vocabulary and previous listening experience; they usually have limited diagnostic significance.

Many patients describe hearing two or more sounds. For example, they might report hearing a low-pitched hum and a high-pitched whistle in the same ear. Interestingly, one of the sounds occasionally will fluctuate while the other may remain constant, or a noise may mask one of the sounds but have no effect on the other. This suggests separate generators for the two sounds.

It is important to distinguish patients who might have a middle-ear tinnitus from those who have sensorineural tinnitus (see Chapter 9). Middle-ear tinnitus resulting from blood-flow abnormalities often result in a pulsing, swooshing, or beating tinnitus. Middle-ear tinnitus resulting from muscle twitching might result in a "twitching" or "clicking" tinnitus. The use of these descriptors should alert the clinician to the possibility of a vascular or muscular tinnitus. However, these sounds may also occur with sensorineural tinnitus.

PERCEPTUAL LOCATION

Patients perceive their tinnitus in one ear; in both ears; at the back, middle, side, and front of the head; and occasionally, outside of the head (see Chapter 1). For example, Stouffer and Tyler (1990a) reported that 52 percent reported bilateral tinnitus, 37 percent unilateral, 10 percent in the head, and less than 1 percent outside the head. Meikle and Griest (1992) report 61 percent bilateral

Table 6-1. Patients' responses to the question "Which of all of these qualities best describes your tinnitus?" Responses were obtained from 528 tinnitus patients. (Adapted from Stouffer & Tyler, 1990a).

Description	Percent of Males (%)	Percent of Females (%)	Percent of Total (%)
Ringing	41.3	32.8	37.5
Buzzing	7.8	15.3	11.2
Cricket	7.5	9.8	8.5
Hissing	9.2	6.0	7.8
Whistling	9.2	3.4	6.6
Humming	4.1	6.8	5.3
Roaring	4.4	4.7	4.5
Musical note	5.1	3.0	4.2
Steam whistle	4.4	3.4	4.0
Pulsing	2.0	6.0	3.8
Rushing	2.0	3.0	2.5
Crackling	0.3	2.6	1.3
Throbbing	0.7	0.9	0.8
Whooshing	0.3	0.9	0.6
Clicking	0.3	0.9	0.6
Pounding	0.7	0.0	0.4
Clanging	0.0	0.9	0.4
Popping	0.3	0.0	0.2
Total	100	100	100

tinnitus, 23 percent unilateral, 6 percent in the head, and multiple or other locations in the remainder.

Erlandsson, Hallberg, and Axelsson (1992) noted that unilateral tinnitus was more prominent in female subjects. People who perceived their tinnitus as having multiple locations were older and had more sleep problems than people who localized their tinnitus to only one ear.

At present, this information has limited diagnostic importance and may be misleading. A tinnitus perceived in only one ear can be masked as effectively in the ear contralateral to the tinnitus (Tyler & Conrad-Armes, 1983b). This suggests the masking is occurring centrally. In some patients, when a tinnitus perceived in one ear is masked by a noise in the same ear, a "new" tinnitus can appear in the opposite ear, perhaps indicating that tinnitus was present in the contralateral ear all along but at a lower level. Thus a distinction between peripheral and central tinnitus cannot be made based on the patient's report of tinnitus location. Interestingly, Meikle and Griest (1992) noted that 9 percent of their tinnitus patients reported that their tinnitus location was currently variable, and 19 percent noted that it was in a different position from where it had been in the past. They noted that a common trend is for the tinnitus to initially be audible in one ear and then later to appear bilaterally (see also Meikle, 1995).

PITCH

The Interpretation of Pitch

Pitch perception is thought to be coded by both place of stimulation and rate of temporal activity. For example, high-pitch sounds stimulate basal cochlear regions. This tonotopicity is maintained throughout the auditory system. Low-pitch tinnitus might correspond to low rates of neural activity (see Chapter 4), or activity of specific neurons that normally respond to low-frequency acoustic tones. Changes in tinnitus pitch might correspond to changes in place of stimulation or specific nerve fibers, or changes in the temporal firing patterns within or across neurons.

Subjective Pitch Estimates

When patients are asked to rate their tinnitus pitch on subjective scales, they typically rate their tinnitus as being high pitched. For example, Stouffer and Tyler (1990a) noted that the average rating on a 10-point scale was 7.12 (S.D. = 2.3), and that 65 percent of patients rated their tinnitus as a 7 or higher (see also Slater & Terry, 1987). This tendency is consistent with the preponderance of high-frequency pitch matches. There are patients, on the other hand, who describe and rate their tinnitus as low pitch.

Pitch Matching

Although patients do not usually describe their tinnitus as tonal, most patients are able to equate the pitch elicited by a pure tone with the *most prominent pitch* of their tinnitus. Even when the tinnitus is described as a low-frequency hum and a high-pitched screech, most patients can focus on their most prominent tinnitus pitch. For example, Meikle reported that 92 percent of 1,033 patients could complete a pitch match.

Pitch-Matching Protocols

Several protocols are available for the estimation of tinnitus pitch.

In the method of limits (see Small, 1973), the patient might be asked whether his tinnitus has a higher or lower pitch than that of a pure tone. The average of a series of pairs of ascending and descending trials is considered the pitch-match frequency. Another variation is to present two tones of different frequency (f1 and f2, where f1<f2), and then ask the patient which is closer in pitch to the tinnitus. For example, if the patient judges the pitch of the higher tone (f2) to be closer in pitch to the tinnitus, then the next two tones are f2 plus a higher tone, f3. Again, a series of runs that begin below and above the pitch-match frequency are combined. These procedures can be used with most clinical audiometers, depending on the desired resolution.

In the method of adjustment, the patient manipulates the frequency of a tone until its pitch is about equal to the most prominent pitch of the tinnitus. The starting frequency is alternated between positions that represent frequencies above and below the pitch-match frequency.

In adaptive methods, often under computer control, the patient is presented with a tone and asked whether their tinnitus is higher or lower in pitch. Depending on the patient's response, the next stimulus presentation will bracket the tinnitus pitch. Different strategies are available regarding the step sizes, rules for changing frequency, and calculation of the pitch-match frequency (Penner & Klafter, 1992; Henry, Meikle & Gilbert, 1999; Mitchell, Vernon & Creedon, 1993). Penner and Bilger (1992) found lower-variability with a "double-staircase" adaptive procedure compared to the method of adjustment. Cacace et al. (1999) has put the protocol to good clinical use. Figure 6-1 shows the consistency of one patient measures at two intervals eight weeks apart.

In all these pitch-matching procedures, it is desirable that the loudness of the pure tone be similar to the loudness of the tinnitus across all frequencies tested. Generally, stimulus intensity can alter the pitch of a pure tone in normal listeners by about

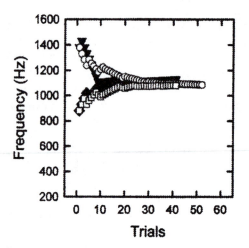

FIGURE 6-1. Consistency of adaptive pitch-matching trials of one patient measured at two intervals eight weeks apart. Closed symbols are from the first test session. Open symbols are from the second test session. Ascending (diamonds and squares) and descending (triangles and circles) trials are shown. (Adapted from Cacace et al., 1999.)

5 percent (Terhardt, 1974). It is important to keep the intensity of the pure tone above threshold and at a similar loudness throughout the frequency region as the frequency is varied. When necessary, a graphic equalizer (between the tone generator and the earphones) can be used to facilitate the maintenance of a similar loudness percept across frequency.

Penner (1980) used a unique technique for determining the spectral locus of the tinnitus. Patients were required to adjust the low-frequency cutoff frequency of a high-pass noise—fixed spectrum sound pressure level (SPL) of 43 dB—until it just masked the tinnitus. Then the high-frequency cutoff frequency of a low-pass noise was similarly adjusted. The frequency region common to both was called the "masking interval" and was related to the spectral region and bandwidth of the tinnitus.

Ohaski et al. (1990) provided some pilot data using musical scales for pitch matching, which could allow for more accurate or reliable measures in patients with musical training.

Penner (1993) required patients to "synthesize" their tinnitus by combining different sine waves (see also Hazell, 1981). Patients judged the combined sine waves as being more similar to their tinnitus than a pure tone.

Pitch-Matching Results

In most patients the tinnitus pitch is matched to a high-frequency tone. For example, in Chapter 8 and Reed, (1960) both noted that the most common frequency matched is about 3,000 Hz. Vernon (1987) reported that about 83 percent of their patients have a pitch-match frequency above 3,000 Hz. Meikle (1995) reported that 33 percent of 646 patients matched their tinnitus to a tone between 3,500 and 6,499 Hz. The high-frequency locus of tinnitus is likely related to the notion that most patients with tinnitus often have high-frequency hearing loss, many caused by noise exposure (see Chapter 1).

Reliability

Some patients show good test-retest reliability for pitch matching whereas others show poor reliability. Tyler and Conrad-Armes (1983a) noted that some patients' pitch matches covered a range of one octave. They also had three of their subjects return three to four months later, and pitch matches were all within one-third of an octave. Burns (1984) found that pitch matching to tinnitus could be ten or twenty times larger than to pure tones (see also Penner, 1983a, who used binaural stimuli). Penner and Saran (1994) have tried various adaptive procedures to limit variability. They note that attending to pitch shifts that result from loudness differences across frequency could be important.

Some clinicians have reported that pitch matches are distributed in two clusters, about one octave in frequency apart (Fowler, 1942; Graham & Newby, 1962). These "octave confusions" could be identified by asking the patient if a tone one octave higher or one octave lower than the frequency selected is closer to the tinnitus pitch. However Penner (1983a) obtained over eighty matches per subjects in three subjects, and did not observe octave confusions. Tyler and Conrad-Armes (1983a) failed to observe any octave confusions when the acoustic tone was in the ear ipsilateral to the tinnitus. If octave confusions do occur, they could be of important theoretical interest. A close examination of octave confusions needs to be evaluated in more patients. A careful examination of the distribution of many replications is best approach.

Penner (1986b) noted that the psychometric function (a graph of signal delectability versus level) is flatter in the region of the tinnitus pitch-match frequency. She interpreted this as indicating that the "unstable" (as evidence from pitch matching) tinnitus acts as a source of internal noise. Mineau and Schlauch (1997) found that, on average, pulse tones are more difficult to detect than continuous tones for tinnitus patients. They interpreted this as being inconsistent with Penner's hypothesis.

The ear chosen for the test stimuli also may influence the results. A different pitch-match frequency may be obtained depending upon which ear receives the tone (Tyler & Conrad-Armes, 1983a). If the tinnitus and the tone are in the same ear, then the tone may change the tinnitus in some way. When binaural diplacusis is present and the tinnitus and tone are in different ears, inaccurate matches can result. Binaural presentation of the tone may be confounded by both effects, and the patient may "listen" with different ears on different trials.

Stability of Pitch Over Time

Pitch-matching reliability varies widely across patients. This is actually consistent with the reports that in about one in every two patients with tinnitus, the pitch can vary from day to day or within a day (Stouffer & Tyler, 1990a). Furthermore, in one of every

five patients, the tinnitus pitch increased over time. Even when the tinnitus pitch is reported to be stable, some patients will have difficulty providing an accurate pitch match. This requires that several replications of the pitch match must be obtained.

Pitch and Etiology

Stouffer and Tyler (1990a) noted very small differences between subjective pitch ratings among groups with different etiologies. The ratings ranged from 7.0 for patients with middle-ear tinnitus to 7.5 for patients with noise-induced tinnitus. Few studies have examined the relationship between etiology of the hearing loss and tinnitus pitch-match frequency.

Henry and Meikle et al. (1999) found that 6 percent of males and 15 percent of females had pitch matches below 1,500 Hz. The gender differences might be attributable to higher proportion of noise exposure in the male population.

Douek and Reid (1968) performed pitch matching on patients and reported results from different groups. In general, pitch matches were as follows:

- Ménière's disease   125 to 250 Hz
- Middle-ear tinnitus   250 to 2,000 Hz
- Noise induced   2,000 to 8,000 Hz
- Presbyacusis   2,000 to 8,000 Hz

Reed (1960), Graham and Newby (1962), and Nodar and Graham (1965) also studied patients with different etiologies. In general, the pitch-match frequency is not pathonomonic of the disease.

Pitch and the Audiogram

Several investigators have noted that tinnitus pitch match often occurs in the frequency region of maximum hearing loss or on the edge of normal hearing and hearing loss. Minton (1923), Fowler (1940), Graham and Newby (1962), and Douek and Reid (1968) reported a decrease in hearing thresholds near the tinnitus pitch-match frequency. Penner (1980) noted that the pitch-match frequency was just below the edge of a precipitous high-frequency noise-induced hearing loss. In contrast, Donaldson (1978) and Tyler and Conrad-Armes (1983a) found that tinnitus pitch was not related to hearing thresholds. Before clear claims can be made about this relationship, it is necessary to carefully measure pitch and the audiogram in large numbers of patients. Henry and Meikle et al. (1999) reported that patients with more low-frequency hearing loss are more likely to have a low-frequency tinnitus.

Clinical Recommendations

If tinnitus pitch is measured, it is important to specify the test ear and record each pitch estimate as well as the mean. Because of the variable nature of pitch matching, at least seven replications are recommended. Giving patients adequate instruction and practice trials can be necessary to produce reliable pitch matches in some patients. Other subjects may simply be unable to provide reliable pitch matches. More than seven replications can be used when large variations are evident across trials. I recommend monaural ipsilateral testing, with the examiner noting the test ear.

LOUDNESS

The Interpretation of Loudness

Loudness perception is normally thought to be coded by both the number of nerve fibers activated and rate of temporal activity. Loud tinnitus might correspond to high rates of neural activity or many nerve fibers active, or both (see Chapter 4). Changes in tinnitus loudness might correspond to changes in the number of nerve fibers involved, or changes in the temporal firing patterns within or across neurons. Both changes in tinnitus pitch and loudness might result from changes in rate of nerve fiber discharge.

Subjective Loudness Estimates

Loudness is typically scaled from soft to loud. Most patients who complain about their tinnitus report that the tinnitus is loud, however, there are many people who experience a soft tinnitus and do not find it disturbing.

Stouffer and Tyler (1990a, b) noted the average loudness rating of 6.3 out of 10 (SD = 2.3). They noted that loudness judgments were greater for patients with Ménière's disease than for other pathologies. Scott, Lindberg, Melin, and Lyttkens (1990) observed that patients who have had tinnitus for a longer period of time tend to perceive their tinnitus as louder than those who experienced their tinnitus for a shorter period of time.

Loudness Matching

Most patients are able to equate the loudness elicited by a pure tone with the *overall loudness* of their tinnitus. Even when the tinnitus is described as containing many sounds, most patients can focus on the overall loudness of their tinnitus.

Loudness Matching Protocols

The loudness of tinnitus has been measured by having the subject adjust the level of a pure tone so that it has about the same loudness as the tinnitus. As with the measurement of tinnitus pitch, variations of the method of limits, the method of adjustment, and adaptive methods can and have been used (Henry & Flick et al., 1999; Henry & Meikle, 1996; 1999; Mitchell, Vernon, & Creedon, 1993; Tyler & Conrad-Armes, 1983b; Penner, 1983a; Burns, 1984; Mortimer, Burr, Wright, & McGarry, 1940).

A different procedure was used by Goodwin and Johnson (1980a, b). They suggested that reaction time could be used as a measure of tinnitus loudness. Reaction times are shorter to the onset of loud sounds than they are to that of soft sounds. Unexpectedly, Goodwin and Johnson found that reaction times were shorter at frequencies close to the tinnitus pitch-match frequency than at other frequencies, even when they were equated in hearing thresholds. The procedure has not found widespread use, in part because of the instrumentation required, and in part because of the additional interpretation required to equate reaction times and loudness.

Loudness Matching Results

Several researchers, including Fowler (1940) and Vernon (1977), have commented that the level of a pure tone equated in loudness to tinnitus is often < 10 dB above threshold, or sensation level, even when the patients complained that their tinnitus was very loud. Although at first, this appears inconsistent, sensation level units are not measurements of loudness; the sensation level in decibels (dB SL) represents the intensity, not loudness, of the signal above threshold. Goodwin and Johnson (1980a, b) realized this difficulty and noted that the loudness match, in dB SL, could be much greater at a frequency with normal hearing than at a frequency with a threshold loss.

Matsuhira and Yamashita (1996b) measured tinnitus loudness at a test frequency where hearing threshold was less than 15 dB HL in 125 patients with various etiolo-

gies. The average loudness match was 13.5 dB SL (s.d. + 10.7 dB).

Figure 6-2 shows the results of loudness matching of two patients. The audiograms (in sound pressure level) are shown, together with loudness matches and uncomfortable loudness levels. For patient 15 (Figure 6-2, left), at the pitch-match frequency, the loudness match is about 2 dB SL, but at 500 Hz, the loudness match is about 50 dB sensation level. For patient 5 (Figure 6-2, right), the corresponding levels are about 3 and 25 dB sensation level.

Tyler and Conrad-Armes (1983a) (see also Penner, 1984; 1986a) calculated the loudness of tinnitus taking into account the threshold loss and loudness recruitment (Figure 6-3) shows their model, which indicates the loudness of a tone in sones (Stevens, 1955), the conventional psychoacoustic units of loudness.

They argued there were three advantages to calculating tinnitus loudness:

- Sones have a communicable meaning. For example, if a patient had a tinnitus loudness of 2 sones, a 50 dB SPL 1,000 Hz tone presented to a normal hearing person would allow them to experience the same loudness.

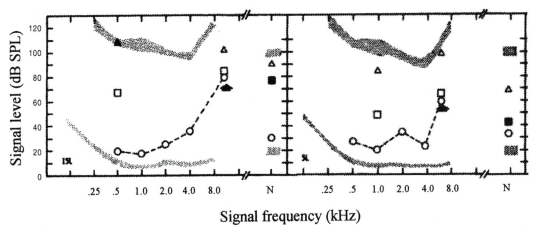

Figure 6-2. Audiogram (in dB SPL) (open circles), tinnitus loudness match (squares), and uncomfortable loudness levels (diamonds) from two patients. The tinnitus pitch-match frequency is identified by the arrow. The hatched areas at the top and bottom represent normal hearing and normal uncomfortable loudness levels, respectively. Measurements to the right of each panel indicate the threshold, equal loudness, and uncomfortable loudness level for broadband noise. (Adapted from Tyler & Conrad-Armes, 1983b.)

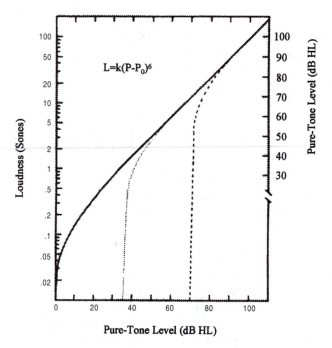

$$L=k(P-P_0)^6$$

FIGURE 6-3. The loudness of tinnitus as predicted from a model of loudness recruitment. The equation predicts tinnitus loudness in sones given the dB sensation level of the loudness match. In normal listeners, a tone of 10 dB sensation level has a loudness of about 0.1 sones. In a listener with a 35 dB HL threshold, a 10 dB sensation level tone has a loudness of nearly 2 sones (20 times louder than normal). (Adapted from Tyler & Conrad-Armes, 1983b.)

■ It allows comparisons across patients. For example, two patients could both have loudness matches of 9 dB SL, but depending on hearing thresholds, the tinnitus loudness could be forty times louder in a patient with a substantial hearing loss.

■ Individuals could be identified who complained of a very loud tinnitus, but whose loudness match suggested a soft tinnitus. These patients might require special counseling.

The equation represented in Figure 6-3 attempts to predict tinnitus loudness given the dB SL loudness match, and the person's equivalent loudness in sones. Although this model is based on an assumed typical recruitment function and therefore may not be precise for each individual, it does illustrate

the severe loudness and thus the disturbing effect of tinnitus (see also Penner, 1984, 1986a, 1988a; and Hinchliffe & Chambers, 1983).

Tyler and Conrad-Armes (1983b) and Penner (1984) also observed patients who had very low dB-SL loudness matches in regions of both normal and abnormal thresholds. Loudness recruitment cannot account for the discrepancy between subjective reports of a loud tinnitus and low dB SL measurements in these patients.

Newman, Wharton, Shivapuja and Jacobson (1994) made several observations in a study relating loudness and handicaps that were consistent with correcting tinnitus loudness for recruitment. These included:

■ Loudness matches reported in sensation level were greater when measured in

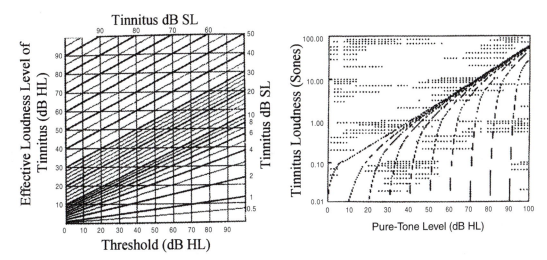

FIGURE **6-4.** Left—Nomogram for converting the sensation level of a loudness match into the "equivalent" hearing level (dB HL) in a normal listener. First, find the signal threshold on x-axis, and the sensation level of the loudness match on the right axis. Follow the curvilinear function from the right axis until it crosses the signal threshold level on the x-axis. Move horizontally to read the equivalent dB HL for a normal listener. (Adapted from Matsuhira, & Yamashita, 1996a.)

Right—Nomogram for converting the sensation level of a loudness match into equivalent sones for a normal listener. First find the signal threshold level on x-axis, and the sensation level of the loudness match on the right axis. Follow the curvilinear function from the right axis until it crosses the signal threshold level on a x-axis. Move horizontally to read the equivalent dB HL for a normal listener. (Adapted from Tyler, Aran, & Dauman, 1992.)

regions of normal hearing than when measured in regions of hearing loss.

■ For a given loudness match reported in sensation level, the greater the hearing loss, the more annoying the tinnitus.

While Tyler and Conrad-Armes (1983b) used "average" loudness growth functions, Jakes, Hallam, Chambers, and Hinchcliffe (1986) proposed measuring the individual loudness growth in each tinnitus patient. These "personal loudness units" were more highly correlated to loudness scales than were other estimates of tinnitus loudness, but also required more time to measure.

Tyler and Conrad-Armes (1983b) also commented that there is a linear relationship between signal level and sones above about 30 dB SPL. Thus, they added dB HL to the upper right axis on Figure 6-3. This enabled a direct conversion from dB SL to the equivalent hearing level in normal listeners. Matsuhira, Yamashita, and Yasua (1992) and Matsuhira and Yamashita

(1996a) took this one step further and provided a nomogram for converting (Figure 6-4, left) loudness matches into equivalent hearing level across a wide range of levels.

Tyler, Aran, and Dauman (1992) also provided a nomogram (Figure 6-4, right). In this case the tinnitus loudness in sones can be converted from the hearing threshold and dB SL of the loudness match. In addition, this could be converted to the equivalent sensation level for a 1,000 Hz tone in a person with normal hearing (at least for tones matched to the tinnitus between 250 and 4,000 Hz). Coles and Baskill (1996) found only small differences in applying the nomograms of Matsuhira and Yamashita (1996a) and Tyler et al. (1992).

Reliability

The variability of loudness adjustments is typically low, but does differ across patients. Although it can be greater than the variability of matching to an external tone, the variability is not as great as with tin-nitus pitch (Bailey, 1979; Burns, 1984; Penner, 1983a). Stouffer and Tyler (1990b) reported that over half of their patients reported that their tinnitus loudness fluctuated while it was present, and half reported that it changed from day to day. In one out of three patients, the tinnitus loudness increases over time. Meikle, Schuff, and Griest (1987) report that approximately four-fifths of the 519 patients that they saw in their clinic indicate that their tinnitus loudness fluctuates. A review of tinnitus loudness estimates is provided in Tyler and Stouffer (1989).

Loudness and Annoyance

Louder sounds are generally more annoying than soft sounds. However, many other factors contribute to annoyance. Although louder tinnitus is generally more annoying than soft tinnitus (particularly when compared within a patient), it should not be surprising that the correlation between loudness and annoyance is not perfect. Annoyance can be influenced by the quality, intermittent or continuous time course, the duration since tinnitus first began (habituation factors), and the "psychological" state of the patient.

Tyler and Conrad-Armes (1983b) found high correlations between the dB SL of noise required to mask tinnitus and tinnitus loudness matches in dB SL. Burns (1984) found no relationship between loudness matching and masking of tinnitus. Tyler and Conrad-Armes (1983b) noted a closer relationship between subjective rating and tinnitus loudness in sones than between tinnitus "loudness" in sensation level.

Stouffer and Tyler (1990b) correlated subjective loudness ratings (1 to 10) to a number of other variables. They found significant correlations among 528 tinnitus subjects and ratings of annoyance (r = .56) and concentration (r = .40). Patients who report a soft tinnitus do not have as many problems

as those who report a loud tinnitus. On the other hand, there are tinnitus patients who report loud tinnitus who develop ways of coping.

Newman et al. (1994) found that the loudness match at the pitch-match frequency was significantly correlated to the self-rated annoyance. Henry and Meikle (1996) failed to find a relationship between loudness ratings and loudness matches. Folmer, Griest, Meikle, and Martin (1999) noted that the tinnitus loudness rating (1 to 10) scale was 7.18 in patients with depression and 6.99 in patients without depression. This difference was not significant in 285 patients.

It is noteworthy that loudness matches and the minimum masking level (see the following) are related, as shown in Figure 6-5 (from Mitchell, Vernon, & Creedon, 1993), suggesting that they both reflect some measure of the tinnitus magnitude.

Andersson and McKenna (1998) compared tinnitus magnitude (as judged by minimum masking levels) and depression. They noted that tinnitus with high depression scores have high minimum masking levels. However, they also observed patients with low tinnitus magnitude and high depression scores. They suggested that these later patients could be more vulnerable, based on a diathesis-stress model. Jastreboff, Hazell, and Graham (1994) also noted that patients who were successful with tinnitus maskers/hearing aids reported an average of 5.3 dB decrease in the broadband noise required to mask their tinnitus, whereas those that were unsuccessfully treated showed an average of 4.25 dB increase in the noise required to mask their tinnitus.

Penner (1996) had patients synthesize their tinnitus with sine waves (also see Penner, 1993) and then the patients and normals ranked the annoyance of the simulation. Both groups ranked the sounds similarly. One implication of this is that the tinnitus itself is critical factor in tinnitus annoyance, not just their individual "psychological" reaction to their tinnitus.

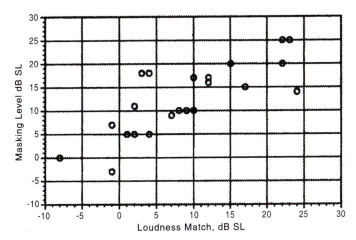

FIGURE 6-5. The relationship between loudness matches (in dB Sensation Level) and the minimum masking level (in dB Sensation Level). (From Mitchell, Vernon, & Creedon, 1993.)

Hyperacusis

Tyler and Conrad-Armes (1983b) observed that several of their tinnitus subjects exhibited reduced uncomfortable loudness levels relative to normal hearing and hearing-impaired listeners. They speculated that the "lesion causing tinnitus could have some direct effect on the loudness perception that leads to a reduced uncomfortable loudness level," or that "having to listen to tinnitus for many years could have rendered some individuals more annoyed by continuous sounds in general" (Tyler & Conrad-Armes (1983b; page 67). Vernon and Meikle (Chapter 14) and Jastreboff (see Chapter 15) now believe that hyperacusis could be intimately linked to tinnitus (see also Tyler, 1999).

Clinical Recommendations

As with tinnitus, pitch is measured when tinnitus loudness is measured. It is important to specify the test ear and to record each loudness estimate. At least five replications are recommended. Report the threshold and loudness match, so that conversions to sones or other estimates of loudness can be obtained. The loudness match in sensation level can be used as an estimate of the magnitude of the tinnitus in an individual patient when the threshold remains stable across time.

MASKING

Masking has been a very powerful tool in the psychophysical investigation of hearing. The fact that masking between two acoustic stimuli occurs at all, and between an acoustic stimulus and tinnitus, are important observations. It is thought that one sound can "mask" (or swamp) another because that masker has rendered the neural channel busy, similar to a busy telephone line (see Moore, 1997). Another explanation is that one sound "suppresses" the neural activity of the other sound (Delgutte, 1990).

In many patients, the presentation of a pure tone or noise can mask tinnitus completely. Vernon (1987) suggests that 91 percent of 491 patients seen in their clinic could be masked completely. The fact that tinnitus can be masked suggests that the tinnitus and the response to the acoustic stimulus share the same neural channels somewhere in the nervous system.

Ipsilateral Tonal Masking

Pure tones can be effective in masking tinnitus, even in a patient whose description of tinnitus is complex. A tinnitus-masking pattern can be measured by determining the minimal level required to mask the tinnitus at several tone frequencies (Bailey, 1979; Formby & Gjerdingen, 1980; Fowler, 1940, 1943; Mitchell, 1983; Burns, 1984; Murai, Ogasawara, Ishikawa, Kusano, & Tsuiki, 1992; Penner, 1987).

Wegel (1931) reported an interesting case whereby a patient's tinnitus could be "canceled" by a tone of slightly higher frequency and level. Both the tinnitus and the tone were inaudible. Wegel (1931) reported a very sharply tuned tinnitus-masking pattern for his own tinnitus.

Feldmann (1971) reported testing about 200 subjects and classified the masking patterns into five broad categories:

- Congruence, in which the tinnitus was masked just above threshold throughout the frequency range
- Distance, in which the tinnitus was masked at high levels throughout the frequency range
- Persistence, in which the tinnitus could not be masked
- Convergence, in which the tinnitus could be masked at high sensation levels at low frequencies and low sensation levels at high frequencies in subjects with a precipitous high-frequency hearing loss
- Divergence, in which the tinnitus could be masked at low sensation levels at low frequencies and high sensation levels at high frequencies in subjects with mild-to-moderate hearing loss

The patients with mild-to-moderate loss were reported to have a low-pitched "whooshing" tinnitus and may have had tinnitus of middle ear origin. Patients with distant, congruent, and convergent types of masking patterns have been observed by others (Mitchell, 1983; Tyler & Conrad-Armes, 1984).

Tyler (1992a) (see Figure 6-6) proposed some alternative descriptors for the categories he observed. These included "low sensation level," "high sound pressure level," "frequency specific," and "unable to mask."

Such tinnitus masking patterns might be useful to establish the site of tinnitus. For example, in the normal ear, a low-level, pure-tone signal excites a small region of the basilar membrane. A second pure tone (a masker) can be introduced that masks the original signal. When this masking occurs, it is assumed that the excitation pattern of the masker has overlapped that of the signal. As the masker frequency gets further and further away from the signal frequency, greater masker intensities are required for the excitation patterns to overlap. When the minimal level required to mask the signal is graphed as a function of masker frequency, then a plot called a psychoacoustic tuning curve is obtained. This represents, at least to a first approximation, the spatial extent of the displacement pattern of signal along the basilar membrane. If tinnitus originated from a localized region of the basilar membrane, we could expect its masking properties to be similar to a low-level pure tone. The broad tinnitus-masking patterns observed by Feldmann (1971) and others, however, had no similarity to the sharply tuned psychoacoustical tuning curves seen in normal listeners.

Since tinnitus patients usually have a threshold loss and since hearing-impaired patients usually exhibit abnormal psychoacoustical tuning curves (Florentine, Buus, Scharf, & Zwicker, 1980; Tyler, Wood, & Fernandes, 1982), comparing psychoacoustical tuning curves and tinnitus masking patterns in the same patient is more appropriate. In this case, the pure-tone signal in the psychoacoustical tuning curves is used to simulate the tinnitus. Thus, Tyler and Conrad-Armes (1984) used tinnitus loudness and pitch matches to determine the signal level and frequency for the psychoacoustical tuning curves. They reported important differences among patients. In

FREQUENCY (HZ)

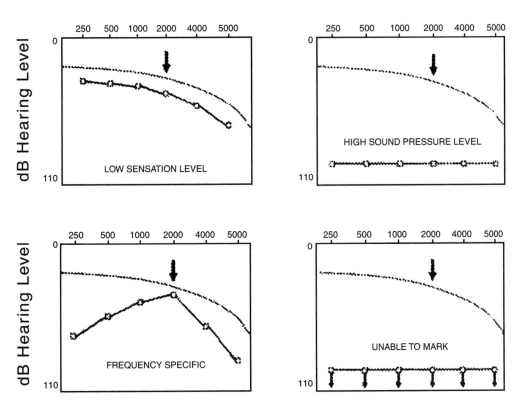

FIGURE 6-6. A schematic representation of tinnitus masking patterns obtained from measuring the lowest level of pure tones required to just mask the tinnitus. The audiograms are shown by the solid lines, and the tinnitus masking patterns are shown with the open circles. (From Tyler, 1992a.)

most cases, the psychoacoustical tuning curve was not similar to the tinnitus-masking pattern. For these individuals, the locus of the tinnitus apparently was not a restricted region along the basilar membrane. In other cases, the shapes of the two functions were similar. This could suggest a peripheral, localized source of the tinnitus. Even in a patient with normal hearing, the tinnitus masking pattern and the psychoacoustic tuning curve was dissimilar (Tyler, 1985).

Burns (1984) also noted a discrepancy in psychoacoustical tuning curves and tinnitus masking patterns in five patients. He grouped his patients into two broad categories: those who required a roughly con-stant SPL masker and those who required a roughly constant sensation level masker to mask the tinnitus.

Penner (1980) observed that lateral suppression mechanisms were impaired in tinnitus patients. Mitchell and Creedon (1995) noted that tinnitus patients with "normal hearing" also had psychophysical tuning curves that had elevated tips and hypersensitive tails compared to nontinnitus normal-hearing listeners.

These observations suggest that the tinnitus does not originate on a single place on the basilar membrane in most cases. The diversity of responses also affirm the likelihood that tinnitus originates in many places in the auditory system.

Noises of Different Bandwidths

Another technique used to measure frequency resolution involves masking by noises of different bandwidths. In normal listeners, the overall level of noise band required to mask a tone is independent of its width at narrow bandwidths. As the masker bandwidth is widened, however, some critical bandwidth is reached beyond which the overall level must be increased in order that the tone be masked. These normal results are shown by the filled circles and dashed line in Figure 6-7.

Shailer, Tyler, and Coles (1981) measured the minimal levels required to mask tinnitus for different bandwidths of noise. The noise level was increased until the tinnitus was masked. In four patients the results resembled those from normal subjects, suggesting that the tinnitus was processed in a discrete frequency channel. In eight other subjects the results are clearly abnormal, suggesting that the tinnitus origin may have a diffuse or central origin (Figure 6-7). When fitting a

tinnitus masker based on the lowest level to mask the tinnitus, careful tailoring of the masker spectrum may be desirable.

In a variation of this strategy, Kitajima, Kitahara, and Kodama (1987) compared the effectiveness of a narrowband masker centered on the tinnitus to an inverse band-reject masker (a broadband masker with the frequency region of the narrowband masker eliminated). They basically found no difference between the conditions. Consistent with tonal masking, frequencies remote from the tinnitus pitch can be effective maskers.

Smith, Parr, Lutmann, and Coles (1991) compared the effectiveness of four different maskers, typically greater than about two octaves bandwidth. Ten patients experienced with tinnitus maskers selected the minimum level required to mask their tinnitus and the level they would "like if the noise was their masker." In four maskers, this later measure was more than 5 dB less than the minimum masking level. There was no single "best" preference among

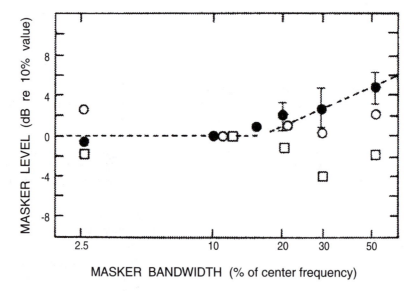

Figure 6-7. The overall level of a noise band required to mask a tone as a function of masker bandwidth for normal listeners (dashed line and filled circles) and tinnitus patients with tonal tinnitus (open circles) and noiselike tinnitus (squares). (From Shailer, Tyler, & Coles; 1981.)

patients and all maskers were about equally as effective. They concluded that complete masking of the tinnitus was not necessary for clinical use and that a general broadband noise masker might be sufficient for most tinnitus patients.

Ipsilateral Broadband Masking

Tinnitus can be masked by a broadband noise presented to the same ear in which the tinnitus is perceived. This is consistent with the observation that pure tones can mask tinnitus. The noise level required to mask the tinnitus should correspond to the "magnitude" of the tinnitus. Thus, the noise required to mask the tinnitus could be an important parameter in quantifying the tinnitus.

Comparing Ipsilateral and Contralateral Broadband Masking

In normal-hearing individuals, a pure tone presented to one ear can be masked most easily by a noise presented to the same ear. A high-intensity noise presented to the opposite ear also masks the tone in the opposite ear. This is achieved by vibrating the skull and thereby stimulating both cochleas. A midfrequency tone in one ear requires at least a 40 dB SPL noise in the other ear to produce this "cross masking" (Liden, Nilsson, & Anderson, 1959).

There is a second mechanism by which a tone can be masked by a noise in the opposite ear. A low-intensity noise presented to one can also raise the threshold of a tone presented to the contralateral ear. The signal threshold can only be increased by a small amount, usually less than 5 dB (Zwislocki, Buining, & Glantz, 1968; Penner, 1987). This is called *central masking*, because the interaction is presumed to occur between the excitation produced by the signal and masker in the central nervous system. Central masking is generally highly frequency specific.

The minimal masking levels of broad-band noise required to mask the tinnitus have been studied for maskers presented to the ipsilateral and contralateral side of the tinnitus (Tyler, Babin, & Niebuhr, 1984; Tyler & Conrad-Armes, 1983b). Surprisingly the masker levels required in the contralateral ears were similar to the levels in the ipsilateral ears indicating that crossover masking was not occurring (Figure 6-8).

Tyler, Babin, and Niebuhr (1984) noted two subjects in whom the tinnitus could not be masked in the ear, which had the loudest tinnitus, but their tinnitus could be masked in the opposite ear (similar findings were reported by Murai, Ogasawara, Saitoh, & Tsuiki, 1987). In these subjects, the masking seemed to occur at levels above the cochlear nucleus, as if the tinnitus contained a major central component, even in those patients who localized their tinnitus to one ear. In some patients, once the unilateral tinnitus was masked, a tinnitus of a similar quality suddenly appeared in the opposite ear, as if the tinnitus were present in both ears all the time, but was lateralized to one ear because of its greater loudness.

Ishikawa, Kusano, Ogasawara, Murai, and Tsuiki (1992) also compared contralateral and ipsilateral broadband noise masking. Correlations were higher when the data were plotted in terms of hearing level (r = 0.67) compared to when they were plotted in dB Sensation Level (r = .56).

The comparison between ipsilateral and contralateral masking suggests that central mechanisms were involved in many patients with tinnitus. They could also help to distinguish patients with peripheral and central components (see the following).

POSTMASKING EFFECTS

Another intriguing characteristic of tinnitus occurs when a masking noise is turned off. In many cases the tinnitus remains inaudible. Feldmann (1971) presented pulsed maskers with long intermasker delays. Between the maskers, patients reported that

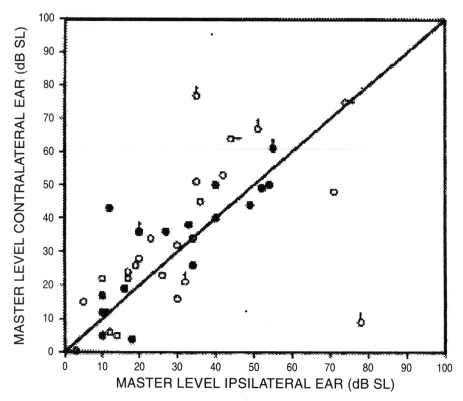

FIGURE 6-8. The minimal masking levels of broadband noise (in sound pressure level) required to mask the tinnitus for maskers presented to the ipsilateral and contralateral side of the tinnitus. Open circles—unilateral tinnitus. Filled circles—bilateral or tinnitus perceived in the head. For the later group, the loudest tinnitus is defined as the ipsilateral ear. (From Tyler, Babin, & Niebuhr, 1984.)

the tinnitus could be completely inaudible. Patients were required to decrease the delay between the maskers until they could no longer hear the tinnitus. In one Ménière's patient, a 0.5 second, 100 dB SPL, one-third octave band noise-masking pulses produced a tinnitus, which was inaudible with a 1.5-second delay between pulses. Bailey (1979) produced dramatic frequency-dependent postmasking effects in one subject using a 30-s, 65-dB SPL masker.

Terry, Jones, Davis, and Slater (1983) measured the postmasking effects of tinnitus in eight patients. After the termination of a single masker, the patients were required: (1) to adjust a dial whose position was to indicate tinnitus loudness, or (2) to balance the loudness of the tinnitus with the loudness of a tone in the contralateral ear. In the second case, the contralateral tone possibly

could have influenced the tinnitus in some way. Both techniques showed reasonable agreement in most cases, indicating that longer duration and high-intensity maskers produced longer relief from tinnitus. The authors reported an absence of postmasking effects when the masker was presented to the ear opposite the tinnitus. They also observed a temporary threshold shift following the masker that appeared to have a similar time course as the reduction in tinnitus.

Tyler, Conrad-Armes, and Smith (1984) studied short-term postmasking effects in ten patients with sensorineural tinnitus. They presented a single, continuous masker (which lasted from 1 to 60 seconds in duration, depending on the experimental condition) and required the patients to indicate when the tinnitus: (1) first returned, and

(2) returned to its normal premasker loudness. Their findings are summarized in Figure 6-9 and show five different types of the postmasking effects. After the termination of the masker, the tinnitus either a) returned to normal loudness immediately, b) returned immediately but initially was softer, c) was absent before gradually returning to normal, d) was absent before abruptly returning to normal, or e) was louder before gradually returning to normal.

Individual differences were large. In some subjects, changing the level over a 30-dB range had little effect, whereas in others it doubled the response time. There were also some unusual observations. One subject reported postmasking "wobbling"; another that the tinnitus changed ears; and in two subjects the tinnitus became audible during the masker (see also Penner, 1988b). Paradoxically, these later subjects were able to detect the offset of the masker and respond when their tinnitus first returned and returned to its normal loudness.

The exacerbation of the tinnitus following the masker was similar to studies of temporary threshold shift that produced tinnitus after high-intensity long-duration tones (Hirsh & Ward, 1952), except that these studies used higher-level tones than presented here. Masker frequency had little effect on the postmasking patterns, except in one of the ten subjects. Increasing masker duration and level typically produced longer effects.

Tyler, Kuk, and Mims (1987) compared postmasking effects with a 5-minute masker which was in either the ear ipsilateral or contralateral to the tinnitus. They required patients to touch a bar on a computer monitor to indicate the tinnitus loudness at about 5- to 10-second intervals. The results from one subject, shown in Figure 6-10, indicate that this procedure is very repeatable. They observed postmasking relief from tinnitus when the masker was presented in either the ipsilateral or contralateral ear to the tinnitus, but it was greater when the masker was presented to the ipsilateral ear.

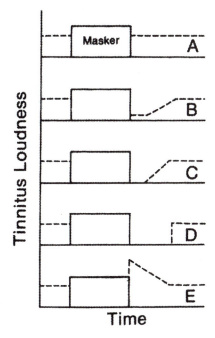

FIGURE 6-9. A schematic representation of the time course of tinnitus loudness before, during, and after the presentation of a noise that masks the tinnitus. After the termination of the masker, the tinnitus either: (a) returned to normal loudness immediately, (b) returned immediately but initially was softer, (c) was absent before gradually returning to normal, (d) was absent before abruptly returning to normal, or (e) was louder before gradually returning to normal. (From Tyler, Conrad-Armes, & Smith; 1984.)

Penner (1988a) also assessed postmasking effects with a 5-minute masker. Subjects judged whether a tone presented 20 ms after the masker was louder or softer than their tinnitus, and subjectively rated whether their tinnitus was louder, softer, or the same compared to its premasker loudness. Three of six subjects reported that their tinnitus had changed but the level of the tone equated in loudness to the tinnitus was not significantly different from a premasker judgment. Penner concluded that the subjective ratings provided by some subjects might reflect the inherent dynamic changes of the tinnitus independent of the influence of the masker. One subject reported that the tinnitus got louder following the masker on some trials and got softer on other trials.

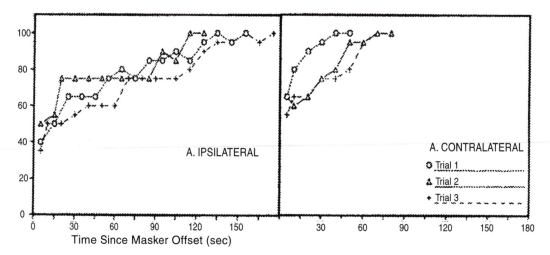

FIGURE 6-10. Postmasking effects obtained with a 5-minute masker presented to either the ear ipsilateral (left) or contralateral (right) to a patient with unilateral tinnitus. The patient was required to rate the tinnitus loudness at serial intervals following the termination of the masker. Three replications are shown. (From Tyler, Kuk, & Mims, 1987.)

Penner also observed that postmasking tinnitus was judged louder when the postmasker tone was presented to ipsilateral ear compared to contralateral presentation.

Vernon and Meikle (1988) have measured postmasking effects in their patients with a 1-minute masker presented at 10 dB above the minimum level required to mask the tinnitus (with a noise band from 3,000 to 12,000 Hz). They reported that 90 percent of their patients demonstrated some form of residual inhibition. Of those that did, 45 percent exhibited partial inhibition, 49 percent demonstrated complete followed by partial, and 6 percent demonstrated complete inhibition. More than half of their patients reported recovered from the inhibition in 2 minutes or less.

Johnson and Sandlin (1996) began some preliminary trials of residual inhibition using tones, noise, and swept-frequency tones. When the stimuli were presented at 10-dB SL, the high-frequency stimuli produced the most inhibition. Swept-frequency tones produced more residual inhibition than noise bands. A few patients also experienced exacerbation of their tinnitus.

Several observations can be drawn from these postmasking effects. They are not likely caused by the same mechanism responsible for temporary threshold shift because the effects can be long duration (several hours) considering they are produced by brief, low-level maskers. The effects seem to be greater for stimuli presented to the ipsilateral tinnitus ear. Finally, such long-term postmasking effects are not observed in auditory-nerve fiber experiments, so they likely involve central mechanisms.

ADAPTATION OF MASKING

If a continuous noise is presented at levels that initially masked the tinnitus, in some patients the tinnitus will reappear after several seconds or minutes. Penner, Brauth and Hood (1981) and Penner (1983a) quantified this effect by requiring the patient to increase the noise level to maintain masking of the tinnitus. Figure 6-11 illustrates this effect for two patients in whom the masker intensity had to be increased; in one by 45

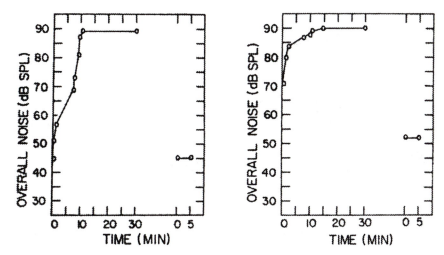

FIGURE 6-11. The level of a continuous broadband noise required to maintain masking of the tinnitus for two different patients. The two data points to the right of each panel represent the noise level required to mask an external tone. (From Penner, Brauth, & Hood, 1981.)

dB over 30 minutes. Forty-five dB is an enormous amount of energy. The authors suggested this effect was caused by the adaptation of the masker, whereas the tinnitus, being processed differently, did not adapt. Another possible explanation is that the masker is exacerbating the tinnitus, and the tinnitus magnitude is increasing over time.

Further work by Penner (1988b) and Penner and Bilger (1989) indicated that in some of the patients, the masker was not adapting, and therefore it seems likely that the tinnitus may be increased by the noise. It seems that the tinnitus and the masker do not share the same neural channels where the adaptation is taking place. Caution should be exercised with this procedure, since the high-level, continuous maskers could have undesirable long-term effects on hearing or on the tinnitus.

BINAURAL MASKING

Because so many psychoacoustical studies suggest central components of tinnitus, binaural masking could play an important role in both understanding the mechanisms and clinical treatments. Binaural phenomenon depends critically on the timing (and phase) relationship between the stimuli at the two ears. For example, when the exact same noise waveform is presented to the two ears, the sound is perceived in the midline. However, the perceptual lateralization within the head can be manipulated by changes in the level or time delay to one ear.

Tyler and Stouffer (1992) evaluated monaural and binaural tinnitus masking, utilizing binaural maskers that were uncorrected, correlated and correlated but time delayed (Figure 6-12). They observed that two uncorrellated maskers were generally the least effective in masking the tinnitus. That is, less masker noise was required to mask the tinnitus with correlated maskers. For a few patients, an additional benefit was observed by delaying the noise to one ear, thereby lateralizing the tinnitus to a certain position within the head. They suggested that binaural tinnitus maskers (or habituation devices) could be more effective clinically (see also Johnson & Hughes, 1992).

This binaural interaction is yet one more example of central components of tinnitus.

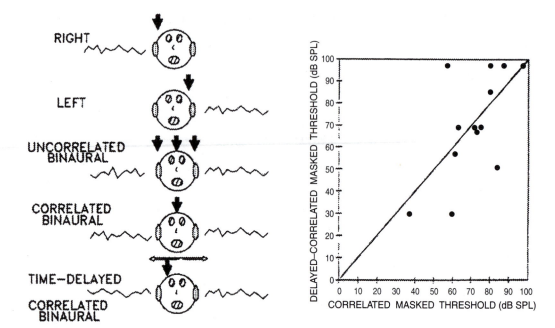

FIGURE 6-12. Left—A schematic representation of monaural and binaural maskers. Binaural maskers were uncorrellated, correlated, and correlated but time delayed. The amount of noise required to mask the tinnitus was measured in each condition. Right—The amount of noise required to mask the tinnitus when the noise was uncorrellated or correlated. (Adapted from Tyler & Stouffer, 1992.)

CLINICAL APPLICATIONS OF MEASUREMENTS

This chapter reviews many of the measurements available to quantify and study tinnitus. But this does not mean it is desirable to perform all these measurements on all patients. Certain "routine" measurements may be desirable on some patients. Additional measures could be helpful in a clinical trial.

Routine Measurements

It is reasonable to perform tinnitus measurements clinically only if they are useful. What is useful will depend on individual needs specific to clinics. Table 6-2 repeats the reasons for measuring tinnitus listed at the beginning of this chapter. It includes measurements that could be useful for each of these goals. These suggestions are intended to reflect only general guidelines.

Clinical Trials

A treatment could change the tinnitus or change the patient's reaction to their tinnitus. A clinical trial should include measurements of both (Tyler, 1992b). Tinnitus disability and handicap questionnaires (Tyler, 1993; see Chapter 11) can be used to measure the patient's reaction to the tinnitus. Psychophysical measures can be used to determine if the tinnitus itself has changed. As described in Table 6-2, to determine if a treatment has had an effect, it can be useful to measure tinnitus loudness and the level of an ipsilateral broadband noise required to mask the tinnitus.

- There is another focus for measuring tinnitus in clinical trials. This includes several issues regarding understanding why a treatment does or does not work.
- The treatment will work for some patients and not others.
- To suggest improvements in treatments.

Table 6-2. Reasons for measuring tinnitus and appropriate measurements

	Reason	*Measurements*
1.	To provide reassurance to the patient that their tinnitus is real.	Pitch and loudness
2.	To be able to reproduce a similar sound to demonstrate to family and significant others some of the characteristics of the tinnitus experienced by the patient.	Pitch and loudness
3.	To provide information that might assist in the determination of site in the auditory system where the tinnitus originates.	Ipsilateral tonal and broadband noise masking, postmasking, ipsilateral versus contralateral masking, binaural masking
4.	To distinguish different subcategories of tinnitus.	Ipsilateral broadband noise masking, tonal masking, postmasking, ipsilateral versus contralateral masking
5.	To determine whether the tinnitus has changed.	Pitch, loudness, ipsilateral masking. Ipsilateral versus contralateral masking
6.	To determine if a treatment has had an effect.	Loudness, ipsilateral broadband noise masking
7.	To provide treatment guidelines.	Ipsilateral broadband noise masking, adaptation of masking
8.	To determine which patients are likely to benefit from some types of treatment.	Ipsilateral broadband noise masking, adaptation of masking
9.	To assist in legal issues.	Pitch and loudness, ipsilateral broadband noise masking, postmasking

These issues are broadly covered under items 3, 4, 7, and 8 mentioned in Table 6-2, and would involve the corresponding measurements. Also noteworthy would be an attempt to distinguish between central and peripheral tinnitus.

There are a few clinical trials, which have used psychoacoustical measurements of tinnitus that have produced some interesting observations.

Several investigators have noted that tinnitus pitch can decrease when there is a relief of symptoms (Tyler, Babin, & Neibuhr, 1984; Donaldson, 1978; Martin & Colman, 1980). Changes in loudness have also been reported (Saito et al., 1999).

Tyler, Babin, and Niebuhr (1984) noted that broadband noise levels required to mask tinnitus followed very closely subjective ratings of loudness and severity. In a double-blind drug tocainide trial, they showed that changes in two subjects' perception of their tinnitus (one who got worse and one who got better) mirrored closely the amount of noise required to mask the tinnitus (Figure 6-13). This was true for both ipsilateral and contralateral noise.

Psychoacoustical measurements should play a critical role in clinical trials.

CENTRAL VERSUS PERIPHERAL TINNITUS

There have been many observations over the years that have suggested that tinnitus is influenced by central mechanisms (Tyler (1981, page 136; Chapters 4, 5, and 9). The following observations are all consistent with central involvement:

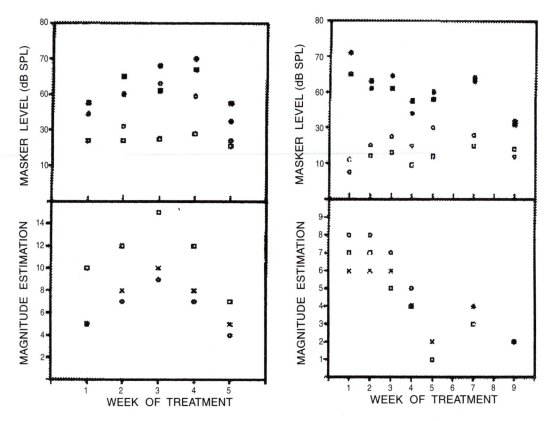

FIGURE 6-13. Noise thresholds, masker levels and subjective ratings as function of week of treatment with the drug tocainide. Left—patient whose tinnitus became worse and the medication was stopped after week 4. Week 1 was a no-treatment control. During weeks 2, 3, and 4, dosages of 400 mg were administered by mouth one, two and three times a day, respectively. Medications were withdrawn the week preceding the measurements at week 5. Right—Patient who completed the trial and whose tinnitus got better. Week 1 was a no-treatment control. During weeks 2, 3, 4, and 5, dosages of 400 mg were administered by mouth one, two, three and four times a day, respectively. Weeks 7 and 9 were double-blind. Week 7 was no treatment and week 9 was 600 mg taken three times per day. (Adapted from Tyler, Babin, & Niebuhr, 1984.)

- Spontaneous activity of auditory nerve fibers is largely unaffected by lesions in animals that often produce tinnitus in humans, such as noise-induced hearing loss.
- Sectioning of the auditory nerve is often ineffective in reducing tinnitus.
- Peripheral degeneration disrupts input to the cochlear nucleus.
- Masking can be effective in either the ipsilateral or contraleral ear.
- There can be frequency independent tonal masking of tinnitus.
- Ipsilateral masking of a unilateral tinnitus can result in the sudden "appearance" of tinnitus in the contralateral ear.

At present, there is no certain test for peripheral, central, or multiple sites of tinnitus. The following observations (see also Tyler, 1999) are generally inconsistent with a central involvement of the mechanisms responsible for tinnitus:

- Tinnitus localized in the one ear.
- Etiologies known to effect the cochlear, such as Ménière's disease, noise-induced hearing loss, and ototoxity (in contrast to hearing losses that are likely to involve the central nervous system as well, such as presbyacusis and head trauma).
- A unilateral sensorineural hearing loss in the ipsilateral tinnitus ear.

- A unilateral tinnitus cannot be masked in the opposite ear.
- Ipsilateral masking effects the tinnitus only in the ipsilateral ear in a patient with binaural tinnitus.
- Frequency dependent tonal masking in the ipsilateral ear.
- A greater postmasking effect in the ipsilateral compared to the contralateral ear.

LEGAL ISSUES

Generally, there are two aspects in which measurements can be useful in a legal case. First, measurements can be used to show that a patient probably has tinnitus. Second, measurements can indicate the magnitude of the impairment, handicap, and/or disability.

Several aspects of legal issues involved with tinnitus are covered in Chapter 17. It is noteworthy that authors have taken quite different perspectives on the usefulness of tinnitus measurements in legal cases. It is likely that individuals whose role is to argue that tinnitus should not be compensated would argue that tinnitus cannot be measured. This is clearly not the case.

A distinction is often made between "subjective" and "objective". Typically an objective test is a physiological measurement in which the patient does not have to respond. Currently, there are no such 'objective' tests for tinnitus (see Chapter 7). It is often implied that objective is preferable because it is independent of potential patient basis. However, most physiological tests require some judgement by the examiner. Therefore, there is a potential for the bias against the tinnitus patient, even for most physiological tests. Actually, what is desirable for both "subjective" and "objective" tests is that the test be valid and reliable. Responses to a questionnaire can be valid if the patient responds truthfully. The questionnaire must also be validated and shown to be reliable. Psychoacoustical measurements of tinnitus can also be valid and reliable.

Tinnitus is Likely Present

Tinnitus is likely present if you can show that it can be reliably measured in the individual. It is presumed here, that a person who is feigning tinnitus would have more difficulty responding in a similar fashion than a patient with a real tinnitus. Similar arguments have been made regarding variability of measurements of hearing loss. Two caveats are needed. As with hearing loss, some feigning patients may be able to reproduce certain tinnitus measurements. In addition, tinnitus can be variable in some patients, thereby variable measurements do not necessarily mean that a tinnitus is being feigned. Test-retest reliability can be measured within or across test sessions.

I suggested in Table 6-2 that measurements of pitch, loudness, ipsilateral broadband noise masking, and postmasking effects could be useful in establishing whether an individual is feigning tinnitus or not. Published data on variability of these procedures can be used provided that instruction and methods are the same. Vernon and Meikle (1988) and Vernon (1996) suggest that the average estimate of tinnitus loudness (based on 5 or 6 trials) repeated "within an hour or so," should be within 3 or 4 dB.

If a patient can make reliable measurements of their tinnitus, it is probable that they have tinnitus.

Magnitude of the Tinnitus Impairment

In cases involving hearing loss, the ability to detect pure tones (or at least thresholds at 500; 1,000; 2,000; and 3,000 Hz) are often used as an indication of the magnitude of the impairment and of the handicap. It is widely acknowledged that this represents a simplification of hearing handicap. For example, thresholds are only one measure of impairment. Other measures include temporal, frequency and intensity distortions. Measuring tinnitus impairment is also not straightforward.

Tyler (1993) has applied the World Health Organizations' (1980) definition of impairment, disability, and handicap to tinnitus (see Table 6-3). Tinnitus disability can be measured with psychoacoustical tests, disability with questionnaires and psychological tests (see Chapters 2 and 11) and handicap with questionnaires.

Specifically, the magnitude of the tinnitus impairment can be measured with estimates of tinnitus loudness and the level of a broadband noise required to mask the tinnitus. Andersson and McKenna (1998) found a statistically significant correlation between the two. Similarly, Mitchell, Vernon, and Creedon (1993) found a very close correspondence between loudness matches and minimum masking levels in twenty-three of twenty-five patients.

Disability is the reduced abilities of a patient and handicap implies a need for extra effort and a lack of independence. Most tinnitus questionnaires (Tyler, 1993, Chapter 11) include measures of both disability and handicap. Some of these tools have been shown to be both valid and reliable and the statistical properties are well defined. To apply these questionnaires to legal cases, it is critical that the patient respond truthfully. This can be difficult to ascertain.

One of the more common areas where tinnitus legal issues arise involves compensation for occupational injury. Each state has its own laws governing this matter. In the state of Iowa, tinnitus is not considered an occupational "hearing loss," and so must be considered with other cases of permanent partial disability to the body (Ehteshamfar v. UTA Engineered Systems Div., 1966). In the case mentioned, the Iowa Industrial Commissioner assessed the disability from tinnitus at 85 percent of the body as a whole.

CONCLUSIONS

There are several reasons for measuring tinnitus. However, it is important to have a clear rationale regarding why they are applied in specific situations. As well as the variability associated with any measurement, tinnitus measurement is complicated because tinnitus often fluctuates and the test stimulus can alter the tinnitus. Care should be taken to use established psychoacoustical procedures and to report variability for individuals. There are several good procedures for measuring tinnitus

Table 6-3. Specification of tinnitus effects based on classification of the World Health Organization (1980). Adapted from Tyler (1993).

	Disorder	Impairment	Disability	Handicap
Definition	Pathology of anatomy and physiology of the auditory system	Dysfunction of auditory system	Reduced abilities of individual	Need for extra effort, reduced independence
Areas affected	Middle ear, inner ear, brain stem, central nervous system	Perception of tinnitus sounds	Concentration, speech perception, localization of sounds, environmental sound perception, sleep	Employment, personal relationships, anxiety, avoiding quiet or noisy situations, annoyance
Measurement	Otoacoustic emissions, imaging studies	Psychoacoustical test, subjective descriptions	Questionnaires, psychological tests	Questionnaires

pitch, loudness, and the masking of tinnitus. There are also important postmasking, adaptation of masking, and binaural masking effects that can be quantified. One of the outstanding characteristics of these measurements is the diverse responses that are observed across patients. This makes these measurements particularly important for routine clinical applications and clinical trials. Some of the measurements strongly suggest either peripheral or central involvement. Finally, the measurements have an important role to play in legal cases.

REFERENCES

Andersson, G., & McKenna, L. (1998). Tinnitus masking and depression. *Audiology, 37,* 174–182.

Bailey, Q. (1979). Audiological aspects of tinnitus. *Australian Journal of Audiology, 1,* 15–18.

Burns, E. (1984). A comparison of variability among measurements of subjective tinnitus and objective stimuli. *Audiology, 23,* 426–440.

Cacace, A. T., Cousins, J. P., Parnes, S. M., Semenoff, D., Holmes, T., McFarland, D. J., Davenport, C., Stegbauer, K., & Lovely, T. J. (1999). Cutaneous-evoked tinnitus: Phenomenology, psychophysics and functional imaging. *Audiology & Neuro-Otology,* 247–257.

Coles, R. R. A., & Baskill, J. L. (1996). Absolute loudness of tinnitus: Tinnitus clinic data. In G. E. Reich and J. A. Vernon (Eds.), *Proceedings of the Fifth International Tinnitus Seminar* (pp. 135–141). Portland, OR: American Tinnitus Association.

Delgutte, B. (1990). Physiological mechanisms of psychophysical masking: Observations from auditory-nerve fibers. *Journal Acoustical Society of America, 87,* 791–809.

Donaldson, I. (1978). Tinnitus: A theoretical view and a therapeutic study using amylobarbitone. *Journal of Laryngology and Otology, 92,* 123–130.

Douek, E., & Reid, J. (1968). The diagnostic value of tinnitus pitch. *Journal of Laryngology and Otology, 82,* 1039–1042.

Ehteshamfar v. UTA Engineered Systems Division, 555 N.W.2d 450 (The Iowa Supreme Court 1996).

Erlandsson, S., Hallberg, L. R. M., & Axelsson, A. (1992). Psychological and audiological correlates of perceived tinnitus severity. *Audiology, 31,* 168–179.

Feldmann, H. (1971). Homolateral and contralateral masking of tinnitus by noisebands and by pure tones. *Audiology, 10,* 138–144.

Florentine, M., Buus, S., Scharf, B., & Zwicker, E. (1980). Frequency selectivity in normally-hearing and hearing-impaired observers. *Journal of Speech and Hearing Research, 23,* 646–669.

Folmer, R. L., Griest, S., Meikle, M. B., & Martin, W. H. (1999). Tinnitus severity, loudness, and depression. *Otolaryngology-Head and Neck Surgery, 121,* 48–51.

Formby, C., & Gjerdingen, D. B. (1980). Pure-tone masking of tinnitus. *Audiology, 19,* 519–535.

Fowler, E. P. (1940). Head noises: Significance, measurement and importance in diagnosis and treatment. *Archives of Otolaryngology—Head and Neck Surgery, 32,* 903–914.

Fowler, E. P. (1942). The illusion of loudness of tinnitus—Its etiology and treatment. *Laryngology, 52,* 275–285.

Fowler, E. P. (1943). Control of head noises: Their illusions of loudness and of timbre. *Otolaryngology—Head and Neck Surgery, 37,* 391–398.

Goodwin, P. E., & Johnson, R. M. (1980a). A comparison of reaction times to tinnitus and nontinnitus frequencies. *Ear and Hearing, 1,* 148–155.

Goodwin, P. E., & Johnson, R. M. (1980b). The loudness of tinnitus. *Acta Otolaryngologica, 90,* 353–359.

Graham, J. T., & Newby, H. A. (1962). Acoustical characteristics of tinnitus. *Archives of Otolaryngology, 75,* 162–167.

Hazell, J. (1981). A tinnitus synthesizer physiological considerations. *Journal of Laryngology and Otology, 4,* 187–195.

Henry, J. A., Flick, C. L., Gilbert, A., Ellingson, R. M., & Fausti, S. A. (1999). Reliability of tinnitus loudness matches under procedural variation. *Journal of the American Academy of Audiology, 10,* 502–520.

Henry, J. A., & Meikle, M. B. (1996). Loudness recruitment only partially explains the small size of tinnitus loudness-matches. In G. E. Reich & J. A. Vernon (Eds.), *Proceedings of the Fifth International Tinnitus Seminar* (pp. 148–157). Portland, OR: American Tinnitus Association.

Henry, J. A., & Meikle, M. B. (1999). Pulsed Versus Continuous Tones for Evaluating the Loudness of Tinnitus. *Journal of American Academy of Audiology, 10,* 261–272.

Henry, J. A., Meikle, M. B., & Gilbert, A. (1999). Audiometric correlates of tinnitus pitch: Insights from the Tinnitus Data Registry. In J. Hazell (Ed.), *Proceedings of the Sixth International Tinnitus Seminar* (pp. 51–57). London: The Tinnitus and Hyperacusis Centre.

Hinchcliffe, R., & Chambers, C. (1983). Loudness of tinnitus: An approach to measurement. *Advances in Oto-Rhino-Laryngology, 29,* 163–173.

Hirsh, I. J., & Ward W. D. (1952). Recovery of the auditory threshold after strong acoustic stimulation. *Journal of the Acoustical Society of America, 24,* 131–141.

Ishikawa, T., Kusano, H., Ogasawara, M., Murai, K., & Tsuiki, T. (1992). Investigation of tinnitus tests: Comparison of ipsilateral and contralateral testing. In J. M. Aran & R. Dauman (Eds.), *Proceedings of the Fourth International Tinnitus Seminar* (pp. 43–48). Amsterdam/ New York: Kugler Publications.

Jakes, S. C., Hallam, R. S., Chambers, C. C., & Hinchcliffe, R. (1986). Matched and self-reported loudness of tinnitus: Methods and sources of error. *Audiology, 25,* 92–100.

Jastreboff, P., Hazel, J. W. P., & Graham, R. L. (1994). Neurophysiological model of tinnitus: Dependence of the minimal masking level on treatment outcome. *Hearing Research, 80,* 216–232.

Johnson, R. M., & Hughes, F. M. (1992). Diotic versus dicotic masking of tinnitus. In J. M. Aran & R. Dounan (Eds.), *Tinnitus 91. Proceedings of the Fourth International Tinnitus Seminar* (pp. 387–390). New York Kugler Publications.

Johnson, R. M., & Sandlin, R. E. (1996). Residual inhibition produced by pure–tone signals and bands of noise. In G. E. Reich, and J. A. Vernon (Eds.), *Proceedings of the Fifth International Tinnitus Seminar* (pp. 167–170). Portland, OR: American Tinnitus Association.

Kitajima, K., Kitahara, M., & Kodama, A. (1987). Can tinnitus be masked by band erased filtered masker? Masking tinnitus with sounds not covering the tinnitus frequency. *American Journal of Otology, 8,* 203–206.

Liden, G., Nilsson, G., & Anderson, H. (1959). Masking in clinical audiometry. *Acta Oto-laryngologica, 50,* 125–136.

Martin, F. W., & Colman, B. H. (1980). Tinnitus: A double-blind cross-over controlled trial to evaluate the use of lignocaine. *Clinical Otolaryngology, 5,* 3–11.

Matsuhira, T., & Yamashita, K. (1996a). Factors contributing to tinnitus loudness. In G. E. Reich & J. A. Vernon (Eds.), *Proceedings of the Fifth International Tinnitus Seminar* (pp. 171–175). Portland, Oregon: American Tinnitus Association.

Matsuhira, T., & Yamashita, K. (1996b). Grading of tinnitus loudness from matching test. In G. E. Reich & J. A. Vernon (Eds.), *Proceedings of the Fifth International Tinnitus Seminar* (pp. 176–179). Portland, OR: American Tinnitus Association.

Matsuhira, T., Yamashita, K., & Yasuda, M. (1992). Estimation of the loudness of tinnitus from matching tests. *British Journal of Audiology, 26,* 387–395.

Meikle, M. B. (1995). The Interaction of Central and Peripheral Mechanisms in Tinnitus. In J. A. Vernon & A. R. Moller (Eds.), *Mechanisms of Tinnitus* (pp. 181–206). Needham Heights, MA: Allyn & Bacon.

Meikle, M. B., & Griest, S. E. (1992). Asymmetry in tinnitus perceptions: Factors that may account for the higher prevalence of left-sided tinnitus. In J. M. Aran & R. Dauman (Eds.), *Tinnitus 91: Proceedings of the Fourth International Tinnitus Seminar* (pp. 231–237). Amsterdam, The Netherlands: Kugler Publications.

Meikle, M. B., Schuff, N., & Griest, S. (1987). Intra-subject variability of tinnitus: Observations from the Tinnitus Clinic. In H. Feldman, (Ed.), *Proceedings of the Third International Tinnitus Seminar* (pp. 175–180). Karlsruhe, Germany: Harsch Verlag.

Mineau, S. M., & Schlauch, R. S. (1997). Threshold measurement for patients with tinnitus: Pulsed or continuous tones. *American Journal of Audiology, 6,* 52–56.

Minton, J. R. (1923). Tinnitus and its relation to nerve deafness with an application to the masking effect of pure tones. *The Physical Review, 22,* 506–509.

Mitchell, C. (1983). The masking of tinnitus with pure tones. *Audiology, 22,* 73–87.

Mitchell, C. R., & Creedon, T. A. (1995). Psychological tuning curves in subjects with tinnitus suggest outer hair cell lesions. *Otolaryngology—Head and Neck Surgery, 113,* 223–233.

Mitchell, C. R., Vernon, J. A., & Creedon, T. A. (1993). Measuring Tinnitus Parameters: Loudness, Pitch, and Maskability. *Journal* of the American Academy of Audiology, 4, 139–151.

Moore, B. C. J. (1997). *An introduction to the psychology of hearing.* San Diego, CA: Academic Press.

Mortimer, H., Burr, E. G., Wright, R. P., & McGarry, E. A. (1940). A clinical method for the localization of tinnitus and the measurement of its loudness level. *TransAmerican Laryngology Rhinology and Otology Society, 46,* 15–31.

Murai, K., Ogasawara, M., Ishikawa, T., Kusano, H., & Tsuiki, T. (1992). Evaluation of tinnitus masking curve measured by Bekesy audiometer. In J. M. Aran & R. Dauman (Eds.), *Proceedings of the Fourth International Tinnitus Seminar* (pp. 61–63). Amsterdam/New York: Kugler Publications.

Murai, K., Ogasawara, M., Saitoh, T, & Tsuiki,T. (1987). An Evaluation of Ipsilateral and Contralateral Masking for Tinnitus. In H. Feldmann (Ed.), *Proceedings of the Third International Tinnitus Seminar* (p. 304). Munster, Germany: Harsch Hverlag Karlsruhe.

Newman, C. W., Wharton, J. A., Shivapuja, B. G., & Jacobson, G. P. (1994). Relationships among psychoacoustic judgments, speech understanding ability and self–perceived handicap in tinnitus subjects. *Audiology, 33,* 47–60.

Nodar, R. H., & Graham, J. T. (1965). An investigation of frequency characteristics of tinnitus associated with Ménière's disease. *Archives of Otolaryngology, 82,* 28–31.

Ohsaki, K., Fujimura, T., Sugiura, T., Tamura, K., Nakagiri, S., Zheng, H. X., Hatano, A., & Kimura, A. (1990). Reproducibility of pitch-matching test for tinnitus, using a heptatonic scale. *Scandinavian Audiology, 19,* 123–126.

Penner, M. J. (1980). Two-tone forward masking patterns and tinnitus. *Journal of Speech and Hearing Research, 23,* 779–786.

Penner, M. J. (1983a). Variability in matches to subjective tinnitus. *Journal of Speech and Hearing Research, 26,* 263–267.

Penner, M. J. (1983b). The annoyance of tinnitus and the noise required to mask it. *Journal of Speech and Hearing Research, 26,* 73–76.

Penner, M. J. (1984). Equal-loudness contours using subjective tinnitus as the standard. *Journal of Speech and Hearing Research, 27,* 274–279.

Penner, M. J. (1986a). Tinnitus as a source of internal noise. *Journal of Speech and Hearing Research, 29,* 400–406.

Penner, M. J. (1986b). Magnitude estimation and the "paradoxical" loudness considering the effects of recruitment. *Journal of Speech and Hearing Research, 29,* 407–412.

Penner, M. J. (1987). Masking of tinnitus and central masking. *Journal of Speech and Hearing Research, 30,* 147–152.

Penner, M. J. (1988a). The effect of continuous monaural noise on loudness matches to tinnitus. *Journal of Speech and Hearing Research, 31,* 98–102.

Penner, M. J. (1988b). Judgements of the loudness of tinnitus before and after masking. *Journal of Speech and Hearing Research, 31,* 582–587.

Penner, M. J. (1993). Synthesizing tinnitus from sine waves. *Journal of Speech and Hearing Research, 36,* 1300–1305.

Penner, M. J. (1996). Rating the annoyance of synthesized tinnitus. *International Tinnitus Journal, 2,* 3–7.

Penner, M. J., & Bilger, R. C. (1989). Adaptation and the masking of tinnitus. *Journal of Speech and Hearing Research, 32,* 339–346.

Penner, M. J., & Bilger, R. C. (1992). Consistent within-session measures of tinnitus. *Journal of Speech and Hearing Research, 35,* 694–700.

Penner, M. J., Brauth, S., & Hood, L. (1981). The temporal course of the masking of tinnitus as a basis for inferring its origin. *Journal of Speech and Hearing Research, 24,* 257–261.

Penner, M. J., & Klafter, E. J. (1992). Measures of tinnitus: Step size, matches to imagined tones, and masking patterns. *Ear and Hearing, 13(6),* 410–416.

Penner, M. J., & Saran, A. (1994). Simultaneous measurement of tinnitus pitch and loudness. *Ear and Hearing, 15,* 416–421.

Reed, G. F. (1960). An audiometric study of 200 cases of subjective tinnitus. *Archives of Otolaryngology, 71,* 84–94.

Saito, T., Manabe, Y., Shibamori, Y., Noda, I., Yamamoto, T., & Saito, H. (1999). Comparison between matched and self-reported change in tinnitus loudness before and after tinnitus treatment. In J. W. P. Hazel (Ed.), *Proceedings of the Sixth International Tinnitus Seminar* (pp. 522–524). Norfolk, UK: Hawthorne Production Services.

Scott, B., Lindberg, P., Melin, L., & Lyttkens, L. (1990). Predictors of tinnitus discomfort, adaptation and subjective loudness. *British Journal of Audiology, 24,* 51–62.

Shailer, M. J., Tyler, R. S., & Coles, R. R. A. (1981). Critical masking bands for sensorineural tinnitus. *Scandinavian Audiology, 10,* 157–162.

Slater, R., & Terry, M. (1987). *Tinnitus: A guide for sufferers and professionals.* London: Croom Helm.

Small, A. M. (1973). Psychoacoustics. In F. D. Minifie, T. J. Hixon, & F. Williams (Eds.), *Normal Aspects of Speech, Hearing, and Language* (pp. 343–420). Englewood Cliffs, NJ: Prentice-Hall, Inc.

Smith, P. A., Parr, V. M., Lutman, M. E., & Coles, R. R. A. (1991). Comparative study of four noise spectra as potential tinnitus maskers. *British Journal of Audiology, 25,* 25–34.

Stevens, S. S. (1955). The measurement of loudness. *Journal of the Acoustical Society of America, 27,* 815–829.

Stouffer, J. L., & Tyler, R. S. (1990a). Characterization of tinnitus by tinnitus patients. *Journal of Speech and Hearing Disorders, 55,* 439–453.

Stouffer, J. L., & Tyler, R. S. (1990b). Subjective tinnitus loudness. *Hearing Instruments, 41,* 17–19.

Terhardt, E. (1974). Pitch of pure tones: Its relationship to intensity. In E. Zwicke & E. Terhardt (Eds.), *Facts and Models in Hearing* (pp. Heidelberg, NY: Springer-Verlag.

Terry, A. M., Jones, D. M., Davis, B. R., & Slater, R. (1983). Parametric studies of tinnitus masking and residual inhibition. *British Journal of Audiology, 17,* 245–256.

Tyler, R. S. (1981). Comments on animal models of tinnitus. In D. Evered & G. Lawernson (Eds.), *Tinnitus* (pp. 136–136). London: Pitman Books Ltd.

Tyler, R. S. (1985). Psychoacoustical measurement of tinnitus for treatment evaluations. In E. Myers (Ed.), *New Dimensions in Otorhinolaryngology—Head and Neck Surgery* Vol 1 (pp. 455–458). Amsterdam: Elsevier Publishing Co.

Tyler, R. S. (1992a). The psychophysical measurement of tinnitus. In J. M. Aran & R. Dauman (Eds.), *Tinnitus 91: Proceedings of the Fourth International Tinnitus Seminar* (pp. 17–26). Amsterdam, The Netherlands: Kugler Publications.

Tyler, R. S. (1992b). Evaluation of tinnitus treatments. In J. M. Aran & R. Dauman (Eds.), *Tinnitus 91: Proceedings of the Fourth International Tinnitus Seminar* (pp. 551–554). Amsterdam, The Netherlands: Karger Publications.

Tyler, R. S. (1993). Tinnitus disability and handicap questionnaires. *Seminars in Hearing, 14,* 377–384.

Tyler, R. S. (1999). The use of science to find successful tinnitus treatments. In J. Hazell, (Ed.), *Proceedings of the Sixth International Tinnitus Seminar* (pp. 3–9). London: The Tinnitus and Hyperacusis Centre.

Tyler, R. S., Aran, J. M., & Dauman, R. (1992). Recent advances in tinnitus. *American Journal of Audiology, 36–44.*

Tyler, R. S., Babin, R., & Niebuhr, D. (1984). Some observations on the masking and postmasking effects on tinnitus. *Journal of Laryngology and Otology, 9,* 150–150.

Tyler, R. S., & Conrad-Armes, D. (1983a). The determination of tinnitus loudness considering the effects of recruitment. *Journal of Speech and Hearing Research, 26,* 59–72.

Tyler, R. S., & Conrad-Armes, D. (1983b). Tinnitus pitch: A comparison of three measurement methods. *British Journal of Audiology, 17,* 101–107.

Tyler, R. S., & Conrad-Armes, D. (1984). The masking of tinnitus compared to the masking of pure tones. *Journal of Speech and Hearing Research, 27,* 106–111.

Tyler, R. S., Conrad-Armes, D., & Smith, P. A. (1984). Postmasking effects of sensorineural tinnitus: A preliminary investigation. *Journal of Speech and Hearing Research, 27,* 466–474.

Tyler, R. S., Kuk, F. K., & Mims, L. A. (1987). Ipsilateral and contralateral postmasking recovery of tinnitus. In H. Feldmann, (Ed.), *Proceedings of the Third International Tinnitus Seminar* (pp. 275–279). Munster: Harsch Verlag Karlsruhe.

Tyler, R. S., & Stouffer, J. L. (1989). A review of tinnitus loudness. *Hearing Journal, 11,* 52–57.

Tyler, R. S., & Stouffer, J. L. (1992). Binaural tinnitus masking with a noise centered on the tinnitus. In J. M. Aran & R. Dauman (Eds.), *Proceedings of the Fourth International Tinnitus Seminar* (pp. 391–394). Amsterdam/New York: Kugler Publications.

Tyler, R. S., Wood, E. J., & Fernandes, M. (1982). Frequency resolution and hearing loss. *British Journal of Audiology, 16,* 45–63.

Vernon, J. (1977). Attempts to relieve tinnitus. *Journal of American Auditory Society, 2,* 124–131.

Vernon, J. (1987). Assessment of the tinnitus patient. In J. Hazell (Ed.), *Tinnitus* (pp. 71–95). Edinburgh: Churchill Livingstone.

Vernon, J. (1996). Is the claimed tinnitus real and is the claimed cause correct? In *Proceedings of the Fifth International Tinnitus Seminar* (pp. 395–396).

Vernon, J., & Meikle, M. B. (1988). Measurement of tinnitus: An update. In M. Kitahara (Ed.), *Tinnitus: Pathophysiology and Management* (pp. 36–52). Tokyo: Igaku–shoin.

Wegel, R. L. (1931). A study of tinnitus. *Archives of Otolaryngology—Head and Neck Surgery, 14,* 158–165.

World Health Organization (1980). *International classification of impairments, disabilities and handicaps—A manual of classification relating to the consequences of disease.* Geneva: World Health Organization.

Zwislocki, J. J., Buining, E., & Glantz, J. (1968). Frequency distribution of central masking. *Journal of the Acoustical Society of America, 43,* 1267–1271.

CHAPTER 7

Physiological Measurement of Tinnitus in Humans

Gary P. Jacobson, Ph.D.

INTRODUCTION

It might be hypothesized that since tinnitus represents the perception of sound when none is present, that this phantom perception of sound should be observable in functional measures of the auditory system. Since the early 1980s, investigators have attempted to identify in electrophysiological recordings from the auditory system the presence or effects of tinnitus on performance measures of auditory function. The purposes of these investigations have been primarily to objectify the tinnitus experience. That is, investigators have employed electrophysiological measures in an attempt to help differentiate those patients complaining of tinnitus who do and do not actually *have* tinnitus. A more important application of these investigations has been the objective quantification of tinnitus. That is, if tinnitus could be observed in electrophysiological recordings, and if the origins of the electrophysiological signals were known, then abnormalities in the results of electrophysiological investigations of tinnitus subjects might provide information

about the origins and mechanisms of tinnitus. It is noteworthy that the National Institutes on Deafness and Other Communication Disorders has identified the "elucidation of tinnitus" as a ". . . promising . . . clinical research opportunity . . . (Snow & Naunton, 1993)." It will be my objective in this review to synthesize the data available that pertains to electrophysiological measures in patients with tinnitus.

Investigators have utilized in tinnitus investigations all available auditory assessment techniques including: spontaneous and evoked transient otoacoustic emissions (see Chapter 8), tympanic electrocochleography, direct VIIIth nerve recording techniques, auditory brain stem responses and both long latency exogenous (obligatory brain responses to sound) and endogenous (brain responses associated with higher level processing of sound) evoked potentials. Inherent to all investigations has been the idea that tinnitus results from a "hyperactive" auditory system (see Chapter 4). This assumption has been supported by the results of recent research showing increased auditory system activity at the level of the dorsal cochlear nucleus in hamsters (Kaltenbach et al., 1996) following noise exposure and at the level of the auditory cortex (Wallhausser-Frank et al., 1996) following salicylate exposure in gerbils. Both signal averaging of auditory-evoked potentials and signal averaging of spontaneous auditory system activity have been used. Inherent to the application of signal averaging of time series data has been the presumption that an evoked potential source involved in tinnitus generation would be (because of the tinnitus) continuously active processing the tinnitus sensation, and thus, unable to respond fully to a competing auditory signal (for example, a click or tone burst). The use of spectral analysis (that is, the display of power by frequency) assumes that the presence of increased spontaneous electrical activity in the auditory system (such as tinnitus) will be revealed as unexplained frequency peaks or an unexplained increase in the overall power spectrum of electrical activity recorded from the cochlea, auditory nerve, brain stem pathways, or auditory cortex.

Despite the ready availability of patients, extremely sensitive recording methods and sophisticated data-processing techniques, the findings reported by investigators to date have been inconclusive. There has not been, as yet, unanimous support for any positive finding. Accordingly, at present, we do not have an objective measure (test) for tinnitus. As a result we have only "hints" of the mechanisms that may be responsible for the tinnitus sensation.

REVIEW OF TECHNIQUES

Otoacoustic Emissions

The area of greatest interest in tinnitus research has been the relationship between otoacoustic emissions and tinnitus (see Chapter 8). Specifically, investigators have attempted to determine: (1) the relationship between spontaneous otoacoustic emissions (SOAEs) and tinnitus, (2) the relationship between parameters of OAE measures and

tinnitus, and, (3) the effectiveness of efferent system suppression of OAEs and the presence of tinnitus. Again, the results of these investigations often have been at odds.

Spontaneous otoacoustic emissions represent low level acoustical signals that are fed back from the cochlea through the middle-ear system to the ear canal. Approximately 30 percent of the normal population have at least one spontaneous OAE and it is possible to have many SOAEs coexisting in one ear. Most often these emissions are of such low amplitude and are steady in frequency (pitch) that, if they are audible, listeners adapt to the signals and they become inaudible unless the emission changes frequency. In this regard, it has been estimated that the average amplitude of SOAEs from twenty-one ears of thirteen normal hearing subjects without tinnitus was −4 dB SPL (Martin et al., 1990). The standard deviation of 20 within session measures of SOAEs has been estimated as 1.16 dB (Frick & Matthies, 1988).

Shortly following the discovery of SOAEs (Kemp et al., 1979) there was great interest in determining whether there was a direct relationship between the frequency/ies of the SOAE and the subjective pitch of a patient's tinnitus. What became clear across at least seventeen studies (Ceranic et al., 1995) was that SOAEs correspond to tinnitus pitch in, at best, approximately 4 to 5 percent of cases. Penner (1990) estimated the incidence of tinnitus related SOAEs as between 1 percent and 9.5 percent (95 percent confidence interval) amongst members of a tinnitus support group.

Penner and Burns (1987a,b) have suggested that before the link between tinnitus and SOAEs, several criteria must be satisfied including: (1) there must be a correspondence between tinnitus pitch and the frequency or frequencies of the SOAE, (2) that suppression of the SOAE by presentation of a lower frequency auditory signal must make the SOAE inaudible, (3) masking of the tinnitus must abolish the SOAE/s, and, (4) pure tone isomasking contours of the tinnitus must demonstrate frequency specificity (that is, there must be "notches" in the masking contours demonstrating effective masking of the tinnitus by a low-intensity pure tone of identical frequency).

Penner (1989a) also presented a case report illustrated with two coexisting types of tinnitus. This patient demonstrated tinnitus in one ear that corresponded to an SOAE on that side (see Figure 7-1). Tinnitus in the other ear was not related to SOAEs. Penner (1989b) and Penner and Coles (1992)

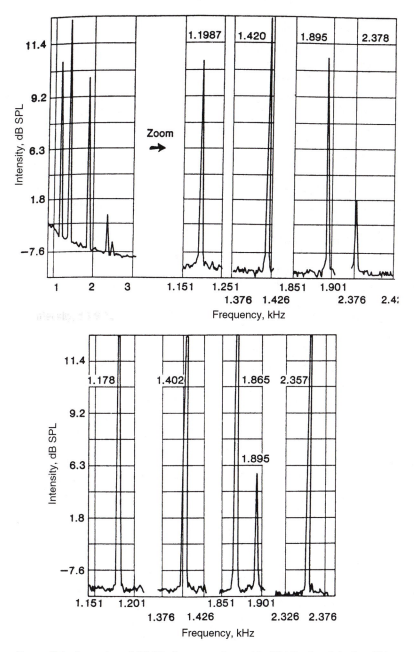

FIGURE 7-1. Examples of SOAEs from a patient with SOAE-related tinnitus. This patient has four SOAEs. All but one of the emissions could be suppressed following the administration of salicylates. From Penner (1989) reproduced with permission.

have reported that salicylates (two 300 mg tablets, administered four times daily) may be used to attenuate SOAEs causing tinnitus. It is ironic that salicylates, that are known to cause reversible tinnitus in normals, actually can attenuate SOAE-related tinnitus if administered in high enough dosages.

Penner (1990) also has reported that SOAEs may be present usually only if hearing sensitivity was better than 20 dB HL. She noted that for SOAE-induced tinnitus, the tone matching frequency was in the 1,000 to 2,000 Hz range instead of the normal 3,000 to 5,000 Hz range for tinnitus not associated with SOAE. Penner and Burns (1987a) discussed reasons for the discordance between the SOAE frequencies and tinnitus pitch match frequencies. Specifically, though tinnitus pitch matches usually equal or exceed 4,000 Hz, few SOAEs exceed 4,000 Hz due to the attenuation effects of the middle ear system (that is, the middle ear system acts as a low pass filter for reverse transfer of frequencies above 4,000 Hz).

Penner (1992) reported that within-session test-retest matches of tinnitus pitch can exceed 1,000 Hz. The reason for this variability is that, for some, the perceived pitch of tinnitus is labile and further SOAE-related tinnitus may have multiple components (frequencies). In this regard, Burns (1989) and Burns and Keefe (1991) demonstrated time-varying SOAE spectra and hypothesized that tinnitus is audible only when changes in SOAE spectra are observed. That is, the auditory system fatigues to SOAE-induced tinnitus of unchanging frequency. However, SOAE-related tinnitus comes back to conscious perception when, and if, the SOAE frequency changes. It is of note that the percentage of normal hearing subjects with SOAE-caused tinnitus has been estimated to be about 8.6 percent (Penner, 1992). Chapter 8 suggests that this percentage may be higher with improved recording techniques.

It has been demonstrated in normals that the introduction of a low-level white noise (for example, 30 dB SL) contralaterally will alter the amplitude of the evoked otoacoustic emission (Collett et al., 1991). This occurs as a function of the medial olivocochlear system. It has been demonstrated in patients with tinnitus that the performance characteristics of the medial olivocochlear system may be normal (that is, > 1 dB suppression of the contralateral transient evoked otoacoustic emission-TEOAE) or deficient as demonstrated in the magnitude of TEOAE suppression following contralateral stimulation. In this regard, Chery-Croze et al. (1993) evaluated thirty-six patients with either unilateral or bilateral tinnitus using TEOAE and distortion product otoacoustic emission (DPOAE) techniques. The investigators reported that some alteration in the function was noted in nineteen of twenty-one patients with unilateral tinnitus and in all sixteen patients complaining of bilateral tinnitus. Generally, for patients with unilateral tinnitus the effects of efferent suppression on the DPOAE were of lesser magnitude for the ear with tinnitus (see Figure 7-2). When looking at this in finer detail using DPOAE techniques, it was observed that efferent suppression was least effective in the region of the tinnitus pitch match frequency for at least one ear. These findings have since been supported by further research in the same laboratory (Chery-Croze et al., 1994a,b) and by others (Graham & Hazell, 1994; Attias et al., 1996). However, contradictory results have been reported by Lind (1996). That is, using TOAE techniques only, the authors found no deficit in efferent suppression for their tinnitus patients. Graham and Hazell (1994) observed that the variability in effects of efferent suppression of TEOAE was greater for patients with tinnitus compared with normal hearing controls. It should be noted that their tinnitus patient sample was older and had hearing loss. This might account for the variability in efferent suppression measures. That is, an older and more impaired system may be expected to demonstrate greater variability in its response characteristics compared to an intact system.

Tinnitus

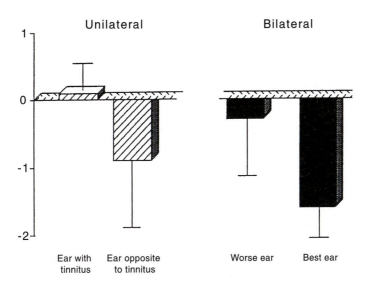

FIGURE 7-2. Summary of data for patients with unilateral (striped bars) and bilateral tinnitus (solid bars). Graph depicts finding that patients with unilateral tinnitus generally show lesser amounts of TEOAE attenuation in the presence of low-level white noise presented contralaterally. The investigators observed that TOAEs recorded from the ear with worst tinnitus in bilateral tinnitus also showed lesser amounts of attenuation in the presence of low-level contralateral broadband noise. From Chery-Croze et al. (1993) reproduced with permission.

Attias et al. (1996a) approached the question of the heterogeneity of an aged subject sample by attempting to control for subject characteristics. That is, their subject samples consisted of: normal hearing—no tinnitus, normal hearing—tinnitus, noise-induced hearing loss—no tinnitus, noise induced hearing loss—tinnitus samples. Also, the age range of the sample was restricted to twenty-six to thirty-seven years of age. The sample consisted of forty-two subjects and fifty-two ears. They evaluated the effects of efferent suppression across five white noise levels from 5 to 45 dB SL in 10 dB increments. The investigators reported that for control subjects without tinnitus (with and without hearing loss) increasing white noise levels resulted in increased efferent suppression of the TEOAE. Alternately, patients with tinnitus (with and without hearing loss), demonstrated paradoxically greater TEOAE levels in the presence of contralateral noise. The effect was most pronounced for patients

with normal hearing and tinnitus. These findings underscored the concept that it might be possible to obtain more consistent findings in OAE research through more stringent control over subject selection.

Direct Recorded VIIIth Nerve Action Potentials

There has been only one report of direct recorded *evoked* VIIIth nerve activity in patients with tinnitus. Moller et al. (1992) recorded compound action potentials to acoustical transients from the exposed VIIIth nerve of nineteen patients (sixteen with hearing loss) undergoing microvascular decompression for intractable tinnitus. These recordings were compared with those obtained from sixteen patients with similar hearing loss undergoing neurovascular decompression of the Vth, VIIth, or IXth cranial nerves. Results revealed large intersubject variability in the shape of the VIIIth nerve compound action potential. There were no between-group differences (patients with hearing loss and tinnitus versus patients with hearing loss and no tinnitus) in compound action potentials (see Table 7-1). No differences were observed in the latencies of peaks of compound action potentials or of peak latencies of waves III and V of ABRs of patients whose tinnitus did improve compared with those whose tinnitus did not improve.

Scalp-Recorded Auditory Brain Stem Response

There have been several reports by investigators who have examined tinnitus patients using auditory brain stem responses (ABR). Both the subject samples and findings have been heterogenous. That is, there have been no consistent changes across investigations observed in ABRs of adults with tinnitus.

Barnea et al. (1990) evaluated the ABR in seventeen subjects with normal pure-tone thresholds and tinnitus and seventeen normal-hearing controls. The investigators found no group differences in ABR latency, amplitude, or interwave intervals. These findings are similar to those reported by Attias et al. (1993) who evaluated the ABR of twelve male patients with noise-induced hearing loss and tinnitus, and twelve tinnitus-free subjects matched for gender, age, and severity and configuration of hearing loss. The investigators evaluated group differences in the latencies and amplitudes of ABR components I, III, and V and interwave intervals I-III, III-V, and I-V. There were no statistically significant group differences. McKee and Stephens (1992) also reported the absence of ABR abnormalities in a group of thirty-seven normal hearing subjects with tinnitus.

In contradiction to these observations, Ikner and Hassen (1990) evaluated the ABR in normal hearing subjects, and hearing loss subjects with and without tinnitus. All subjects had hearing thresholds of less than 25 dB at 1,000 and 2,000 Hz. The investigators matched the samples based upon contra-

Table 7-1. Latencies and amplitudes of direct recorded VIIIth nerve compound action potential (N_1) and following negativity (N_2) in response to condensation and rarefaction click stimulation. Latency values from condensation polarity clicks are denoted with the letter "C." Latency values from rarefaction polarity clicks are denoted with the letter "R."

	N_1		N_2	
	R	**C**	**R**	**C**
Patients with tinnitus and high-frequency hearing loss N = 16 (this study)				
$\bar{x}$	3.10	3.20	4.89	4.72
SD	0.45	0.41	0.82	0.57
Patients with normal hearing N = 16 (from Moller et al.[28])				
$\bar{x}$	2.97	3.02	4.23	4.59
SD	0.12	0.23	0.29	0.33
Patients with high-frequency hearing loss but no tinnitus N = 15 (from Moller and Jho[29])				
$\bar{x}$	3.22	3.16	4.72	4.55
SD	0.42	0.30	0.68	0.56
Hearing loss: difference between patients with tinnitus and patients without tinnitus				
	−0.12	0.04	0.17	0.17

From Moller et al. 1992, reproduced with permission of publisher.

lateral stapedial reflex thresholds, high-frequency pure tone average (average thresholds at 1,000 Hz, 2,000 Hz and 4,000 Hz) and auditory threshold at 4,000 Hz and normal hearing from 1,000 to 4,000 Hz. The investigators reported prolongation of wave I in females with tinnitus compared with females who were tinnitus free. The results suggested to the investigators that the characteristics of wave I could be used as a diagnostic indicator for tinnitus in females. Problems with this investigation included the tinnitus subjects having poorer high-frequency hearing sensitivity, which is known to increase selectively the latency of wave I. This subject-related difference might have accounted for the observed group difference in the latency of wave I of 0.14 ms. Additionally, the authors used only one click polarity. It is known that hearing loss potentiates polarity-dependent changes in ABR latency. Therefore, it is possible that the group differences in wave I latency might have disappeared had the investigators used data obtained from the "best click polarity."

In a much larger series Rosenhall and Axelsson (1994) reported ABR data obtained from fifty-six tinnitus patients with normal hearing or "slight" sensorineural hearing loss, fifty-seven tinnitus patients with moderate-to-"pronounced" sensorineural hearing loss. These data were compared to data collected from a cohort of 220 controls matched for gender, age, and hearing loss. The authors reported two patterns of abnormalities in 10 to 11 percent of the patients with tinnitus, (1) a prolongation (> 2 SD) of wave I accompanied by a prolongation of waves III and V greater than that seen in the controls, and (2) a prolongation of the wave III to V interwave interval.

Jastreboff et al. (1992) reported the results of an investigation where frequency instead of time-domain averaging techniques were employed in an attempt to detect differences in the ABRs of patients with tinnitus. The judge (Jastreboff) was "blinded" in this investigation. He was provided with three diskettes each containing three-channel ABR data (obtained from ipsilateral, contralateral and horizontal electrode derivations) from seven normal subjects (diskette 1), and, from two groups of tinnitus patients (diskettes 2 and 3). Jastreboff performed a frequency analysis on the data and found statistically significant differences between the three groups (corresponding to the three diskettes). Moreover, he was able to differentiate meaningfully the tinnitus from control groups based upon power spectral analysis of data recorded from the horizontal electrode derivation (mastoid to mastoid derivation) at 100 Hz (tinnitus patients having lesser magnitudes), 200 Hz and 600 Hz (tinnitus patients having greater magnitude). Using a time-series analysis the investigator was able to differentiate the tinnitus from control groups using data obtained from all derivations (three orthogonal vectors). The differences in the ABR waveform occurred in the latency region of 7 ms in the ipsilateral recording channel. The investigator interpreted the frequency data as suggestive that tinnitus affected auditory processing at the caudal pontine level. The time series data suggested that the effects of tinnitus modified auditory processing at level of the midbrain (determined on the basis of the group differences observed at 7 ms poststimulus onset). The authors cautioned that these data were suggestive only due to their small subject samples (a total of twenty-one subjects, fourteen with tinnitus). This paper was particularly interesting because it introduced an alternative method to the conventional time series analysis for analyzing the ABR.

Finally, Attias et al. (1996b) compared the ABR of patients with tinnitus and noise-induced hearing loss with an age and hearing loss-matched sample of subjects without tinnitus. The authors utilized both conventional latency and amplitude measures of the ABR as well as parameters derived from three-channel Lissajous trajectory analyses. The authors reported that for their subjects with tinnitus they found an enhanced Wave III amplitude (in the vertex to ipsilateral mastoid electrode derivation—see Figure 7-3). This finding had not been reported previously.

IPSILATERAL

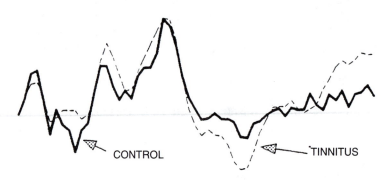

CONTRATERAL   .25 μV

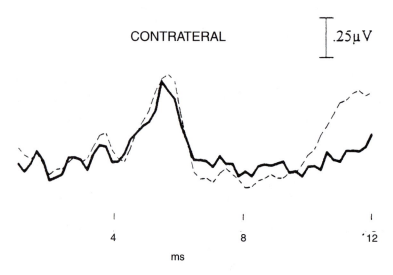

FIGURE 7-3. Time domain, grand averaged ipsilateral and contralateral ABRs in response to 1024 consecutive click stimuli, for the tinnitus and control subjects. Notice the enhancement of wave III amplitude for the tinnitus subjects (dashed lines). This finding was observed only in the ipsilateral recording derivation. Note also the incidental finding of an enhancement of ABR amplitude in the time period following the wave V peak. From Attias et al. (1996) reproduced with permission.

Scalp-Recorded Late Cortical Evoked Potentials N1/P2

It has been hypothesized that constant afferent activity from the periphery representing tinnitus would result in sustained neural activity in cortical receptor areas where the afferent activity is received. This would make those cortical areas less responsive to transient acoustical stimulation and would result in significant differences in cortically generated evoked potentials between those patients with and without tinnitus. In this regard, Hoke et al. (1989) conducted an investigation of long latency evoked magnetic fields N1m and P2m (that is, the magnetic equivalents of evoked potential components N1 and P2) in normals and subjects with tinnitus. The investigators made three recordings using a single-channel neuromagnetometer that is designed to detect and record small magnetic field changes emitted by the brain in response to sound. The auditory signals were 1,000 Hz tone bursts. The authors observed that for normal subjects the P2 component was at least one-half the amplitude of the N1 component (normal P2/N1 amplitude ratio of 0.5 or greater). However, for tinnitus patients N1 was larger and P2 was absent or of very low amplitude. This resulted in a P2/N1 amplitude ratio that was less than 0.5 for patients with tinnitus. Also, the authors reported that P2, when present, was prolonged in latency for the patients with tinnitus. This initial report was followed by a case study by the same group (Pantev et al., 1989). In this investigation the auditory evoked field data was presented from a soldier with tinnitus caused by exposure to gunfire. The authors demonstrated that whereas the P2/N1 amplitude ratio was small initially, the amplitude ratio normalized over a period of 256 days during which the patient became tinnitus-free. It was the investigators' hypothesis that the constant inflow of activity from the periphery served to desynchronize activity for that part of the auditory cortex responsible for the generation of P2. Since P2 and N1 overlap somewhat (resulting in a partial phase cancellation) the loss or reduction of P2 would result in a net increase in the amplitude of N1. The loss of the desynchronizing influence of the tinnitus on P2 with recovery from tinnitus would result in P2 becoming larger and N1 becoming smaller resulting in a normalized P2/N1 amplitude ratio.

Jacobson et al. (1991) sought to extend the observations of Hoke et al. (1989) and Pantev et al. (1989). In this investigation both normal subjects and patients with unilateral tinnitus were evaluated using a stimulating and recording paradigm similar to that used by the previous investigators. For patients with unilateral tinnitus the investigators planned to compare N1 and P2 recorded contralaterally to the tinnitus ear (following stimulation of the ear with tinnitus) with N1 and P2 recorded over the hemisphere contralateral to the normal ear (following stimulation of the normal ear). Unfortunately, the results failed to support the findings of Hoke et al. (1989). Specifically, there was no evidence suggesting that N1 amplitude was larger, P2 latency occurred later or the P2/N1 amplitude ratio was smaller for the patients with tinnitus (see Figure 7-4). Additionally, there were no differences in the amplitudes or latencies of N1 and P2 when results obtained following stimulation of the tinnitus and non-tinnitus ears of tinnitus patients were compared. These findings were supported by the results of a similar investigation conducted by Colding-Jorgenson et al. (1992), and Kristeva et al. (1991) who used a large array, first-order gradiometer magnetoencepholgraphic (MEG) recording system. More recently Attias et al. (1996c) conducted a late evoked potential investigation of N1, P2, and P3 in patients with high-frequency hearing loss and tinnitus and age-matched and hearing loss matched controls without tinnitus. The investigators used both repetitive stimulation (to record N1 and P2) and the conventional "oddball" stimulation paradigm to record P300. The investigators observed a statistically significant increase in N1 latency for tinnitus subjects. The amplitudes of N1 and P2 were smaller overall for subjects with tinnitus although these differences did not reach statistical significance. The authors explained the finding in terms of adaptive processes of the brain in response to chronic internal auditory stimulation (the tinnitus).

The disparities in the results of what appear to be similar investigations need to be viewed critically. There is an impulse to attempt to explain why one group did not observe what another group did in terms of differences in experimental paradigm (active versus passive listening), instrumentation (evoked potentials versus evoked magnetic fields, MEG recorded with first or

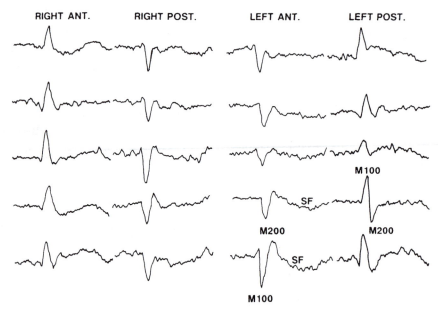

FIGURE 7-4. Auditory evoked cortical responses from five representative normal subjects. Components N1 and P2 are identified. Note that contrary to the findings of Hoke et al. (1989) P2 often was absent in the group of normal subjects. From Jacobson et al. (1991) reproduced with permission.

second-order gradiometers) and subject sample (tinnitus versus bothersome tinnitus; normals versus normals with equivalent hearing loss but without tinnitus). However, it is equally possible that the interstudy variability has occurred because there is no consistent effect of tinnitus on evoked potentials. This might occur because the sources of tinnitus in the cortex are not involved in the generation of long-latency, cortically-generated, auditory evoked potentials to externally presented tones.

Scalp Recorded Endogenous Evoked Potentials Nd and P300

Current hypotheses surrounding tinnitus suggest that, for some, adaptive processes may occur centrally that help "preserve" tinnitus for those patients that attend to it (see Chapter 15). These adaptive processes may be potentiated by the patient's emotional response to the perceived threat represented by the tinnitus. In turn, the per-

ceived threat of the tinnitus might have a predictable influence over the level of attention directed by the patient toward the tinnitus (attention toward the warning stimulus would increase). Thus, attentional mechanisms may have the capability of potentiating the nociceptive effects of tinnitus. Attention toward tinnitus may influence how permanently embedded in the central auditory system is this phantom auditory image. The negative difference wave (Nd) is a late evoked potential elicited in a double oddball paradigm where subjects are instructed to attend to one ear only and respond (for example, by pressing a button) when an occasional target stimulus is presented in a series of frequent stimuli to that ear. The other ear also is presented with frequent and infrequent stimuli, which the listener is instructed to ignore. The paradigm yields four evoked potential traces representing the signal averaged responses to the "attend-frequent," "attend-infrequent (target)," "ignore-frequent," and "ignore-

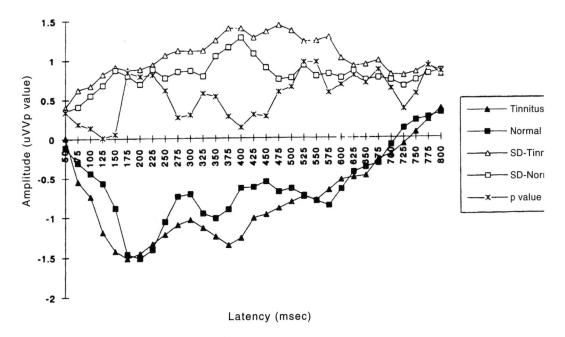

FIGURE 7-5. Time series plot of Nd at 25 ms intervals from 50-800 ms following onset of a frequent tone in the attended channel of normal controls and subjects with tinnitus. Note that significant differences in Nd amplitude occur at the 125 ms time point. From Jacobson et al. (1996) reproduced with permission.

infrequent" stimuli. When the "ignore-frequent" waveform is superimposed upon the "ignore-infrequent" waveform a separation between the tracings can be observed. This separation begins as early as 50 to 70 ms poststimulus onset and appears as a negative bias in the "attend-frequent" tracing. The effects of attention can be isolated from N1 and P2 by subtracting the "ignore-frequent" from the "attend-frequent" tracing. The derived waveform is called the Nd (see Figure 7-5) and is believed to "index" a person's ability to attend selectively to one channel and ignore others. That is, the larger the Nd wave, the stronger the selective attention.

Jacobson et al. (1996) conducted a series of investigations in an attempt to determine whether selective auditory attentional processes differed between normals and patients with bothersome tinnitus. Specifically, the investigators evaluated differences between groups in the exogenous N1, P2 components and the endogenous negative differ-

ence wave (Nd). Subjects were thirty-seven adults with tinnitus and high-frequency hearing loss and fifteen subjects who were audiometrically and otologically normal. Stimuli were 500 and 1,000 Hz tone bursts presented at a rate of 3 Hz with infrequent and frequent stimuli having a probabilities of occurrence of 10 percent and 90 percent respectively. Subjects were instructed to press a button when they detected the target in the attended channel. The results suggested that an electrophysiological index of early selective auditory attention (the negative difference wave, Nd) was of greater magnitude in tinnitus patients (see Figure 7-5). Also, the cortical N1 component occurred significantly later in the presence of selective attention in tinnitus subjects only (see Figure 7-6).

In a similar vein, Attias et al. (1996c) evaluated the effects of tinnitus on auditory and visual long-latency responses. Listeners were engaged in both auditory, and separately, visual oddball paradigms. Subjects

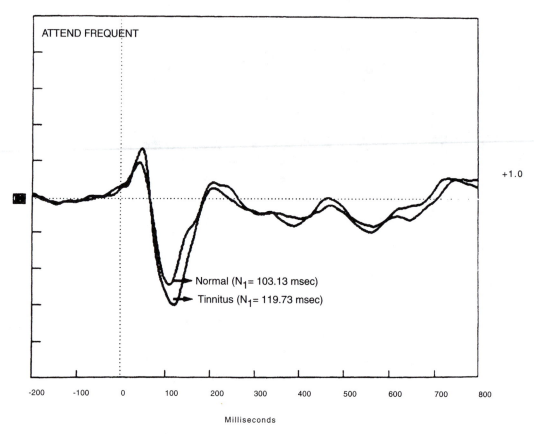

FIGURE 7-6. Superimposition of grand-averaged (normal versus tinnitus) N1 waveforms following stimulation with frequent tones in the attended ear. Notice the difference in the peak latency of N1 between the two groups. From Jacobson et al. (1996) reproduced with permission.

were twenty-one patients with tinnitus due to noise exposure. These subjects were compared with age and hearing-loss matched controls. The results of this investigation showed that the N1, N2, and P3 components evoked by the "standard" or "frequent" stimuli were longer in latency for the patients with tinnitus. Further, the auditory P3 component was smaller for the tinnitus patients. This trend occurred for visual evoked potentials recorded using a similar oddball paradigm (see Figure 7-7). Thus, the results of this investigation were important since they demonstrated the possibility that tinnitus or the response to tinnitus had affected general changes in the manner by which the brain processes sensory stimuli.

The findings of investigations conducted by both Jacobson et al. (1996) and Attias

et al. (1996) have suggested that bothersome tinnitus may act as a well-rehearsed, internally generated, phantom auditory signal that is often associated with a strong affective response and is capable of imparting a potent attentional trace. The persistence of this significant phantom signal and the attention drawn toward it by the patient may have lasting effects on the degree to which other channel-specific signals are analyzed. This view is supported in both investigations by the delayed N1 response in the "attended" channel and evidence from the Jacobson et al. (1996) study suggesting an enhanced Nd wave for subjects with intrusive bothersome tinnitus.

Both Attias et al., (1996) and Jacobson et al., (unpublished data) have tested the hypothesis that a "simulated tinnitus" (for

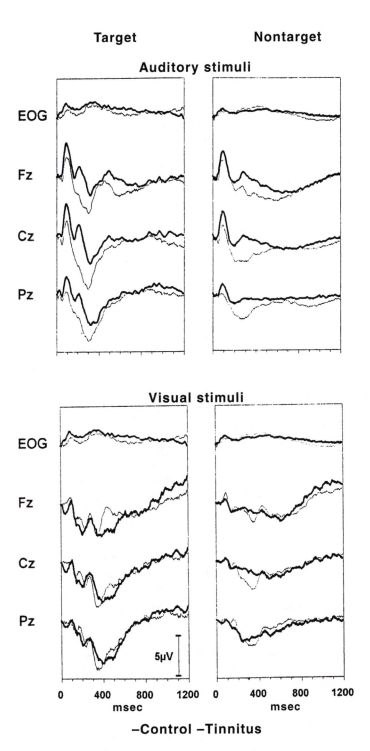

FIGURE 7-7. Grand-averaged evoked potentials in response to target (infrequent) and nontarget (frequent) stimuli for individuals engaged in both auditory (top) and visual (bottom) oddball paradigm. Data were recorded from midline frontal, central and parietal electrodes. Notice that the late positive component (i.e. P300) is smaller and later for subjects with tinnitus regardless of sensory modality. From Attias et al. (1996) page 331, reproduced with permission of Williams and Wilkins publishers.

example, continuous tone or noise band) superimposed on an evoking stimulus would affect changes in the auditory-evoked cortical potentials and auditory-evoked fields like those seen in tinnitus patients. Both investigators have failed to produce differences like those reported for patients with tinnitus. Accordingly, it appears that tinnitus differs from other steady auditory signals in that it is a source of great salience, which results in a strong negative affective response.

Spontaneous Direct-Recorded VIIIth Nerve Activity

A series of investigators have evaluated the effects of salicylates (known to induce tinnitus in humans when given in large dosages) on central auditory system function in animals (Evans et al., 1981; Jastreboff & Sasaki, 1986; Schreiner & Snyder, 1987). All investigators have observed increases in electrical activity at the level of the VIIIth nerve (Evans et al., 1981; Schreiner & Snyder, 1987) and midbrain (Jastreboff & Sasaki, 1986) following administration of the salicylates. Further, Schreiner and Snyder (1987) conducted a spectral analysis of the spontaneous electrical recorded from the auditory nerves of treated animals. Following treatment the authors noted a peak in the amplitude spectrum that was centered at 200 Hz. This peak disappeared when the animals were infused with lidocaine. The investigators suggested that this 200 Hz peak in the spectrum might have represented tinnitus since high doses of aspirin in humans is known to cause tinnitus. Martin and colleagues have extended these observations in both animals (Martin et al., 1993) and humans (Martin et al., 1996). The investigators first recorded spontaneous activity from both the round window and exposed VIIIth nerve of cats. The baseline recordings were obtained and then the animals were infused with either sodium salicylate (150 mg/kg) or saline as a control (20 ml). Recordings of the spontaneous activity were

made 2 to 3 hours post infusion. In their animals that survived the salicylate infusion, they found only a peak at 200 Hz in the averaged spectrum of the spontaneous activity. The peak frequency varied over time in one animal (Figure 7-8). The authors interpreted the 200 Hz peak as representing the electrophysiological "footprint" of tinnitus. What was not clear was why the peak frequency in the averaged spectrum was 200 Hz when tinnitus in humans often is pitch matched to tones in excess of 4,000 Hz. The authors suggested that the 200 Hz peak could represent in increase in the total number of units firing at 200 Hz or an increase in the synchronization of already active units. It also possible that the 200 Hz peak could be coding a signal higher in frequency than 200 Hz (that is, frequency coding by the "volley" theory). This investigation was followed by a report demonstrating that the 200 Hz peak was present as well in humans with tinnitus. The investigators recorded spontaneous activity from the exposed auditory nerve, and from the round window of patients undergoing neurosurgical and otologic surgical procedures. Twelve of fourteen subjects undergoing the neurosurgical procedures demonstrated the 200 Hz spectral peak in the spontaneous activity. All but one of those patients had tinnitus. The two patients not showing the 200 Hz peak also did not have tinnitus. Of the seventeen subjects undergoing middle-ear procedures the 200 Hz peak could be recorded in only three cases and all three had tinnitus at least some of the time. Unfortunately, there were four patients with tinnitus who failed to show the 200 Hz peak. This investigation was significant because: (1) the 200 Hz peak was demonstrated for the first time in humans, and, (2) that no tinnitus-free patients demonstrated the 200 Hz peak, and therefore, the 200 Hz peak has high specificity. The authors suggested that the low incidence of the 200 Hz peak in the round window recordings may have occurred due to the unfavorable signal-to-noise ratio for those recordings.

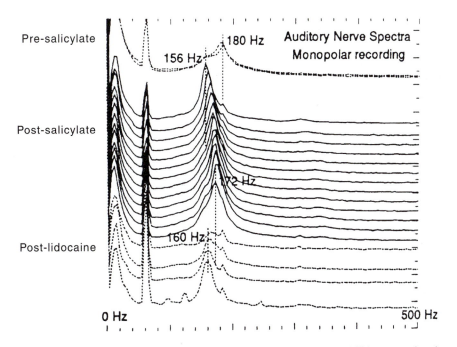

FIGURE 7-8. Power spectra of spontaneous activity recorded from the VIIIth nerve showing changes in the center frequency of peak activity as a function of time. Notice that following salicylate injection there is a large peak in the spectrum occurring at 156 Hz. This amplitude peak shifts upward in frequency. It is almost totally abolished following the administration of lidocaine. From Martin et al. (1993) reproduced with permission of the publisher and the Triological Society.

SUMMARY

A summary of representative investigations designed to identify in electroacoustical or electrophysiological recordings the effects of tinnitus is shown in Table 7-2. It can be observed from the review of these investigations that there have been many attempts to confront what seems to be a logical assumption. If a patient hears an internal auditory signal, then it should be trivial to, in some manner, verify the patient's perception using electrophysiological techniques. Unfortunately, attempts to prove this point have been inconclusive. One must ask then why chasing this phantom has been so difficult. There probably are several reasons why it has been difficult to find objective evidence of tinnitus in electrophysiological recordings of auditory system function in humans: (1) the recording methods may not have been sensitive, (2) the location of the injury resulting in tinnitus is distant from our recording electrodes, (3) tinnitus may be generated in more rostral structures of the auditory nervous system (numbers 1 through 3 from Moller et al., 1992). I would add to this list: (4) the neurophysiological mechanisms responsible for tinnitus perception may be a distributed phenomenon (for example, throughout the central nervous system) and not a focal phenomenon, and, (5) the origins of acute and chronic tinnitus may differ. The origins of the tinnitus occurring acutely may be circumscribed and analogous to those effects observed with direct round window and VIIIth nerve recordings in animals following noise and salicylate exposure. Chronic tinnitus may involve adaptive processes in either or both subcortical and cortical auditory areas.

It is interesting to note that theories about tinnitus generation have been advanced with

Table 7-2. Summary of representative investigations designed to evaluate whether tinnitus can be demonstrated in electroacoustical or electrophysiological measures

Investigation	Type	N	Comments
Penner (1989)a	SOAE	1	Patient with tinnitus in both ears. For one ear the pitch corresponded to the SOAE frequency. In the other ear the SOAE frequency was unrelated to the pitch of the tinnitus.
Penner (1989b)	SOAE	1	SOAEs were recorded before and following salicylate treatment of tinnitus. Aspirin abolished the SOAE and the tinnitus.
Penner and Coles (1992)	SOAE	1	Placebo controlled investigation of relationship between SOAE suppression and tinnitus suppression. Suppression of SOAE with aspirin resulted in the disappearance of tinnitus.
Chery-Croze et al. (1993)	DPOAE suppression	36 (16 bilateral/ 20 unilateral tinnitus)	No efferent suppression, or, enhancement of OAE for the ear with contralateral noise.
Lind (1996)	TEOAE suppression	20 (12 left tinnitus/ 8 right tinnitus)	TEOAE was smaller in tinnitus ear in the 10 to 15 ms post-stimulus interval. No difference in contralateral suppression found for ears with and without tinnitus.
Attias et al. (1996a)	TEOAE suppression	42 divided into 4 groups, normal hearing with tinnitus (11), NIHL (9), NIHL with tinnitus (14)	Tinnitus patients had greater TEOAEs in the presence of contralateral white noise than those without tinnitus.
Moller et al. (1992)	Dir. VIIth nerve and ABR	19 (16 with hearing loss) undergoing NVD for intractable tinnitus and 16 without tinnitus undergoing NVD of other cranial nerves	No group differences were observed in compound action potential latencies/amplitudes or those of waves III and V.
Barnea et al. (1990)	ABR	34 normal hearing (17 with and 17 without tinnitus.	No group differences in ABR component measures were observed.
Ikner and Hassen (1990)	ABR	35 with tinnitus, 35 without tinnitus matched for age, gender, and hearing loss	Wave I was prolonged in females with tinnitus compared with females who were tinnitus-free.

continues

Table 7-2 *continued*

Investigation	Type	N	Comments
Attias et al. (1993)	ABR	24 (12 with high frequency sensorineural hearing loss and tinnitus and 12 age and hearing loss matched controls without tinnitus)	No group differences were observed in the latencies or amplitudes of ABR.
Jastreboff et al. (1992)	ABR	21 (3 groups of 7 subjects, 2 groups with tinnitus, one group without)	Investigator was able to differentiate groups based upon frequency analysis of ABR data.
Rosenhall and Axelsson (1994)	ABR with spectral analysis	113 tinnitus patients with hearing loss of various degrees, 220 controls	ABR was abnormal for 10 to 11% of patients.
Attias et al. (1996b)	ABR with 3 CLT analysis	13 with high frequency, sensorineural hearing loss and 11 matched controls without tinnitus	Reported enhanced wave III amplitude in vertex-ipsilateral mastoid electrode derivation.
Hoke et al. (1989)	LLAEF (N1/P2)	40 normals and 25 tinnitus patients	Cortically generated P2 generally was reduced in amplitude or absent for tinnitus patients resulting in a P2/N1 amplitude ratio that was < 0.5 for tinnitus patients.
Pantev et al. (1989)	LLAEF (N1/P2)	1	Case report showing normalization of P2/N1 amplitude ratio as tinnitus resolved for a patient with noise-induced tinnitus.
Jacobson et al. (1991)	LLAEF (N1/P2)	25 normals, 14 patients with unilateral tinnitus with normal hearing to 1,500 Hz	Could not replicate the findings of Hoke et al. (1989).
Colding-Jorgenson et al. (1992)	LLAEF (N1/P2)	14 tinnitus patients and 14 sex- and age-matched controls	Could not replicate the findings of Hoke et al. (1989).
Attias et al. (1996c)	LLAEF (N1/P2)	24 (12 with high frequency sensorineural hearing loss and tinnitus and 12 age- and hearing loss-matched controls without tinnitus)	Slight increase in N1 latency and decrease in P2 latency for tinnitus patients. Amplitudes of N1 and P2 were smaller for patients with tinnitus.

continues

Table 7-2 *continued*

Investigation	Type	N	Comments
Jacobson et al. (1996)	Nd	67 (30 normals and 37 tinnitus patients with normal hearing to 1,500 Hz)	Early Nd was larger for tinnitus patients. N1 latency was longer for tinnitus patients.
Attias et al. (1996c)	LLAEP (N1, N2, P3), VEP	19 with NIHL matched for hearing loss with group of 19 subjects from previous investigation	AEP and VEP latencies were longer for tinnitus subjects. P3 was smaller for tinnitus subjects.
Martin et al. (1993)	SA round window, VIIIth nerve	10 cats following salicylate exposure	200 Hz peak occurred following treatment and was eliminated following administration of lidocaine.
Martin et al. (1996)	SA round window, VIIIth nerve	14 humans undergoing neurosurgical procedures	12 out of 14 patients showed the 200 Hz peak. These patients had tinnitus. Two patients not showing 200 Hz peak did not have tinnitus.

SOAE = Spontaneous otoacoustic emission

TEOAE = Transient (click) evoked otoacoustic emission

DPOAE = Distortion product otoacoustic emission

Direct VIIIth nerve = Direct electrode recording from the exposed VIIIth nerve

LLAEP = Long-latency auditory evoked potentials

LLAEF = Long-latency auditory evoked magnetic field recordings

Nd = Negative difference wave attention-related endogenous evoked potential

SA = Spectral analysis from exposed VIIIth nerve, and/or, round window

3CLT = Three-channel Lissajous pattern recordings of the ABR

P3 = P300 endogenous evoked potential

NIHL = noise-induced hearing loss

NVD = neurovascular decompression surgery

the addition of each new audioelectrodiagnostic technique. That is, with the addition of each new technique investigators have attempted to demonstrate group differences in measurement parameters between those with and without tinnitus. Some of these investigations have been flawed by the mixing of hearing-impaired and nonhearing-impaired samples. Additionally, some investigators have used unconventional stimulating and recording methods. It must be mentioned that the origins of tinnitus are many and diverse. Accordingly, it is possible that the causes and sites of injury to the auditory system may differ within a subsample of tinnitus patients. For these reasons it is not surprising that there has been a lack of consistency in the findings of audioelectrodiagnostic measures for any sample of tinnitus patients.

Future studies most likely will involve a combination of electrophysiological and functional imaging techniques such as PET, SPECT, and functional MRI where it might be expected that metabolic activity would increase in temporal lobe areas for tinnitus subjects (see Chapter 5). In this regard, both Sataloff et al. (1996) and Arnold et al. (1996) using PET ([18F] deoxyglucose) have reported findings in ten patients with tinnitus (ten = six with tinnitus in the left ear, two with tinnitus in the right ear, and two with tinnitus centered at midline). Nine patients had significantly increased metabolic activity in the left and one patient in the right primary auditory cortex (Brodmann area 41). One patient was evaluated on three occasions corresponding to times when tinnitus was low and high in severity. The investigators reported predictable increases in activation of the primary auditory cortex during periods when tinnitus severity was severe.

The electrophysiological investigations of auditory function in humans has yielded a patchwork quilt of findings none of which has reached unanimity. That is, with the exception of electroacoustical measures of SOAEs that coincide with tinnitus pitch

matches, and, the recording of spontaneous 200 Hz activity from the VIIIth nerve, the sensitivity of electrophysiological measures for the detection of tinnitus has been low. Also, it should be noted that although some of the investigations reviewed have demonstrated group differences on electrophysiological measures, few have been replicated. Finally, with few exceptions, differences between tinnitus and no tinnitus samples have represented group and not individual differences. Accordingly, none of the electrophysiological techniques have provided a means to identify the presence of tinnitus in a single patient. Accordingly, at present, there is no auditory electrophysiological technique (that is, test) that can be used (for example, for medical-legal purposes—see Chapter 17) to objectify tinnitus. These electrophysiological tools, however, have been useful for the development of hypotheses and theories that help explain how tinnitus is generated, and further, what causes this low level auditory "signal" to persist at the conscious level when we are able to habituate successfully to constant auditory signals in the environment that are of greater intensities. There seems to be sufficient evidence supporting the contention that tinnitus is accompanied by increases in spontaneous electrophysiological activity at the periphery. There is evidence that some of this spontaneous activity may represent dynamic processes in the cochlea (that is, spontaneous otoacoustic emissions). There is some evidence that the continuous stream of heightened afferent activity may modify the processing of auditory signals in, at least, the pontine auditory pathway. There is evidence that once this correlated auditory activity reaches the cortex, adaptive changes may occur that modify how the auditory cortex responds to other external sounds. Also, it appears that the magnitude of energy that is spent listening to tinnitus not only has an effect on the handicapping effects of tinnitus but also may result in a bias for the auditory system to gate preferentially auditory signals ascending in that channel (ear).

It is hoped that in the future the combined evaluation of auditory processes using functional imaging and electrophysiological techniques will provide us with greater insights into the physiological processes underlying the perception of tinnitus.

REFERENCES

Arnold, W., Bartenstein, P., Oestreicher, E., Romer, W., & Schwaiger, M. (1996). Focal metabolic activation in the predominant left auditory cortex in patients suffering from tinnitus: A PET study with [18F] deoxyglucose. *Journal of Oto-Rhino-Laryngology and Its Related Specialties, 58,* 195–199.

Attias, J., Bresloff, I., & Furman, V. (1996a). The influence of the efferent auditory system on otoacoustic emission in noise-induced tinnitus: Clinical relevance. *Acta Otolaryngologica, 116,* 534–539.

Attias, J., Bresloff, I., Furman, V., & Urbach, D. (1995). Auditory event related potentials in simulated tinnitus. *Journal of Basic and Clinical Physiology and Pharmacology, 6,* 173–183.

Attias, J., Pratt, H., Reshef, I., Bresloff, I., Horowitz, G., Polyakov, A., & Shemesh, Z. (1996b). Detailed analysis of auditory brain stem responses in patients with noise-induced tinnitus. *Audiology, 35,* 259–270.

Attias, J., Furman, V., Shemesh, Z., & Bresloff, I. (1996c). Impaired brain processing in noise-induced tinnitus patients as measured by auditory and visual event-related potentials. *Ear and Hearing, 17,* 327–333.

Barnea, G., Attias, J., Gold, S., & Shahar, A. (1990). Tinnitus with normal hearing sensitivity: Extended high frequency audiometry and auditory nerve brain-stem evoked responses. *Audiology, 29,* 36–45.

Burns, E. M. (1989). Alternate-state OAEs as a basis for episodic intermittent tinnitus. *Journal of the Acoustical Society of America, 85,* S35.

Burns, E. M., & Keefe, D. H. (1992). Intermittent tinnitus resulting from unstable otoacoustic emissions. In J. M. Aran & R. Daumann (Eds.), *Tinnitus 91. Proceedings of the Fourth International Tinnitus Seminar* (pp. 89–94). Amsterdam: Kugler Publications.

Ceranic, B. J., Prasher, D. K., & Luxon, L. M. (1995). Tinnitus and otoacoustic emissions. *Clinical Otolaryngology, 20,* 192–200.

Chery-Croze, S., Collet, L., & Morgon, A. (1993).

Medial olivo–cochlear system and tinnitus. *Acta Otolaryngologica, 113,* 285–290.

Chery-Croze, S., Moulin, A., Collet, L., & Morgon, A. (1994a). Is the test of medial efferent system function a relevant investigation in tinnitus? *British Journal of Audiology, 28,* 13–25.

Chery-Croze, S., Truy, E., & Morgon, A. (1994b). Contralateral suppression of transiently evoked otoacoustic emissions and tinnitus. *British Journal of Audiology, 28,* 255–266.

Colding-Jorgenson, E., Lauritzen, M., Johnsen, N. J., Mikkelsen, K. B., & Saermark, K. (1992). On the evidence of auditory evoked magnetic fields as an objective measure of tinnitus. *Electroencephalography and Clinical Neurophysiology, 83,* 322–327.

Collet, L., Morgon, A., Veullet, E., & Gartner, M. (1991). Noise and medial olivocochlear system in human. *Acta Otolaryngologica, 110,* 231–233.

Evans, E. F., Wilson, J. P., & Borerwe, T. A. (1981). Animal models of tinnitus. In *CIBA Foundation 85: Tinnitus* (pp. 108–138). London: Pitman.

Frick, L. R. & Matthies, M. L. (1988). Effects of external stimuli on spontaneous otoacoustic emissions. *Ear and Hearing, 9,* 190–197.

Graham, R. L., & Hazell, J. W. (1994). Contralateral suppression of transient evoked otoacoustic emissions: Intra–individual variability in tinnitus and normal subjects. *British Journal of Audiology, 28,* 235–245.

Hoke, M., Feldman, H., Pantev, C., Lutkenhoner, B., & Lehnertz, K. (1989). Objective evidence of tinnitus in auditory evoked magnetic fields. *Hearing Research, 37,* 281–286.

Ikner, C. L., & Hassen, A. H. (1990). The effects of tinnitus on ABR latencies. *Ear and Hearing, 11,* 16–20.

Jacobson, G. P., Ahmad, B. K., Moran, J., Newman, C. W., Tepley, N., & Wharton, J. (1991). Auditory evoked cortical magnetic field (M100/M200) measurements in tinnitus and normal groups. *Hearing Research, 56,* 44–52.

Jacobson, G. P., Calder, J. A., Newman, C. W., Peterson, E. L., Wharton, J. A., & Ahmad, B. K. (1996). Electrophysiological indices of selective auditory attention in subjects with and without tinnitus. *Hearing Research, 97,* 66–74.

Jastreboff, P. J., Ikner, C. L., & Hassen, A. (1992). An approach to the objective evaluation of tinnitus in humans. In J. M. Aran & R. Dauman (Eds.), *Proceedings of the Fourth International Tinnitus Seminar: Tinnitus 91* (pp. 331–339). Amsterdam: Kugler.

Jastreboff, P. J., & Sasaki, C. T. (1986). Salicylate-induced changes in spontaneous activity of single units in the inferior colliculus of the guinea pig. *Journal of the Acoustical Society of America, 80,* 1384–1391.

Kaltenbach, J. A., & McCaslin, D. (1996). Increases in spontaneous activity in the dorsal cochlear nucleus following exposure to high intensity sound: A possible neural correlate of tinnitus. *Auditory Neuroscience, 3,* 57–78.

Kemp, D. T. (1979). Evidence of mechanical non-linearity and frequency selective wave amplification in the cochlea. *Annals of Otology Rhinology Laryngology, 224,* 37–45.

Kristeva, R., Lutkenhoner, B., Ross, B., Elbert, T., Kowalik, Z., Hampson, S., Hoke, M., & Feldman, H. (1992). The amplitude ration M200/M100 of the auditory evoked magnetic field in normal hearing subjects and tinnitus patients. In J. M. Aran & R. Dauman (Eds.) *Proceedings of the Fourth International Tinnitus Seminar: Tinnitus 91* (pp. 327–329). Amsterdam: Kugler.

Lind, O. (1996). Transient-evoked otoacoustic emissions and contralateral suppression in patients with unilateral tinnitus. *Scandinavian Audiology, 25,* 167–172.

Martin, G. K., Probst, R., & Lonsbury-Martin, B. L. (1990). Otoacoustic emissions in human ears: Normative findings. *Ear and Hearing, 11,* 106–120.

Martin, W. H., Schwegler, J. W., Scheibelhoffer, J., & Ronis, M. L. (1993). Salicylate-induced changes in cat auditory nerve activity. *Laryngoscope, 103,* 600–604.

Martin, W. H., Schwegler, J. W., Shi, Y-b, Pratt, H., & Adler, S. (1996). Developing an objective measurement tool for evaluating tinnitus: Spectral averaging. In G. E. Reich & J. A. Vernon (Eds.), *Proceedings of the Fifth International Tinnitus Seminar* (pp. 127–134). Portland, OR: American Tinnitus Association.

McKee, G. J., & Stephens, S. D. G. (1992). An investigation of normally hearing subjects with tinnitus. *Audiology, 31,* 313–317.

Moller, A. R., Moller, M. B., Jannetta, P. J., & Jho, H. D. (1992). Compound action potentials recorded from the exposed eighth nerve in patients with intractable tinnitus. *Laryngoscope, 102,* 187–197.

Pantev, C., Hoke, M., Lutkenhoner, B., Lehnertz, K., & Kumpf, W. (1989). Tinnitus remission objectified by neuromagnetic measurements. *Hearing Research, 40,* 261–264.

Penner, M. J. (1989a). Empirical tests demonstrating two coexisting sources of tinnitus: A case study. *Journal of Speech and Hearing Research, 32,* 458–462.

Penner, M. J. (1989b). Aspirin abolishes tinnitus caused by spontaneous otacoustic emissions. *Archives of Otolaryngology Head and Neck Surgery, 115,* 871–875.

Penner, M. J. (1990). An estimate of the prevalence of tinnitus caused by spontaneous otacoustic emissions. *Archives of Otolaryngology Head and Neck Surgery, 116,* 418–423.

Penner, M. J. (1992). Linking spontaneous otacoustic emissions and tinnitus. *British Journal of Audiology, 26,* 115–123.

Penner, M. J., & Burns, E. M. (1987a). The dissociation of SOAEs and tinnitus. *Journal of Speech and Hearing Research, 30,* 396–403, 1987.

Penner, M. J., & Burns, E. M. (1987b). Five empirical tests for a relation between SOAEs and tinnitus. In H. Feldman (Ed.), *Proceedings of the Third International Tinnitus Seminar* (pp. 82–85). Harsch Verlag Karlsruhe.

Penner, M. J. & Coles, R. R. (1992). Indications for aspirin as a palliative for tinnitus caused by SOAEs: A case study. *British Journal of Audiology, 26,* 91–96.

Rosenhall, U., & Axelsson, A. (1994). Auditory brain stem response latencies in patients with tinnitus. *Scandinavian Audiology, 24,* 97–100.

Sataloff, R. T., Mandel, S., Muscal, E., Park, C. H., Rosen, D. C., Kim, S. M., & Spiegel, J. R. (1996). Single-photon-emission computed tomography (SPECT) in neurotologic assessment: A preliminary report. *American Journal of Otology, 17,* 909–916.

Schreiner, C. E., & Snyder, R. L. (1987). A physiological animal model of peripheral tinnitus. In H. Feldmann (Ed.), *Proceedings of the Third International Tinnitus Seminar* (pp.100–106). Harsch Verlag Karlsruhe.

Snow, J. B. Jr., & Naunton, R. F. (1993). Research in the auditory and vestibular systems. The recommendations of the National Institute on Deafness and Other Communication Disorders National Strategic Research Plan. *Journal of Oto-Rhin-Laryngology and its Related Specialties, 55,* 154–158.

Wallhausser-Franke, E., Braun, S., & Langner, G. (1996). Salicylate alters 2-DG uptake in the auditory system: A model for tinnitus? *NeuroReport, 7,* 1585–1588.

Zwicker, E. (1987). Objective otoacoustic emissions and their uncorrelation to tinnitus. In H. Feldman (Ed.) *Proceedings of the Third International Tinnitus Seminar* (pp. 75–81). Harsch Verlag Karlsruhe.

CHAPTER 8

Spontaneous Otoacoustic Emissions and Tinnitus

M. J. Penner

INTRODUCTION

The inner ear sometimes acts as a sound generator continuously producing sounds called spontaneous otoacoustic emissions (SOAEs) that may be recorded when a sensitive miniature microphone is inserted into the ear canal. Although most individuals are unaware of their own SOAEs, some SOAEs—especially those that fluctuate—may cause tinnitus (that is, be audible and annoying). Clinically, the SOAE-tinnitus link may be important because aspirin generally abolishes SOAEs and could therefore provide a palliative for such tinnitus. In this chapter, we discuss issues in the measurement of SOAEs, present some case studies in which the subject appeared to have tinnitus caused by SOAEs, and discuss the prevalence of SOAE-caused tinnitus. Finally, because measurement considerations indicate that it is unlikely that all internal cochlear tones manifest themselves as SOAEs, it is possible that tinnitus may have a cochlear origin even when SOAEs cannot be measured. Data consistent with this speculation are also presented.

Although the physiological basis of tinnitus is generally unknown, a major advance in understanding one form of tinnitus was made when some cases of tinnitus were linked to spontaneous otoacoustic emissions (SOAEs), acoustic energies that may be detected when a sensitive miniature microphone is inserted into the ear canal (Burns & Keefe, 1992; Penner, 1988; 1989a, b; 1992; Plinkert, Gitter, & Zenner, 1990). In this chapter, we present archival data and theory preceding the discovery of SOAEs which indicate the ear itself generated more tones that could cause tinnitus, discuss the issues involved in measurement of SOAEs, review data connecting some tinnitus to SOAEs, and explore the possibility that tinnitus may be caused by idiotones (Flottorp, 1953; Ward, 1952, 1955), internal tones of presumed cochlear origin that may exist even when SOAEs cannot be measured.

ARCHIVAL DATA AND THEORY

Historical Perspective

In 1948, Gold (1948) postulated that the ear not only received sounds but could generate them as well. His reasoning was based on his mathematical model of cochlear function, but for thirty years thereafter, his prediction remained merely a hypothetical possibility.

During this extensive gap between theoretical prediction and unambiguous empirical verification by measurement of low-level sounds in the ear canal, there were a series of experimental results that could have been taken as supporting his hypothesis. Unfortunately, these results came from endeavors so far removed from Gold and his proponents (Pumphrey & Gold, 1948) that it would be surprising if the cognoscenti in the two areas even read each other's papers.

One piece of evidence supporting Gold's (1948) speculation had actually preceded his publication. In 1931, Wegel (1931) reported that his tinnitus could beat with external tones. Beating is typically produced by the waxing and waning of the amplitude of two external pure tones whenever these tones are near each other in frequency and amplitude. If internally generated tinnitus beat with a single external tone, then the tinnitus could be caused by an internal cochlear tone. The existence of such internally generated tones is the core of Gold's (1948) model.

Other evidence favoring tinnitus generated by internal tones originating in the cochlea was published in the 1950s. Both Flottorp (1953) and Ward (1952, 1955) reported on a phenomenon that has subsequently become known as diplacusis. Diplacusis, double (di) hearing (acusis), is a condition in which a pure tone does not sound pure to the listener, but instead elicits the sensation of beats experienced by Wegel (1931), or roughness or multiple tones, or possibly an aftertone. The phenomenon of diplacusis led to the hypothesis that the ear produced internal tones or idiotones, thereby providing additional empirical data strengthening Gold's (1948) theory. By the early 1950s, then, it seemed clear that the ear could generate sound, at least in rare pathological conditions for a subject with abnormal hearing and tinnitus (Wegel, 1931) and, in some presumed infre-quent cases, for normal hearing subjects (Flottorp, 1953; Ward, 1952; 1955).

In the 1950s, the inference that low-level idiotones existed depended on the psychophysical measures of a scant number of subjects' sensations. It came as no small surprise therefore when clinical data appeared indicating that some subjects' ears generated sounds that were so *intense* that they were undeniably audible to surrounding persons (Citron, 1969; Coles, Snashell, & Stephens, 1975; Glanville, Coles, & Sullivan, 1971; Huizing & Spoor, 1973).

In one remarkable study (Glanville et al., 1971), these sounds were attributed to genetic transmission by the father. Both he and two of his children had high-pitched externally audible whistling sounds emanating from their ears. The spectrum of these sounds indicated that the frequency of the emitted tones was about 6 kHz.

This family was studied in the early 1970s and nearly a decade later by Wilson and Sutton (1983) who reported the appearance of emissions in addition to those noted by Glanville et al. (1971). Remarkably, none of the patients whose ears generated audible sounds heard them. However, one child in the Glanville et al. (1971) report did remark that he heard the recorded version of the emission belonging to his right ear when it was played so that he could hear it in his left ear. Nonetheless, there was no evidence that high-level externally audible tones caused bothersome tinnitus. However, the patent presence of loud sounds emanating from the ear was again consistent with Gold's (1948) hypothesis that the ear itself could generate sound.

Although detailed description is beyond the scope of this chapter, in Gold's (1948) model, the internal generation of sound could arise whenever the posited feedback grew too large. In particular, Gold wrote that, "A sensitive instrument may be able to pick up these oscillations . . ." No such instrument was available in 1948. It was not until the 1970s that direct tests of Gold's (1948) hypothesis became technically feasible and SOAEs were discovered.

MEASUREMENT OF SOAEs

Kemp (1978) was the first to demonstrate that acoustic energies could be recorded in the ear canal using a miniature microphone and special methods to analyze the output of the microphone. Acoustic energies measured in the ear canal in the absence of auditory input are currently called SOAEs. As the lengthily time between the hypothesis that SOAEs existed and their successful measurement suggests, the technology involved in ascertaining that these low-level sounds are real is intricate.

Measurement of SOAEs depends on the characteristics of the microphone, on the procedure employed to classify a spectral peak as an SOAE, and on the spectral characteristics which are used to analyze the data and reduce the noise floor.

Microphone Sensitivity

The microphone typically used the measure SOAEs is an ER-10A manufactured by Etymotic Research. Occasionally, other microphones are employed, but these microphones typically have slightly higher noise floors and consequently fewer SOAEs are detected (Cerniac, Prasher, & Luxon, 1997).

One way to determine the effect of a more intense noise floor (that is, of a less sensitive microphone) on the prevalence of SOAEs, is to estimate the prevalence as the signal-to-noise ratio required for labeling a spectral peak as an SOAE changes. For example, Penner, Glotzbach, and Huang (1993) noted that the prevalence of SOAEs in females would drop from 75 percent to 60 percent if the ratio increased by 3 dB (if the noise floor of the microphone were 3 dB larger). Thus, if the noise floor of the microphone exceeded that in the ear canal, it is theoretically possible that a more sensitive microphone would lead to measurement of additional SOAEs.

Classification of Spectral Peaks as SOAEs

In most studies, peaks in a spectral floor were identified as SOAEs based on visual inspection or on an arbitrary designation that any peak exceeding the noise floor by a certain number of db was an SOAE. For large peaks, the procedure undoubtedly works because large deviations from the noise floor are statistically unlikely to be caused by a single aberrantly large frequency component of the noise floor. However, because of fluctuations in the noise floor itself, a small peak may correspond to an SOAE or merely to a fluctuation in the noise floor.

To distinguish between a fluctuation in the noise floor and an SOAE, investigators have typically selected a criterion for designating a peak as an SOAE. Typically the criterion is the ratio of the level of a peak to the level of the surrounding noise floor. As the ratio declines, it is possible that some peaks labeled as SOAEs may not in fact be SOAEs. As the ratio increases, it is possible that some fluctuations thought to belong to the noise floor might really be SOAEs.

Penner et al. (1993) were the first to point out that detecting a spectral maximum (an SOAE) embedded in a noise floor (of the ear or of the microphone) was conceptually similar to a yes-no task in which a signal embedded in noise is to be detected. The analogy applies to what psychophysicists call a yes-no task, in which a subject must decide whether a clearly demarcated sound contained a signal embedded in noise or was merely the noise alone. The task gets its name because the subject responds "yes" whenever he thinks the signal was present and "no" if he thinks the signal was not present. For detecting SOAEs in noise, the experimenter must decide whether a clearly demarcated interval in time contained an SOAE embedded in noise or the noise alone.

In either a yes-no task or in the detection of SOAEs, the detection process could be completely described if two independent outcomes, the hit and false alarm rates, were known. When detecting external signals (Green & Swets, 1966), the hit rate (the probability of saying yes given a signal was presented) is typically graphed as a function of the false alarm rate (the probability of saying yes given that no signal was presented). This graph is called a receiver operating characteristic (ROC).

An ROC cannot be obtained for detecting SOAEs because the hit rate (the probability of concluding that a subject has an SOAE given the presence of an SOAE) is unknown (that is, the presence or absence of SOAEs is neither known nor controlled by the experimenter). The false alarm rate, on the other hand, depends on the measurement system and may be estimated.

The measurement system includes the microphone, the details of the spectral analyses, and the algorithm for labeling a spectral maximum as an SOAE. To estimate the false alarm rate, the output from a 0.5 cc syringe, used to simulate the volume of the ear canal, may be recorded and analyzed. A spectral peak recorded from the syringe labeled as an SOAE by the measurement system constitutes a false alarm. After hundreds of recordings from the syringe are analyzed, it is possible to calculate the false alarm rate for the measurement system. The false alarm rate varies as the criterion for labeling a peak as an SOAE is varied.

Figure 8-1 displays the estimated prevalence of SOAEs as a function of the false alarm rate for the measurement system and employed in our laboratory (Penner et al., 1993). Each false alarm corresponds to a different criterion as labeled on the upper part of the figure. For females, prevalence estimates ranged from 75 percent to 100 percent as the false alarm rate increased from 0 percent to 35 percent. Similarly, for males, the prevalence increased from 58 percent to 100 percent as the false alarm rate increased from 0 percent to 57 percent. With false alarm rates of about 14 percent, gender differences in the prevalence of SOAEs disappear.

One inference from Figure 8-1 is that some SOAEs could fail to be detected, especially when the false alarm rate is near zero. That is, some idiotones of presumed cochlear origin could fail to manifest themselves as measurable SOAEs when the false alarm rate is zero. To avoid problems of failing to

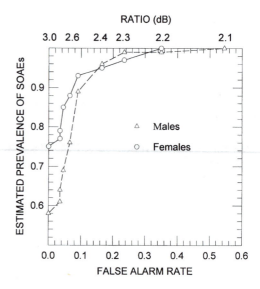

FIGURE 8-1. Estimates of the prevalence of SOAEs for females (circles) and males (triangles) as a function of the false alarm rate (bottom axis). Note that the estimated prevalence of SOAEs increases as the false alarm rate increases. (Reprinted with permission of *Hearing Research*).

detect an SOAE, it is possible to increase the false alarm rate. However, as the false alarm rate increases, peaks labeled as SOAEs might merely correspond to increments in the noise floor. Thus, SOAEs could be judged to be present if the false alarm rate exceeded zero even though there was no underlying SOAE.

Estimates of the false alarm rate depend on the sensitivity of the microphone, on the spectral analyses techniques, and on the level required for labeling a peak as an SOAE.

Spectral Analysis Techniques

Although the contribution of the choice of data analysis to the measurement of SOAEs has been implicitly recognized, most investigators have simply selected a fixed number of spectral averages and one frequency resolution and measured the resulting SOAEs (Bargones & Burns, 1988; Burns, Arehart, & Campbell, 1992; Dallmayr, 1985; Hammel, 1983; McFadden & Loehlin, 1995;

Moulin, Collet, Delli, & Morgon, 1991; Probst, Lonsbury-Martin, & Martin, 1991; Wier, Norton, & Kincaid, 1984; Zurek, 1981). Reasons for the choice of a single set of analysis parameters differed somewhat, but in the majority of the cases the signal was not digitized and was measured on a real-time spectrum analyzer. Therefore, to perform multiple analyses, the subject would have to remain in the booth while the spectrum resulting from each selection of FFT parameters was determined. Changes in subsequent spectra could be attributed to changes in the SOAE itself or could reflect changes in the spectral analysis. With the advent of digitization of the ear's output, storage of the output on a floppy disc, and subsequent computer analysis of the stored recording, it became possible to examine many spectral representations of the stored data.

The importance of the spectral analysis parameters can be easily conceptualized. First, however, it is necessary to note that a given spectral analysis depends on the frequency resolution and the number of spectra that are averaged to produce the final frequency spectrum.

To begin, consider the effect of the resolution of the measurement system. If SOAEs differ somewhat in bandwidth, then the spectral analysis parameters might best be tailored to match the bandwidth of a specific SOAE. If the bandwidth of an SOAE exceeds the frequency resolution, the power of the SOAE is split into two or more frequency bins. On the other hand, if the bandwidth of the SOAE is less than the frequency resolution, the power of the SOAE is combined with that of the surrounding noise floor, thereby generally decreasing the ratio of the power in that bin to the power in nearby frequency bins. Therefore, there exists an optimal frequency resolution for each specific SOAE bandwidth.

To emphasize the importance of the frequency resolution, consider the example in Figure 8-2. The subject whose data appear in this figure had multiple SOAEs. The figure presents the average level of some of

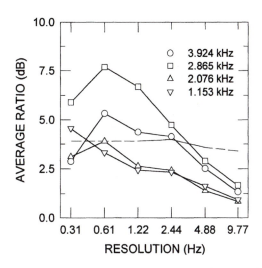

FIGURE 8-2. The peak-to-trough ratio as a function of frequency resolution with sixteen spectral averages. Each symbol represents one of the subject's SOAEs that were at the nominal frequencies labeled in the figure. The dashed line is the ratio for which no false alarms were observed during 200 recordings with no input to the microphone. (Reprinted with permission from *Hearing Research*).

this subject's SOAEs for sixteen spectral averages. The dashed line is the ratio required for a peak to be labeled as an SOAE, as discussed later.

In Figure 8-2, the peak at a nominal frequency of 1.153 kHz exceeded the criterion for labeling a peak as an SOAE only with a resolution of 0.305 Hz, while other peaks at nominal frequencies of 3.924 kHz and 2.076 kHz would only have been labeled as SOAEs with other resolutions. Thus, maximal detection of SOAEs did not appear at a fixed resolution for all peaks for this subject.

To emphasize the importance for spectral averages, consider the example in Figure 8-3 which consists of the same subject's data as shown in Figure 8-2. Figure 8-3 presents a measure of the level of this subject's SOAEs with various numbers of averages to produce the resulting spectrum. The dashed line is the ratio required for a peak to be labeled as an SOAE, as discussed later.

In Figure 8-3, one peak at a nominal frequency of 1.723 kHz would be identified as an SOAE for any number of averages

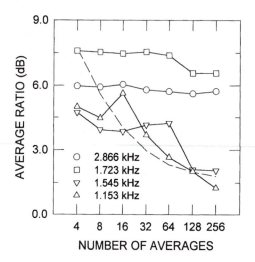

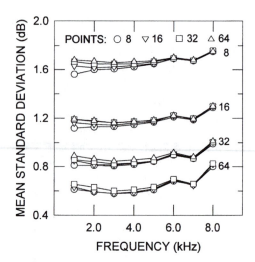

FIGURE 8-3. The peak-to-trough ratio as a function of the number of averages (resolution of 2.44 Hz). Each symbol represents one of the subject's SOAEs that were at nominal frequencies as labeled in the figure. The dashed line is the ratio for which no false alarms were observed with 200 recordings with no input to the microphone. (Reprinted with permission from *Hearing Research*).

FIGURE 8-4. The mean standard deviation of the noise floor as a function of the frequency and number of averages to produce a spectrum. From left to right, the symbols above all the curves represent the number of points per Fast Fourier Analysis (FFT) divided by 1,024. Note that the standard deviation was essentially independent of frequency, irrespective of the number of points per FFT. From top to bottom, the data clusters represent the number of averages (8, 16, 32, or 64) to produce a spectrum. (Reprinted with permission from *Hearing Research*).

employed, whereas other peaks required eight or more averages (2.865 kHz) or sixteen or more averages (1.153 and 1.545 kHz). Even though most peaks were identified as SOAEs with 256 averages, many of the SOAEs were identifiable with far fewer averages.

Increasing the number of averages affects the variability of the noise floor. In order to empirically verify these effects, we placed an ER-10A microphone in a 0.5 cc syringe (to simulate the volume of the ear canal) and performed 200 spectral analyses on the output of the microphone. In this way, we were able to observe changes in the noise floor as the number of spectral averages increased. The standard deviation (SD) within 3.5 percent of numerous center frequencies was computed. As seen in Figure 8-4 the SD of the noise floor decreased as the number of spectral averages increased, and the SD was nearly independent of frequency if the number of averages was constant. Further, the SD decreased as the square root of the number of averages.

One important factor in identifying peaks is the value of the SD of the noise floor because a peak is basically defined as an excursion several SDs above the noise floor. As seen in Figure 8-4, nearly the same SD is obtained at each frequency if the number of averages is constant. It follows that the false alarm rate of the system is independent of frequency and thus the same criterion may be used to identify SOAEs independent of the frequency of the SOAE.

The dependence of the SD on the number of averages does, however, mean that the criterion for identifying a peak as an SOAE depends on the number of averages as seen in Figure 8-5. For example, a zero false alarm rate was obtained here with a peak-to-noise ratio of about 5 dB or about 2.5 dB depending on the number of averages. Thus, intermittent SOAEs or those that fluctuate in level (such as those in Figure 8-2) could be identified as SOAEs only when some spe-

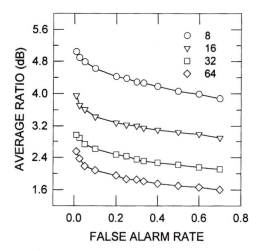

FIGURE 8-5. The peak-to-alps ratio as a function of the false alarm rate of the system. The symbol in the figure represents the number of averages with 16,384 points per FFT. (Reprinted with permission from *Hearing Research*).

cific number of spectra were averaged but not with other numbers of averages.

The data presented in Figures 8-3 to 8-5 suggest that the magnitude of a peak depends on the spectral resolution as well as on the number of spectra averaged. It is therefore possible to improve the estimate of the prevalence of SOAEs or the measurement of a specific SOAE by using many different spectral resolutions and numbers of averages.

One example of such multiple analyses revealed a prevalence of 83 percent in females and 62 percent in males with a false alarm rate of less than 3.9 percent (Penner & Zhang, 1997). For the same data, a single spectral analysis revealed a prevalence as low as 64 percent for females and 39 percent for males.

Measurement of SOAEs is an evolving field. New techniques to reduce the noise floor and to maximize detection of spectral peaks are being undertaken in numerous laboratories (Cheng, 1994; 1997; Zhang & Penner, in preparation). It would not be surprising if the prevalence of SOAEs increased dramatically as measurement techniques continue to improve. One meaningful consequence of this prediction is that extant estimates of the prevalence of SOAE-caused tinnitus could represent only a small portion of the actual cases. Before considering this implication, however, data linking SOAEs and tinnitus need to be examined.

LINKING SOAEs AND TINNITUS

Measurable SOAEs have not frequently been linked to tinnitus. One aspect of the low correspondence between the frequency of the SOAEs and the frequency of the pure tone that matches the pitch of the tinnitus is the fact that, even for recent studies of the prevalence of SOAEs which employ a sensitive microphone and considerable spectral averaging, relatively few SOAEs have been measured at frequencies above 4 kHz (Dallmayr, 1985; Penner et al., 1993; Talmadge, Long, Murphy, & Tubis, 1992) where the majority of the frequencies said to match the pitch of the tinnitus lie (Penner, 1990; Reed, 1960).

The scarcity of SOAEs above 4 kHz may simply reflect the severe high-frequency attenuation by the middle ear of the retrograde wave from the (presumed) cochlear site of the SOAE rather than the actual paucity of idiotones above 4 kHz. Thus, part of the reason for the low correspondence for SOAEs and tinnitus may be that although idiotones exist, they do not always manifest themselves as measurable SOAEs.

Another aspect of the low correspondence among the frequencies of SOAEs and the frequency of a tone said to match the pitch of the tinnitus is related to the difficulty in determining the composition of the tinnitus (see Chapter 7). Unfortunately, the composition of the tinnitus cannot often be definitively assessed from masking or matching paradigms. Masking tinnitus with external pure tones does not usually yield the frequency-specific masking patterns (such as psychophysical tuning curves) associated with the masking of low-level narrow-band external stimuli (Burns, 1984; Feldmann, 1971; Penner, 1987; Tyler & Conrad-Armes, 1983). Because the masking patterns of tinnitus are often flat (the masker level may be independent of masker frequency), they do not define the spectrum of the tinnitus.

Matching the tinnitus with external pure tones does not provide a conclusive definition of the tinnitus because matches are frequently unreliable (Burns, 1984; Penner, 1983; Tyler & Conrad-Armes, 1983) or reliable only because all but one component of the tinnitus is ignored (Penner, 1993; Penner & Bilger, 1992; Penner & Klafter, 1992). Variations of several octaves in the matching tone are not uncommon (Burns, 1984; Penner, 1983). The evanescent nature of the pitch matches made to tinnitus using the method of adjustment could arise because the tinnitus is labile or because it is a multicomponent broadband signal, and the subject is uncertain about which component of the tinnitus is to be matched (Penner, 1993; Hazell, 1981), or both. In any event, tinnitus should probably be represented by a range of frequencies rather than by a single frequency. If so, SOAEs in a broad region of frequencies bracketing the tinnitus could be viewed as corresponding to it. However, Penner and Burns (1987) argue that the correspondence of the SOAE frequency and the frequency of a tone matching the pitch of the tinnitus, or even the frequency region bracketing the tinnitus, does not necessarily link the two phenomena because association does not prove causation.

Tests Linking SOAEs and Tinnitus

The difficulties in measuring SOAEs and the problem of associating even measurable SOAEs with tinnitus raise the important issue of determining which empirical tests can link the two phenomena.

Tests to address the SOAE-tinnitus link focus on the differences between the psychophysical behavior of tinnitus and that of SOAEs. For example, an SOAE will actually disappear in the presence of a suitably chosen low-level external tone whereas such a tone has no effect on tinnitus which is not caused by SOAEs. The disappearance of the SOAE is referred to as suppression. Suppression is the basis for a test used to demonstrate that SOAEs may cause tinnitus. Specifically, Penner and Burns (1987) argue that if SOAEs can be suppressed without affecting the tinnitus, and if tinnitus can be masked without affecting the SOAEs, then the tinnitus and SOAEs are likely to be physiologically independent.

An example of the masking/suppression demonstration is seen in Figure 8-6. In the first panel, two SOAEs at 1.375 and 2.4 kHz are detected. In the second panel, a 4.3 kHz tone was presented and it was reported to mask the tinnitus, yet the SOAEs are clearly visible. In the third panel, two SOAE suppressors were presented, yet the subject's tinnitus was still audible and unchanged in pitch. Thus, for this subject, SOAEs did not seem to be the cause of tinnitus.

Although the masking/suppression demonstration is conclusive, the psychophysical armamentaria of tests linking SOAEs and tinnitus may be expanded to include a converging series of psychophysical tests. In addition to the masking/suppression demonstration, isomasking contours (masker level as a function of masker frequency) obtained using tinnitus as the signal may be contrasted with suppression tuning curves (STCs) (suppressor level as a function of suppressor frequencies) for the SOAEs. Because STCs are frequency-specific (Schloth & Zwicker, 1983) whereas tinnitus masking patterns are not (Feldmann, 1971; Penner, 1987), differences in these functions also provide circumstantial evidence that the tinnitus is not an SOAE.

Other psychophysical tests are also feasible. For example, because SOAEs which are shifted by mechanical forces become momentarily audible (Schloth & Zwicker, 1983), SOAEs that fluctuate spontaneously may also be audible. Hence, fluctuant SOAEs may provide circumstantial evidence favoring the SOAE-tinnitus link. In addition, the frequencies of SOAEs change systematically throughout the menstrual cycle (Bell, 1992). Therefore, if the frequency of a tone matching the pitch of the tinnitus also changed

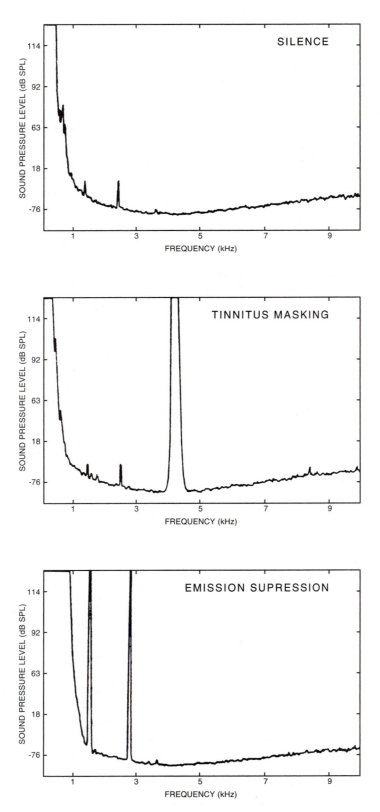

FIGURE 8-6. The SOAEs for one subject. The ordinate represents the level in dB SPL. The abscissa represent frequency (in kHz). See text for explanation. (Reprinted with permission from the *Journal of Speech and Hearing Research*).

systematically throughout the menstrual cycle, additional support for the SOAE-tinnitus link could be garnered. In the following cases reported, these tests and others tailored to the specific subject serve as the basis for inferring an SOAE-tinnitus link.

In addition to the following cases, interested readers are referred to Burns & Keefe (1991), Hammel (1983), Hazell (1984), Plinkert et al. (1990), and Sutton and Wilson (1987).

Cases of SOAE-Caused Tinnitus

Case 1: Fluctuant SOAEs cause tinnitus.

In the first well-documented case of SOAE-caused tinnitus (Penner, 1988) discussed here, the subject was a 26-year-old woman who had a twenty-three month history of tinnitus (Penner, 1988). The tinnitus was reported to be binaural but worse in her right than in her left ear. The presence of the cacophonous internal sound made her "irritable and nervous, interfered with concentration, and made it difficult to be quiet."

The threshold sensitivities for this subject were nearly normal while her SOAEs fluctuated in level. The tests linking SOAEs and tinnitus for this subject demonstrated that: (1) when SOAEs were suppressed, the tinnitus was inaudible, (2) the SOAEs were somewhat variable in frequency, (3) pitch matches to tinnitus corresponded to the lowest frequency SOAE, which was relatively stable, and, finally, (4) the SOAEs were more intense and there were more SOAE components in the right than in the left ear, as seen in Figure 8-7, corresponding to the subject's report that the tinnitus was binaural but worse in her right ear. These results are consistent with the conclusion that the subject had SOAE-caused tinnitus.

Case 2: Two coexisting causes of tinnitus.

The second subject (Penner, 1989a) was a 38-year-old female who had a ten-year history of tinnitus. She had been to an otolaryngologist to complain about her tinnitus which was described by the subject as ringing and changing tones. The tinnitus was reported to be irritating, causing moderate interference with work, slightly disrupting her sleep, and in her left ear only.

Her threshold sensitivities were not normal. The hearing in her right ear was better than that in the left ear and the threshold at 8 kHz in the left ear exceeded 90 dB SPL, the maximum level the local Institutional Review Board permits in testing subjects. The subject had a single SOAE in her right ear. No SOAEs were found in her left. During eight experimental sessions, the level of the SOAE in her right ear fluctuated by only 3.2 dB.

Because the SOAE was relatively stable, it was surprising to find that it was part of the tinnitus. Indeed, the masking/suppression demonstration indicated that the tinnitus was reported to be masked only when a continuous masker was presented in the left ear and a suppressor was in the right ear. No other combination of the masker and suppressor was reported to mask the tinnitus. The fact that tinnitus could only be masked when two contralateral tones were presented simultaneously might be interpreted as indicating that the tinnitus was binaural even though the subject reported it to be monaural.

Evidence favoring the binaural nature of the tinnitus was also obtained from iso-masking contours and from matches of external tones to the pitch of the tinnitus. In the presence of a continuous suppressor in her right ear, the subject adjusted a tone in her left ear so that it masked the tinnitus. The tinnitus isomasking contour was flat. In contrast, with a masker in her left ear, the tinnitus isomasking contour was frequency-specific. Further, the frequency of a tone said to match the pitch of the tinnitus in her right ear was stable (SD of 0.036 kHz) whereas that in her left ear was quite variable (SD of 0.128 kHz).

Taken together, the data indicate that this subject had two coexisting sources of tinnitus: one in her right ear caused by an SOAE, and one in her left accompanying her sensorineural hearing loss.

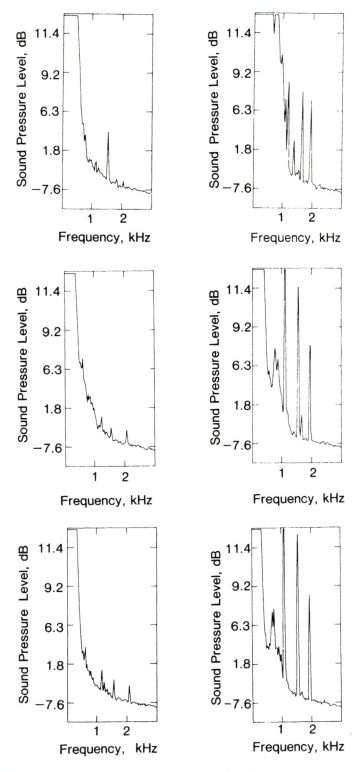

FIGURE 8-7. SOAEs in the subject's right and left ears during three sessions. Note that there were more fluctuant SOAEs in her right than in her left ear. The tinnitus was reported to be in her right ear. (Reprinted with permission from *Archives of Otolaryngology*).

Case 3: Menstrual rhythms and SOAE-caused tinnitus.

Two interesting publications (Bell, 1992; Haggarty, Lusted, & Morton, 1993) present data showing that the frequencies of most SOAEs display menstrual rhythms. Although the effect is small (about 1 percent), SOAE frequencies generally decline before the onset of menstruation. It follows that the predominant pitch of SOAE-caused tinnitus and the frequency of the associated SOAE should co-vary.

In order to explore this co-variation, data were collected from one normal hearing subject who had SOAE-caused tinnitus (Penner, 1994). In particular, the subject had binaural tinnitus which was perceived principally as being in her right ear where the majority of her fluctuant SOAEs were observed. Data were collected for forty-four days. Because there are circadian rhythms in SOAE frequencies (Bell, 1992; Haggerty et al., 1993), the SOAEs measure were made at nearly the same time each day.

A total of twenty-one different SOAEs were measured during the forty-four days with as many as nineteen SOAEs and as few as seven SOAEs appearing in a single session. In the left ear, the SOAEs were independent. In the right ear, the SOAEs displayed two types of interactions.

First, some SOAEs interacted to produce cubic distortion product SOAEs. SOAEs arise when two independent SOAEs interact, as would two external tones, to produce a third SOAE. The SOAE cannot be suppressed with a tone at a nearby frequency, but can be suppressed if one of the original tones is.

Second, some SOAEs were alternate-state SOAEs. That is, the presence of some SOAEs occurred only in the absence of others (the SOAEs alternated). It seems likely that alternate-state SOAEs are variable enough to draw the subject's attention to the SOAEs thereby causing tinnitus.

Figure 8-8 shows the frequency variations for the stable SOAEs in the right and left ears during one menstrual cycle. In order to enable fluctuations of these SOAEs to appear

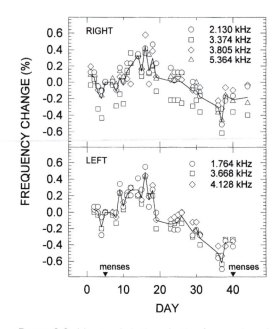

FIGURE 8-8. Menstrual rhythms in the frequencies of the unremitting SOAEs in the right (top graph) and left (bottom graph) ears. The solid line represents the average of the percent frequency change for all the SOAEs graphed. (Reprinted with permission from the *Archives of Otolaryngology*).

in one figure, the ordinate represents the percent by which the SOAEs shifted in frequency regarding the first day of menses, day 5. For the menstrual cycle in this graph, a local minimum in the frequencies of the SOAEs occurred near the onset of menstruation.

The salient issue here is whether the fluctuations in the tinnitus pitch followed the fluctuations in the SOAEs. The subject was able to match external tones to the highest and lowest components of her tinnitus, but not to the intervening ones. Therefore the pitch matching data are necessarily restricted to these components.

Figure 8-9 displays the frequency of the SOAE that was typically associated with the predominant pitch of the tinnitus and the frequency of the nearby SOAE. Local minima in the frequency of both the SOAE and the frequency of the tone matching the tinnitus pitch appear before menstruation, and

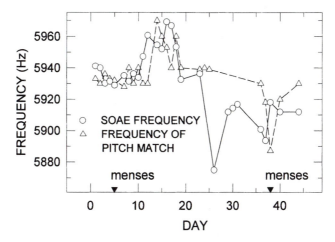

FIGURE 8-9. Menstrual rhythm of the frequency of the tone matching the predominant pitch of the tinnitus (triangles) and the frequency of the associated SOAE (circle). (Reprinted with permission from the *Archives of Otolaryngology*).

the maxima for both frequencies is reached after the onset of menses.

For two of the days (24 and 25), the tinnitus pitch was matched to a frequency of about 5.90 kHz, which did not correspond to a measurable SOAE on that day. One interpretation is that the nearby SOAE had fluctuated in level and had reappeared when the matches to the tinnitus were made. Another interpretation is that the subject was merely matching to the remembered pitch. An argument against this is that the subject did not always match to the same pitch. In particular, on four days (26, 29, 30, and 31), the frequencies of the matches to tinnitus averaged 5.372 kHz. For these four testing sessions, there was an associated SOAE with an average frequency of 5.364 kHz and these days the level of the SOAE at 5.364 kHz was significantly greater than that of the SOAE at a nominal frequency of 5.490 kHz. It is possible that the SOAE at the lower frequency might have governed the tinnitus percept during these sessions. Thus, co-variation of SOAE frequency and the frequency of the tone matching the tinnitus pitch provide another piece of circumstantial evidence linking SOAEs and tinnitus.

Case 4: Aspirin may abolish SOAE-caused tinnitus. Because aspirin abolishes most SOAEs (Long & Tubis, 1988; McFadden & Plattsmeir, 1984), perhaps the most conclusive test for linking SOAEs would be provided if aspirin abolished both the SOAEs and the tinnitus. One problem with this approach is that aspirin may abolish the SOAE-caused tinnitus while producing other forms of tinnitus.

The only successful attempt to abolish SOAE-caused tinnitus was reported in 1992 (Penner & Coles, 1992). The aspirin dose employed was 600 mg per day. As seen in Figure 8-10, when the aspirin abolished the SOAE, the tinnitus was not audible. Thus there is some hope that aspirin may provide a palliative for tinnitus in rare cases.

Prevalence of SOAE-Caused Tinnitus

Given that SOAEs may cause tinnitus, how often do they do so? Of ninety-six subjects tested (Penner, 1990), 4.1 percent were judged to have SOAE-caused tinnitus using the masking/suppression demonstration. The 95 percent confidence limits for this estimate are 1.1 percent and 9.05 percent.

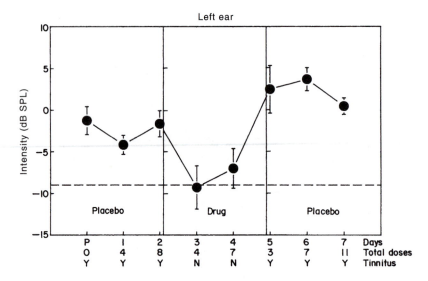

FIGURE 8-10. Average level of the subject's SOAE. The dashed line indicates the average level of the noise floor at 0.5 kHz during the preliminary testing session labeled P. The abscissa information presents the day of the trial, the total number of doses consumed prior to testing, and the patient's report concerning tinnitus (Y, tinnitus present; N, tinnitus absent). The vertical bars represent the standard deviation of the level of the SOAE for the day labeled on the abscissa. (Reprinted with permission from the *British Journal of Audiology*).

More recently, Dr. Coles (personal communication) found that 4.5 percent of the patients in his tinnitus clinic had SOAE-caused tinnitus.

One important question emerging from this prevalence study involves the identification of the characteristics of subjects who are likely to have SOAE-caused tinnitus. At present, the scarcity of such subjects probably precludes generalizations. However, the prevalence data provide several hints. It may be that the typical person with SOAE-caused tinnitus will be a normal-hearing woman who matches the tinnitus pitch with tones in the 1 to 2 kHz region. The reason for this suggestion is that SOAEs are much more likely to occur in women than in men, that SOAEs do not occur at frequencies for which there is a hearing loss (Moulin, Collet, Delli, & Morgon, 1991) and most SOAEs occur in the 1 to 2 kHz region whereas tinnitus not caused by SOAEs is frequently higher in pitch.

IDIOTONES AND TINNITUS

The 4 percent estimate for the prevalence of SOAE-caused tinnitus requires the measurement of SOAEs. As already discussed, the measurement of SOAEs depends on the sensitivity of the microphone, on the procedure employed to classify a spectral peak as an SOAE, and on the spectral characteristics used to analyze the data and to reduce the noise floor. In addition, the attenuation characteristics of the middle ear and the stiffness of the tympanic membrane also affect the appearance of spectral peaks (Wiederhold, 1990). Given such intricacies, it seems likely that not all tones manifest themselves as SOAEs. The issue then is whether internally generated tones that do not manifest themselves as SOAEs could cause tinnitus.

There is a long history of psychophysicists postulating the existence of tones based on the interaction of the presumed internal and external tones. The interaction produces a variety of perceptions known collectively as monaural diplacusis.

As discussed earlier, monaural diplacusis is said to occur if a pure tone does not sound pure but elicits sensations of beats, roughness, multiple tones or an area of silence and possibly an aftertone. The simplest explanation of the phenomena of diplacusis is that two tones, an internal and external tone, sound different from an external tone. More accurately, the interaction of two tones produces distortion products that may underlie monaural diplacusis.

In five articles (Bacon & Viemeister, 1985; Flottorp, 1953; Formby & Gjerdignen, 1981; Ward, 1952, 1955), the phenomenon of monaural diplacusis has been viewed as evidence favoring the existence of internal tones when SOAEs were not detected. Is it possible that idiotones that do not produce measurable emissions cause tinnitus?

Some data from a subject of Penner (1986) are of interest in this regard. Thus far the results of three psychophysical tests are consistent with his having idiotones that cause tinnitus.

First, the subject (number 7 in Penner, 1986) reliably matched the pitch of the tinnitus with a pure tone. The standard deviation of the matches for this subject was 1.96 percent. This is smaller than Burns (1984) obtained for any of the eight subjects he studied and is markedly different from the several hundred standard deviation obtained from most subjects. The standard deviation of the pitch matches made by Subject 7 is, in fact, the smallest ever reported for repeated between-session matches to the pitch of tinnitus which is not known to be caused by SOAEs.

Second, the slope of this subject's psychometric function (the probability of correctly detecting an external tone as a function of the level of the external tone) was the same in the tinnitus region as above and below it whereas that of nine other tinnitus sufferers was flatter in the tinnitus region. According to the theory of signal detection

(Green & Swets, 1966), the slope of the psychometric function flattens as the variability of the background noise increases. Thus, if tinnitus served as a source of internal noise, the psychometric function in the region containing the tinnitus could be flatter than in the region above or below it.

The third unusual result is that the subject had monaural diplacusis in the neighborhood of 2.463 kHz, which was the average frequency matched to the pitch of tinnitus. It was the presence of monaural diplacusis that first induced speculation that idiotones existed. In a similar manner, monaural diplacusis in the frequency region of tinnitus would seem to suggest that idiotones might be irritating.

These three psychophysical results are consistent with the behavior of a tone generated in the cochlea. The inference is that, if tinnitus behaves as would an external tone, then it might be generated by an internal tone originating in the cochlea even if SOAEs are not apparent. In other words, psychophysically similar tones may have a common origin. The logic has historical precedent: because SOAEs behave like external tones, they are thought to be generated in the cochlea (Kemp, 1978). By analogy, if sounds with similar psychophysics have a common origin, then some cases of tinnitus may be caused by idiotones even when SOAEs cannot be measured. Thus, the existence of this last subject raises the question of whether tinnitus may be caused by idiotones when SOAEs are not detected and what sort of psychophysical measures could be used to establish that idiotones cause tinnitus.

DISCUSSION AND CONCLUSION

Because most normal-hearing men and women have SOAEs and yet do not have tinnitus, the link between SOAEs and troublesome tinnitus must be relatively infrequent, as the data show. Indeed, SOAEs are seldom even audible. On the other hand, not all idiotones manifest themselves as measurable SOAEs and techniques for detecting SOAEs are evolving, so it may be that the SOAE-tinnitus connection will occur a bit more frequently than is currently suspected.

The majority of SOAEs that cause tinnitus are fluctuant. Although many SOAEs are stable, Schloth and Zwicker (1983) remarked that one of their subjects had erratic emissions. Kohler et al. (1986) also mentioned that an intense emission at 11 dB SPL was not present all the time. Burns et al. (1984) noted that some emissions are linked so that the presence of one set of SOAEs precluded the presence of another. Subjective reports suggest that when an SOAE is released from suppression, it is heard as a decaying tone. Thus, if an SOAE were to fluctuate, it might be heard and be annoying.

In conclusion, the evolution of techniques for analyzing digitized recordings from the ear canal is far from complete. A glance at the literature on auditory brain stem response (for example, a review by Hall, 1992) reveals a progression in measurement techniques following the discovery of the original phenomenon. Comparable development in the measurement of SOAEs has not yet occurred. There is presently no agreed upon method for measuring SOAEs or even upon the criterion for evaluating the measurement system. Therefore, it is expected that the association of SOAEs and tinnitus will also evolve and that current estimates of the prevalence of SOAE-caused tinnitus are too low. Future research will test the veracity of this expectation.

REFERENCES

Bacon, S. P., & Viemeister, N. F. (1985). A case study of monaural diplacusis. *Hearing Research, 19,* 46–56

Bargones, J. Y, & Burns, E. M. (1988). Suppression tuning curves for spontaneous otoacoustic emissions in infants and adults. *Journal of the Acoustical Society of America, 83,* 1809–1816.

Bell, A. (1992). Circadian and menstrual rhythms in frequency variations of spontaneous otoacoustic emissions. *Hearing Research, 58,* 91–100.

Burns, E. M. (1984). A comparison of the variability among measurements of subjective tinnitus and objective stimuli. *Audiology, 23,* 426–440.

Burns, E. M., Arehart, K., & Campbell, S. L. (1992). Prevalence of spontaneous otoacoustic emissions in neonates. *Journal of the Acoustical Society of America, 19,* 1571–1575.

Burns, E. M., & Keefe, D. H. (1991). Unstable spontaneous otoacoustic emission as a cause of tinnitus. *Abstracts of the Association for Research in Otolaryngology, 239.*

Burns, E. M., Strickland, E. A., Tubis, A., & Jones, K. (1984). Interactions among spontaneous otoacoustic emissions I. Distortion products and linked emissions. *Hearing Research, 16,* 271–278.

Cerniac, B. J., Prasher, D. K., & Luxon, L. M. (1997). *Changes in cochlear micromechanics due to noise exposure and its relevance to tinnitus.* Paper presented at the Second European Conference on Protection Against Noise, Barbican Centre, London.

Cheng, J. (1994). Time frequency analysis of transiently evoked otoacoustic emissions via a smoothed pseudo Wigner distribution. *Scandinavian Journal of Audiology, 24,* 91–96

Cheng, J. (1997). *Spectral estimation of spontaneous otoacoustic emissions.* Paper presented at the Second European Conference on Protection Against Noise, Barbican Centre, London.

Citron, L. (1969). *Observations on a case of objective tinnitus.* Paper presented at Medical International Congress (p. 91). Amsterdam, Excerpta Medica Int. Cong. Ser. 189, 91.

Coles, R. R. A., Snashell, S. E., & Stephens, S. D. G. (1975). Some varieties of objective tinnitus. *British Journal of Audiology, 9,* 1–6.

Dallmayr, C. (1985). Spontane oto-akustische emissionen: Statistik und reaktion auf akustische stortone (Spontaneous oto-acoustic emission: Statistics and reaction to suppression tones). *Acoustica, 59,* 67–75.

Feldmann, H. (1971). Homolateral and contralateral masking of tinnitus by noise bands and by pure tones. *Audiology, 10,* 138–244.

Flottorp. G. (1953). Pure–tone tinnitus evoked by acoustic stimulation: the idiophonic effect. *Acta Otolaryngologica, 43,* 396–415.

Formby, C., & Gjerdignen, D. B. (1981). Some systematic observations on monaural diplacusis. *Audiology, 20,* 219–233.

Glanville, J. D., Coles, R. R. A., & Sullivan, B. M. (1971). A family with high-tonal objective tinnitus. *Journal of Laryngology and Otology, 85,* 1–10.

Gold, T. (1948). Hearing II: The physical basis of the action of the cochlea. *Proceedings of the Royal Society of London* (pp. 492–498).

Gold, T., & Pumphrey, R. J. (1948). Hearing I. The cochlea as frequency analyzer. *Proceedings of the Royal Society of London* (pp. 462–491).

Green, D. M. & Swets, J. (1966). *Signal detection theory and psychophysics.* New York: Wiley and Sons.

Haggarty, H. S., Lusted, H. S., & Morton, S. C. (1993). Statistical quantification of 24-hour and monthly variation of spontaneous otoacoustic emission frequency in the human ear. *Hearing Research, 70,* 31–49.

Hall, J. W. III (1992). *Handbook of auditory evoked response.* Boston: Allyn and Bacon.

Hammel, D. R. (1983). *The frequency of occurrence of spontaneous otoacoustic emissions in normal-hearing young adults.* Unpublished master's thesis, University of Illinois, Urbana-Champaign, Illinois.

Hazell, J. W. P. (1981). A tinnitus synthesizer: Physiological considerations. In Shulman, A. (Chairman), *Proceedings of the First International Tinnitus Seminar* as published in the *Journal of Laryngology and Otology* (pp. 187–195).

Hazell, J. W. P. (1984). Spontaneous otoacoustic emissions and tinnitus: Clinical experience in the tinnitus patient. *Journal of Laryngology and Otology, 9,* 106–110.

Huizing, E. H., & Spoor, A. (1973). An unusual type of tinnitus. *Archives of Otolaryngology, 98,* 134–136.

Kemp, D. T. (1978). Stimulated acoustic emissions from the human auditory system. *Journal of the Acoustical Society of America, 64,* 1386–1391.

Kohler, W., Fredriksen, E., & Fritze, W. (1986). Spontaneous otoacoustic emissions: A comparison of the left versus the right ear. *Archives of Otorhinolaryngology, 243,* 43–46.

Long, G. R., & Tubis, A. (1988). Modification of spontaneous and evoked emissions and associated psychoacoustic microstructure by aspirin consumption. *Journal of the Acoustical Society of America, 84,* 1343–1353.

McFadden, D. (1982). *Tinnitus: Facts, theories and treatments.* Washington, DC: National Academy Press.

McFadden, D., & Loehlin, J. C. (1995). On the heritability of spontaneous otoacoustic emissions: A twin study. *Hearing Research, 85,* 181–198.

McFadden, D., & Plattsmeir, H. S. (1984). Aspirin abolishes spontaneous otoacoustic emissions. *Journal of the Acoustical Society of America, 76,* 443–448.

Moulin, A., Collet, L., Delli, D., & Morgon, A. (1991). Spontaneous otoacoustic emissions and sensori–neural hearing loss. *Acta Otolaryngology* (Stockholm), *111,* 835–841.

Penner, M. J. (1983). Variability in matches to subjective tinnitus. *Journal of Speech and Hearing Research, 26,* 263–267.

Penner, M. J. (1986). Tinnitus a source of internal noise. *Journal of Speech and Hearing Research, 29,* 400–406.

Penner, M. J. (1987). The masking of tinnitus and central masking. *Journal of Speech and Hearing Research, 26,* 147–152.

Penner, M. J. (1988). Audible and annoying spontaneous otoacoustic emissions: A case study. *Archives of Otolaryngology, 114,* 150–153.

Penner, M. J. (1989a). Two coexisting sources of tinnitus: A case study. *Journal of Speech and Hearing Research, 32,* 458–461.

Penner, M. J. (1989b). Aspirin abolishes tinnitus caused by spontaneous otoacoustic emissions. *Archives of Otolaryngology, 115,* 871–875.

Penner, M. J. (1990). An estimate of the prevalence of SOAE–caused tinnitus. *Archives of Otolaryngology, 116,* 428–432.

Penner, M. J. (1992). Linking spontaneous otoacoustic emissions and tinnitus. *British Journal of Audiology, 26,* 115–123.

Penner, M. J. (1993). Synthesizing tinnitus from sine waves. *Journal of Speech and Hearing Research, 36,* 1300–1305.

Penner, M. J. (1994). Covariation of tinnitus pitch and the associated emission: A case study. *Otolaryngology—Head and Neck Surgery, 110,* 304–309.

Penner, M. J., and Bilger, R. C. (1992). Consistent within-session measures of tinnitus. *Journal of Speech and Hearing Research, 30,* 396–403.

Penner, M. J., & Burns, E. M. (1988). The dissociation of SOAEs and tinnitus. *Journal of Speech and Hearing Research, 36,* 1300–1304.

Penner, M. J., & Coles, R. R. A. (1992). Indications for aspirin as a palliative for SOAE-caused tinnitus. *British Journal of Audiology, 26,* 91–96.

Penner, M. J., Glotzbach, L., & Huang, T. (1993). Spontaneous otoacoustic emissions: Measurement and data. *Hearing Research, 68,* 229–237.

Penner, M. J., & Klafter, E. J. (1992). Measures of tinnitus: Step size, matches to imagined tones, and masking patterns. *Ear and Hearing, 6,* 410–416.

Penner, M. J., & Zhang, T. (1997). Prevalence of spontaneous otoacoustic emissions in adults revisited. *Hearing Research, 103,* 28–34.

Plinkert, P., Gitter, A., & Zenner, H. (1990). Tinnitus associated spontaneous otoacoustic emissions. *Acta Otolaryngologica, 110,* 342–347.

Probst, R., Lonsbury-Martin, B. L. & Martin, G. K. (1991). A review of otoacoustic emissions. *Journal of the Acoustical Society of America, 89,* 2027–2067.

Reed, G. F. (1960). An audiometric study of two hundred cases of subjective tinnitus. *Archives of Otolaryngology, 71,* 94–104.

Schloth, E., & Zwicker, E. (1983). Mechanical and acoustical influences on spontaneous otoacoustic emissions. *Hearing Research, 11,* 285–293.

Strickland, E. A., Burns, E. M., & Tubis, A. (1985). Incidence of spontaneous otoacoustic emissions in children and infants. *Journal of the Acoustical Society of America, 78,* 931–935.

Sutton, G. J., & Wilson, J. P. (1987). Spontaneous otoacoustic emissions in a tinnitus population. *British Journal of Audiology, 21,* 313–314.

Talmadge, C. L., Long, G. R., Murphy, W. J., & Tubis, A. (1993). New off–line method for detecting spontaneous otoacoustic emissions in human subjects. *Hearing Research, 71,* 170–182.

Tyler, R. S., & Conrad-Armes, D. (1983). Tinnitus pitch: A comparison of three measurement methods. *British Journal of Audiology, 17,* 101–107.

Ward, W. D. (1952). A case of tonal unilateral diplacusis. *Journal of the Acoustical Society of America, 24,* 449.

Ward, W. D. (1995). Tonal monaural diplacusis. *Journal of the Acoustical Society of America, 27,* 365–372.

Wegel, R. (1931). A study of tinnitus. *Archives of Otolaryngology—Head and Neck Surgery, 14,* 160–165.

Wiederhold, M. (1990). Effects of tympanic membrane modification on distortion product otoacoustic emissions in the cat ear canal. In P. Dallos, C.D. Geisler, J. W. Matthews, M. Ruggero, & C. R. Steels (Eds.), *Mechanics and biophysics of hearing* (pp. 251–258). New York: Springer Verlag.

Wier, C. C., Norton, S. J., & Kincaid, G. E. (1984). Spontaneous narrow-band otoacoustic signals emitted by human ears: A replication. *Journal of the Acoustical Society of America, 76,* 1248–1250.

Wilson, J. P., & Sutton, G. J. (1983). A family with high tonal objective tinnitus. In D. Evered & G. Lawrenson (Eds.), *Tinnitus* (pp. 82–107). London: Pitman.

Zurek, P. M. (1981). Spontaneous narrowband acoustic signals emitted by human ears. *Journal of the Acoustical Society of America, 69,* 514–523.

CHAPTER 9

Medical and Surgical Evaluation and Management of Tinnitus

Brian P. Perry, M.D.
Bruce J. Gantz, M.D.

INTRODUCTION

This chapter focuses on the medical evaluation of tinnitus patients, including both radiological and laboratory testing, as well as medical and surgical management. Often, treatment of the underlying pathologic condition, or withdrawal from the offending medication, will alleviate the symptom of tinnitus. In this chapter, common causes of tinnitus will be discussed, in addition to their treatment. Tinnitus that is the result of sensorineural hearing loss (no matter what the etiology), and its management, will be discussed in later chapters.

HISTORY

Obtaining a thorough history is perhaps the most important aspect of the initial encounter with a patient complaining of tinnitus. The most important information to obtain is an accurate description of the symptom. The etiology is at first an assumption based upon available information; the most common causes being noise exposure, presby-cusis, acoustic tumors, and vascular anomalies (Table 9-1). The character of the symptom can be described as ringing, buzzing, roaring, or pulsating, and may be in one or both ears. When bilateral, the tinnitus may be either symmetrical or different in each ear. Often, directed questions regarding frequency are needed: is the sound constant or intermittent with the pulse or in conjunction with chewing? Bilateral pulsatile symptoms are unlikely to be associated with vascular malformations or tumors; while aggravation of the symptom by chewing and swallowing may alert the clinician to an etiology such as palatal myoclonus. Having the patient characterize the pitch as either high or low may aid in the eventual diagnosis (Ménière's disease has a characteristic low-pitched roaring tinnitus). Vertigo, hearing loss, and other cranial nerve deficits (especially IX, X, XI, and XII) should be elicited during the interview as well.

The past medical, social, and family histories are equally important in uncovering the cause of the patients' tinnitus. Pertinent historical information regarding infections and their subsequent treatments, medical

Table 9-1. Tinnitus classification

Objective Tinnitus	Subjective Tinnitus
Pulsatile	Presbycusis
Neoplasm	
Glomus tumor	Noise exposure/trauma
Meningioma	Whiplash injury/cochlear concussion
Adenoma	
Hemangioma	Pharmacologic agents
Vascular lesions	Nonototoxic drugs
Acquired arterial alteration (carotid	Ototoxic drugs
or vertebral artery)	Ménière's disease
stenosis	
totuosisty	Cerebellopontine angle tumors
dissection	Acoustic neuroma
aneurysm	Meningioma
Congenital arterial alteration	
persistant stapedial artery	Middle ear disease
aberrant internal carotid	Acute otitis media
dural or cervical arteriovenous	Serous otitis media
malformation (AVM)	Chronic otitis media
Congenital venous anomalies	
high jugular bulb	Temporal bone neoplasm
jugular diverticulum	
jugular bulb dehiscence	
enlarged jugular vein	
Acquired venous processes	
dural arteriovenous fistula (AVF)	
extracranial avf	
stenotic transverse sinus	
Benign intracranial hypertension	
Great vessel bruits	
High cardiac output	
Nonpulsatile	
Palatal myoclonus	
Temporomandibular joint dysfunction	
Tensor tympani muscle spasm	

conditions, surgical procedures, and medications must be attained. In addition, a review of the patients' noise exposure history (both recreational and occupational), social habits (smoking, drinking, diet), and previous trauma should be pursued. A family history of hearing loss, tinnitus and medical illnesses should be sought. It has been shown that up to 50 percent of glomus tumors are familial, inherited by a mutation on chromosome 11; these tumors often present with pulsatile tinnitus (van der Mey, 1989; Baysal, 1997).

A key component of a complete history, and one often forgotten, is an adequate review of systems. These item lists can be filled out by the patient prior to clinician evaluation for expediency. Essential questions for tinnitus evaluation include hearing loss, dizziness, and aural fullness to rule out otologic disease. Visual changes and headaches are important to uncover because of their association with arteriovenous malformations and fistulas. Prior transient ischemic attacks, syncopy, and paresthesias can lead to the diagnosis of carotid athero-

Table 9-2. Key aspects of the patient's history

Key Features of the Patient History	
Chief Complaint:	Unilateral or bilateral, symmetrical, or asymmetrical
History of Present Illness:	Duration, character, pulsatile or tonal, constant or intermittent, associated vertigo and/or hearing loss
Past Medical History:	Head trauma, medications, medical illnesses, and treatments
Past Surgical History:	Prior otologic surgery
Social History:	Tobacco and alcohol usage, noise exposure (occupational/ recreational)
Family History:	Tinnitus, hearing loss, tumors
Review of Systems:	Visual changes, headaches (arteriovenous fistula); transient ischemic attacks, syncopy, paresthesias (carotid atherosclerotic disease); polyuria, polydipsia (diabetes mellitus); temperature intolerance (thyroid dysfunction); diarrhea, anxiety, palpitations (glomus tumor)

sclerotic disease. Endocrine dysfunction can also cause tinnitus; diabetes mellitus will often present with polydipsia and polyuria, while temperature intolerance and anxiety are often seen with thyroid dysfunction. Each of these findings may lead the physician to diagnostic possibilities (especially those of a systemic nature) and to focused laboratory and imaging procedures. Table 9-2 lists the critical items ascertained from the history.

Special consideration must be given to the child who presents with the complaint of tinnitus, since children infrequently complain about this problem (see Chapter 10). Open-ended questions without cues are important, because children are prone to try and please the examiner with positive responses (Black & Lilly, 1996). The same detailed account of the symptom is necessary; however, information will need to come from both the parent, and child without prompting. A review of middle ear infections and serous otitis media will be particularly relevant in this population.

PHYSICAL EXAMINATION

A complete head, neck and neuro-otologic examination is always required when evaluating a new patient with tinnitus. The tympanic membranes should be carefully evaluated with otomicroscopy, with special emphasis on movements with respiration (patulous eustachian tube), or myoclonic activity (palatal myoclonus); both of which can produce tinnitus, and may be present on the tympanogram. The middle ear space may demonstrate an aberrant carotid artery or jugular vein, as well as vascular tumors and otospongiotic focci. Glomus tumors often demonstrate blanching of the tumor with positive pressure (Brown's sign); whereas Schwartze's sign is a red hue overlying the promontory and stapes in active otosclerosis that does not blanch with pneumo-otoscopy. Tuning fork evaluation may uncover either a sensorineural or conductive hearing loss, confirming audiologic testing. Unsuspected neurological abnormalities and skull base tumors can be uncovered by carefully testing each of the cranial nerves, including neuromas, meningiomas and multiple sclerosis. Neuromas of cranial nerves IX, X, and XI can cause pulsatile tinnitus by disturbing flow through the jugular bulb within the jugular foramen. Fundoscopic examination is critical for identifying benign intracranial hypertension in young, obese females with papilledema, and elevated cerebral spinal fluid pressure, without neurological deficits (Sismanis, 1990), which might otherwise be overlooked.

The oral cavity should be inspected closely during a tinnitus evaluation. Palpation of the temporomandibular joint (TMJ) and inspection of the dentition and occlusion can be helpful in finding a cause for the patient's complaint. TMJ syndrome and malocclusion are potential causes of tinnitus secondary to increased tension within the pterygoid musculature (Gelb & Bernstein, 1983). Observation of the palate during symptomatic periods may demonstrate myoclonic activity, consistent with the diagnosis of palatal myoclonus.

Auscultation of the ear canal, pre- and postauricular regions, the orbit and neck are also routine aspects of the tinnitus work-up. Carotid bruit, jugular venous hum, arterio-venous malformation (AVM) thrill, and myoclonic clicks are all detectable to the attentive examiner using either a diaphragm/bell stethoscope, or a double armed stethoscope (Tewfik, 1984). Gentle occlusion of the ipsilateral (to the side of the tinnitus) internal jugular vein may reduce or abolish the tinnitus produced by a flow disturbance in the jugular bulb or by benign intracranial hypertension, as may turning the head from side to side (Hazell, 1988). This maneuver does not decrease the sound produced by carotid atherosclerotic disease, AVMs, or glomus tumors.

DIAGNOSTIC CLASSIFICATION

After a complete history and physical examination, with the additional information provided by the audiogram, the clinician can separate the patient's tinnitus into one of two categories. The first broad tinnitus division includes those sounds generated by para-auditory structures (vascular or myoclonic), whereas, the second is generated by the auditory system itself (Tyler & Babin, 1993). Those entities of vascular and muscular origin typically cause pulsatile tinnitus; whereas, the sounds generated by the auditory system are nonpulsatile. In this chapter, those entities causing pulsatile tinnitus are referred to as objective tinnitus; whereas, nonpulsatile tinnitus is referred to as subjective tinnitus. Although this classification system is dependent on a second party's ability to hear the perceived sound; an accurate description of the sound itself will often suffice.

RADIOLOGICAL EVALUATION

The decision to pursue further testing is made when there is a reasonable chance that a correctable cause for the otologic symptom exists. In those patients with a history of noise exposure, bilateral nonpulsatile tinnitus (sensorineural), and a consistent audiogram, no further testing need be performed. If, on the other hand, the patient has unilateral tinnitus and an asymmetrical audiogram, a magnetic resonance imaging (MRI) scan with Gadolinium contrast agent is the study of choice to evaluate the possibility of a retrocochlear lesion (Jackler, 1990; House, Waluch, & Jackler 1986). Table 9-3 lists the most common retrocochlear lesions.

When the patient presents with pulsatile (objective) tinnitus, without evidence of myoclonus, or eustachian tube dysfunction on exam or audiogram, an imaging study is necessary. Both computerized tomography (CT) and MRI should be obtained if a retrotympanic mass is identified on otoscopic examination (Brunberg, 1995). Axial and coronal CT images correctly characterize glomus tumors, middle ear adenomas, and congenital arterial anomalies (Hasso, 1994); additionally, CT is better for identifying an aberrant carotid artery or enlarged

Table 9-3. Differential diagnosis of cerebellopontine angle lesions

Cerebellopontine Angle Lesions
Acoustic neuroma
Arachnoid cyst
Ceruminoma
Chondroma/chondrosarcoma
Chordoma
Dermoid
Epidermoid (cholesteatoma)
Lipoma
Meningioma
Metastases
Paraganglioma
Schwannoma of cranial nerve V, IX, X
Teratoma

jugular vein. Gadolinium enhanced MRI will easily demonstrate the size and extent of glomus tumors of the middle ear, jugular foramen, and vagus nerve (paraganglioma) (Dietz et al., 1994), as well as neuromas of cranial nerves nine through twelve. Small ventricles and an empty sella tursica can be seen on MRI in those persons with benign intracranial hypertension (Sismanis, Stamm, & Sobel, 1994). Magnetic resonance angiography (MRA) is useful in evaluating the vascular causes of pulsatile tinnitus, including both arterial (AVF, AVM, aberrant or stenotic carotid, aneurysm, fibromuscular dysplasia), and venous (although CT is better) etiologies (high or dehiscent jugular bulb, diverticulum) (Dietz, 1994). Dural AVFs and glomus tumors are the two most common causes of pulsatile tinnitus; therefore, a protocol of both MRI and MRA should be performed (Dietz, 1994). Small dural AVMs of the skull base have been missed by MRI/MRA protocols, however, primarily due to volume averaging and slow, turbulent flow through these vessels (Koenigsberg, 1996). If MRI/MRA fail to demonstrate a lesion in a patient with troublesome pulsatile tinnitus, then carotid arteriography should be utilized, albeit with a known risk of stroke (Lo, 1991). Carotid arteriography can also help predict which patients should undergo repair or embolization to prevent intracranial hemorrhage (Brown, Wiebers, & Nichols, 1994). Increased risk of hemorrhage is seen in those patients with an AVF of the straight and petrosal sinuses, an associated venous varix on the draining vein, and drainage into a leptomeningeal vein (Brown, 1994).

LABORATORY EVALUATION

Nonpulsatile bilateral tinnitus will rarely require an imaging study, however, depending on the history and physical exam, laboratory studies may be indicated. If the history is suggestive of a metabolic derangement, then appropriate blood work should be performed. This may include a complete blood count (anemia), chemistry panel (renal disease), blood glucose (diabetes), and lipid panel (Seidman & Jacobson, 1996). For potential endocrinopathies, thyroid function testing should be assessed, whereas, screens for ototoxic drugs and pollutants (solvents, heavy metals, carbon monoxide) should be ordered for patients with acute or chronic occupational exposure (Morris, 1969). Syphilis serology should be obtained in any patient with an unexplained, rapidly progressive hearing or balance disorder (House & Derebery, 1995). In a patient with bilateral hearing loss of unknown etiology, an autoimmune workup, including blood work for antibody to nuclear antigen (ANA), rheumatoid factor, C reactive protein and Western blot immunoassay for serum antibody to inner ear antigens is performed (Harris & Sharp, 1990). Although each of the disease processes listed earlier has been associated with tinnitus (as have numerous others), a shotgun approach to laboratory evaluation is not recommended, as it will rarely yield diagnostic information without a relevant historical or physical finding.

DISEASES AND DISORDERS ASSOCIATED WITH TINNITUS

Subjective (Nonpulsatile) Tinnitus

Endolymphatic Hydrops

Prosper Ménière (1861) first characterized a disease process characterized by recurrent, spontaneous episodes of vertigo, fluctuating hearing loss, aural fullness and tinnitus. The pathophysiology of hydrops was not identified until 1938 when Hallpike and Cairns identified dilation of the saccule and scala media within the cochlea (Hallpike & Cairns, 1938). The cause of Ménière's disease is unknown, however many disease processes (Table 9-4) can lead to endolymphatic hydrops, yielding similar clinical findings: systemic infectious diseases (syphilis, mumps, measles), autoimmune mediated diseases (Cogan's syndrome) (Schwaber & Whetswell, 1997). Since endolymphatic hydrops can be produced experimentally by blocking or obliterating the endolymphatic sac, abnormal absorption of endolymph is considered the etiology (Kimura, 1967; 1965).

Although primarily a clinical diagnosis, Ménière's disease must be differentiated from a retrocochlear lesion (that is, acoustic tumor) radiographically. A gadolinium contrast MRI scan should be ordered to rule out an acoustic neuroma prior to making the diagnosis of hydrops; up to 10 percent of patients with this tumor initially present with complaints suggestive of endolymphatic hydrops (Sheehy, 1979; Jackler et al., 1990). Although unnecessary to make the diagnosis, caloric responses in the affected ear are often reduced compared to the opposite healthy ear (Jongkees, 1964). The audiogram will demonstrate fluctuations in speech reception threshold and speech discrimination scores during, and between attacks. Over the course of the disease, a characteristic low-frequency sensorineural hearing loss usually develops (Antoli, Candela, 1976).

The medical management of these dis-

Table 9-4. Differential diagnosis of endolymphatic hydrops

Etiology of endolymphatic hydrops

Noise trauma

Autoimmune inner ear disease
  Sudden sensorineural hearing loss
  Cogan's syndrome

Chronic otitis media
  Otic capsule fenestration

Congenital deafness

Labyrinthine concussion
  Surgical
  Traumatic

Systemic illness
  Letterer-Siwe disease
  Leukemia
  von Hipple-Lindau disease

Congenital inner ear dysplasia
  Mondini
  Alexander
  Scheibe

Bone disease
  Otosclerosis
  Paget's disease

Labyrinthitis
  Serous
  Viral
  Bacterial

Systemic infection
  Syphilis
  Mumps
  Measles

Temporal bone trauma

---

ease processes is aimed at decreasing the amount of endolymph in the inner ear (Rauch, Merchant, & Thedinger, 1989) so as to reduce the number of vertiginous spells. A low sodium diet (< 1,800 mg/day) and a diuretic (dyazide taken twice a day) are the mainstays of medical therapy; the intention being a reduction in the endolymph volume (Rauch, 1989). The majority of patients will demonstrate a reduction or elimination of vertiginous episodes, however tinnitus, hearing loss and aural fullness are not significantly affected (Klockhoff, Lindblom, & Stahle, 1974). Failure of the vertigo to respond to this treatment regiment could lead to one of several surgical options (endolymphatic shunt, labyrinthectomy, or vestibular nerve section) based on the patients' hearing status and general health. Successful control of the audiovestibular complaints will occasionally, but not reliably, lead to a reduction in the level of tinnitus for these patients (Hazell, 1988).

Dandy (1941) sectioned the acoustic nerve in over 400 patients with Ménière's disease, and reported that 50 percent of patients had an improvement in their tinnitus, similarly poor results have been reported for labyrinthectomy (House & Derebery, 1995).

Cerebellopontine Angle Tumors

Unilateral tinnitus should always be evaluated thoroughly, due to the possibility of an acoustic tumor. The vestibular schwannoma is the most common CPA tumor (Figure 9-1), and usually presents with asymmetric

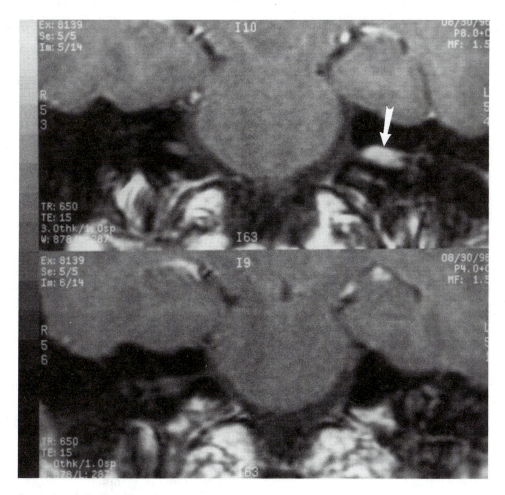

FIGURE 9-1. MRI (T1 with gadolinium) of an intacanalicular acoustic neuroma on the left (arrow). Note marked enhancement of the left internal auditory canal (top image) compared to the right side (bottom image).

hearing loss and unilateral, high-pitched tinnitus (Brackman & Bartels, 1980). Other benign tumors affecting the eighth nerve include meningiomas, hemangiomas, and chondromas; malignant forms of these also occur, but are less common (Table 9-3). Characteristically, speech discrimination is reduced disproportionately compared to the speech reception threshold and pure tone average, usually occurring over many years. In up to 25 percent of patients the hearing loss may be of sudden onset and is confused with an idiopathic or viral etiology (Higgs, 1973; Pensak et al., 1985; Selesnick & Jackler, 1993). Either tumor infiltration/compression of the eighth nerve, or vascular compression by the growing tumor is thought responsible for the hearing loss. High-pitched, unilateral tinnitus is also a common finding with an acoustic tumor and may occur with or without associated hearing loss (Parving, 1992). Other signs and symptoms of these tumors include vertigo, disequilibrium, and dysmetria.

In any patient who presents with the above clinical and audiological findings, a search for a retrocochlear etiology should be performed. MRI with gadolinium enhancement will demonstrate any of the CPA lesions clearly (Figure 9-1), and delineate the extent of tumor involvement of the internal auditory canal, brain stem, and CPA (Jackler, 1990).

Surgical resection of these tumors can be done in one of several ways depending on the hearing status of the patient. The translabyrinthine approach is used for tumors that are in contact with the brain stem, when the hearing is poor and when the patient is over age 65 years (Brackman, 1992; Giannotta, 1992). This approach necessarily results in complete loss of hearing. The middle cranial fossa and retrosigmoid approaches are employed in an attempt to preserve hearing in small tumors occurring in younger patients who can tolerate either temporal lobe or cerebellar retraction (Gantz, Parnes, Harker, & McCabe, 1986; Brackman, 1992; Cohen, 1992). Henrich, McCabe and

Gantz (1995) found that of those patients who had tinnitus preoperatively, it was eliminated completely in 45 percent, lessened in 17 percent, unchanged in 30 percent, and greater in 8 percent after surgical excision. Among patients without preoperative tinnitus, 10 to 17 percent report tinnitus postoperatively (Henrich, 1995; Berliner, Shelton, Hitselberger, & Luxford, 1992).

Temporomandibular Joint Syndrome

There have been numerous reports of successful resolution of tinnitus concomitant with treatment of TMJ (Gelb & Arnold, 1959; Gelb & Bernstein, 1983; Koskinen et al., 1980). Symptoms of the temporomandibular joint syndrome include pain, crepitus, joint locking, tinnitus, aural fullness, vertigo, hyper- or hypoacusis, blurred vision, hoarseness and orofacial dysesthesia (Chan & Reade, 1994). Signs of the disorder primarily involve pain at the joint with either palpation or movement, malocclusion and jaw deviation with excursion (Chan & Reade, 1994). Dental pulpagia has also been reported to cause bilateral preauricular pain and tinnitus which resolved with treatment of the offending tooth (Wright & Gullickson, 1996). Numerous theories have arisen attempting to explain the underlying cause of tinnitus in the TMJ syndrome: shared ligaments between the joint and the malleus, common trigeminal nerve supply, and muscular fatigue (Chan & Reade, 1994; Wright & Gullickson, 1996). None of these have been proven with placebo-controlled studies; however, it is commonly seen that treatment of TMJ syndrome results in a subjective improvement of tinnitus (Chan & Reade, 1994; Gelb & Bernstein, 1983). What has not been addressed, is whether or not the tinnitus is caused by the high doses of aspirin and NSAIDS that are prescribed for the disease, and the relief of symptoms brought about by the discontinuation of these medicines after successful rehabilitation (Campbell, 1993).

Sensorineural Hearing Loss

Pharmacology. Many different disease processes lead to sensorineural hearing loss and tinnitus, including presbycusis, ototoxicity and noise exposure. The amount of tinnitus does not correlate with either the degree or type of hearing loss. Numerous medical treatments have been tried and touted as successful, however, for the most part, they lack placebo-controlled trials (Murai, Tyler, Harker, & Stouffer, 1992). Agents that have been used fall into several categories: anesthetics, anticonvulsants, tranquilizers, barbiturates, and antidepressants. Lidocaine, a local anesthetic agent is the most successful drug at relieving tinnitus, unfortunately it has a very short half-life (Hartigh et al., 1993), which makes it useless clinically. Temporary relief is seen in as many as 89 percent of patients after IV administration of lidocaine (Shea & Harell, 1978), the effect is short-lived however. Oral forms of similar agents (tocainide) have not been successful at relieving tinnitus, and have many cardiovascular side effects (Murai et al., 1992).

Another class of drugs that have been tried, in an attempt to alleviate tinnitus, are the anticonvulsants. Preliminary studies using carbamazepine suggested promise (Shea & Harell, 1978), however, placebo-controlled trials were unfavorable (Donaldson, 1981). Similarly, Amino oxyacetic acid and primidone (both oral antiseizure medications) have been used with some success in poorly controlled trials (Reed et al., 1985; Melding & Goodey, 1979).

Treatment of tinnitus with antidepressant medications is of benefit in some patients. Although the tinnitus is not relieved, the overall well-being of the patient has improved (Dobie et al., 1993). Nortriptyline, given to tinnitus patients with marked depressive symptoms, has improved tinnitus-related disability, possibly related to its effect on improved sleep (Sullivan et al., 1993). Probably by the same mechanism, improved sleep, barbiturates have shown some promise (Donaldson, 1978); however,

controlled studies failed to show a significant benefit over placebo (Marks, Karl, & Onisiphorou, 1981).

Benzodiazepines are mild tranquilizer/anxiolytic agents whose exact method of action is unknown; it is thought to be due to an effect on the inhibitory neurotransmitter gamma-aminobutyric acid (GABA). Several of these agents have been used for the treatment of tinnitus. It has been demonstrated in one clinical trial, that both clonazepam and oxazepam relieved tinnitus significantly in up to 69 percent of patients (Lechtenberg & Shulman, 1984). Recent studies point to a reduction in the hyperexcitability of the inferior colliculus, as a possible explanation for this effect (Szczepaniak & Moller, 1996). This same study revealed that baclofen (a GABA analog, used in the treatment of trigeminal neuralgia) reversed the hyperexcitability of the inferior colliculus in a dose-dependent manner (Szczepaniak & Moller, 1996). Despite these results, clinical trials with baclofen have not shown any benefit over placebo (Westerberg, Robertson, & Stach, 1996). Johnson (1993) reported that of seventeen patients receiving alprazolam, thirteen had a reduction in the loudness of their tinnitus after twelve weeks of therapy; whereas, only one out of nineteen patients receiving placebo had a similar reduction. Although the alprazolam study is double blinded, critics state that it is at best an open label trial demonstrating activity and that further controlled crossover studies are needed (Huynh & Fields, 1995).

Numerous additional agents have been tried for the relief of tinnitus, without success. These include calcium channel blocking agents, intratympanic injections of adrenaline, steroids, and muscle relaxants. Tinnitus associated with sensorineural hearing loss probably has multiple etiologies; therefore, no single agent will ever be effective in all patients. Nonpharmacologic therapy has also been investigated, including electromagnetic stimulation of the cochlea (Roland et al., 1993), hypnotherapy (Marks, 1985), acupuncture (Marks, Emery, & Onisiphorou, 1984), and biofeedback (House,

Miller, & House, 1977). Of these, only biofeedback has been shown superior to placebo in controlled studies. As with pharmacologic therapy, depressed and anxious patients show the most benefit from biofeedback training; certain studies demonstrate a 70 percent improvement (House & Derebery, 1995; House, 1977). Tinnitus masking, psychological therapies and habituation are discussed in other chapters of this book.

Surgery. Surgical management of sensorineural (subjective) tinnitus has also been performed with variable success. Two types of procedures are described: vascular decompression and cochlear neurectomy. Vascular compression syndrome is used to describe a condition presumed to be caused by compression of a cranial nerve by a vessel, which causes focal axon degeneration. Secondary changes at the brain stem nuclei level lead to hyperfunction and excitability of the nerve (Schwarber & Whetswell, 1992). Microsurgical vascular decompression (MVD) of the eighth nerve in the CPA has been performed since the 1970s to relieve vertigo, disequilibrium, sensorineural hearing loss, and more recently, tinnitus (Jannetta, 1975, 1984; Moller, MB., Moller, MR., Jannetta, Jho, 1993; Brookes, 1996). Results of MVD for tinnitus relief demonstrate a complete abolition rate of 18 percent (13/72), and improvement in another 22 percent (16/72) for an overall success rate of 40 percent (Brookes, 1996). Results vary according to author and selection criteria, from 40 to 77 percent improvement (Brookes, 1996; Moller, 1993).

Cochlear neurectomy for debilitating tinnitus has been performed with variable success, ranging from 50 to 75 percent improvement (Dandy, 1941; Fisch, 1976; Silverstein, 1976; House & Brackman, 1981). Pulec (1995) presented a large series (151 patients) of intractable tinnitus sufferers, without serviceable hearing, who had failed medical management and then went on to cochlear neurectomy. Complete relief of tinnitus was achieved in 101 patients (67 percent) and improvement noted in an additional 43 patients; in 7 patients there was no improvement (Pulec, 1995). Recently Wazen, Foyt, and Sisti (1997) reported the results of two patients who underwent selective cochlear neurectomy with preservation of the vestibular nerves. Both patients noted significant relief of tinnitus, without postoperative vertigo, nausea and vomiting that are characteristic of a non-selective eighth nerve section (Wazen, 1997). Candidates for such surgery must have no serviceable hearing in the affected ear, failed medical management, and understand that the results of surgery are unpredictable.

Objective (Pulsatile) Tinnitus

Myoclonus

Myoclonic activity of the tensor and levator veli palatini muscles, salpingopharyngeus, and superior constrictor muscle, can give rise to involuntary movement of the soft palate at a rate of 40 to 240 beats per minute (Saeed & Brookes, 1993). Although rare, it can lead to "clicking" tinnitus, presumably due to forceful closure of the eustachian tube, associated with the contractions. Although the precise etiology is unknown, experimental lesions of the inferior olive have produced the myoclonic activity in monkeys (Fitzgerald, 1984). Palatal myoclonus has also been identified after viral encephalitis, malaria, syphilis, demyelinating diseases, and vascular infarction (Saeed & Brookes, 1993). Similar agents have been used for the treatment of palatal myoclonus, as for nonpulsatile tinnitus (anxiolytics, barbiturates, and so forth), without much success. The use of clostridium botulinum toxin, injected into the soft palate, has provided complete resolution of the tinnitus in preliminary reports (Saeed & Brookes, 1993).

Middle ear myoclonus has also been reported to cause pulsatile tinnitus, due to the activity of the tensor tympani and stapedius muscles (Badia, Parikh, & Brookes, 1994). Characteristically, the tinnitus is described as rhythmic clicking or buzzing, which is usually unilateral. The sound produced could be caused by the propagation of muscle contraction noise, or vibration of the tympanic membrane during clonic activity (Kirikae, 1960). To date, the only successful treatment appears to be surgical section of the tensor tympani and stapedial tendons through a tympanotomy incision (Badia & Brookes, 1994).

Vascular

The complaint of pulsatile tinnitus should initiate an extensive search to uncover a vascular abnormality, or a skull base tumor. There are numerous vascular causes of pulsatile tinnitus; the most common of which are arteriovenous malformations (AVM) and fistulas (AVF). Carotid abnormalities (atherosclerotic disease, fibromuscular dysplasia, and aneurysms) can also cause the sensation of pulsating tinnitus. The physical examination of the patient will direct the radiologic evaluation. A red hue behind an intact tympanic membrane, which blanches with pneumo-otoscopy (Brown's sign), is indicative of a glomus tumor. An aberrant carotid artery or "high-riding" jugular bulb can also be identified behind the tympanic membrane, but will not blanch with positive pressure. Recently, benign intracranial hypertension has been increasingly reported as a major cause of pulsatile tinnitus in women, which can be identified by papilledema on fundoscopic exam.

Dural Arteriovenous Malformation (AVM)

Dural arteriovenous malformations account for 10 to 15 percent of intracranial AVMs and most commonly present with pulsatile tinnitus (Newton & Cronqvist, 1969; Hernesniemi, Saari, & Puranen, 1994). The most frequently involved vessels are the transverse, cavernous and sigmoid sinuses, with communication to the occipital and great auricular arteries (Arenberg & McCreary, 1972). The AVM can be either congenital, or acquired secondary to trauma, infection, intracranial surgery and pregnancy; they do

not usually present until the fourth decade (Lasjaunias & Bernstein, 1987; Sismanis, 1997). Dural AVMs are thought to arise secondary to venous obstruction, which causes enlargement of naturally occurring microarteriovenous shunts within the dura mater (Lasjaunias & Bernstein, 1987).

Dural AVMs can often be heard by the examiner with auscultation over the retro-auricular region (Brown, 1994). Evaluation of this lesion is best accomplished by MRI/MRA, which has both high sensitivity and specificity for dural AVMs and AVFs (Dietz, 1994). If the source of the tinnitus is not identified, strong consideration should be given to carotid arteriography which remains the gold standard in detecting these and other arterial anomalies (Koenigsberg, 1996). Once the diagnosis is established, surgical resection or embolization is indicated, due to the 3 percent risk of subarachnoid hemorrhage if left untreated (Brown, 1994). Treatment of the AVM by either surgery or embolization generally relieves the pulsating tinnitus (Kurl, Vanninen, & Saari, 1996).

Dural Arteriovenous Fistula (AVF)

Dural arteriovenous fistulas comprise about 15 percent of all intracranial vascular malformations, and most commonly involve the transverse and sigmoid sinuses (Newton & Cronqvist, 1969; Aminoff, 1973). The arterial feeding vessels generally arise from branches of the external carotid artery, although internal carotid involvement has been described (Schievink, Piepgras, & Nichols, 1995) (Figure 9-2). The primary difference between an AVF and an AVM is the lack of a vascular mass connecting the arterial and venous flow, which is seen in the latter (Garretson, 1985). The etiology for the two abnormalities is the same (venous obstruction), and pulsatile tinnitus is the most common symptom for both entities (Garretson, 1985). AVFs are more prone to severe sequela, such as intracranial hemorrhage and progressive neurological sequela (Aminoff, 1973; Ishii et al., 1987; Brown, 1994).

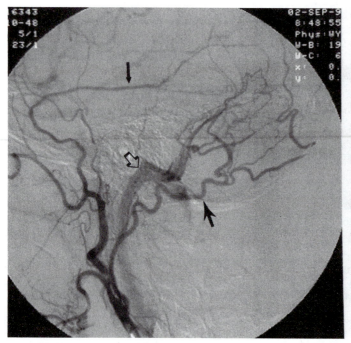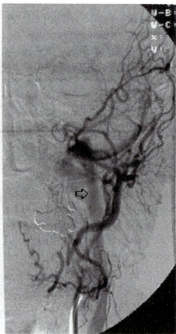

FIGURE 9-2. Cerebral arteriogram demonstrating a dural arteriovenous fistula. The feeding vessels from the occipital (arrow) and middle meningeal (arrowhead) arteries, are shown to empty into the sigmoid sinus (white arrow).

Identification of a dural AVF is often preceded by the recognition of pulsatile tinnitus (65 percent), visual changes (25 percent), headache (18 percent), or mental status change (5 percent) (Brown, 1994). MRA has been shown to be a reliable test for these lesions, while carotid angiography remains the gold standard for diagnosis (Figure 9-2) (Dietz, 1994). Ligation of the involved vessels is the treatment of choice if easily accessible, otherwise selective embolization of the feeding vessels is the preferred treatment (Brown, 1994; Sonier et al., 1995).

Carotid Abnormalities

Carotid artery pathology can also cause pulsatile tinnitus. The more common clinical conditions are atherosclerosis, aberrance, aneurysm, and fibromuscular dysplasia. The tinnitus is probably related to turbulence within the vessel secondary to caliber change near the skull base (Dietz, 1994).

Evaluation of the carotid artery and its tributaries has classically been performed using arteriography; unfortunately, there is a small risk of stroke associated with this procedure. Recently, the combination of MRI and MRA has been used to evaluate the cerebral circulation. MRA has been shown to markedly enhance the ability to diagnose arterial lesions, including those that cause pulsatile tinnitus (Dietz, 1994). In those cases where MRA is negative, and the patient's symptoms are suggestive of a lesion, then carotid arteriography can be performed.

Atherosclerotic carotid artery disease (ACAD) should be suspected in an individual with appropriate risk factors: hypertension, hypercholesterolemia, diabetes, smoking. A carotid bruit is usually identified on physical examination of these patients, and the pulsatile tinnitus does not resolve with light ipsilateral neck compression (Sismanis, 1994). Pulsatile tinnitus in these patients is a result of turbulent blood flow produced by the atheromatous plaque, which is transmitted to the skull base. The diagnosis of ACAD can be confirmed with vascular flow mapping (duplex carotid ultrasound). Evaluation by a vascular surgeon to determine the need for carotid endarterectomy is performed if signs or symptoms of cerebrovascular ischemia are present (Sismanis, 1994). Treatment of the ACAD by either carotid endarterectomy or ligation eliminates the tinnitus; these are rarely indicated however (Carlin, McGraw, & Anderson, 1997; Sismanis, 1994).

An aberrant carotid artery can occasionally be seen in the mesotympanum as a red, pulsating mass, which does not blanch with pneumo-otoscopy. This anomaly is due to absence of the bony plate between the carotid canal and tympanic cavity; it has an incidence of about 1 percent in the general population (Anderson, Stevens, Sundt, Stockard, & Pearson, 1983). High resolution CT scanning demonstrates these lesions to be a well-defined soft tissue mass in the hypotympanum with an associated defect in the posterolateral bony margin of the carotid canal (Swartz et al., 1985). MRI may not delineate the problem secondary to poor contrast between the flow void of the artery and the surrounding bone (Ashikaga, Araki, & Ishida, 1995). An aberrant carotid artery is treated conservatively with reassurance.

Fibromuscular dysplasia is an idiopathic angiopathy, which commonly affects the carotid artery, and is associated with multiple constrictions and aneurysmal dilatations (Sismanis, 1997). The most frequent symptom is pulsatile tinnitus, along with headache, vertigo and transient ischemic attacks (Wells & Smith, 1982). MRI/MRA has been used to diagnose this lesion, however the sensitivity and specificity is unknown (Heiserman, Drayer, Fram, & Keller, 1992). Lack of findings on MRI/MRA is an indication to pursue an angiogram on patients with these symptoms (Dietz, 1994). Fibromuscular dysplasia is treated with balloon angioplasty; the patient's degree of symptomatology dictates when this procedure should be performed (Wells & Smith, 1982).

Jugular Vein

The jugular bulb is usually separated from the hypotympanum by a plate of bone. Occasionally this bony partition may be deficient, leading to a high riding jugular vein within the middle ear space. Pulsatile tinnitus may occur secondary to turbulent flow within the vein (Smythe, 1975), especially in young athletes with a high cardiac output. Diagnosis of this condition can be made during otoscopy, where one sees a blue mass in the posterior-inferior quadrant of the middle ear. Either CT or MRI scanning (Figure 9-3) will confirm the diagnosis (Dietz, 1994). For symptomatic patients, the floor of the hypotympanum can be created with mastoid cortical bone (Glasscock, Dickens, & Jackson, 1980). Most patients respond to conservative reassurance.

Turbulent blood flow through a normal internal jugular vein can also cause pulsatile tinnitus; this condition is often referred to as a venous hum (Chandler, 1983). Prior to making this diagnosis however, all other causes of pulsatile tinnitus should be ruled out with appropriate imaging studies, especially benign intracranial hypertension. An asymptomatic venous hum can be identified in up to 57 percent of normal subjects (Cutforth, Wiseman, & Sutherland, 1970). Movement of the neck causes the jugular vein on the opposite side to bend over the transverse process of the atlas, leading to turbulent flow (Ward, Babin, Calcaterra, & Konrad, 1975). Simple patient reassurance is generally all that is needed in terms of therapy; for significant symptoms (of this or any vascular lesion) a tinnitus masker should be offered. (Masking devices are discussed elsewhere.) Ligation of the internal jugular vein has been proposed as an effective cure for this condition (Nehru, Al-Khaboori, & Kishore, 1993), however, cases have been reported to recur (Ward, 1975). Although not advocated, if ligation is pursued, an angiogram is essential to rule out benign

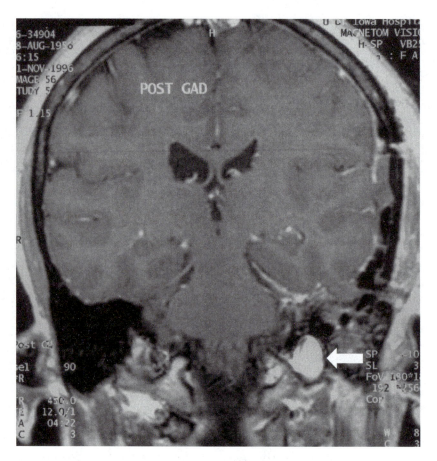

FIGURE 9-3. MRI (T1 with gadolinium) demonstrating left-sided, high-riding jugular bulb (arrow).

intracranial hypertension, vascular pathology, and to document a normal jugular vein on the opposite side (Holgate, Wortzman, & Noyek, 1977).

Skull Base Neoplasms

Paragangliomas (glomus tumors, chemodectomas) are the most common vascular neoplasms of the skull base, frequently presenting with pulsatile tinnitus, with, or without hearing loss (Spector, Ciralsky, & Ogura, 1975). Glomus tympanicum tumors arise from the chemoreceptor cells found along Jacobson's (cranial nerve IX) and Arnold's (cranial nerve X) nerves; whereas, glomus jugulare tumors originate in the adventitia of the jugular bulb. These are the most common tumors of the middle ear

and jugular bulb respectively. The average age at presentation is around 50 years old, with a 6 to 1 female preponderance (Batsakis, 1975). Multiple tumors are seen in 10 percent of cases, and an autosomal dominant inheritance pattern can occasionally be found (Horn & Hankinson, 1994). Approximately 10 percent of the tumors secrete vasoactive amines causing hypertension, pallor, tachycardia, sweating, and fatigue. The metastatic potential is low, estimated to be 3 percent or less (Batsakis, 1975).

Symptoms of a glomus tumor are usually mild early on, however, with growth of the tumor, cranial nerve deficits are likely to appear. The most common presenting symptom is conductive hearing loss, which occurs in 80 percent, followed by pulsatile

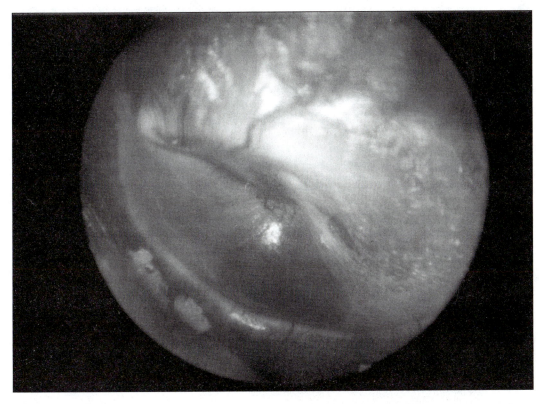

FIGURE 9-4. Endoscopic view of left tympanic membrane reveals a vascular tumor in the hypotympanum consistent with a glomus tympanicum.

tinnitus in 60 percent of patients (Horn & Hankinson, 1994). A red tympanic mass that blanches upon placement of positive pressure (Browns' sign) is classic (Figure 9-4). A CT scan is critical in this evaluation to differentiate between a glomus jugulare and tympanicum, as well as to identify various tumors and carotid abnormalities (Sismanis, 1994). Motheaten bony erosion of the jugular foramen by a soft tissue mass is seen on CT. MRI is also necessary to determine the extent of intracranial involvement (Figure 9-5) (Horn & Hankinson, 1994).

The pulsatile tinnitus in these patients may be caused by the formation of microvascular shunts within the tumor mass (Sismanis, 1997). Treatment involves complete surgical resection of the tumor, while preserving vital structures nearby (cranial nerves, hearing, cerebral arteries). A middle ear and mastoid approach is useful for tumors confined to the middle ear; however, skull base techniques are utilized if the tumor extends to the jugular foramen and upper neck (Horn & Hankinson, 1994). Preoperative angiography (Figure 9-6) and embolization of the primary vasculature is essential to reduce the massive blood loss that can occur at surgery for glomus jugulare tumors (Horn & Hankinson, 1994).

In addition to glomus tumors, other skull base tumors are capable of causing pulsatile tinnitus; these include acoustic neuroma, meningioma, and hemangioma. It has been shown that a cost-effective way to evaluate skull base neoplasms is to proceed with MRI/MRA when no tympanic mass is identified; this provides excellent localization of these tumors, without the risk of CVA associated with carotid arteriography (Dietz, 1994). When further bony detail is required, as when contemplating surgery, a high resolution CT scan of the skull base is warranted (Dietz, 1994).

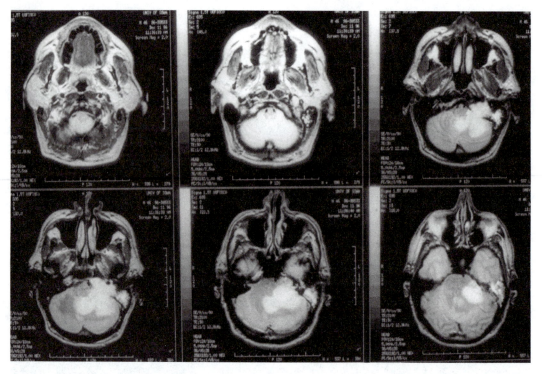

FIGURE 9-5. MRI (T1 with gadolinium) reveals a glomus jugular tumor with extensive intracranial involvement. Note involvement of jugular foramen, mastoid, and middle ear.

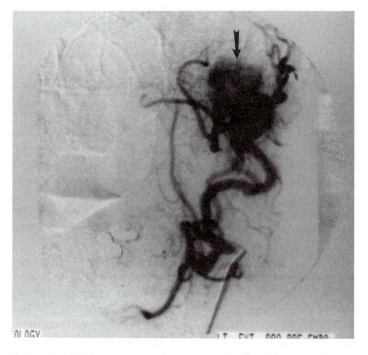

FIGURE 9-6. Carotid arteriogram demonstrates hypervascular tumor (arrow) at the skull base with feeding vessels from both the internal and external carotid arteries.

Benign Intracranial Hypertension (BIH)

Pseudotumor cerebri, or "benign intracranial hypertension," is a syndrome complex consisting of increased intracranial pressure without neurological deficits; a diagnosis which can only be made after a space-occupying lesion, and meningitis has been ruled out (Sorensen, Krogsaa, & Gjerris, 1988). In most patients the syndrome is self-limited, however in up to 25 percent of patients the disease becomes chronic (Sorensen, 1988). Although usually idiopathic, certain disease processes can cause the syndrome, including obesity, pregnancy, thyroid dysfunction, vitamin deficiency, anemia, and Cushing's syndrome (Sismanis, 1987). In addition, medications can also be responsible for the symptom complex of benign intracranial hypertension: oral contraceptives, indomethacin and certain antibiotics (Sismanis, 1987). The exact pathophysiology of the disease is unknown, recent evidence suggests that elevated intra-abdominal pressure leads to decreased venous return from the brain, with subsequent cerebral edema (Josephs, Este-McDonald, Birkett, & Hirsch, 1994).

In some series, benign intracranial hypertension is the most common cause of pulsatile tinnitus, often associated with headaches, visual disturbances, dizziness, and aural fullness (Sismanis, 1994). Obesity and papilledema are often present, with a normal CT and MRI scan. Diagnosis rests on an elevated CSF opening pressure (>200 mm water), without evidence of meningitis (Sismanis, 1987). Treatment involves elimination of any inciting disease process or offending medication, weight reduction, and diuresis. Acetazolamide given three times per day at a dose of 250 mg, and furosamide 20 mg twice a day, are commonly used agents that are thought to reduce the production of CSF, as well as provide adequate diuresis (Sismanis, 1994). Failure to respond to this regiment, or progression of papilledema necessitates lumbar-peritoneal shunting (Sismanis, 1987).

Systemic disease

Treatment of hypertension with either calcium channel blocking agents, or angiotensin converting enzyme inhibitors can lead to a hyperdynamic state, with subsequent pulsatile tinnitus (Sismanis, 1994). Reduction in dosage, or changing to a different class of drug is usually effective (Sismanis, 1994).

Both Paget's disease and otosclerosis have been shown to cause pulsatile tinnitus, probably due to the neovascularization of the newly formed bone (Gibson, 1973). The formation of small temporal bone arteriovenous fistulae may also be responsible for this symptom in these disease processes (Sismanis, 1994; Gibson, 1973).

CONCLUSIONS

Tinnitus is a somewhat terrifying chronic symptom that can be disabling to the patient. It is important to rule out significant medical etiologies as outlined previously. For many patients, reassurance that there are no underlying tumors or impending medical emergencies can reduce their anxiety and symptoms. A thorough medical evaluation must accompany the management of tinnitus, as underlying medical etiologies of tinnitus may go undiagnosed for years with increased morbidity.

REFERENCES

Aminoff, M. J. (1973). Vascular anomalies in the intracranial duramater. *Brain, 96,* 601–612.

Anderson, J. M., Stevens, J. C., Sundt, T. M., Stockard, J. J., & Pearson, B. W. (1983). Ectopic internal carotid artery seen initially as middle ear tumor. *Journal of the American Medical Association, 149,* 2228-2230.

Antoli, Candela, F. (1976). The histopathology of Ménière's disease. *Acta Otolaryngologica* (Stockholm), *340,* 1–42.

Arenberg, I. K., & McCreary, H. S. (1972). Objective tinnitus aurium and dural arteriovenous malformations of the posterior fossa. *Annals of Otology, Rhinology, and Laryngology, 80,* 111.

Ashikaga, R., Araki, Y., & Ishida, O. (1995). Bilateral aberrant internal carotid arteries. *Neuroradiology, 37*, 655–657.

Badia, L. B., Parikh, A., & Brookes, G. B. (1994). Management of middle ear myoclonus. *Journal of Laryngology and Otology, 108*, 380–382.

Batsakis, J. G. (1975). Chemodectomas. In J. G. Batsakis (Ed.), *Tumors of the head and neck* (pp. 280–284). Baltimore: William and Wilkins.

Baysal, B. E. (1997). Fine mapping of an imprinted gene for familial nonchromaffin paragangliomas on chromosome 11q23. *American Journal of Human Genetics, 60*, 121–132.

Berliner, K. I., Shelton, C., Hitselberger, W. E., & Luxford, W. M. (1992). Acoustic tumors: Effect of surgical removal on tinnitus. *American Journal of Otology, 13*, 13–17.

Black, O. F., & Lilly, D. J. (1996). Tinnitus in children. In C. D. Bluestone and S. E. Stool (Eds.), *Pediatric otolaryngology* (3rd ed., pp. 302–311). Philadelphia: W. B. Saunders.

Brackman, D. E. (1992). Middle fossa approach for acoustic tumor removal. *Clinical Neurosurgery, 38*, 603–618.

Brackman, D. E., & Bartels, L. J. (1980). Rare tumors of the cerebello-pontine angle. *Otolaryngology Head Neck Surgery, 88*, 555–559.

Brackman, D. E., & Green, J. D. (1992). Translabyrinthine approach for acoustic tumor removal. *Otolaryngology Clinics of North America, 25*, 311–329.

Brookes, G. B. (1996). Vascular decompression surgery for severe tinnitus. *American Journal of Otology, 17*, 569-576.

Brown, R. D., Wiebers, D. O., & Nichols, D. A. (1994). Intracranial dural arteriovenous fistulae: Angiographic predictors of intracranial hemorrhage and clinical outcome in nonsurgical patients. *Journal of Neurosurgery, 81*, 531–538.

Brunberg, J. A. (1995). Letter to Editor. *American Journal of Radiology, 226*.

Campbell, K. (1993). Tinnitus and Vertigo [Letter to the editor]. *Archives of Otolaryngology Head Neck Surgery, 119*, 474.

Carlin, R. E., McGraw, D. J., & Anderson, C. B. (1997). Objective tinnitus resulting from internal carotid artery stenosis. *Journal of Vascular Surgery, 25*, 581–583.

Chan, S. W. Y., & Reade, P. C. (1994). Tinnitus and temporomandibular pain-dysfunction disorder. *Clinical Otolaryngology, 19*, 370–380.

Chandler, J. R. (1983). Diagnosis and cure of venous hum tinnitus. *Laryngoscope, 93*, 892–895.

Cohen, N. L. (1992). Retrosigmoid approach for acoustic tumor removal. *Otolaryngology Clinic of North America, 25*, 295–310.

Cutforth, R., Wiseman, J., & Sutherland, R. D. (1970). Genesis of cervical venous hum. *American Heart Journal, 80*(4), 488–492.

Dandy, W. E. (1941). Surgical treatment of Ménière's disease. *Surgical Gynecology and Obstetrics, 72*, 421–425.

Dietz, R. R., Davis, W. L., & Harnsberger, H. R., et al. (1994). MR Imaging and MR Angiography in the Evaluation of Pulsatile Tinnitus. *American Journal of Neuroradiology, 15*, 879–889.

Dobie, R. A., Sakai, C. S., & Sullivan, M. D., et al. (1993). Antidepressant treatment of tinnitus patients: Report of a randomized clinical trial and clinical predication of benefit. *American Journal of Otology, 14*, 18–23.

Donaldson, I. (1978). Tinnitus: A theoretical view and a therapeutic study using amylobarbitone. *Journal of Laryngology and Otology, 92*, 123–130.

Donaldson, I. (1981). Tegretol: A double blind trial in tinnitus. *Journal of Laryngology and Otology, 95*, 947–951.

Fisch, U. (1976). Surgical treatment of vertigo. *Journal of Laryngology and Otology, 1990*, 75–86.

Fitzgerald, D. C. (1984). Palatal Myoclonus-case report. *Laryngoscope, 94*, 217–219.

Gantz, B. J., Parnes, L. S., Harker, L. A., & McCabe, B. F. (1986). Middle cranial fossa acoustic neuroma excision: Results and complications. *Annals of Otology, Rhinology, and Laryngology, 95*, 454–459.

Garretson, H. D. (1985). Intracranial arteriovenous malformation. In R. H. Wilkins & S. S. Rengachary (Eds.), *Neurosurgery* (pp. 1448–1458). New York: McGraw-Hill.

Gelb, H., & Arnold, G. E. (1959). Syndromes of the head and neck of dental origin. *Archives of Otolaryngology Head and Neck Surgery, 70*, 681–691.

Gelb, H., & Bernstein, I. (1983). Clinical evaluation of two hundred patients with temporomandibular joint syndrome. *Journal of Prosthetic Dentistry, 49*, 234–243.

Gelb, H., & Bernstein, I. M. (1983). A comparison of three different populations with TMJ pain dysfunction syndrome. *Dental Clinics of North America, 27*, 495.

Giannotta, S. L. (1992). Translabyrinthine approach for removal of medium and large tumors of the cerebellopontine angle. *Clinical Neurosurgery, 38*, 589–602.

Gibson, R. (1973). Paget's disease of the temporal bone. *Acta Otolaryngologica, 87*, 299–301.

Glasscock, M. E., Dickens, J. R. E., & Jackson, C. G., et al. (1980). Vascular anomalies of the middle ear. *Laryngoscope, 90*, 77–78.

Hallpike, C. S., & Cairnes, H. (1938). Observations on the pathology of Ménière's syndrome. *Journal of Laryngology and Otology, 53*, 625.

Harris, J. P., & Sharp, P. (1990). Inner ear autoantibodies in patients with rapidly progressive sensorineural hearing loss. *Laryngoscope, 97*, 63–76.

Hartigh, J. D., Carina, G. J. M., & Hilders, M. S., et al. (1993). Tinnitus suppression by intravenous lidocaine in relation to its plasma concentration. *Clinical Pharmacology and Therapeutics, 54*, 415–420.

Hasso, A. N. (1994). Imaging of pulsatile tinnitus: Basic examination versus comprehensive examination package. *American Journal of Neuroradiology*, 890–892.

Hazell, J. W. P. (1988). Tinnitus. In P. W. Alberti, & R. J. Ruben (Eds.), *Otologic medicine and surgery* (pp. 1605–1622). New York: Churchill Livingstone.

Heiserman, J. E., Drayer, B. P., Fram, E. K., & Keller, P. J. (1992). MR angiography of cervical fibromuscular dysplasia. *American Journal of Neuroradiology, 13*, 1454–1457.

Henrich, D. E., McCabe, B. F., Gantz, B. J. (1995). Tinnitus and acoustic neuromas: Analysis of the effect of surgical excision on postoperative tinnitus. *ENT Journal, 74*(7), 462–466.

Hernesniemi, J., Saari, T., & Puranen, M. (1994). Treatment of 23 dural AVMs located at the transverse and sigmoid sinuses. In A. Pasqualin & R. Da Pian (Eds.), *New trends in management of cerebrovascular malformations* (pp. 273–315). Heidelburg: Springer.

Higgs, W. A. (1973). Sudden deafness as the presenting symptom of acoustic neuroma. *Archives of Otolaryngology, 98*, 73–76.

Holgate, R. C., Wortzman, G., & Noyek, A. M. (1977). Pulsatile tinnitus: The role of angiography. *Journal of Otolaryngology, 6*(3), 49–63.

Horn, K. L., & Hankinson, H. (1994). Tumors of the jugular foramen. In R. K. Jackler & D. E. Brackman (Eds.), *Neurotology* (pp. 1059–1064). New York: Mosby.

House, J. W., & Brackman, D. E. (1981). Tinnitus: Surgical management. *Ciba Foundation Symposium, 85*, 204–216.

House, J. W., & Derebery, M. J. (1995). Tinnitus: Evaluation and Treatment. In F. E. Lucente (Ed.), *Highlights of the instructional courses* (Vol. 8, pp. 293–296). Saint Louis: Mosby.

House, J. W., Miller, L., & House P. R. (1977). Severe tinnitus: Treatment with biofeedback training (results in 41 cases). *Transamerican Academy of Ophthalmology and Otolaryngology, 84*, 697–703.

House, J. W., Waluch, V., & Jackler, R. K. (1986). Magnetic resonance imaging in acoustic neuroma diagnosis. *Annals of Otology, Rhinology, and Laryngology, 95*, 16.

Huynh, L., & Fields, S. (1995). Alprazolam for Tinnitus. *Annals of Pharmacology, 29*, 311–312.

Ishii, K., Goto, K., & Ihara, K., et al. (1987). High risk dural arteriovenous fistula of the transverse and sigmoid sinuses. *American Journal of Neuroradiology, 8*, 113–1120.

Jackler, R. K., et al. (1990). Gadolinium-DTPA enhanced magnetic resonance imaging in acoustic neuroma diagnosis and management. *Otolaryngology Head and Neck Surgery, 102*, 670.

Jannetta, P. J. (1975). Neurovascular cross compression in patients with hyperactive dysfunction of the eighth cranial nerve. *Surgery Forum, 26*, 467–469.

Jannetta, P. J., Moller, M. B., & Moller, A. R. (1984). Disabling positional vertigo. *New England Journal of Medicine, 310*, 1700–1705.

Johnson, R. M., Brummett, R., & Schleuning, A. (1993). Use of Alprazolam for relief of Tinnitus: A double blind study. *Archives of Otolaryngology Head and Neck Surgery, 119*, 842–845.

Jongkees, L. B. W., & Philipszoon, A. J. (1964). The caloric test in Ménière's disease. *Acta Otolaryngologica* (Stockholm), *230*, 5–9.

Josephs, L. G., Este-McDonald, J. R., Birkett, D. H., & Hirsch, E. F. (1994). Diagnostic laparoscopy increases intracranial pressure. *Journal of Trauma, 36*, 815–819.

Kimura, R. S. (1967). Experimental blockage of the endolymphatic duct and sac and its effect on endolymphatic hydrops. *Annals of Otology, Rhinology, and Laryngology, 76*, 664–687.

Kimura, R. S., & Schuknecht, H. (1965). Membranous hydrops in the inner ear of the guinea pig after obliteration of the endolymphatic sac. *Practical Otology, Rhinology, and Laryngology, 27*, 343.

Kirikae, L. (1960). *The structure and function of the middle ear.* Tokyo: University of Tokyo Press, 129–130.

Klockhoff, I., Lindblom, U., & Stahle, J. (1974). Diuretic treatment of Ménière's disease. *Archives of Otolaryngology, 100*, 262.

Koenigsberg, R. A. (1996). Spontaneous pulsatile tinnitus secondary to a dural malformation not visualized by magnetic resonance angiography. *Clinical Imaging, 20*, 95–98.

Koskinen, J., Paavolainen, M., & Raivio, M., et al. (1980). Otological manifestations in temporomandibular joint dysfunction. *Journal of Oral Rehabilitation, 7*, 249–254.

Kurl, S., Vanninen, R., Saari, T., & Hernesniemi, J. (1996). Development of right transverse sinus dural arteriovenous malformation after embolization of a similar lesion on the left. *Neuroradiology, 38*, 386-388.

Lasjaunias, P., & Bernstein, A. (1987). Surgical neuroangiography. Berlin: Springer, 273–315.

Lechtenberg, R., & Shulman, A. (1984). Benzodiazepines in the treatment of tinnitus. *Journal of Laryngology and Otology, 9*(Suppl.), 271–276.

Lo, W. M. (1991). Vascular Tinnitus. In P. M. Som, & R. T. Bergeson (Eds.), *Head and neck imaging* (pp. 1108–1115). St. Louis: Mosby.

Marks, N. J., Emery, P., & Onisiphorou, C. (1984). A controlled trial of acupuncture in tinnitus. *Journal of Laryngology and Otology, 98*, 1103–1109.

Marks, N. J., Karl, H., & Onisiphorou, C. A. (1985). Controlled trial of hypnotherapy in tinnitus. *Clinical Otolaryngology, 10*, 43–46.

Marks, N. J., Onisiphorou, C., & Trounce, Jr. (1981). The effect of single doses of amylobarbitone sodium and carbamazepine in tinnitus. *Journal of Laryngology and Otology, 95*, 941–945.

Melding, P. S., & Goodey, R. J. (1979). The treatment of tinnitus with oral anticonvulsants. *Journal of Laryngology and Otology, 93*, 111–122.

Ménière, P. (1861). Congestions cerebrales apoplectiformes. *Gaz md Paris, 16*, 55.

Moller, M. B., Moller, A. R., Jannetta, P. J., & Jho, H. D. (1993). Vascular decompression surgery for severe tinnitus: Selection criteria and results. *Laryngoscope, 103*, 421–427.

Morris, T. M. O. (1969). Deafness following acute carbon monoxide poisoning. *Journal of Laryngology and Otology, 83*, 219–225.

Murai, K., Tyler, R. S., Harker, L. A, & Stouffer, J. L. (1992). Review of pharmacologic treatment of tinnitus. *American Journal of Otolaryngology, 13*, 454–464.

Nehru, V. I., Al-Khaboori, M. J. J., & Kishore, K. (1993). Ligation of the internal jugular vein in venous hum tinnitus. *Journal of Laryngology and Otology, 107*, 1037–1038.

Newton, T. H., & Cronqvist, S. (1969). Involvement of the dural arteries in intracranial arteriovenous malformations. *Radiology, 93*, 1071–1078.

Parving, A. (1992). Tinnitus before and after surgery for an acoustic neuroma. In M. Tos & J. Thomsen (Eds.), *Proceedings of the First International Conference on Acoustic Neuroma* (pp. 891–894). Amsterdam: Kugler.

Pensak, M. L., et al. (1985). Sudden hearing loss and cerebellopontine angle tumors. *Laryngoscope, 95*, 1188–1193.

Pulec, J. L. (1995). Cochlear nerve section for intractable tinnitus. *Ear Nose Throat Journal, 74*, 468–476.

Rauch, S. D., Merchant, S. M., & Thedinger, B. A. (1989). Ménière's syndrome and endolymphatic hydrops—double blind temporal bone study. *Annals of Otology, Rhinology, and Laryngology, 98*, 873–883.

Reed, H. T., Meltzer, J., Crews, P., et al. (1985). Amino-oxyacetic acid as a palliative in tinnitus. *Archives of Otolaryngology Head Neck Surgery, 111*, 803–805.

Remley, K. B., Coit, W. E., & Harnsberger, H. R., et al. (1990). Pulsatile tinnitus and the vascular tympanic membrane: CT, MR, and angiographic findings. *Radiology, 174*, 383–389.

Roland, N. J., Hughes, J. B., & Daley, M. B., et al. (1993). Electromagnetic stimulation as a treatment of tinnitus: A pilot study. *Clinical Otolaryngology, 18*, 278–281.

Saeed, S. R., & Brookes, G. B. (1993). The use of clostridium botulinum toxin in palatal myoclonus. A preliminary report. *Journal of Laryngology and Otology, 107*, 208–210.

Schievink, W. I., Piepgras, D. G., & Nichols, D. A. (1995). Spontaneous carotid-jugular fistula and carotid dissection in a patient with multiple intracranial arachnoid cysts and hemifacial atrophy: A generalized connective tissue disorder? *Journal of Neurosurgery, 83*, 546–549.

Schwaber, M. K. (1997). Vestibular Disorders. In G. B. Hughes & M. L. Pensak (Eds.), *Clinical Otology* (2nd ed., 24, pp. 345–365), New York: Thieme.

Schwaber, M. K., & Whetswell, W. O. (1992). Cochleovestibular nerve compression syndrome. II. Histopathology and theory of pathophysiology. *Laryngoscope, 102*(9), 1030–1036.

Seidman, M. D., & Jacobson, G. P. (1996). Update on Tinnitus. *Otolaryngology Clinics of North America, 29*(3) 455–465.

Selesnick, S. H., & Jackler, R. K. (1993). Atypical hearing loss in acoustic neuroma patients, *Laryngoscope, 103,* 437–441.

Shea, J. J, & Harell, M. (1978). Management of tinnitus aurium with lidocaine and carbamazepine. *Laryngoscope, 88,* 1477–1484.

Sheehy, J. L. (1979). Neuro-otologic evaluation. In House Wand Luetje, (Eds.), *Acoustic tumors,* (Vol. 1, diagnosis, p. 199). Baltimore: University Park Press.

Silverstein, H. (1976). Transmeatal labyrinthectomy with and without cochleovestibular neurectomy. *Laryngoscope, 86,* 1777–1791.

Sismanis, A. (1987). Otologic manifestations of benign intracranial hypertension syndrome: Diagnosis and management. *Laryngoscope, 97*(Suppl. 42), 1–17.

Sismanis, A. (1990). Otologic manifestations of benign intracranial hypertension syndrome: Diagnosis and management. *Laryngoscope, 100,* 33–36.

Sismanis, A. (1997). Pulsatile tinnitus. In G. B. Hughes & M. L. Pensak (Eds.), *Clinical Otology* (2nd ed., pp. 445–460). New York: Thieme.

Sismanis, A., & Smoker, W. R. K. (1994). Pulsatile tinnitus: Recent advances in diagnosis. *Laryngoscope, 104,* 681–687.

Sismanis, A., Stamm, M. A., & Sobel, M. (1994). Objective tinnitus in patients with atherosclerotic carotid artery disease. *American Journal of Otology, 15*(3), 404–407.

Smythe, G. O. (1975). A case of protruding jugular bulb. *Laryngoscope, 75,* 669–672.

Sonier, C. B., De Kersaint-Gilly, A., & Viarouge, M. P., et al. (1995). Fistules durales de la loge caverneuse. *Journal of Neuroradiology, 22,* 289–300.

Sorensen, P. S., Krogsaa, B., & Gjerris, F. (1988). Clinical course and prognosis of pseudotumor cerebri: A prospective study of 24 patients. *Acta Neurology Scandinavia, 77,* 64–172.

Spector, G. J., Ciralsky, R. H., & Ogura, J. H. (1975). Glomus tumors in the head and neck. III. Analysis of clinical manifestations. *Annals of Otology, Rhinology, and Laryngology, 84,* 73–79.

Sullivan, M., Katon, W., & Russo, J., et al. (1993). A randomized trial of Nortriptyline for severe chronic tinnitus. *Archives of Internal Medicine, 153,* 2251–2259.

Swartz, J. D., Bazarnic, M. L., & Naidich, T. P, et al. (1985). Aberrant internal carotid artery lying within the middle ear: High resolution CT diagnosis and differential diagnosis. *Neuroradiology, 27,* 322–326.

Szczepaniak, W. S., & Moller, A. R. (1996). Effects of (-) baclofen, clonazepam, and diazepam on tone exposure-induced hyperexcitability of the inferior colliculus in the rat: Possible therapeutic implications for pharmacological management of tinnitus and hyperacusis. *Hearing Research, 97,* 46–53.

Tewfik, S. (1984). Phonocephalography: An objective diagnosis of tinnitus. *Journal of Laryngology, 88,* 869.

Tyler, R. S., & Babin, R. W. (1993). Tinnitus. In C. W. Cummings (Ed.), *Otolaryngology—Head and Neck Surgery* (2nd ed., pp. 3031–3053). New York: Mosby.

van der Mey, A. G. L., Maaswinkel-Mooy, P. D., Cornelisse, C. J., Schmidt, P. H., & van de Kamp, J. J. (1989). Genomic imprinting in hereditary glomus tumors: Evidence for new genetic theory. *Lancet, 2,* 1291–1294.

Ward, P. H., Babin, R., Calcaterra, T. C., & Konrad, H. R. (1975). Operative treatment of surgical lesions with objective tinnitus. *Annals of Otology, Rhinology, and Laryngology, 84,* 473–482.

Wazen, J. J., Foyt, D., & Sisti, M. (1997). Selective cochlear neurectomy for debilitating tinnitus. *Annals of Otology, Rhinology, and Laryngology, 106,* 568–570.

Wells, R. P., & Smith, R. R. (1982). Fibromuscular dysplasia of the internal carotid artery: A long followup. *Neurosurgery, 10,* 39–43.

Westerberg, B. D., Robertson, J. B Jr., & Stach, B. A. (1996). A double-blind placebo controlled trial of Baclofen in the treatment of tinnitus. *American Journal of Otolaryngology, 17,* 896–903.

Wright, E. F., & Gullickson, D. C. (1996). Dental pulpalgia contributing to bilateral preauricular pain and tinnitus. *Journal of Orofacial Pain, 10*(2), 166–168.

CHAPTER 10

Tinnitus in Children

Joseph L. Hegarty, M.D.
Richard J. H. Smith, M.D.

TINNITUS IN CHILDREN WITH "NORMAL" HEARING

The first study to investigate childhood tinnitus was reported in 1972. Nodar (1972) examined over 2,000 rural United States children between ages 11 and 18 (grades 5 to 12) for three years and found that 13.3 percent who passed a school audiometric screen reported "noises" in their ears when specifically questioned. In contrast, those children who failed this screening test reported "noise" in their ears 58.6 percent of the time. After suggesting "ringing, buzzing or clicking" as examples of tinnitus, children most often described their aural sensation as "ringing" (52 percent). The age group most commonly reporting tinnitus was 13 to 15 years old.

This study served to demonstrate that tinnitus does affect the pediatric population, but occurs much more commonly in children with hearing impairments. A later report by Mills et al. (1986) found a 29 percent prevalence of "noises" in the ears of 93 normal-hearing British children between ages 5 and 16; the most common description was "buzzing" (55 percent). Stouffer et al.

(1992) reported tinnitus in 36 percent of a population of normal hearing (< 15 dB HL) Canadian children between ages 7 and 10 years. The occurrence of pediatric tinnitus reported by these two studies is similar to the occurrence of tinnitus reported in adults in the United States (32 percent of the population) and Great Britain (17 percent of the population) (McFadden, 1982). To control for a child's desire to give affirmative responses in order to please an investigator, a reliable response-consistency measure was employed this time, revealing only 6 percent of the 140 normal-hearing children with tinnitus (Stouffer et al., 1992). Their tinnitus was most often described as "beeping" or "buzzing." Interestingly, only 3 percent of children without hearing impairment volunteer a complaint of tinnitus when compared to the approximately one-third of children who admit tinnitus after direct questioning (Mills et al., 1984; Graham et al., 1995). This underscores the fact that children will rarely offer a complaint of tinnitus without being prompted but when directly questioned can potentially overreport it, making the study of tinnitus in children especially challenging.

Tinnitus in Children Presenting for Evaluation of Tinnitus

Children who present for medical evaluation complaining of tinnitus appear to represent a different group of children when compared to those only reporting tinnitus after questioning. In children who present with a chief complaint of tinnitus, approximately 50 percent have normal hearing and will typically describe their tinnitus as a "high-pitched noise" or "whistle" (Martin, 1994). Martin and Snashall also report significant correlation between the level of hearing and the timing of tinnitus (Martin, 1994). In the "normal-hearing, constant tinnitus" group, the majority of children (83 percent) report considerable disturbance related to their tinnitus, compared with the "hearing-impaired, intermittent tinnitus" group, where few (9.6 percent) are bothered by their tinnitus. Thus, at least one subpopulation may exist in childhood tinnitus that appears to mimic the disturbing pattern seen in adulthood.

TINNITUS IN HEARING-IMPAIRED CHILDREN

Tinnitus in Association with Conductive Hearing Loss

Mills and Cherry (1984) reported that 44 percent of sixty-six children 5 to 15 years of age with middle-ear disease (primarily serous otitis media) had tinnitus when specifically asked. However, only 3 percent of these children with documented ear disease *spontaneously* reported tinnitus, similar to children without any hearing impairment (Mills et al., 1992; Graham et al., 1995). Similarly, adult patients with conductive hearing losses (due to otitis and otosclerosis) report spontaneous tinnitus 10 percent of the time (Hazell et al., 1985). These statistics indicate that even though conductive hearing loss (due to middle ear effusion) has a considerably higher prevalence in the pediatric age group, children complain of auditory disturbances less frequently than do adults. Moreover, a history of recurrent otitis media does not appear to be a significant factor in the pathogenesis of tinnitus in children. No statistical correlation could be found when evaluating children with and without tinnitus and the presence or absence of prior otitis media (Viani et al., 1989). The conductive hearing loss may merely unmask "physiologic tinnitus" normally masked by environmental sounds (Mills et al., 1986).

Tinnitus in Children with Moderate-Severe Sensorineural Hearing Loss

Present data suggest that tinnitus occurs more frequently in the hearing-impaired pediatric population when compared to normal-hearing or profoundly deaf children. Graham (1981) surveyed seventy-four children (ages 12 to 18 years) with moderate-to-severe sensorineural hearing loss (mean pure tone average for 250; 500; 1,000; 2,000 Hz–52.5 dB HL) and found that 66 percent reported "noises" in their ears. However, only 13 percent of this hearing-impaired group of children spontaneously complained about it prior to evaluation (Graham, 1995; Viani, 1989). Stouffer et al. (1992) studied twenty-one children who failed audiometric screening at 15 dB HL and found that 76 percent had tinnitus. Using controlled, consistency-based questioning, however, 24 percent of hearing-impaired children reliably reported tinnitus ≥ 5 minutes in duration (Stouffer et al., 1992). Their tinnitus was characterized as intermittent in 97.5 percent, > 5 minutes in duration in 52 percent, associated with dizziness in 55 percent, and associated with headache in 20 percent (Graham, 1981). Of children with unilateral tinnitus and moderate asymmetric sensorineural hearing loss, 89 percent reported tinnitus in their better hearing ear (Graham, 1982). Children with a moderate degree of hearing loss using a unilateral hearing aid reported tinnitus in the aided ear 70 percent of the time (Graham, 1981).

Tinnitus in Children with Severe-profound Sensorineural Hearing Loss

Interestingly, children with profound deafness report tinnitus much less often than children with only moderately impaired hearing. It has been suggested that the quality of sound perceived by children with profound hearing loss is so poor that tinnitus may be actually interpreted as distorted environmental sounds (Hazell, 1987). In the largest study to date, 30 percent of 331 profoundly deaf children (ages 6 to 18 years) reported tinnitus when not using hearing aids (Drukier, 1989). In two other studies, tinnitus was reported in 29 percent of sixty-six children (Graham, 1981) and 23 percent of 102 children (Viani, 1989) with profound hearing loss (mean pure tone average of 95 dB HL for 250; 500; 1,000; 2,000 Hz). A fourth study reported a 35 percent tinnitus prevalence in thirty-seven children with severe-to-profound hearing loss (70 to 110 dB HL pure tone average) (Nodar et al., 1984).

Although only 3 percent of children with severe-to-profound sensorineural hearing loss complained of tinnitus before being questioned (Viani, 1989)—an incidence similar to that in normal-hearing children—when specifically questioned, 61 percent (Drukier, 1989) to 82 percent (Graham, 1981) reported some degree of annoying tinnitus. In addition, 47 percent (Graham, 1981) to 70 percent (Drukier, 1989) reported difficulty understanding speech with tinnitus present. These figures suggest that tinnitus may contribute to poor attentiveness and poor school performance in this already challenged population.

Like children with partial hearing impairments, children with severe-to-profound hearing loss characterize their tinnitus as intermittent (80 percent), lasting seconds to minutes (48 percent [Graham, 1981] to 62 percent [Drukier, 1989]), and associated with dizziness (32 percent) (Graham, 1981) or headaches (26 percent) (Graham, 1981). Four of six children with unilateral tinnitus and profound, but asymmetric sensorineural hearing loss reported tinnitus in their better hearing ear (Graham, 1981). Children with profound hearing loss using a unilateral hearing aid reported tinnitus in the aided ear 50 percent (Drukier, 1989) to 80 percent (Graham, 1981) of the time, suggesting that the use of a hearing aid may not influence the side on which tinnitus occurs (Viani, 1989). Reported as "very loud" in up to 30 percent (Drukier, 1989; Graham, 1981) and as a "high annoyance" in 37 percent (Graham et al., 1984), tinnitus can be as disturbing to children as it is to adults.

DIFFERENCES BETWEEN CHILDREN AND ADULTS

The most notable difference between tinnitus in children and adults is that, unlike adults, children will complain only rarely of tinnitus. It is thought that children with hearing loss (often congenital or acquired early in life) may have continuously experienced tinnitus, and therefore are not disturbed by such a long-standing sensation. In contrast, tinnitus in adults is usually acquired, most often the result of a high-frequency sensorineural hearing loss associated with age and/or noise exposure. It is this change in aural sensation that prompts medical evaluation. Children have a less well-developed body image (Leonard et al., 1983), are more easily distracted (Viani, 1989), and may accept more easily an aural sensation as being normal (Mills, 1984). These factors may contribute to an infrequent complaint of tinnitus in the pediatric population.

Another major difference between tinnitus in hearing-impaired children and adults is its reported duration. Hearing-impaired children nearly always report *intermittent* tinnitus whereas hearing-impaired adults often report *constant* tinnitus. Interestingly, children with "normal" hearing often will report constant tinnitus (Martin, 1994). In a study of adult tinnitus patients, tinnitus was reported to be constant in 91 percent of patients (Meikle et al., 1987). In contrast, tinnitus was described as intermittent in

94 to 100 percent of hearing-impaired children (Graham, 1981; Mills et al., 1987; Nodar et al., 1984; Viani, 1989). Graham (1995) proposes that congenitally hearing-impaired children do not perceive constant tinnitus because aberrant afferent neural activity remains below threshold for conscious perception in children. This aberrant neural activity usually is acquired in adults with tinnitus, surpassing their threshold of perception. Another explanation why hearing-impaired children report intermittent tinnitus more frequently than constant tinnitus is that the former may be more distracting than the latter (Viani, 1989).

Otitis media is one of the most common health care problems in the pediatric age group. Two-thirds of children are diagnosed with otitis media by age 2, and 40 percent of those children have a persistent middle ear effusion after one month (Paparella et al., 1991). Conductive hearing loss has been thought to unmask "physiologic tinnitus" (Leonard et al., 1983), bringing it to the attention to those who had not previously noticed it. In general, however, tinnitus is associated most frequently with sensorineural hearing loss and less frequently with conductive hearing loss. In adults with middle-ear disease however, 51 percent will report tinnitus (Venters, 1953). Similarly, 44 percent of children with serous otitis media report tinnitus when specifically questioned (Mills, 1984). Since children are considerably more afflicted with middle-ear disease than adults, if otitis media does not result in physiologic tinnitus, most children largely ignore their tinnitus.

Adults often report that hearing aids mask tinnitus and occasionally afford hours of tinnitus relief after their removal, a phenomenon known as residual inhibition (Vernon & Meikle, 1998; and Chapter 14). Unlike tinnitus in hearing-impaired adults, tinnitus in children does not appear to be suppressed with extrinsic noise (Graham, 1981; Viani, 1989). Children report suppression of tinnitus with hearing aids less often than adults (Viani, 1989), possibly related to the more significant degree of hearing loss

in children. There are children, however, who have benefited from tinnitus maskers to such a degree that their pure tone audiograms have improved markedly during periods of residual inhibition (Graham et al., 1984; and Chapter 9).

SENSORINEURAL TINNITUS IN CHILDREN

Ototoxic Drugs

Neonates are particularly susceptible to bacterial infection (for example, coliform meningitis) and frequently are placed on prolonged courses of ototoxic intravenous antibiotics, including gentamycin and kanamycin. Few prospective studies address the long-term effects of ototoxic antibiotics on the cochleovestibular systems of these children, and none address tinnitus *per se*. Because no measurable cochleovestibular symptoms have been found up to five years after treatment (Finitzo-Hieber et al., 1979), it is generally thought that these antibiotics are safe. However, since clinical audiometry tests hearing only up to 8,000 Hz, it is possible that selective hair cell losses in the basal turn of the cochlea may not be apparent with routine testing. In support of this hypothesis, children will occasionally describe high-pitched tinnitus that may reflect a very high-frequency sensorineural hearing loss (that is, 13,000 Hz) (Fausti et al., 1984).

Studies using auditory brain stem response latencies show a statistically significant prolongation of wave V in neonates receiving intramuscular gentamycin or tobramycin (5 to 7.5 mg/kg/day divided in two daily doses) when compared to age-matched controls (Bernard, 1981), suggesting that these antibiotics are not innocuous. These latency delays can be noted as early as five days, with the average length of therapy being 8.7 days. Using gentamycin-treated kittens, similar wave V prolongation can be noted at day 10 of treatment, with histopathologic confirmation of outer hair cell damage in the basal turn of the cochlea (Bernard, 1981). Adult cats in identical protocols show no evidence of ABR or histopathologic abnormalities, offering support that neonatal cats are particularly susceptible to aminoglycosides during the period auditory maturation (Bernard, 1981). Human auditory maturation is not complete until the end of the first year of life (Starr et al., 1977), and if histopathologic correlation of wave V prolongation and outer hair cell damage holds true for neonates as for kittens, the risk-benefit ratio of instituting aminoglycosides should be carefully considered.

Recently, familial aminoglycoside-induced deafness (occurring at therapeutic levels) has been linked to a mutation in the small ribosomal RNA gene (12S rRNA) of the human mitochondria (1555 A-to-G substitution) (Bacino et al., 1995; Cortopassi et al., 1994; Prezant et al., 1993). This maternally-inherited point mutation makes the mitochondrial rRNA structurally more similar to its bacterial counterpart which, in turn, renders the mitochondria-rich hair cell highly susceptible to the cytotoxic effects of the antibiotic. It is likely that genetic screening will become available in the future to allow us to identify susceptible individuals before initiating aminoglycoside therapy.

Ménière's Disease in Children

Ménière's disease is defined as fluctuating sensorineural hearing loss, tinnitus and episodic vertigo lasting 20 minutes to several hours. It is usually only seen in the adult population and is most commonly diagnosed in the fifth to sixth decades of life (Cawthorne, 1954). Ménières' first description of this "apoplectiform" disorder was, however, in a child (Ménière, 1861). Although children represent only 1 to 3 percent of all Ménière's patients, the auditory and vestibular symptoms typically are as severe as those found in adults (Hausler et al., 1987; Meyerhoff et al., 1978). Although usually diagnosed in children aged 10 to 19 years, cases have been reported as early as age 4 (Parving, 1976; Simonton, 1940). Over one-

third of affected children have a history of an inner ear insult, either from mumps, meningitis, temporal bone fractures or congenital hyperbilirubinemia, typically 5 to 11 years before the onset of symptoms (Hausler et al., 1987). The remaining children have no other otologic insults or abnormalities, suggesting that both secondary and idiopathic Ménière's syndrome is found in children.

Perilymph Fistula

A perilymph fistula is an abnormal communication between the inner and middle ear, typically occurring at the oval and/or round windows. It is often associated with Mondini dysplasia (a bony and membranous labyrinthine malformation), inner ear microtrauma from straining, barotrauma, and head injury. Because of the variety of auditory and vestibular symptoms produced, perilymph fistulae often masquerade as other inner ear disorders. Definitive diagnosis is made at the time of surgical exploration.

In a retrospective review by Parnes and McCabe, nine of sixteen children complained of tinnitus preoperatively when a perilymph fistula was confirmed surgically (Parnes et al., 1987). Nearly all had associated hearing loss and one-half had vestibular symptoms. Tinnitus was relieved in four of nine children after repair of the fistula. Vestibular symptoms also typically abated, although improvement of auditory symptoms was less predictable.

Noise Exposure

In adults, prolonged and repeated noise exposure, in addition to presbycusis, results in bilateral high frequency sloping sensorineural hearing loss typically in the 2,000 to 8,000 Hz range (Feldman, 1995). If testing is continued beyond 8,000 Hz, detection of sensorineural losses may be dramatic. This may be especially true when there is a history of exposure to cochlear ototoxic agents (gentamycin, cisplatin) or high-frequency noise exposure. A neural derangement in the middle turn of the cochlea also may show no audiometric abnormality (that is, a hidden "dip") if the lesion lies between two tested octaves (Black et al., 1996). It is therefore important to test beyond 8,000 Hz or between octaves to help explain some patients' tinnitus.

Society is becoming increasingly complacent regarding excessive recreational noise exposure during childhood. Most rock concerts produce > 100 dB SPL (Yassi et al., 1993), and portable stereo headphones can produce output in excess of 120 dB SPL (Katz et al., 1982). The Occupational Safety and Health Administration (OSHA) allows no more than 85 dBA for an 8-hour exposure period. With each subsequent 5 dB increase in intensity, exposure time must be halved. For example, a 100 dB noise exposure must be limited to 1 hour, a duration typically exceeded at the average rock concert.

Sound pressure levels > 140 dB are thought to cause irreparable permanent threshold shifts (Consensus National Conference, 1990). Temporary threshold shifts are reversible increases in hearing thresholds after loud noise exposure and are generally thought to lead to permanent threshold shifts following accumulated inner ear microtrauma. The National Academy of Science recommends that the temporary threshold shift at 2 minutes not exceed 20 dB at 3,000 Hz (Moody et al., 1978). An average rock concert will sustain >100 dB SPL (with up to 130 dB peaks) for up to 3 hours (Yassi et al., 1993). A temporary threshold shift of 10 to 20 dB at 4,000 Hz has been detected audiometrically in over 80 percent of all concert goers, with 40 percent of concert-goers having a measurable temporary threshold shift at 2 minutes > 20 dB (Yassi et al., 1993). Sixty percent are aware of subjective tinnitus immediately after leaving the concert, and 44 percent notice a change in their hearing thresholds, emphasizing the serious nature of seemingly harmless entertainment (Yassi et al., 1993). The use of portable stereo headphones at an output of > 100 dB SPL for 3 hours has been shown to produce a temporary thresh-

old shift of 30 dB at 4,000 Hz (Lee et al., 1985), clearly in excess of safe limits. Reduction to an output of 90 dBA for 3 hours, however, produces no temporary threshold shift (Lee et al., 1985). Unknowingly, children use portable headsets at excessive volumes, suggesting that output limits may be necessary to ensure minimal acoustic trauma.

Pharmacological Agents

Children frequently are subjected to drug treatments that cause tinnitus. Although the number of drugs that elicit tinnitus is significant, those most frequently implicated are salicylate analgesics, nonsteroidal anti-inflammatory drugs, certain antibiotics (aminoglycosides, doxycycline, ciprofloxin), quinine and related antimalarials, cardiac medications (quinidine, propanolol) and the "loop-inhibiting" diuretics (furosemide) (Shulman, 1991). Chemotherapeutic agents, such as cisplatin, also produce sensorineural hearing loss and tinnitus (Black, 1996).

RARER CAUSES OF TINNITUS IN CHILDREN

Acoustic Neuromas

Vestibular schwannomas, in the absence of associated neurofibromatoses, are rare in children. To date, less than twenty sporadic acoustic neuromas have been described between ages 1 and 14 years (Chen et al., 1992). Although 80 percent of adults with acoustic neuromas complain of tinnitus associated with a unilateral sensorineural hearing loss at the time of diagnosis (Sheehy, 1979), children rarely report any symptoms and these tumors are often discovered during evaluation of an asymmetric screening audiogram or found incidentally during brain stem imaging for an unrelated reason. Since children generally do not complain of hearing abnormalities, tumor size in these rare cases is often large, precluding preservation of serviceable hearing.

Children with neurofibromatosis type I (von Reckinghausen's disease) appear to be at no higher risk than the general pediatric population of developing acoustic tumors, however children with neurofibromatosis type II, an autosomal dominant disease which gives rise to multiple schwannomas and meningiomas of the central nervous system, are afflicted with bilateral acoustic neuromas. Usually the diagnosis is made in the early 20s and is associated with *cafe au lait* spots (43 percent), cataracts (38 percent) and skin tumors (68 percent) (Evans et al., 1992). Hearing loss and tinnitus are present in approximately 50 percent of patients (Evans et al., 1992).

Congenital Neurosyphilis

Tinnitus is present as the initial symptom of congenital neurosyphilis in one-third of patients and is noted in 80 percent of patients at some time during the course of the disease (Skeckelberg et al., 1984). Often referred to as the "great imitator" because of its protean cochleovestibular symptoms, patients with lues usually have bilateral sensorineural hearing loss, multiple vestibular complaints and roaring tinnitus (Skeckelberg et al., 1984). The mean age at diagnosis is in the fourth decade, although the youngest child reported with congenital syphilis was only 12 years old. Associated findings, such as interstitial keratitis and a positive FTA-ABS, are helpful in establishing the diagnosis and initiating appropriate treatment.

Blood Dyscrasias

Subjective tinnitus has been associated with blood dyscrasias that result in anemia. Children with sickle cell disease have an associated sensorineural hearing loss and tinnitus, presumably from altered blood flow within the cochlea following a "crisis" (Shulman, 1991). Sluggish blood flow associated with polycythemia vera and leukemia also have been associated with tinnitus (Shulman, 1991).

Middle-ear tinnitus in children

Graham (1981) reported that approximately one-quarter of hearing-impaired children have pulsatile tinnitus. Of these children, only 23 percent had middle-ear disease. If pulsatile tinnitus is reported, a thorough evaluation to rule out potentially lethal disorders such as glomus tumors and vascular malformations is indicated (Table 10-1).

Venous Hums

The diagnosis of a venous hum is made most commonly in childhood. The associated tinnitus usually is described as low-pitched and pulsatile, and is thought to be due to turbulent blood flow in the internal jugular vein perhaps caused by vessel impingement at the second cervical vertebra (Cutforth et al., 1970) or increased intracranial pressure (Meador, 1982). Light pressure over the ipsilateral internal jugular vein or turning the head to the uninvolved side will reduce the tinnitus both subjectively and objectively, and is diagnostic of a venous hum.

Although usually benign and self-limiting, disabling tinnitus can be treated by ligating the internal jugular vein high in the neck or by ablating the transverse sinus (Tyler & Babin, 1993). The potentially life-threatening high flow arteriovenous fistula must be considered in the diagnosis and if necessary, an arteriogram or magnetic resonance angiogram should be performed.

Table 10-1. Pulsatile, middle ear tinnitus in children

Venous hums

Transmitted bruits

Glomus tumors

Hydrocephalus

Vascular malformations
  Dural arteriovenous fistulae
  Dehiscent jugular bulb
  Aberrant carotid artery
  Persistent stapedial artery

Transmitted Bruit

Vascular abnormalities distant from the ear can cause pulsatile tinnitus (Levine et al., 1987; Sismanis et al., 1994). Fibromuscular dysplasia of the carotid or vertebral arteries, intracranial or extracranial arterial dissections, high grade carotid stenosis or even a loud cardiac murmur may transduce turbulent flow through the vasculature to be heard as pulse synchronous tinnitus. Increased cardiac output, associated with anemia or thyrotoxicosis, and Paget's disease of the bone also have been reported to cause pulsatile tinnitus (Levine et al., 1987).

Glomus Tumors

Glomus tumors (also known as paragangliomas, chemodectomas, receptomas, and glomerocytomas) are the most common primary neoplasms of the middle ear, usually occurring in adult females in their fourth decade. Pulse-synchronous tinnitus, a red retrotympanic mass that blanches with positive pneumotoscopy (Brown's sign), and a high-resolution CT of the temporal bone that confirms a middle ear mass are diagnostic. Glomus tumors that arise from branches of the IX (Jacobson's) or X (Arnold's) cranial nerves but do not erode the bony septum between the hypotympanum and the jugular fossa are known as glomus tympanicum tumors; tumors with bone destruction usually arise from glomus bodies in the adventitia of the jugular bulb are known as glomus jugulare tumors.

In contrast to over 1,000 reported cases in adults (Zak et al., 1982), glomus tumors in the pediatric population are exceedingly rare. Only sixteen cases have been reported in children less than fourteen years of age (Bartels, et al., 1988; Jackson et al., 1996; Jacobs et al., 1994; Magliulo et al., 1996; Thompson et al., 1989), the youngest patient being six months old (Jacobs et al., 1994). Although similar histopathologically to their adult counterparts, pediatric glomus jugulare tumors tend to be more aggressive and carry an approximate 50 percent mortality rate compared to a 5 to 13 percent mortality rate in adults (Green et al., 1994). Children also have a higher incidence of multicentricity (20 percent [Bartels et al., 1988] versus 10 percent of adults [Green et al., 1994]) and vasoactivity (40 percent [Bartels et al., 1988] versus 4 percent of adults [Green et al., 1994]). Due to obstructive middle-ear symptoms in the face of a hypervascular tympanic membrane, glomus tympanicum tumors are diagnosed earlier than glomus jugulare and carry a 0 percent mortality rate (Green et al., 1994).

Up to 50 percent of cases of glomus tumors are thought to be familial (van der Mey et al., 1989), with up to 33 percent multicentricity in certain families (Green et al., 1994). These heritable glomus tumors appear to be autosomal dominant (from carrier fathers only) with an age-dependent penetrance. Current research has localized this genetic mutation to chromosome 11q23 (Baysal, 1997).

Hydrocephalus

Pulsatile tinnitus can be the first sign of increased intracranial pressure. A benign form of intracranial hypertension known as pseudotumor cerebri has been described in young, overweight females (Sismanis et al., 1990). This pulse-synchronous tinnitus is thought to be due to vascular pulsations in the cerebrospinal fluid transiently compressing the dural venous sinuses resulting in turbulent blood heard by the patient. Symptoms are relieved by lowering the cerebrospinal fluid pressure. Arnold-Chiari malformation and stenosis of the Sylvian aqueduct also have been reported to result in pulsatile tinnitus (Wiggs et al., 1996). A history of pulsatile tinnitus in a child with developmental delay should prompt a neurologic evaluation, including computed tomography of the cranium.

VASCULAR MALFORMATIONS OF THE MIDDLE EAR

Dural Arteriovenous Fistulae

A dural arteriovenous fistula is one of the more common causes of pulsatile tinnitus accompanying a normal-appearing tympanic membrane (Willinsky, 1992). Most commonly branches of the occipital artery aberrantly communicate with the transverse or sigmoid sinus (Arenberg et al., 1972). These fistulae have been reported following middle ear or intracranial infections, after temporal bone surgery, and after head trauma, although in the majority of patients, no antecedent event can be documented.

A dural sinus thrombosis is often found prior to development of a fistula and a partial thrombus may be discovered within the fistula, suggesting a causal relationship. Possibly, a preexisting venous thrombus enlarges normally present arteriovenous shunts by overwhelming normal autoregulatory mechanisms until significant flow is produced, resulting in symptoms of pulse-synchronous tinnitus confirmed by auscultation over the mastoid. Venous hypertension also may play a role in dilatation of these arteriovenous shunts (Halbach et al., 1987).

Symptoms of a dural arteriovenous fistula in children include a heart beat sound in the ear worsened by activity or certain head positions, headaches, and visual changes. The clinical diagnosis can be made using a Toynbee stethoscope to listen to the pulse in the ear of the patient, while trying to abolish the tinnitus with ipsilateral carotid artery compression. If the offending arterial vessel can be palpated in the mastoid region (occipital artery), firm pressure will eliminate the tinnitus. Definitive diagnosis is made by selective arteriography or magnetic resonance angiography. Children with grade I and II (no cortical venous flow) flow have a 0 percent chance of intracranial bleeding; those with grade III and IV (cortical venous flow present) flow have a 31 percent and 100 percent chance, respectively (Lalwani et al., 1993).

Treatment depends on the grade of flow identified (Lalwani et al., 1993). Children with grade I and II arteriovenous fistulae may be observed or offered compressive therapy (that is, compression of the occipital artery 30 minutes many times a day), which induces thrombosis and symptom relief in one-quarter of patients (Halbach et al., 1987). With grade III and IV arteriovenous fistulae, superselective embolization without or with surgical excision is required. It is important for children with low-grade fistulae flow to monitor the quality of their tinnitus. Any changes in the loudness or quality should prompt reevaluation since this could indicate that a thrombus is enlarging, resulting in increased cortical venous drainage (Halbach et al., 1987).

Dural arteriovenous fistulae have been reported in at least fourteen infants and children one day to twenty-three months of age (Cataltepe et al., 1993), nearly half of whom died. There is a suggestion that congenital infections associated with vasculitic changes, like toxoplasmosis, play a role in venous sinus thrombosis and result in arteriovenous fistulae formation (Cataltepe et al., 1993). Prompt diagnosis and treatment is therefore indicated.

Dehiscent Jugular Bulb

The high riding or dehiscent jugular bulb is the most common cause of diagnosable pulsatile tinnitus. A 6 percent incidence of jugular bulb extension above the inferior rim of the bony annulus has been noted in adult temporal bone specimens (Overton et al., 1973), compared with a 7 percent incidence of bony dehiscence over the jugular bulb (Graham, 1977). A high jugular bulb in proximity to the internal auditory canal also has been shown in 6 percent of children < 6 years of age (Rauch et al., 1993). For the most part, however, a dehiscent jugular bulb is asymptomatic. If symptoms do occur, they usually include pulsatile tinnitus and/or conductive hearing loss following the obstruction of the round window niche (Suarez et al., 1993). Dehiscence is more common in the right ear, a bias that can be attributed to the larger size of the right transverse/sigmoid sinus in 75 percent of the population (Robin , 1972).

Children with craniofacial dysostoses have a higher incidence of jugular bulb dehiscence than the general population, although whether the incidence of pulsatile tinnitus is higher is unknown. In a study by van Die et al. (1995), four of eleven children with Crouzon syndrome were noted to have high jugular bulbs in at least one ear when evaluated with temporal bone computed tomography, and two of four had partial or complete bony dehiscence of the jugular bulb. In a study by Gould et al. (1982), six patients with Apert syndrome underwent exploratory tympanotomy for conductive hearing loss, and in two, a dehiscent jugular bulb was found. These groups of children have poor eustachian tube function and often require myringotomy and tympanostomy, theoretically posing a risk of hemorrhage during myringotomy. Consideration of anterior-superior placement of a tympanostomy tube in this patient population may minimize surgical risk to a dehiscent jugular bulb.

Aberrant Carotid Artery

An internal carotid artery aberrantly located in the middle ear is defined as extension beyond Lapayowker's "vestibular line" (a vertical line drawn through the lateral part of the vestibule on an anteroposterior arteriogram [Lapayowker et al., 1971]). This congenital middle ear vascular anomaly has been reported in less than fifty cases (Glasscock et al., 1993). Although many theories exist to explain this aberrancy (Glasscock et al., 1993), it is most probably due to abnormal involution of the dorsal aorta cranial to the third aortic arch. As a result of this vascular interruption, blood flows through the second branchial arch

vasculature to a more distal portion of the internal carotid artery. The aberrancy around the middle ear involves the ascending pharyngeal artery leading to its inferior tympanic branch, then into the caroticotympanic artery that ultimately rejoins the internal carotid artery in the petrous portion of the temporal bone (Glasscock et al., 1993). The vertical carotid canal fails to remain canalized due to the absence of blood flow, which can be confirmed radiologically.

High-resolution temporal bone computed tomography not only reveals an absent vertical segment of the internal carotid artery, but also an enlarged inferior tympanic canaliculus, an enhancing hypotympanic mass and a bony dehiscence of the internal carotid artery in the middle ear (Anand et al., 1991). The diagnosis can be confirmed with an arteriogram, which has the appearance of a number "7" (the "7" sign) compared to the normal side (Figure 10-1). This diagnosis must be anticipated in every middle-ear surgery, since approximately 25 percent of patients will suffer a devastating neurologic event if the lumen is violated (Anand et al., 1991). Confirmation of an aberrant internal carotid artery can be made safely using a 27-gauge needle to aspirate blood, confirming its arterial nature with a blood gas analysis (Anand et al., 1991). Additionally, for patients with significant complaints of pulsatile tinnitus, coverage of an exposed internal carotid artery may control symptoms.

Persistent Stapedial Artery

Even though the first case of persistent stapedial artery described by Hyrtl in 1836 was noted to cause tinnitus (Pahor et al., 1992), the majority of diagnoses are made incidentally during exploratory tympanotomy. To date, only approximately fifty cases of persistent stapedial artery have been reported (Govaerts et al, 1993). Persistent stapedial arteries in children occasionally are associated with other congenital anomalies, such as anencephaly, trisomy 13–15 and thalidomide sequelae (Marion et al.,

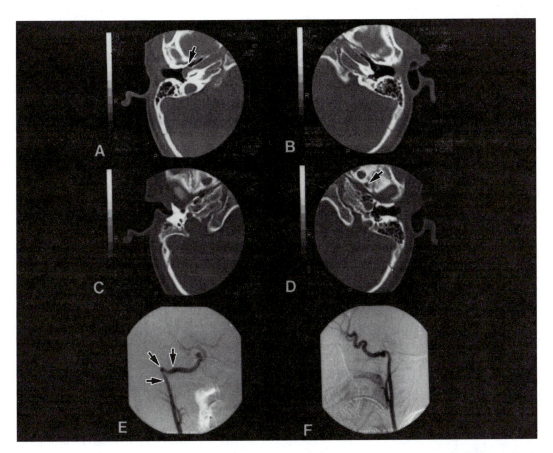

FIGURE 10-1. Aberrant carotid artery with persistent stapedial artery. Axial CT scan and carotid arteriography of right aberrant carotid artery. A, B—the aberrantly located internal carotid artery extends into the middle ear space (arrow, A). C,D—there also is an absence of the foramen spinosum (through which the middle meningeal artery would normally course) on the right side, indicating the probable presence of a persistent stapedial artery. The foramen spinosum is seen in its usual location on the left side (arrow, D). E, F—selective internal carotid arteriography reveals the aberrant course of this vessel through the temporal bone, resulting in the typical "7 sign," so named because the vessel takes the shape of an inverted number seven. The internal carotid artery is seen in its usual position on the patient's left side (F).

1985), but most often are not associated with any other craniofacial abnormality. On occasion, a persistent stapedial artery can be associated with an aberrant carotid artery, perhaps by "tethering" the internal carotid artery in the middle ear space (Suarez et al., 1993). Radiologic characteristics of the persistent stapedial artery include an absent foramen spinosum (since the middle meningeal artery originates from the internal carotid artery rather than the external carotid artery) and an enlarged anterior tympanic segment of the fallopian canal adjacent to

the cochleariform process (Pahor et al., 1992) (Figure 10-1).

The incidence of persistent stapedial artery varies from 1:5,000 to 10,000, as noted during routine stapedectomy (Schuknecht, 1974), to 1:200, as noted during temporal bone histopathologic review (Moreano et al., 1994). The stapedial artery originates at the hyoid artery, an embryonic branch of the internal carotid artery. It then passes between the stapedial crura forming lower (maxillomandibular) and upper (supraorbital) divisions, the latter becoming the middle meningeal artery. The fixed intra-crural space eventually limits the blood supply to the growing face and the ventral pharyngeal artery (an external carotid artery branch) assumes primary blood supply to the head, leaving the stapedial artery to involute by the tenth embryonic week (Marion et al., 1985). Unlike its usual external carotid artery origin, in the case of a persistent stapedial artery, the middle meningeal artery derives from the internal carotid artery's persistent stapedial branch. Surgical dogma is to leave the blood supply of the persistent stapedial artery undisturbed since it may be the sole blood supply to the pyramidal tract, medial lemniscus and trapezoid body. Vascular injury could theoretically result in hemiplegia and hearing loss (Hogg et al., 1972), although practically, when the persistent stapedial artery has been ligated, no neurologic sequelae have been identified (Govaerts et al., 1993). Therefore, it appears to be safe to interrupt a persistent stapedial artery if it is symptomatic or interferes with middle ear surgery.

NONPULSATILE, MIDDLE-EAR TINNITUS

Palatal Myoclonus

Palatal myoclonus is a rare extrapyramidal disorder involving the cerebellum, resulting in the loss of inhibition of both cranial nerve nuclei and lower motor neurons (Lyons et al., 1975). It is characterized by rhythmic, involuntary contractions of the soft palate, usually bilateral and occurring 10 to 200 times per minute. Tinnitus is thought to be the result of the snapping open of the eustachian tube orifice, occurring as a result of tensor veli palatini contraction. The diagnosis is established by observing the soft palate in the presence of a Toynbee tube between the patient's and the observer's ears, visualizing palatal movement with each ear click. Often, a widely opened mouth will suppress the palatal contractions and a nasopharyngeal view of the soft palate is necessary. A tympanogram will show click-associated waveforms, associated with changes in the middle-ear impedance following eustachian tube closure.

Patients with a diagnosis of palatal myoclonus generally fall into two categories—"symptomatic" (73 percent) or "essential" (27 percent) groups (Deuschl et al., 1990). The "symptomatic" group represents patients with central nervous system disorders, such as cerebrovascular diseases, multiple sclerosis, brain stem tumors, encephalitis, trauma or hydrocephalus resulting in an abnormal brain stem or cerebellar exam. These disorders are thought to lead to lesions in the Guillian-Mollaret triangle, the area defined between the red nucleus, dentate nucleus, and inferior olivary nucleus (Kim et al., 1994). The inferior olivary nucleus subsequently hypertrophies, revealing the characteristic inferior olive enlargement seen on magnetic resonance imaging.

The "essential" group of myoclonic patients is seen mostly commonly by the otologist. These children have no abnormal neurologic findings except for palatal myoclonus and have normal magnetic resonance imaging. The "essential" group can be differentiated from the "symptomatic" group in that they are younger (25 ± 13 years compared to 45 ± 17 years in the symptomatic group), have a normal neurologic exam, and nearly always present with ear clicking as their chief complaint (90 percent compared to 7.6 percent in the symptomatic group) (Deuschl et al., 1990).

Treatment of palatal myoclonus involves decreasing the ability of the eustachian tube orifice to move. Successful medical treatment has included the use of anticonvulsants (phenytoin, valproic acid and carbamazepine [Deuschl et al., 1990]), benzodiazepines (clonazepam [Bakheit et al., 1990]) and anticholinergics (trihexyphenidyl [Jabbari et al., 1989]). Successful surgical treatments have included hamulus fracture, dislocation of the tensor veli palatini tendon from the hamulus, tensor veli palatini paralysis using botulinum toxin (Saeed et al., 1993; Varney et al., 1996), sectioning of the tensor tympani (Badia et al., 1994) and/or stapedial muscle in the middle ear (Williams, 1980) and tympanostomy tube placement (Kwee et al., 1972).

Middle-ear Myoclonus

The presence of objective, nonpulsatile tinnitus in the absence of palatal movement suggests a diagnosis of middle-ear myoclonus. This rare disorder is thought to be due to tensor tympani and/or stapedial muscle contractions, and tenotomy of both muscles provides effective relief of symptoms (Badia et al., 1994). A jet of cool air onto the cornea also has been shown to abolish ear clicking in a 6-year-old boy who noticed the tinnitus immediately after a bee flew into his external ear canal (Quarry, 1972). This corneal stimulation presumably abolished the hypersensitive reflex arc of repeated tensor tympani contractions. Stapedial muscle spasm has been described in association with facial nerve paralysis, especially with eyelid-blinking (Watanabe et al., 1974). This noise is often described as a buzzing and is thought to be associated with early return of facial nerve function. High power otomicroscopy reveals tympanic membrane mobility associated with the tinnitus; stapedial tenotomy usually is curative (Badia et al., 1994; Hazell, 1987). Interestingly, placement of a tympanostomy tube has been reported to exacerbate the tinnitus associated with stapedial muscle spasm (Badia et al., 1994).

Patulous Eustachian Tube

The patulous eustachian tube, with symptoms of autophony, aural fullness, and ear click associated with swallowing, is uncommon in the pediatric population, but has been reported as complication following adenoidectomy (Kavanagh et al., 1988). Symptoms are transiently improved with head hanging, engorging the venous plexus of the tubal mucosa. The diagnosis is confirmed using otomicroscopy, visualizing tympanic membrane mobility associated with respiration. This disorder has been associated with rapid weight loss, especially in young adults or older children with anorexia or bulimia. Many treatments have been directed at augmenting the peritubal tissue (that is, Teflon injections [Pulec, 1967]) or reducing the lumen size of the eustachian tube (silver nitrate cautery), although weight gain alone may improve this problem considerably.

Temporomandibular Joint Disorders

Temporomandibular joint disorders are frequently thought of as the "great impostors" (Morgan, 1987). Costen's syndrome (temporomandibular joint neuralgia) has a 20 percent reported prevalence in the adult population, although it is rarely reported in the pediatric population. Auditory symptoms (clicking, popping, snapping, tinnitus) are present in 25 percent of those afflicted (Myrhang, 1964; Ren and Isberg, 1995).

Familial Tinnitus

A family with nonpulsatile objective tinnitus was reported in 1971 (Glanville et al., 1971) in which the father and two of his three children had loud, high-frequency noises emitting from their ears (see Chapter 9). The noises were heard up to 4 feet away, measured at approximately 50 dB SPL and were characterized by tones at 5,650 and 7,650 Hertz in left and right ears. Intraoperatively, a stapedial tenotomy did not abolish the tinnitus but intravenous succinylcholine did. Head position also resulted in transient abolition of the tinnitus. The etiology was presumed to be vascular.

Table 10-2. Non-pulsatile, middle ear tinnitus in children

Palatal myoclonus

Middle-ear myoclonus

Patulous eustachian tube

Temporomandibular joint disorders

Familial tinnitus

EVALUATION OF THE CHILD WITH COMPLAINTS OF TINNITUS

History

Sensorineural Tinnitus

Since children rarely volunteer the symptom of tinnitus, serious evaluation of their complaint is indicated. The assessment of the quality of the tinnitus should proceed similar to that in adults (see Chapter 9). Anticipating that children are often eager to please an examiner, questions should be worded so that they are nonleading and open. This format allows the child to describe his ear noise by comparing it to sounds with which he is most familiar. Important aspects of the history involve questions regarding loudness, pitch, temporal characteristics, localization, annoyance, psychological influences, and effects of environmental noise (Black et al., 1996).

Middle-ear Tinnitus

The early differentiation between sensorineural and middle-ear tinnitus in children is of considerable importance since the latter category could represent an aggressive glomus tumor, a dural arteriovenous fistula, or a central nervous system disorder with resultant palatal myoclonus or hydrocephalus. Middle-ear tinnitus should be characterized as fully as possible by the child, again with as little prompting as possible to avoid misleading data. Most importantly is the early establishment of pulsatile versus nonpulsatile middle-ear tinnitus. On investigating pulsatile tinnitus the history should include questions that identify a conductive hearing loss (possibly, a recent otitis media or a history of middle-ear cholesteatoma), which can unmask a "physiologic" tinnitus. A history of bloody otorrhea, otalgia, paroxysms of hypertension, and sweating suggest a diagnosis of a glomus tumor. If the tinnitus is clearly not associated with a pulse yet heard by the child or his parents, a diagnosis of palatal myoclonus is suggested. An occasional patient will notice rhythmic palatal contractions associated with the ear click. The history should always include any neurologic changes, seizures, or changes in personality, since approximately three-quarters of patients with palatal myoclonus are found to have a central nervous system disease (Deuschl et al. 1990).

Physical Examination

Meticulous microscopic examination of tympanic membrane is performed to evaluate the status of the tympanic membrane and middle ear. Serous fluid, cholesteatoma or poor mobility of the tympanic membrane suggest a cause for conductive hearing loss. A red mass with margins completely visualized suggests a glomus tympanicum tumor, whereas a similar appearing mass incompletely visualized in its inferior extent suggests a glomus jugulare tumor. Both of these masses reveal their vascular nature when blanching is noted with positive pressure pneumatic otoscopy (Brown's sign). Pneumotoscopy in the absence of a retrotympanic mass is important in diagnosing a perilymph fistula, with vertigo and nystagmus accompanying positive pressure. A pale red mass located anteriorly suggests an aberrant carotid artery whereas a dark blue mass located posteriorly suggests a dehiscent jugular bulb. Palpitation of the child's pulse while he verbally mimics the sound confirms the vascular nature of the middle ear abnormality. A Toynbee tube also allows objective assessment of pulsatile tinnitus. Careful auscultation of the heart, neck, mastoid, cranium, and orbits will evaluate para-auditory pulsatile tinnitus resulting from transmitted arterial or venous flow abnormalities.

Examination of the soft palate in children with tinnitus is essential to verify rhymthic palatal myoclonus. A nasopharyngeal view is often desirable since wide mouth opening may transiently suppress palatal contractions. Evaluation of eustachian tube orifi can sometimes reveal palatal-associated movement in palatal myoclonus or an abnormally widened orifice in a patulous eustachian tube.

Cranial nerve exam, especially palatal elevation, vocal cord mobility, and shoulder/neck movement is important to rule out involvement of the jugular foramen by a glomus jugulare tumor. A fundoscopic exam may establish increased intracranial pressure, and a general neurologic testing is useful to evaluate causes of palatal myoclonus.

Audiologic Evaluation

Every child with complaints of tinnitus should have an audiogram and tympanometry. Like adults, tinnitus is most frequently associated with sensorineural hearing loss. The high frequency range should be extended as much as possible, especially if there is a history of ototoxic agent exposure associated with high-pitch tinnitus. Tympanometry helps establish the presence of conductive hearing loss and also can reveal palatal myoclonus, rhythmically changing the impedance of the ossicular chain with each contraction of the tensor tympani muscle. Abnormalities in audiometric studies should lead to further diagnostic testing to identify the source of the tinnitus. Otoacoustic emissions can confirm the integrity of the outer hair cells, while auditory brain stem response testing can identify pathology located more centrally.

Radiologic Evaluation

Any child with a normal otoscopic and audiometric evaluation who complains of tinnitus deserves consideration for an imaging study, especially if the tinnitus has a pulsatile component. Nonpulsatile tinnitus with bilateral or unilateral hearing loss may suggest a congenital defect in cochleovestibular development, such as cochlear dysplasia, and may indicate the need for computed tomography of the temporal bone. In the absence of developmental deformities, tinnitus associated with unilateral or bilateral hearing loss may suggest

the need for magnetic resonance imaging of the brain stem. This test will diagnose a sporadic acoustic neuroma or bilateral acoustic neuromas associated with neurofibromatosis type II. Pulsatile tinnitus in the presence of a normal audiometic and otomicroscopic exam should be evaluated with a computed tomogram of the head to rule out hydrocephalus, followed by a cerebral arteriogram or magnetic resonance angiogram if physical examination supports the diagnosis of a dural arteriovenous fistula. If a retrotympanic mass is visualized in a child with tinnitus, a temporal bone tomogram should be performed, whether the quality is pulsatile or nonpulsatile. Nonpulsatile tinnitus suggests the retrotympanic mass may be a cholesteatoma, especially with a history and physical exam findings that suggest this diagnosis. Diagnoses confirmed by temporal bone imaging when pulsatile tinnitus is associated with a retrotympanic mass include glomus tumors, aberrancy of the internal carotid artery, persistence of a stapedial artery, and a high-riding jugular bulb (Willinsky, 1992).

Counseling/treatment Options for Children

Children rarely complain of tinnitus, and when they do it does not appear to have the debilitating effects it has on adults. When children do complain of tinnitus, however, they should be taken seriously as it is likely particularly disturbing to them. Since tinnitus is most often a symptom of an underlying disease, an accurate diagnosis must first be established before attempting treatment. Once all treatable causes (medically and surgically) of tinnitus have been excluded, treatment should be directed by symptoms. Tinnitus may contribute to behavioral problems in children, in particular, distracting them while in school (Graham et al., 1993). Successful use of tinnitus maskers has been reported in children with tinnitus resulting from sensorineural hearing loss, palatal myoclonus and venous hum (Graham et al., 1993). Hearing aids alone may be effective tinnitus maskers, as many children report that their tinnitus is only noticeable after removing their aids (Graham et al., 1983). Effective treatment also involves counseling for the child and his/her parents and offering reassurance that tinnitus is typically associated with otologic disease and infrequently has adverse sequelae (Mills et al., 1986).

REFERENCES

Anand, V. K., Casano, P. J., & Flaiz, R. A. (1991). Diagnosis and treatment of the carotid artery in the middle ear. *Otolaryngology Head and Neck Surgery, 105*(5), 743–747.

Arenberg, I. K., & McCreary, H. S. (1972). Objective tinnitus aurium and dural arteriovenous malformations of the posterior fossa. *Annals of Otology, Rhinology and Laryngology, 80,* 111.

Bacino, C., Prezant, T. R., Bu, X., Fourhier, P., & Fischel-Ghodsian, N. (1995). Susceptibility mutations in the mitochondrial small ribosomal RNA gene in aminoglycoside induced deafness. *Pharmacogenetics, 5*(3), 165–172.

Badia, L., Parikh, A., & Brookes, G. B. (1994). Management of middle ear myoclonus. *Journal of Laryngology and Otology, 108,* 380–382.

Bakheit, A., & Behan, H. (1990). Palatal myoclonus successfully treated with clonazepam. *Journal of Neurology, Neurosurgery and Psychiatry, 53,* 806.

Bartels, L. J., & Gurucharri, M. (1998). Pediatric glomus tumors. *Oto-HNS, 99*(4), 392–395.

Baysal, B. E. E. A. (1997). Fine mapping of an imprinted gene for familial nonchromaffin paragangliomas, on chromosome 11q23. *American Journal of Human Genetics, 60,* 121–132.

Bernard, P. A. (1981). Freedom from ototoxicity in aminoglycoside treated neonates: A mistaken notion. *Laryngoscope, 91*(12), 1985–1994.

Black, O. F., & Lilly, D. J. (1996). Tinnitus in Children. In B. C. E. Al. (Ed.), *Pediatric otolaryngology* (3rd ed., pp 302–311). Philadelphia: W. B. Saunders.

Cataltepe, O., Berker, M., Gurcay, O., & Erbengi, A. (1993). An usual dural arteriovenous fistula in an infant. *Neuroradiology, 35*(5), 394–397.

Cawthorne, T. (1954). Modern trends in diseases of the ear, nose and throat. In M. Ellis (Ed.), *Aural Vertigo* (p. 13). London.

Chen, T. C., Maceri, D. R., Giannotta, S. L., Shih, L., & McComb, J. G. (1992). Unilateral acoustic neuromas in childhood without evidence of neurofibromatosis: Case report and review of the literature. *American Journal of Otology, 13* (4), 318–322.

Consensus National Conference. (1990). Noise and hearing loss. *Journal of the American Medical Association, 263,* 3185–3190.

Cortopassi, G., & Hutchin, T. (1994). A molecular and cellular hypothesis for aminoglycoside-induced deafness. *Hearing Research, 78*(1), 27–30.

Cutforth, R., Wiseman, J., & Sutherland, R. D. (1970). The genesis of cervical venous hum. *American Heart Journal, 80,* 488.

Deuschl, G., Mischke, G., Schenck, E., Schulte-Monting, J., & Lucking, C.H. (1990). Symptomatic and essential rhythmic palatal myoclonus. *Brain, 113,* 1645–1672.

Drukier, G. (1989). The prevalence and characteristics of tinnitus with profound sensorineural hearing impairment. *AAD,* Oct, 260–264.

Evans, D. G., Huson, S., Donnai, D., Neary, W., Blair, V., Newton, V., & Harris, R. (1992). A clinical study of type 2 neurofibromatosis. *Quarterly Journal of Medicine, 84*(304), 603–618.

Fausti, S. A., Rappaport, B. Z., & Schecter, M. A. (1984). Detection of aminoglycoside ototoxicity by high frequency auditory evaluation: Selected case studies. *American Journal of Otolaryngology, 5,* 177.

Feldman, H. (1995). *Mechanisms of tinnitus.* J. A. Vernon & A. R. Moller (Eds.), Needham Heights: Simon & Schuster, 263.

Finitzo-Hieber, T., McCracken, G. H., Jr., Roeser, R. J., Allen, D. A., Chrane, D. F., & Morrow, J. (1979). Ototoxicity in neonates treated with gentamicin and kanamycin: Results of a four-year controlled follow-up study. *Pediatrics, 63* (3), 443–449.

Glanville, J. D., Coles, R. R. A., & Sullivan, B. M. (1971). A family with high-tonal objective tinnitus. *Journal of Laryngology and Otology, 85,* 1–10.

Glasscock, M. E., Seshul, M., & Seshul, M. B. (1993). Bilateral Aberrant Internal Carotid Artery—Case Presentation. *Archives of Otolaryngology Head and Neck Surgery, 119,* 335–339.

Gould, H. J., & Caldarelli, D. D. (1982). Hearing and Otopathology in Apert Syndrome. *Archives of Otolaryngology, 108,* 347–349.

Govaerts, P. J., Marquet, T. F., Cremers, W. R., & Offeciers, F. E. (1993). Persistent stapedial artery: Does it prevent successful surgery? *Annals of Otology, Rhinology and Laryngology, 102,* 724–728.

Graham, M. D. (1977). The jugular bulb: Its anatomic and clinical considerations in contemporary otology. *Laryngoscope, 87,* 105–125.

Graham, J. (1981). Pediatric tinnitus. *Journal of Laryngology and Otology, 4,* 117–120.

Graham, J. (1981). Tinnitus in children with hearing loss. In *CIBA Foundation Symposium* (85, pp. 172–192). London: Pitman Books Ltd.

Graham, J., & Butler, J. (1984). Tinnitus in children. In A. S. J. Ballantyne (Ed.), *Proceedings of the Second International Tinnitus Seminar,* New York, 10 and 11, June 1983 (pp. 236–241). Ashford: Headley Brothers Ltd.

Graham, J. M. (1995). Tinnitus in children with hearing loss. In J. A. Vernon & A. R. Moller (Eds.), *Mechanisms of tinnitus* (pp. 51–56). Needham Heights: Simon & Schuster.

Green, J. D., Brackmann, D. E., Nguyen, C. D., Arriaga, M. A., Telischi, F. F., & De la Cruz, A. (1994). Surgical management of previously untreated glomus jugulare tumors. *Laryngoscope, 104,* 917–921.

Halbach, V. V., Higashida, R. T., Hieshima, G. B., Goto, K., Norman, D., & Newton, T. H. (1987). Dural fistulas involving the transverse and sigmoid sinuses: Results of treatment in 28 patients. *Radiology, 163,* 443–447.

Hausler, R., Toupet, M., Guidetti, G., Basseres, F. & Montandon, P. (1987). Ménière's disease in children. *American Journal of Otolaryngology, 8,* 187–193.

Hazell, J. (1987). *Tinnitus.* J. Hazell (Ed.), New York: Churchill Livingstone, 207.

Hazell, J. W. P., Wood, S. M., Cooper, H. R., Stephens, S. D., Corcoran R. R., Baskill J. C., & Sheldrake, J.B. (1985). A clinical study of tinnitus maskers. *British Journal of Audiology, 19,* 65–146.

Hogg, I. D., Stephens, C. B. & Arnold, G. E. (1972). Theoretical anomalies of the stapedial artery. *Annals of Otology, Rhinology, and Laryngology, 81,* 860–870.

Jabbari, B., Scherokman, B., & Gunderson, C. H. (1989). Treatment of movement disorders with trihexyphenidyl. *Movement Disorders, 4,* 202–212.

Jackson, C. G., Pappas, D. G., Jr., Manolidis, S., Glasscock, M. E., Von Doersten, P. G., Hughs, C.A., & Marrero, R. J. (1996). Pediatric neurotologic skull base surgery. *Laryngoscope, 106,* 1205–1209.

Jacobs, I. N., & Potsic, W. P. (1994). Glomus Tympanicum in Infancy. *Archives of Otolaryngology Head and Neck Surgery, 120,* 203–205.

Katz, A. E., Gerstman, H. I., Sanderson, R. G., & Buchanan, R. (1982). Stereo earphones and hearing loss. *New England Journal of Medicine, 307,* 1460–1461.

Kavanagh, K. T., & Beckford, N. S. (1988). Adenotonsillectomy in children: Indications and contraindications. *Southern Medical Journal, 81* (4), 507–514.

Keeling, S. D., McGorray, S., Wheeler, T. T., & King, G. L. (1994). Risk factors associated with temporomandibular joint sounds in children 6 to 12 years of age. *American Journal of Orthodontics and Dentofacial Orthopedics, 105*(3), 279–287.

Kim, S. J., Lee, J. H. & Suh, D. C. (1994). Cerebellar MR changes in patients with olivary hypertrophic degeneration. *American Journal of Neuroradiology, 15,* 1715–1719.

Kwee, H. L., & Sturben, W. H. (1972). Tinnitus and myoclonus. *Journal of Laryngology and Otology, 86,* 237.

Lalwani, A. K., Dowd, C. F., & Halbach, V. V. (1993). Grading venous restrictive disease in patients with dural arteriovenous fistulas of the transverse/sigmoid sinus. *Journal of Neurosurgery, 79,* 11–15.

Lapayowker, M. S., Liebman, E. P., Ronis, M. L., & Safer, J. N. (1971). Presentation of the internal carotid artery as a tumor of the middle ear. *Radiology, 98,* 293–297.

Lee, P. C., Senders, C. W., Gantz, B. J., & Otto, S. R. (1985). Transient sensorineural hearing loss after overuse of portable headphone cassette radios. *Otolaryngology Head and Neck Surgery, 93*(5), 622–625.

Leonard, G., Black, F. O., & Schramm, V. L. (1983). Tinnitus in children. In C. D. Bluestone & S. E. Stool (Eds.), *Pediatric otolaryngology* (pp. 271–277). Philadelphia: W. B. Saunders.

Levine, S. B., & Snow, J. B. (1987). Pulsatile tinnitus. *Laryngoscope, 97,* 401–406.

Lyons, G. D., Melancon, B.B., Kearby, N.L., Zimmy, M. (1976). The otological aspects of palatal myoclonus. *Laryngoscope, 86*(7), 930–936.

Magliulo, G., Cristofari, P., & Terranova, G. (1996). Glomus tumor in pediatric age. *International Journal of Pediatric Otorhinolaryngology, 38*(1), 77–80.

Marion, M., Hinojosa, R., & Khan, A. A. (1985). Persistence of the stapedial artery: A histopathologic study. *Otolaryngology Head and Neck Surgery, 93*, 298–312.

Martin, K. & Snashall S. (1994). Children presenting with tinnitus: A retrospective study. *British Journal of Audiology, 28*, 111–115.

McFadden, D. (1982). *Tinnitus: Facts, theories, and treatments.* Washington: National Academy Press.

Meador, K. J. (1982). Self-heard venous bruit due to increased intracranial pressure. *Lancet, 1*, 391.

Meikle, M., Schuff, N., & Griest, S. (1987). Intrasubject variability of tinnitus: Observations from the tinnitus clinic. In H. Feldmann (Ed.), *Proceedings of the Third International Tinnitus Seminar.* Munster, 1987. Karlsruhe: Harsch Verlag.

Ménière, P. (1861). Pathologie auriculaire: Mémoire sur des lésions de l'oreille interne donnant lieu á des symptômes de congestion cérébrale apoplectiforme. *Gazette Méd de Paris, 38*, 597–601.

Meyerhoff, W. L., Paparella, M. M., & Shea, D. (1978). Ménière's disease in children. *Laryngoscope, 88*, 1504–1511.

Mills, R. P., Albert, D. M., & Brain, C. E. (1986). Tinnitus in childhood. *Clinical Otolaryngology 11*, 431–434.

Mills, R. P., & Cherry, J. R. (1984). Subjective tinnitus in children with otological disorders. *International Journal of Pediatric Oto-Rhino-Laryngology, 7*, 21–17.

Moody, D. B., Stebbins, W. C., Hawkins, J. E., Jr., & Johnsson, L. G. (1978). Hearing loss and cochlear pathology in the monkey (macaca) following exposure to high levels of noise. *Archives of Otorhinolaryngology, 220*, 47–72.

Moreano, E. H., Paparella, M. M., Zelterman, D., & Goycoolea, M. V. (1994). Prevalence of facial canal dehiscence and of persistent stapedial artery in the human middle ear: A report of 1,000 temporal bones. *Laryngoscope, 104*, 309–321.

Morgan, D. H. (1987). My experience with the TMS, tinnitus and related symptoms. In *ATA Newsletter*, 2–4.

Myrhang, H. (1964). The incidence of ear symptoms in cases of malocculsion and temporomandibular joint disturbances. *British Journal of Oral Surgery, 2*, 28–32.

Nodar, R. (1972). Tinnitus aurium in school age children: A survey. *Journal of Auditory Research, 12*, 133–135.

Nodar, R. H., & LeZak, M. H. W. (1984). Pediatric tinnitus (a thesis revisited). *Journal of Laryngology and Otology, 9*(Suppl.), 234–235.

Overton, S. B., & Ritter F. N. (1973). A high-placed jugular bulb in the middle ear. A Clinical and temporal bone study. *Laryngoscope, 83*, 1986–1991.

Pahor, A. L., & Hussain, S. S. M. (1992). Persistent stapedial artery. *Journal of Laryngology and Otology, 106*, 254–257.

Paparella, M. M., Jung, T. T. K., & Goycoolea, M. V. (1991). Otitis media with effusion. In M. M. Paparella (Ed.), *Otolaryngology* (p. 1317). Philadelphia: W. B. Saunders.

Parnes, L., & McCabe, B. F. (1987). Perilymph fistula: An important cause of deafness and dizziness in children. *Pediatrics, 80*, 524.

Parving, A. (1976). Ménière's disease in childhood. *Journal of Laryngology and Otology, 90*, 817–821.

Prezant, T. R., Agapian, J. V., Bohlman, M. C., Bu, X., Oztas, S., & Qiu, W. Q. (1993). Mitochondrial ribosomal RNA mutation associated with both antibiotic-induced and non-syndromic deafness. *Nature Genetics, 4*(3), 289–294.

Pulec, J. L. (1967). Abnormally patent eustachian tubes: Treatment with injection of poly-tetra-fluoroethylene (teflon) paste. *Laryngoscope, 77*, 1543–1554.

Quarry, J. G. (1972). Unilateral objective tinnitus. *Archives of Otolaryngology, 96*, 252–253.

Rauch, S. D., Xu, W.–Z., & Nadol, Jr., J. B. (1993). High jugular bulb: Implications for posterior fossa neurotologic and cranial base surgery. *Annals of Otology, Rhinology and Laryngology, 102*, 100–107.

Ren, Y.-F., Isberg, A. (1995). Tinnitus in patients with temporomandibular joint internal derangement. *Journal of Craniomandibular Practice, 13*, 75–80.

Reuland, P., Overkamp, D., Aicher, K. P., Bien, S., Muller-Schaunburg, W., & Feine, U. (1996). Catacholamine secreting glomus tumor detection by iodine-123-MIBG scinitigraphy. *Journal of Nuclear Medicine*, 463–465.

Robin, P. E. (1972). A case of upwardly situated jugular bulb in left middle ear. *Journal of Laryngology and Otology, 86*, 1241–1246.

Saeed, S. R., & Brookes, G. B. (1993). The use of clostridium botulinum toxin in palatal myoclonus. A preliminary report. *Journal of Laryngology and Otology, 107*(3), 208–210.

Schuknecht, H. (1974). *Pathology of the ear.* Cambridge: Harvard University Press.

Sheehy, J. L. (1979). Neurotologic evaluation. In W. J. House & C. M. Leutje (Eds.) *Acoustic tumors,* 199–208. Baltimore: University Park Press.

Shulman, A. (1991). *Tinnitus: Diagnosis/Treatment,* A. Shulman (Ed.), Philadelphia: Lea & Febiger.

Simonton, K. M. (1940). Ménière's symptom complex: Review of the literature. *Annals of Otology, 60,* 610.

Sismanis, A., Butts, F. M., & Hughes, G. B. (1990). Objective tinnitus in benign intracranial hypertension: An update. *Laryngoscope, 100,* 33–36.

Sismanis, A., & Smoker, W. R. K. (1994). Pulsatile tinnitus: Recent advances in diagnosis. *Laryngoscope, 104,* 681–688.

Skeckelberg, J. M., & McDonald, T. J. (1984). Otologic involvement in late syphilis. *Laryngoscope, 94,* 753–757.

Starr, A., Amlie, R., & Martin, M. (1977). Development of auditory function in newborn infants revealed by auditory brainstem potentials. *Pediatrics, 60,* 831–839.

Stouffer, J. L., Tyler, R. S., Both, J. C., & Buckrell, B. (1992). Tinnitus in normal-hearing and hearing-impaired children. In J.-M. Aran & R. Dauman (Eds.), *Tinnitus 91* (pp. 255–259). Amsterdam/New York: Kugler.

Suarez, P. A., & Batsakis, J. G. (1993). Nonneoplastic vascular lesions of the middle ear. *Annals of Otology, Rhinology and Laryngology, 102,* 738–740.

Thompson, J. W., & Cohen, S.R. (1989). Management of bilateral carotid body tumors and a glomus jugular tumor in a child. *International Journal of Pediatric Otorhinolaryngology, 17,* 75–87.

Tyler, R. S., & Babin, R. W. (1993). Tinnitus. In C. W. Cummings (Ed.), *Otolaryngology—Head and Neck Surgery* (2nd ed., pp. 3031–3053). St. Louis: Mosby-Year Book.

van der Mey, A. G. L., Maaswinkel-Mooy, P. D., Cornelisse, C. J., Schmidt, P. H., & van de Kamp, J. J. (1989). Genomic imprinting in hereditary glomus tumors: Evidence for new genetic theory. *Lancet, 2,* 1291–1294.

van Die, A., de Groot, J. A., Zonneveld, F. W., Vaandrager, J. M., & Beck, F. J. (1995). Dehiscence of the jugular bulb in Crouzon's disease. *Laryngoscope, 105,* 432–435f.

Varney, S. M., Demetroulakos, J. C., Fletcher, M. H., McQueen, W. J., & Hamiton, M. K. (1996). Palatal myoclonus: Treatment with clostridium botulinum toxin injection. *Otolaryngology Head and Neck Surgery, 114,* 317–320.

Venter, R. (1953). Discussion on tinnitus aurium. *Proceedings of the Royal Society of Medicine, 46,* 825–829.

Viani, L. (1989). Tinnitus in children with hearing loss. *Journal of Laryngology and Otology, 103,* 1142–1145.

Watanabe, I. U., Kumagami, H., & Tsuda, Y. (1974). Tinnitus due to abnormal contraction of stapedial muscle. *Otology, Rhinology and Laryngology, 36,* 217–226.

Wiggs, W. J., Sismanis, A., & Laine, F. J. (1996). Pulsatile tinnitus associated with congenital central nervous system malformations. *American Journal of Otology, 17,* 241–244.

Williams, J. D. (1980). Unusual but treatable cause of fluctuating hearing loss. *Annals of Otology, Rhinology and Laryngology, 89,* 239–240.

Willinsky, R. A. (1992). Tinnitus: Imaging algorithms. *Canadian Association of Radiologists Journal, 43*(2), 93–99.

Yassi, A., P. N., Tran, N., & Cheang, M. (1993). Risks to hearing from a rock concert. *Canadian Family Physician, 39,* 1045.

Zak, F. G., & Lawson, W. (1982). Glomus jugulare tumors. In Bergstedt & Low (Eds.), *The Paraganglionic Chemoreceptor System,* 339–391. New York: Springer-Verlag.

CHAPTER 11

Psychological Management of Tinnitus

Peter H. Wilson, Ph.D.
Jane L. Henry, Ph.D.

BACKGROUND

The aim of this chapter is to provide an overview of the contributions that psychological approaches can offer in the assessment and management of tinnitus. When other treatments have failed or are judged to be unlikely to be effective, many patients with tinnitus are told that they will have to "learn to live with the problem." In practice, learning to live with tinnitus involves dealing with the consequences of the problem, such as the negative emotional states of depression, anxiety and anger, sleep difficulties, and interference with social, employment, and other enjoyable activities (see Chapter 2). The distinction between tinnitus as a sensory experience and as a sensation to which an individual responds with their attentional, perceptual, and emotional processes needs to be kept in mind. Thus, tinnitus is both a medical and a psychological phenomenon. In this respect, there is a good deal of similarity between tinnitus and chronic pain (Tonndorf, 1987). Both pain and tinnitus may have a chronic

course, with relatively small fluctuations in severity over time. Many different types of medical and nonmedical treatments have been employed in the management of both problems but most treatments are effective for a relatively small proportion of patients. The consequences of chronic pain and tinnitus are similar: emotional effects, reduced involvement in work-related activities, interpersonal problems, and decreased opportunities to engage in previously enjoyable activities. Both tinnitus and pain patients report that other people do not understand them because there is no obvious external evidence of the problems they experience. As with pain, a great deal has been learned about the psychological aspects of tinnitus over recent years and some very promising steps forward have been made with respect to the development of interventions that can have a marked impact on the well-being and quality of life of those people who are affected by the problem.

The aim of psychological treatment is to improve the ability of the individual to reduce the impact of tinnitus on their well-being and lifestyle. Various psychological approaches have been suggested as a means of achieving this outcome, including biofeedback (see Chapter 12), relaxation training, hypnosis, and cognitive therapy (see Chapter 13). It is commonly stated that psychological approaches are designed to assist people in *coping* with tinnitus. In this context, the term "coping" refers to the use of behaviors and cognitive processes to deal effectively with a problematic event or situations such as the hearing of tinnitus sounds. Some ways of coping may be more adaptive, leading to the amelioration of distress, whereas other ways of coping may be ineffective, failing to reduce the distressing impact of an aversive event. In this sense, the term "coping" is entirely neutral, referring either to good or poor coping. The judgment about the adequacy of coping is based on the outcome that is achieved when the person employs whatever coping strategies are available to them. Learning to live with tinnitus refers to the use of good coping skills or adapting to the tinnitus in spite of its continued presence. It is important that therapists discuss with patients the ways in which they might improve their ability to cope with tinnitus without inducing further negative emotional states such as guilt and depression about their apparent failure to cope successfully with the problem in the past.

It is apparent that not all people who experience tinnitus have difficulty in coping with it. Various processes have been suggested to account for poor coping, such as a failure to habituate (Hallam, Rachman, & Hinchcliffe, 1984) or lack of control over the sound (Jakes, Hallam, Rachman, & Hinchcliffe, 1986). Anxiety and depression appear to be the most common psychological responses to tinnitus (see Kirsch, Blanchard, & Parnes, 1989; Halford & Anderson, 1991a). As with most medical problems, it is understandable that people are initially anxious about the significance of the symptoms and the future course that the tinnitus might take. Following a period of medical consul-

tations, people may either be reassured on these issues or become depressed as a result of developing thoughts with themes of helplessness, victimization, catastrophization, and hopelessness about the future (Hallam, Jakes, & Hinchcliffe, 1988). In other words, people who cope less well with tinnitus are likely to engage in thoughts such as "tinnitus is the worst thing that could happen to me" or "my life will be never be the same because of the tinnitus," or "my tinnitus will just get worse and worse until I will not be able to stand it any longer."

ASSESSMENT OF PSYCHOLOGICAL ASPECTS OF TINNITUS

The aim of this section is to provide an overview of the psychological factors which a clinician needs to consider when interviewing a person about their tinnitus. The format of a comprehensive interview will be presented and the range of available self-report measures will be discussed. A thorough assessment of a person who experiences tinnitus should result in detailed information concerning: (1) history and descriptive characteristics of the tinnitus; (2) specific behavioral and cognitive features of the reaction to the tinnitus; and (3) factors which may exacerbate the tinnitus itself, or may lead to an increase in the person's tinnitus-related distress. The aim is not to investigate the specifically medical aspects of the tinnitus (see Chapter 9), as this can be accomplished better by a physician, but to arrive at an understanding of the nature of the tinnitus problem and to identify the causes of distress or impairment for each individual. Tinnitus patients should be referred to an otolaryngologist or other specialists for additional investigations. Of course, referral to an audiologist will be necessary in order to obtain an evaluation of the pitch and loudness of the tinnitus and the extent of any hearing impairment (see Chapter 6). The clinician also needs to be aware that, although people may complain of tinnitus, other problems may also be contributing to any negative emotional states that they report. For example, a coexistent hearing impairment or balance problems may contribute to the person's difficulties. Other life stressors may also have an impact on the person's ability to cope with the tinnitus at certain times although some people may incorrectly attribute their feelings of depression and anxiety entirely to the tinnitus. Keefe, Salley, and Lefebvre (1992) have drawn attention to this point in relation to chronic pain, by stating that "one might expect that the pain experience is the primary stressor with which the pain patient must cope. In most patients, however, multiple stressors (such as loss of income, confinement, and marital discord) are present and different sources of stress interact" (p. 131). It is useful to know the extent to which other sources of environmental stress are responsible for the person's current state and whether they exacerbate the person's reactions to their tinnitus. One aim of the initial assessment is to disentangle the important causal connections between tinnitus, other difficulties, and emotional states. This analysis is bound to occupy a lengthy period of time and draws upon general expertise in psychological assessment that goes well beyond the field of hearing impairment.

The interviewer needs to pose questions concerning the history and development of the tinnitus itself, together with basic features of the tinnitus (perceived loudness, type of sounds, location of sound, and so forth). An overview of the content of the interview is provided in Table 11-1. These questions provide an opportunity to understand how the patient views the problem. A thorough assessment of the qualitative features of the tinnitus may lead to the use of more individually tailored assessment monitoring tasks (such as the self-recording of dizziness, headaches, or insomnia). The tinnitus patient will gain greater confidence in the skills of the therapist if there has been an

Table 11-1. Content of interview for tinnitus

Description of current tinnitus
  – types of sounds, loudness, pitch, location, variability

History of tinnitus
  – duration, possible origin, treatments received

Other hearing problems
  – balance problems, dizziness

Other problems such as headaches, facial pain

Effect of tinnitus on sleep (falling asleep, staying asleep)

Effect of tinnitus on
  – work
  – participation in enjoyable activities
  – social interaction (with friends, family, partner)

Cognitive reactions to tinnitus
  – thoughts noticed when tinnitus is at its worst
  – thoughts noticed when trying to fall asleep

Behavioral aspects
  – avoidance of situations

Factors that appear to increase or decrease loudness

Factors that worsen or alleviate distress

Sources of stress in person's life
  – common daily hassles
  – major life events

Effect of daily stressors on tinnitus perception and distress

Effect of major life events on tinnitus perception and distress

Current depression and anxiety levels

Disentangling causal connection between tinnitus distress, other stressors, and emotional states (such as depression, anxiety and anger)

Risk of suicide
  – effects of tinnitus on mood and view of the future
  – does the person ever have thoughts about committing suicide?
  – frequency, recency, and controllability of suicidal thoughts
  – analysis of any previous attempts (how recent, means used, what prevented it)
  – current availability of means of committing suicide (such as pills, firearms)
  – look for themes of "hopelessness" or "sense of burden on others"

opportunity to describe the symptoms in detail. Thus, any assessment of tinnitus needs to commence with a thorough analysis of the experience of tinnitus by the patient.

Questions that revolve around the search for sources of stress are particularly important. It is often quite useful to discuss the concept of stress with the patient, pointing out that stressors may not necessarily be major catastrophes, but may be relatively minor, frequent hassles such as being interrupted when one is trying to complete some important work; getting caught in a traffic jam; dealing with difficult people; or rushing to the supermarket at the last moment to buy ingredients for a dinner party. A good deal of the interview should be directed towards understanding how the tinnitus affects the individual. It is important to investigate the nature of the cognitive appraisals that are made by the person when the tinnitus is especially troublesome, and to examine the impact of tinnitus on the person's work, sleep, social relations, and general lifestyle.

Another important area of investigation concerns the risk of suicide. The clinician should be particularly alert to cognitions with a theme of hopelessness, such as "my life will be ruined because of the tinnitus" or "I will never be able to experience any pleasure again in life because of this unbearable noise." People may contemplate suicide as a means of escaping from their unrelenting tinnitus. Rather than avoiding asking questions about suicide, the clinician should address the issue directly, commencing with questions about the effect of tinnitus on the person's mood, their view of the future, and leading on to more direct questions such as: "Does the tinnitus ever lead you to think about ending your own life"? The frequency, recency, and controllability of such thoughts should be assessed, together with more specific questions about previous attempts, the likely means of attempting suicide and the current availability of those means (such as access to a gun, possession of tablets such as antidepressant medication, and so on). A crisis form of cognitive therapy can be utilized in an attempt to

decrease the strength of suicidal feelings until the difficulties can be addressed in a more intensive fashion. In using cognitive therapy with suicidal people, the aim is to identify the most salient thoughts that lead the person to feelings of deep despair (often thoughts of hopelessness), the specific reasons for contemplating suicide, and the possible reasons for not committing suicide. These three areas can form the basis for challenging the existing beliefs and attitudes, at least to the point that the strength of the suicidal thoughts is decreased. From an international study of suicide in tinnitus patients, Lewis, Stephens, and McKenna (1994) identified the following risk factors for suicide: male; older age; social isolation; current depression and suicidal attempts in previous year. These factors, which are similar to those reported in other studies of suicide, need to be evaluated when assessing the likely risk of suicide. Of course, the clinician will need to consider the appropriateness of taking immediate steps to reduce the potential for self-harm by contacting other professionals or authorities, arranging for admittance to hospital, referral to other specialists and so forth. The precise steps that would be taken are beyond the scope of the present chapter and will depend upon the severity of suicidal risk and the training and professional expertise of the clinician.

Specific Assessment of Tinnitus

The most commonly employed tinnitus assessment device that is helpful in a psychological approach consists of a tinnitus monitoring form. Ratings of self-reported loudness, annoyance, interference, and sleep disturbance can be employed as a measure of treatment outcome, and as a means to identify temporal or other patterns of tinnitus occurrence. Patients can be asked to record any possible antecedent or consequential events on the tinnitus monitoring form once they have been trained to identify such events in the therapy sessions.

Apart from the interview and daily monitoring, the clinician may wish to administer one of the formal psychometric assessment devices that are now available. These measures include the Tinnitus Reaction Questionnaire (Wilson, Henry, Bowen, & Haralambous, 1991), Tinnitus Handicaps Questionnaire (Kuk, Tyler, Russell, & Jordan, 1990), Tinnitus Effects Questionnaire (Hallam, Jakes, & Hinchcliffe, 1988; Hallam, 1996) and the Tinnitus Cognitions Questionnaire (Wilson & Henry, 1998). The characteristics and uses of these measures are displayed in Table 11-2.

The Tinnitus Reaction Questionnaire was developed by Wilson et al. (1991) to measure psychological distress that is related to tinnitus. The scale consists of twenty-six items each of which is rated on a 5-point scale. The Tinnitus Reaction Questionnaire appears to have good psychometric properties, including a high degree of internal consistency (Cronbach's alpha = .96) and good test-retest stability (r = .88). The scale appears to be a valid device for the assessment of tinnitus-related psychological distress as revealed by generally moderate to high correlations with measures of depression and anxiety (Wilson et al., 1991). The Tinnitus Reaction Questionnaire is also significantly correlated with other measures to be described below (Henry & Wilson, 1998a), including the Tinnitus Handicaps Questionnaire (r = 0.76) and the Tinnitus Effects Questionnaire (r = 0.75). These findings all provide support for the construct validity of the Tinnitus Reaction Questionnaire. In a principal components factor analysis, two factors were identified: a general factor and a second factor which was interpreted as reflecting avoidance of and interference with activities. The Tinnitus Reaction Questionnaire may be a useful assessment device in clinical practice as a measure of psychological distress before and after treatment. The main value of the Tinnitus Reaction Questionnaire is in obtaining a global measure of the degree of distress experienced by the individual.

The Tinnitus Handicap Questionnaire was developed by Kuk et al. (1990) as a measure of the perceived degree of handi-

Table 11-2. Psychological measures related to tinnitus

Tinnitus Reaction Questionnaire (Wilson, Henry, Bowen, & Haralambous, 1991)
  – 26 items
  – measure of general distress related to tinnitus
  – best to use total score

Tinnitus Effects Questionnaire (Hallam, Jakes, & Hinchcliffe, 1988; Hallam, 1996)
  – 52 items
  – five subscales:
    – sleep disturbance
    – emotional distress
    – auditory-perceptual difficulties
    – intrusiveness
    – somatic complaints
  – best to use subscale scores

Tinnitus Handicap Questionnaire (Kuk, Tyler, Russell, & Jordan, 1990)
  – 27 items
  – three subscales:
    – emotional, social and physical effects
    – effects on hearing and communication
    – appraisal of the tinnitus

Tinnitus Severity Scale (Halford & Anderson, 1991b)
  – 16 items
  – measure of general distress related to tinnitus
  – best to use total score

Tinnitus Cognitions Questionnaire (Wilson & Henry, 1998)
  – 26 items (13 negative, 13 positive)
  – measure of thoughts about tinnitus
  – yields 3 scores: negative, positive, and total

Tinnitus Coping Style Questionnaire (Budd & Pugh, 1996)
  – 40 items
  – measures types of coping strategies

---

cap associated with tinnitus. The questionnaire consists of twenty-seven items such as "the general public does not know about the devastating nature of tinnitus" and "tinnitus causes me to feel depressed." Kuk et al (1990) report high internal consistency (Cronbach alpha = .95) and good test-retest reliability (r = 0.89) for the total scale. Henry and Wilson (1998a) also report in good test-retest reliability (r = 0.84 over six to eight weeks) and internal consistency (Cronbach alpha = 0.89) in an Australian sample. Both Kuk et al. (1990) and Henry and Wilson (1998a) report similar factorial solutions. The three factors can be interpreted as: (1) the emotional, social, and physical sequelae of tinnitus; (2) effects of tinnitus on hearing acuity and communication; (3) and appraisal of tinnitus. The first two factors also have good internal consistency and test-retest reliability (Kuk et al., 1990; Newman, Wharton, & Jacobson, 1995).

The Tinnitus Effects Questionnaire (sometimes called simply the Tinnitus Questionnaire) was developed by Hallam et al. (1988) as a measure of dimensions of complaints about tinnitus. For each of the fifty-two items respondents are asked to indicate their agreement by circling one of the three response alternatives—"True," "Partly true" or "Not true." Examples of items include: "I can sometimes ignore the noises even when they are there"; "your attitude to the noise makes no difference to how it affects you"; "it takes me longer to get to sleep because of the noises" and "I am a victim of my noises." Hallam et al. (1988) identified three factors as reflecting "sleep disturbance," "emotional distress," and "auditory perceptual difficulties." An earlier factor analysis (Jakes et al., 1985) had led to the identification of a factor which was described as "intrusiveness" which consisted of items reflecting self-report of loudness, and self-report of the tinnitus being distracting, unpleasant and resulting in inability to cope. In the comprehensive manual, Hallam (1996) reports that the test consists of these four subscales plus "somatic complaints." Evidence of good psychometric properties is presented, including high internal consistency for each of the subscales. Henry and Wilson (1998a) also report on the psychometric properties of Tinnitus Effects Questionnaire. Cronbach's alpha was found to be 0.91, indicating very good internal consistency. The test-retest correlation was 0.91 (n = 32; retest period six to eight weeks) which indicates very good stability over time. Factor analyses revealed five factors.

Factor 1 accounted for 21.0 percent of the variance and consisted of items which represent coping orientations to the problem of tinnitus, negative *cognitions or irrational beliefs* associated with tinnitus, and the emotional sequelae of tinnitus and effect on mood. Factor 2 accounted for 6.9 percent of the variance and consisted of items that tend to reflect the loudness/unpleasantness of the noise and its *persistence/intrusiveness.* Factor 3 accounted for 5.8 percent of the variance and consisted of items that reflect the effect of *tinnitus on communication* and hearing acuity, together with the general effect of the tinnitus on confidence and concentration. Factor 4 accounted for 4.4 percent of the variance and consisted of items which all tend to reflect the impact of tinnitus on *sleep.* Factor 5 accounted for 4.1 percent of the variance and consisted of items that reflect the effect of tinnitus on *physical well-being,* although some emotional effects and coping orientation items also load on this Factor. Hiller and Goebel (1992) have also reported the results of a factor analysis of a German translation of the Tinnitus Effects Questionnaire. They identified four factors that they interpreted as representing cognitive and emotional distress, intrusiveness, auditory-perceptual difficulties, and sleep disturbance. A fifth factor was interpreted as reflecting bodily complaints of the head and neck (headache, pain, tension). Hiller, Goebel, and Rief (1993) found high test-retest reliabilities for the full scale and the subscales. Overall, the results of the various factor analyses are remarkably similar. The practical implications of these results is that five subscale scores might be extracted for use in the assessment of patients with tinnitus. It is possible that different treatments may have differential impact on some of these subscales. Thus, evaluations of treatments, either in research or clinical contexts, might be conducted using these subscale scores as outcome measures.

Several other scales are worthy of brief mention at this point. The Subjective Tinnitus Severity Scale (Halford & Anderson,

1991b) is a sixteen-item scale which is designed to provide a general index of psychological distress. The Tinnitus Cognitions Questionnaire is a self-report scale which was designed by Wilson and Henry (1998) to assess the kinds of cognitions in which people report that they engage in relation to their tinnitus. The twenty-six items of the Tinnitus Cognitions Questionnaire consist of thirteen negative thoughts and thirteen positive thoughts are each rated on a five-point scale. For each item, respondents are asked to "indicate how often you have been aware of thinking a particular thought on occasions when you have noticed the tinnitus." The Tinnitus Cognitions Questionnaire may be a useful measure of the reported cognitive responses to tinnitus. For additional information on a tinnitus handicap/support scale the reader is also referred to Erlandson, Hallberg, and Axelsson (1992) and Tyler (1993). As can be seen from this overview, there are now quite a number of tinnitus-specific instruments that may be useful for the clinician to administer as part of a comprehensive assessment of patients with tinnitus.

Several other measures may be useful as part of a broad assessment of the individual. The Beck Depression Inventory (Beck, Ward, Mendelson, Mock, & Erbaugh, 1961) is the most widely used and well-validated self-report scale for the assessment of severity of depressive symptoms. The Beck Hopelessness Scale is a short instrument that can be used to assess the strength of feelings of hopelessness which have been found to be related to suicidal risk (Beck, Weissman, Lester, & Trexler, 1974). Both these questionnaires, together with individual items related to suicide on the specific tinnitus measures can be used to alert the clinician to the possibility of suicidal ideation. While we have not focused on audiological assessment in this chapter, it should be noted that a portable tinnitus matching device has been developed which, combined with daily-monitoring data, might prove to be a valuable additional assessment technique (Lindberg, Scott, Melin, & Lyttkens, 1995).

Information from the interviews, daily monitoring and the various self-report scales should enable the therapist to formulate a view about the nature of the difficulties experienced by the particular individual, the person's coping responses, their resources to deal with the problem, the influences on their perceptions of the tinnitus, the consequences of the tinnitus for the person's lifestyle, social relationships, and so forth. From this formulation, a specific treatment program may be developed which is likely to be effective for that individual.

PSYCHOLOGICAL TREATMENTS

Relaxation Methods

The earliest psychological approaches employed some form of relaxation training, including biofeedback. It needs to be recognized that biofeedback is simply a form of relaxation training in which a physiological response (such as muscle tension or skin temperature) is presented to the person in the form of a simple signal such as a tone which varies in intensity (pitch or loudness) as the response changes, assisting the person to learn ways to control their arousal level (Chapter 12). This approach may have a place in the treatment of tinnitus in people who have difficulty learning to achieve states of relaxation through less expensive, conventional methods.

Relaxation techniques have been widely employed in the management of health-related problems such as headaches or hypertension. It is generally thought that biofeedback and relaxation training achieve their effects through induction of a state of relaxation. There are several forms of relaxation training, but the commonly used method is referred to as progressive muscular relaxation (Bernstein & Borkovec, 1973). In this approach, the patient is shown how to decrease muscular tension through a series of structured exercises in which the therapist instructs them how to sequentially tense and relax various muscle groups.

Specific muscle groups include the forearms, upper arms, upper back, lower back, thighs, calves, feet, neck, shoulders, and various muscles in the face. A small amount of tension is often applied initially in order for the person to isolate the muscle in question more easily and to provide a means of learning to discriminate between tension and relaxation.

Although several sessions may be spent on showing the person the basic technique, an essential component of relaxation training consists of home practice on a daily basis. Although audiotapes may be a useful adjunct to treatment, they are seldom of much therapeutic value on their own. People are encouraged to view relaxation as a skill that needs to be practiced in order to be successfully acquired. The muscle groups are gradually amalgamated into larger units of the body, and the person moves from practice in comfortable settings to practice in real-life settings such as sitting on a bus, driving a car, doing the shopping, making a telephone call. The aim is to help the person to achieve states of relaxation in very brief periods of time, almost automatically as a response to detecting small levels of tension. Relaxation techniques may be helpful in assisting people to learn a way of coping either with the tension and anxiety caused by the tinnitus or in reducing their reactivity to nontinnitus sources of stress. In regard to the latter use, it has sometimes been suggested that stress may exacerbate tinnitus or lead a person to experience the tinnitus as louder, and that a reduction in stress levels may therefore reduce the annoyance of the tinnitus. Some specific benefits may be obtained from relaxation methods by those tinnitus patients who have sleep difficulties. When used as part of a program that is designed to decrease sleep difficulties, the person is instructed to practice the relaxation techniques when trying to fall asleep. Relaxation training has long been employed by psychologists as a means of reducing insomnia (see Morin, Culbert, & Schwartz, 1994). For patients

with severe sleep difficulties, training in relaxation techniques may provide some benefit with this particular problem. Our own impression from our clinical experience and the research literature is that biofeedback and/or relaxation training are of limited usefulness for most tinnitus patients *when used as the sole psychological treatment*. Nevertheless, a small proportion of tinnitus patients may derive some benefit from relaxation training, particularly as a means of coping with stressful situations.

Cognitive Therapy

Cognitive therapy will be described in some detail since this approach has emerged as the main psychological technique that may be helpful for tinnitus patients. A distinction needs to be made between two different types of cognitive therapy (see also Chapter 13). One form of cognitive therapy aims to assist the person to control the direction of attention (for example, imagery and attention-focus techniques). We will employ the term "attention-control" to refer to these approaches. The other cognitive techniques have the aim of altering the actual content of thoughts (cognitive restructuring). The two approaches share a similar overall philosophy in providing people with ways to manage their tinnitus by bringing cognitive processes under self-control.

Cognitive therapy was developed in the 1970s by Beck (Beck, Rush, Shaw, & Emery, 1979), Meichenbaum (1977), Mahoney (1974), and Bandura (1977), among others, as a treatment for emotional states such as depression and anxiety. Cognitive therapy techniques have been shown to be particularly effective as a treatment for depression (Hollon, Shelton, & Davis, 1993). Beck's cognitive theory asserts that the influence of a situation or event experienced by a person is through the way a person appraises an event. According to cognitive theory, the emotions that a person experiences is the result of the appraisals which are made of the event, not the event itself.

As described by Wilson and Henry (1993):

> Cognitive therapy involves the identification of dysfunctional beliefs and recurrent, persistent negative thoughts which occur in reaction to significant life events or daily stressors. People are taught methods to challenge those thoughts, and to substitute their catastrophic, unrealistic thoughts with more constructive ones, an approach known as cognitive restructuring. This is different from a simple "positive thinking" approach because the therapist and patient collaborate to identify particularly salient, idiosyncratic thoughts, to construct appropriate alternatives to such thinking, and to challenge dysfunctional beliefs. Although Beck has not written specifically about tinnitus, his theoretical stance would suggest that the source of distress for the tinnitus patient is the way in which the person perceives the tinnitus. The person may have negative thoughts such as "How can I live my life with this noise," "The noise is making my nerves bad," and "This is the worst thing to happen to anyone." Alternatively, a good coper might think: "The noise won't hurt me," "It has been as bad as this before, but it generally gets better after a while," and "If I do something enjoyable, I probably won't notice it as much." It would also be expected that people who have a certain set of beliefs that were held even before the tinnitus began, would be particularly likely to engage in these negative thoughts. For example, a person who believes that "it is it is essential for my satisfaction to have a perfectly healthy body," or that "any bodily ailment is a sign of deterioration or weakness," or "people will not like or respect me if I have any disability" would be especially prone to depression as a result of the development of tinnitus or other chronic health problems. (Wilson & Henry, 1993, p. 299).

Cognitive therapy involves a detailed examination of the content of thoughts that the person experiences when they are aware of or bothered by the tinnitus. Using cognitive restructuring techniques, the therapist helps the patient to identify the thoughts that commonly occur, to challenge the validity of these thoughts, and to learn ways to substitute more constructive thoughts. Cognitive therapy is a collaborative approach in which the client and therapist identify dysfunctional thoughts (beliefs, attitudes, or attributions) and to develop hypotheses which can be tested in relation to these thoughts. The therapist helps the client to challenge (or test) the validity of the thoughts as a description of themselves, the world or future events. The client is assisted in using such challenges in their natural environment through carefully constructed between-session assignments. Cognitive therapy is usually conducted in an intensive phase of treatment (such as weekly sessions for two to three months), sometimes followed by sessions that may be spaced out over longer intervals if it is considered that there is a high risk of relapse (see Wilson, 1992).

Cognitive therapy has been applied to chronic pain and other aversive medical problems (Nicholas, Wilson, & Goyen, 1991; Nicholas, Wilson, & Goyen, 1992; Turk Meichenbaum, & Genest, 1983; Turner & Clancy, 1988; Turner, Clancy, McQuade, & Cardenas, 1990). In the early 1980s, researchers and clinicians began extending the work on cognitive therapy into the area of tinnitus. The literature on cognitive therapy for tinnitus is now growing steadily. Several groups of researchers have been developing and refining the techniques, and conducting evaluations of the effects of treatment. These groups include Hallam, Jakes, and their colleagues in London; Lindberg, Scott, and colleagues in Uppsala; Henry, Wilson, and others in Australia; and Hiller and Goebel in Prien, Germany.

Attention Control Techniques

Mention has been made of the existence of attention-control approaches that aim to alter attentional processes through imagery or redirection of attention. For example, a person may be asked to imagine that the tinnitus is masked by the sound of a fountain or waterfall, or to imagine that they are lying down on a sloping, grassy hill, surrounded by trees in which insects are making a noise. In these imagery exercises, tinnitus is either masked ("waterfall") or incorporated into what may be a pleasant scene for some people (trees with insects). In another exercise, people may be asked to imagine controlling the direction of their attention to and from the tinnitus, perhaps alternating between the tinnitus sensations and the feelings in their feet or hands. The use of the word "control" here is quite deliberate. In other words, the aim is not just to learn to divert attention (although this might also be achieved), but to help the person to learn that they can control the direction of their attention. Switching to and from the tinnitus serves to illustrate that tinnitus is something which is part of one's body and need not be avoided. In fact, fighting against the tinnitus may only serve to maintain the focus on the sounds. Attentional and imagery techniques were originally developed for use in the management of chronic low back pain (Turk, Meichenbaum, & Genest, 1983), and have been adapted for use by tinnitus patients. In practice, these approaches are rarely used as the sole therapeutic method, but are incorporated into relaxation training or cognitive restructuring interventions. A relatively smooth transition can be made from relaxation techniques to attention control techniques because relaxation is itself a form of self-directed control. The cues to use the basic approach can also be placed on audiotapes so that the home practice of the technique can be facilitated and the most useful variant can be identified by the patient following a period of use over several weeks.

Several techniques are often integrated into the one therapeutic program. For example, Scott, Lindberg, Melin, and Lyttkens (1985) evaluated a cognitive technique that involved training subjects to "transfer their attention from their tinnitus to something unrelated to this phenomenon" (p. 227). Lindberg, Scott, Melin, and Lyttkens (1988) also describe a comprehensive approach that includes information, behavioral analy-

sis, relaxation training, and cognitive techniques. Similarly, Jakes, Hallam, Rachman, and Hinchcliffe (1986) employed a combined relaxation/attention-switching training preceded by an orientation phase involving education, and discussion of attitudes towards tinnitus. While it is possible to distinguish between these techniques, as we illustrate in Table 11-3, it is common to combine the approaches and to suggest to tinnitus patients that they should try a number of techniques and discover which ones work best for them.

OUTCOME OF THERAPY

Over the last fifteen years there has been a steady flow of research studies on the effectiveness of psychological methods to help people to manage their tinnitus. Early studies tended to focus on the efficacy of progressive muscular relaxation training

Table 11-3. Cognitive and behavioral techniques

Relaxation Training
 — Information about relaxation
 — Identification of stressors
 — Link between stressors and tension
 — Discussion of tinnitus as a stressor
 — Relaxation of each major muscle group
 — Home practice
 — Use of relaxation in real-life situations

Cognitive Therapy
 — Identification of negative, maladaptive thoughts and beliefs
 — Thought monitoring
 — Challenging of unhelpful cognitions
 — Substituting with constructive thoughts
 — Applying the challenging in real life settings

Attention Control
 — Learning to direct attention to and from tinnitus
 — Applying the attention control in real life settings

Imagery Training
 — Absorbing the tinnitus sound into image (for example, rushing sound into waterfall)
 — Using pleasant visual imagery
 — Applying the imagery training in real-life settings

(Ireland, Wilson, Tonkin, & Platt-Hepworth, 1985) or biofeedback (Borton & Clark, 1988; Borton, Moore, & Clark, 1981; Elfner, May, Moore, & Mendelson, 1981; Erlandsson, Carlsson, & Svensson, 1989; Grossan, 1976; Haralambous, Wilson, Platt-Hepworth, Tonkin, Hensley, & Kavanagh, 1987; House, 1978; Kirsch, Blanchard, & Parnes, 1987; Svihovec & Carmen, 1982; Walsh & Gerley, 1985; White, Hoffman, & Gale, 1986). These studies have produced mixed results. From our own research, we concluded that neither relaxation training nor electro-myographic biofeedback, when delivered alone, has a beneficial effect on tinnitus (Haralambous et al. 1987; Ireland et al., 1985). On the other hand, Scott et al. (1985) evaluated a treatment that involved both relaxation training and cognitive coping techniques. They randomly assigned subjects to either this type of treatment or to a no-treatment control condition and found that patients who received treatment improved significantly more than the waiting-list controls on measures of depression, subjective tinnitus loudness, and tinnitus-discomfort. The effects on tinnitus discomfort were maintained at a nine-month follow-up (Lindberg, Scott, Melin, & Lyttkens, 1987). In a later study, Lindberg, Scott, Melin, and Lyttkens (1989) compared three groups: relaxation training with direct exposure to tinnitus-provoking auditory stimulation; relaxation with distraction/imagery methods; and a waiting list control. In comparison to the waiting-list control group, both treatments resulted in improvement on measures of subjective loudness, discomfort from tinnitus, and ability to control the discomfort from tinnitus. Subsequently, in a large study that involved seventy-five patients, Lindberg et al. (1988) reported the results of a comprehensive cognitive-behavioral therapy that included information, behavioral analysis, relaxation training, and cognitive techniques. At the three-month follow-up, 75 percent of subjects reported improvements in their tinnitus complaints. Although there was no control group in this study, the results are suggestive of the im-

portance of psychological factors in the amelioration of tinnitus-related distress.

As with the Australian and Swedish groups, relaxation training figured prominently in the initial work which was conducted in the United Kingdom by Hallam, Jakes and their colleagues (Jakes et al., 1986). They compared the effects of two treatments: (1) relaxation training and (2) a combined relaxation/attention-switching training. Both treatments were preceded by an orientation phase that involved education, and a discussion of attitudes towards tinnitus that resembles cognitive therapy. The attention-switching consisted of learning to shift attention from tinnitus during relaxation to distracting stimuli such as "external background sounds or pleasant images" (p. 499) while being relaxed. Although there were no differences in effectiveness between the two modes of treatment, there were significant reductions in annoyance, distress, insomnia, depression, and interference with daily activities. Jakes et al. report that treatment was clinically significant in nine of the twenty-four patients.

In view of the success of cognitive approaches in the treatment of depression, the presence of catastrophic and other negative cognitions in tinnitus patients, and the frequent co-existence of depression with tinnitus, we designed several experiments to evaluate the efficacy of cognitive therapy in the management of tinnitus. In the most important of these studies (Henry & Wilson, 1996), sixty people with tinnitus were randomly allocated to either cognitive/educational therapy, an education only program, or a waiting-list control condition. The cognitive therapy that was employed in this study involved a combination of both the cognitive restructuring methods and the attention-diversion approach. Henry and Wilson (1996) found that the cognitive/educational treatment was more effective than either of the other groups in reducing tinnitus-related distress (that is, lowering scores on the Tinnitus Reaction Questionnaire, Tinnitus Handicap Questionnaire and the emotional distress subscale of the Tinnitus

Effects Questionnaire), and decreasing reported engagement in dysfunctional cognitions (as measured by the Tinnitus Cognitions Questionnaire). The lack of improvement in the educational program or waiting-list control suggests that the effects of treatment cannot be attributed to either nonspecific treatment factors nor natural remission processes. Thus, the results of this experiment provide the clearest support to date for the efficacy of a cognitive approach to the management of tinnitus-related distress. Admittedly, we have expressed a need for caution about the interpretation of this study because only about half the sample achieved a clinically significant result and, while the effects were well-maintained up to eight months, a notable relapse had occurred by the twelve-month assessment session.

Several other smaller studies are worthy of comment here. Henry and Wilson (1998b) compared: (1) cognitive restructuring, (2) attention control and imagery training, (3) the combination of the two techniques, and (4) a waiting-list control condition. The results revealed some effects in favor of the cognitive restructuring and combined approaches although subjects who received the combined treatment improved more than subjects in the single treatments on the Tinnitus Reaction Questionnaire. It should also be noted that the best clinical effects have been found in our studies in which treatment continued for from eight to ten sessions with a combination of individual and group formats (Wilson, Bowen, & Farag, 1992).

The group in the United Kingdom has also explored the efficacy of cognitive therapy (Jakes, Hallam, McKenna, & Hinchcliffe, 1992). In this study, subjects were randomly allocated to one of five groups: (1) cognitive therapy, (2) masker, (3) cognitive therapy plus masker, (4) placebo masker, or (5) a waiting-list control. The results of this study are less clear cut. While there was no indication of differential effectiveness of the various treatments at the end of treatment, some modest effects in favor of cognitive

therapy were found at a three-month follow-up on the emotional distress subscale of the Tinnitus Effects Questionnaire. However, it should be noted that the length of therapy in this study was fairly brief and that, as a result, there was fairly limited time for the implementation of each of the components.

In one of the most recent studies to have appeared, Davies, McKenna, and Hallam (1995) compared individual cognitive therapy with applied relaxation training and passive relaxation training. The applied relaxation training included some of the cognitive control procedures that were mentioned previously (reinterpreting tinnitus as pleasant interpretations of the sounds such as "wind in the trees"). Subjects in the applied relaxation training were taught to use the relaxation methods in individually identified problematic situations. Passive relaxation simply involved learning to relax without specific instructions about using the techniques in everyday situations. The cognitive therapy involved the cognitive restructuring procedures in which maladaptive thoughts were identified and ways to challenge these thoughts were developed. A total of thirty subjects completed the treatment to which they had been randomly allocated. Because of a high discontinuance rate in the passive relaxation training group (54 percent), the main comparisons were limited to the other two treatments. Cognitive therapy and applied relaxation training were both associated with significant improvements on the Tinnitus Effects Questionnaire and measures of depression and anxiety, but there were no differences between the treatments in the amount of improvement on these measures. The applied relaxation training appeared to have a more positive impact on ratings of annoyance although this effect was not maintained at a four-month follow-up. In general, the positive initial effects were not maintained, as judged from the standardized measures, although a blind assessor judged only 2/26 patients to be in need of further therapy at follow-up. The disappointing results at follow-up, at least on the self-report measures, are in contrast to previous findings by this group of researchers. The authors suggest that the group version of the cognitive therapy that had been used in previous studies may actually be more beneficial than the individual version which was used in this study.

Kroner-Herwig, Hebing, Van Rijn-Kalkmann, Frenzel, Schilowsky, and Esser (1995) compared cognitive-behavioral group training, yoga and a self-monitoring control condition with a sample of forty-three tinnitus patients. The cognitive-behavioral approach was found to produce greater reductions in difficulties associated with tinnitus than either of the other conditions on measures that included the Tinnitus Effects Questionnaire and a number of other indices of improvement. Treatment effects were maintained at a three-month follow-up.

Collectively, the results of the studies that have been cited in the previous section suggest that psychological approaches, particularly those that involve cognitive methods hold great promise for people who experience distress related to their tinnitus. Cognitive therapy needs to be delivered in a sufficiently intense format in order to produce clinically beneficial results. The authors would argue that multiple components (such as cognitive restructuring, attention control, imagery training, and relaxation methods) are probably necessary in order to obtain the best results. This is hardly surprising, given the complex nature of the tinnitus-related distress. There is a need for sufficient time to be allowed for each component to be introduced and to permit practice to take place between sessions. Many of the published studies involve treatment in a group format (the Swedish studies are an exception to this observation). This approach is presumably helpful for some people, who come into contact with other people who have experienced similar difficulties and provide some opportunities for modeling, but may be less helpful to other people who do not fully engage in the group process. The studies

that have been conducted to date have helped to identify some of the potentially important components of treatment. There is now a need for research to be undertaken which is capable of identifying those people who display the best response to treatment so that they can be selected for future applications of these approaches in community and hospital settings. More research will need to be conducted in order to identify the reasons for failure to respond to these approaches in that subset of people who do not currently benefit from psychological approaches. This research will involve making predictions from existing theoretical positions about the nature of coping with chronic aversive stimuli and including appropriate measures at the pretreatment assessment session so that these measures can be used to identify subsequent responders and nonresponders to treatment. Variables of interest would include pretreatment level of depression, duration of the tinnitus, sense of control over the tinnitus, and optimism. The authors would predict that the less successful candidates for treatment are those who: (1) continue to search for a medical cure or have unrealistic expectations that psychological treatment will remove their tinnitus, (2) maintain a high level of anger about the origin of their tinnitus and the failure of researchers and medical practitioners to find a solution, and (3) have multiple stressors in their lives, especially those who misattribute their emotional distress to the tinnitus when the other sources of emotional difficulty should be more directly addressed.

Another area that deserves greater attention is the maintenance of treatment effects for long periods after initial treatment. Booster sessions may assist people in maintaining the effects of treatment (see Lindberg et al., 1988). Other more specific methods that have been developed for use with depressed patients may also be adapted for tinnitus patients (Wilson, 1992). Given the promising results from studies of the initial cognitive-behavioral interventions, attention could usefully shift towards the evaluation of relapse-prevention programs for tinnitus. One such study has recently being conducted by the authors in Australia (Henry & Wilson, 1999). Following an initial eight-week treatment phase, the responders received either: (1) relapse-prevention; (2) regular, non-structured contact; or (3) no further contact during the follow-up period (twelve months). The relapse-prevention involved a structured program in which a number of specific relapse prevention strategies were included such as: preparing for future life-stressors; increasing engagement in pleasant activities; identifying and dealing with situations that place the person at high risk for relapse; coping with future negative emotional states, and developing appropriate responses to any subsequent relapse. This study produced a high response rate for the initial treatment program (approximately 74 percent), a result that was largely maintained in the longer term, irrespective of the type of contact that occurred during the follow-up period.

Overview of Ideal Intervention Program

What should be included in an ideal psychological program for tinnitus patients? At the outset, there is a need for a careful analysis of the problem as there are wide individual variations in the ways in which people are affected by tinnitus. In a group program, this analysis can still be achieved by a separate initial assessment session and by individualizing the treatment components based on this information. The assessment devices that have been described earlier can be administered at this stage in order to more systemically gather information about the level of distress experienced by the person (especially on the Tinnitus Reaction Questionnaire or the Tinnitus Severity Scale), and a more detailed analysis of the components of the person's difficulties (on the Tinnitus Effects Questionnaire or the Tinnitus Handicaps Questionnaire). Some form of daily monitoring is also useful at this stage (monitoring of self-

perceived loudness, mood, sleep difficulties). It is particularly important to assess the presence of diagnosable disorders such as depression and anxiety and to evaluate the risk of suicide. Clearly, if severe levels of depression are present, or if suicidal risk is judged to be high, referral for more immediate attention from an appropriately qualified specialist is necessary. The initial session should also provide an opportunity to present information on tinnitus, the ear structure and hearing processes, and to reassure the person that there is hope for a better future. It is important that the patient understands the role of psychological assistance with the problem. Patients often misperceive the referral to a psychologist as indicating that others believe that their tinnitus is not real—that they are imagining the sounds. Little will be achieved unless the patient understands that the aim is to assist the person to enjoy a high-quality lifestyle despite tinnitus and that there is much that they can achieve by understanding their reaction to the tinnitus and gaining control over their emotional states.

As part of the assessment process the therapist needs to choose the best component with which to commence therapy. Starting with relaxation training often has the advantage that the person can quickly gain a sense of control over their body. This sense of control can increase the person's confidence that something can be achieved from attending the sessions and may provide a basis for moving on to the attention control components. The cognitive therapy procedures can be incorporated into the treatment in parallel with the other approaches. It generally takes some time for people to gain control over their cognitive reactions to the tinnitus, and there is some advantage to be gained from commencing this process at an early stage. Monitoring of thoughts about tinnitus on a daily basis can generate useful material for discussion. The monitoring will often help to increase the person's awareness about the content of their thoughts so that the therapist can begin to identify any common themes. Challenging the thoughts, which is necessarily a collaborative effort between the therapist and the client, can gradually be extended to occupy increasing amounts of time in the sessions. It is extremely important that therapists who have not been trained in these techniques are aware that cognitive therapy does not simply involve replacing negative thoughts with positive thoughts, but is an active process through which the client learns: to identify maladaptive thought content; to challenge those thoughts; and to develop idiosyncratic constructive responses to these thoughts. Home practice in real-life situations is an important part of this process. Over time, like relaxation, this process should ideally become more or less automatic.

CONCLUSION

In this chapter we have attempted to identify the contribution that can be made by psychological approaches to the assessment and management of tinnitus. As stated at the outset, the aim of psychological approaches is not to "treat" the tinnitus, but to help people to enjoy a greater quality of life and achieve a sense of well-being despite the presence of the tinnitus. Of course, when people can employ these psychological techniques successfully and automatically, it is quite likely that the person will notice their tinnitus less often and will be less bothered by it. Following a thorough assessment of the patient via an interview and administration of a number of specific self-report measures, the clinician can select treatments or tailor the components of treatment according to the results of this initial analysis. A number of controlled studies have revealed significant treatment effects for cognitive therapy, including cognitive restructuring and attentional control approaches. Multiple treatment components, such as combined cognitive therapy, attention control and relaxation training, appear to produce the most consistent positive results. Relaxation training may be useful as a vehicle for teaching some of the cognitive attention control methods, for helping people with sleep problems, or for reducing general reactivity to stress. There is a need to build upon the knowledge that we have now gained and to develop additional therapeutic procedures to increase the proportion of patients who benefit and subsequently maintain the initial improvements after treatment.

REFERENCES

Bandura, A. (1977). Self-efficacy: Toward a unifying theory of behavioral change. *Psychological Review, 84,* 191–215.

Beck, A. T., Rush, A. J., Shaw, B. F., & Emery, G. (1979). *Cognitive therapy of depression.* New York: Guilford.

Beck, A. T., Ward, C. H., Mendelson, M., Mock, J., & Erbaugh, J. (1961). An inventory for measuring depression. *Archives of General Psychiatry, 4,* 561–571.

Beck, A. T., Weissman, A., Lester, D., & Trexler, L. (1974). The measurement of pessimism: The Hopelessness Scale. *Journal of Consulting and Clinical Psychology, 42,* 861–865.

Bernstein, D. A., & Borkovec, T. D. (1973). *Progressive relaxation training: A manual for the helping professions.* Champaign, IL: Research Press.

Borton, T. E., & Clark, S. R. (1988). Electromyographic biofeedback for treatment of tinnitus. *The American Journal of Otology, 9,* 23–30.

Borton, T. E., Moore, W. H., & Clark, S. R. (1981). Electromyographic feedback treatment for tinnitus aurium. *Journal of Speech and Hearing Disorders, 46,* 39.

Budd, R. J., & Pugh, R. (1996). Tinnitus coping style and its relationship to tinnitus severity and emotional distress. *Journal of Psychosomatic Research, 4,* 327–335.

Davies, S., McKenna, L., & Hallam, R. S. (1995). Relaxation and cognitive therapy: A controlled trial in chronic tinnitus. *Psychology & Health, 10,* 129–144.

Elfner, L. F., May, J. G., Moore, J. D., & Mendelson, J. H. (1981). Effects of EMG and thermal feedback training on tinnitus: A case study. *Biofeedback and Self-Regulation, 6,* 517–521.

Erlandsson, S., Carlsson, S. G., & Svensson, A. (1989). Biofeedback in the treatment of tinnitus: A broadened approach. *Goteborg Psychological Reports, 19*, 6:1–6:12.

Erlandsson, S. I., Hallberg, L., & Axelsson, A. (1992). Psychological and audiological correlates to perceived tinnitus severity. *Audiology, 31*, 168–179.

Grossan, M. (1976). Treatment of subjective tinnitus with biofeedback. *Ear, Nose, Throat Journal, 55*, 22–30.

Halford, J. B. S., & Anderson, S. D. (1991a). Anxiety and depression in tinnitus sufferers. *Journal of Psychosomatic Research, 35*, 383–390.

Halford, J. B. S., & Anderson, S. D. (1991b). Tinnitus severity measured by a subjective scale, audiometry and clinical judgement. *Journal of Laryngology and Otology, 105*, 89–93.

Hallam, R. S. (1996). *Manual of the Tinnitus Questionnaire (TQ).* The Psychological Corporation, Harcourt Brace & Co.

Hallam, R. S., Jakes, S. C., & Hinchcliffe, R. (1988). Cognitive variables in tinnitus annoyance. *British Journal of Clinical Psychology, 27*, 213–222.

Hallam, R. S., Rachman, S. J., & Hinchcliffe, R. (1984). Psychological aspects of tinnitus. In S. J. Rachman (Ed.), *Contributions to medical psychology* (Vol. 30). New York: Pergamon Press.

Haralambous, G., Wilson, P. H., Platt-Hepworth, S., Tonkin, J. P., Hensley, V. R., & Kavanagh, D. J. (1987). EMG biofeedback in the treatment of tinnitus: An experimental evaluation. *Behaviour Research and Therapy, 25*, 49–55.

Henry, J. L., & Wilson, P. H. (1996). The psychological management of tinnitus: Comparison of a combined cognitive educational program, education alone and a waiting-list control. *International Tinnitus Journal, 2*, 9–20.

Henry, J. L., & Wilson, P. H. (1998a). The psychometric properties of two measures of tinnitus complaint and handicap. *International Tinnitus Journal, 4*, 114–121.

Henry, J. L., & Wilson, P. H. (1998b). An evaluation of two types of cognitive intervention in the management of chronic tinnitus. *Scandanavian Journal of Behaviour Therapy, 27*, 156–166.

Henry, J. L., & Wilson, P. H. (2000). Comprehensive cognitive-behaviour therapy for tinnitus: Effects of initial treatment and relapse prevention. (in preparation).

Hiller, W., & Goebel, G. A. (1992). A psychometric study of complaints in chronic tinnitus. *Journal of Psychosomatic Research, 36*, 337–348.

Hiller, W., Goebel, G., & Rief, W. (1994). Reliability of self-rated distress and association with psychological symptom patterns. *British Journal of Clinical Psychology, 33*, 231–239.

Hollon, S. D., Shelton, R. C., & Davis, D. D. (1993). Cognitive therapy for depression: Conceptual issues and clinical efficacy. *Journal of Consulting and Clinical Psychology, 61*, 270–275.

House, J. W. (1978). Treatment of severe tinnitus with biofeedback training. *Laryngoscope, 88*, 406–412.

Ireland, C. E., Wilson, P. H., Tonkin, J. P., & Platt-Hepworth, S. (1985). An evaluation of relaxation training in the treatment of tinnitus. *Behaviour Research and Therapy, 23*, 423–430.

Jakes, S. C., Hallam, R. S., McKenna, L., & Hinchcliffe, R. (1992). Group cognitive therapy for medical patients: An application to tinnitus. *Cognitive Therapy and Research, 16*, 67–82.

Jakes, S. C., Hallam, R. S., Rachman, S., & Hinchcliffe, R. (1986). The effects of reassurance, relaxation training and distraction on chronic tinnitus sufferers. *Behaviour Research and Therapy, 24*, 497–507.

Keefe, F. J., Salley, A. N., & Lefebvre, J. C. (1992). Coping with pain: Conceptual concerns and future directions. *Pain, 51*, 131–134.

Kirsch, C. A., Blanchard, E. B., & Pares, S. M. (1989). Psychological characteristics of individuals high and low in their ability to cope with tinnitus. *Psychosomatic Medicine, 51*, 209–217.

Kroner-Herwig, B., Hebing, G., Van-Rijn-Kalkmann, U., Frenzel, A., Schilowsky, & Esser. (1995). The management of chronic tinnitus: Comparison of a cognitive-behavioural group training with yoga. *Journal of Psychosomatic Research, 39*, 153–165.

Kuk, F. K., Tyler, R. S., Russell, D., & Jordan, H. (1990). The psychometric properties of a Tinnitus Handicap Questionnaire. *Ear and Hearing, 11*, 434–442.

Lewis, J. E., Stephens, S. D. G., & McKenna, L. (1994). Tinnitus and suicide. *Clinical Otolaryngology, 19*, 50–54.

Lindberg, P., Scott, B., Melin, L., & Lyttkens, L. (1987). Long-term effects of psychological treatment of tinnitus. *Scandinavian Audiology, 16*, 167–172.

Lindberg, P., Scott, B., Melin, L., & Lyttkens, L. (1988). Behavioral therapy in the clinical management of tinnitus. *British Journal of Audiology, 22*, 265–272.

Lindberg, P., Scott, B., Melin, L., & Lyttkens, L. (1989). The psychological treatment of tinnitus: An experimental evaluation. *Behaviour Research and Therapy 27*, 593–603.

Lindberg, P., Scott, B., Melin, L., & Lytkkens, L. (1995). Matching tinnitus in natural environments with portable equipment. *Journal of Audiological Medicine, 4*, 143–159.

Mahoney, M. J. (1974). *Cognition and behaviour modification.* Cambridge, Mass.: Ballinger.

Meichenbaum, D. H. (1977). *Cognitive behaviour modification.* New York: Plenum Press.

Morin, C. M., Culbert, J. P., & Schwartz, S. (1994). Nonpharmacological interventions for insomnia: A meta-analysis of treatment efficacy. *American Journal of Psychiatry, 151*, 1172–1180.

Newman, C. W., Wharton, J. A., & Jacobson, G. P. (1995). Retest stability of the Tinnitus Handicap Questionnaire. *Annals of Otology, Rhinology, and Laryngology, 104*, 718–723.

Nicholas, M. K., Wilson, P. H., & Goyen, J. (1991). An evaluation of cognitive and behavioural treatments for chronic low back pain, with and without relaxation training. *Behaviour Research and Therapy, 29*, 225–238.

Nicholas, M. K., Wilson, P. H., & Goyen, J. (1992). Comparison of cognitive-behavioral group treatment and an alternative, non-psychological treatment for chronic low back pain. *Pain, 48*, 339–347.

Scott, B., Lindberg, P., Melin, L., & Lyttkens, L. (1985). Psychological treatment of tinnitus: An experimental group study. *Scandinavian Audiology, 14*, 223–230.

Svihovec, D., & Carmen, R. (1982). Relaxation-biofeedback treatment for tinnitus. *Hearing Instruments, 33*, 32.

Tonndorf, J. (1987). The origin of tinnitus—A new hypothesis: An analogy with pain. *Proceedings of the Third International Tinnitus Seminar.* Munster, Harsch Verlag Karlsruhe, 70–74.

Turk, D. C., Meichenbaum, D. H., & Genest, M. (1983). *Pain and behavioral medicine: A cognitive-behavioral perspective.* New York: Guilford Press.

Turner, J. A., & Clancy, S. (1988). Comparison of operant behavioral and cognitive-behavioral group treatment for chronic low back pain. *Journal of Consulting and Clinical Psychology, 56*, 261–266.

Turner, J. A., Clancy, S., McQuade, K. J., & Cardenas, D. D. (1990). Effectiveness of behavioral therapy for chronic low back pain: A component analysis. *Journal of Consulting and Clinical Psychology, 58*, 573–579.

Tyler, R. S. (1993). Tinnitus disability and handicap questionnaires. *Seminars in Hearing, 14*, 377– 384.

Walsh, W. M., & Gerley, P. P. (1985). Thermal biofeedback and the treatment of tinnitus. *Laryngoscope, 95*, 987–989.

White, T. P., Hoffman, S. R., & Gale, E. N. (1986). Psychophysiological therapy for tinnitus. *Ear and Hearing, 7*, 397–399.

Wilson, P. H. (Ed.) (1992). *Principles and practice of relapse prevention.* New York: Guilford Press.

Wilson, P. H., Bowen, M., & Farag, P. (1992). Cognitive and relaxation techniques in the management of tinnitus. In *Proceedings of the Fourth International Tinnitus Conference* (Bordeaux, France).

Wilson, P. H., & Henry, J. L. (1993). Psychological approaches in the management of tinnitus. *Australian Journal of Otolaryngology, 1*, 296–302.

Wilson, P. H., & Henry, J. L. (1998). Tinnitus Cognitions Questionnaire: Development and psychometric properties of a measure of dysfunctional cognitions associated with tinnitus. *International Tinnitus Journal, 4*, 23–30.

Wilson, P. H., Henry, J. L., Bowen, M., & Haralambous, G. (1991). Tinnitus Reaction Questionnaire: Psychometric properties of a measure of distress associated with tinnitus. *Journal of Speech and Hearing Research, 34*, 197–201.

CHAPTER 12

Biofeedback Training in the Treatment of Tinnitus

David W. Young, M. A.

INTRODUCTION

This chapter provides an introduction to biofeedback, an overview of its history, concepts, and methods, and a review of its applications to tinnitus. Biofeedback has been classified as a component of behavioral medicine (Friedman, Sedler, Myers, & Benson, 1997). Grounded in notions of patient responsibility and self-care, biofeedback training can assist the individual in making changes to improve health. Its techniques, as with other behavioral medicine approaches, are objective and standardized. While it addresses the psychosocial nature of illness, it is intended to elicit changes in physical symptomology through self-regulation of the autonomic nervous system. While it has at times been considered as an alternative medical treatment, it stands apart from those alternative approaches that lack rigorous scientific foundation. Biofeedback is based on demonstrable physiological principles and, in recent years, has been submitted to the scientific method with ever-increasing frequency.

CONCEPTS, HISTORY, AND APPLICATIONS

Overview

Biofeedback training is used in learning to control physiological processes associated with the stress response. Biofeedback instruments monitor these processes and present this information to the individual in auditory or visual form. The person learns to control the auditory or visual signals as a step toward influencing blood pressure, vasodilation and peripheral skin temperature, muscle tension, and brainwave activity. The goal in biofeedback treatment is to reduce symptomology by moderating stress or tension and to increase the patient's capacity to manage despite the presence of illness.

The modalities used in biofeedback may include electromyography, peripheral skin temperature training, electrodermal activity, heart rate, blood volume, respiration, and electroencephalography. Instruments are used to closely monitor physiological processes associated with each of these modalities. For example, the electrical activity evident in muscle tissue are monitored in electromyography. With peripheral skin temperature training, skin temperature is monitored as a reflection of vasodilation or vasoconstriction. The feedback provided can be visual, auditory, or sometimes kinesthetic and has inherent reinforcing properties. In the treatment process, the therapist assumes the role of "coach" or trainer as the person receives information from the instruments. The therapist's goal is to encourage self-regulation without the biofeedback instruments and assist the person in transferring skills learned in biofeedback training to everyday life.

The metaphor of a "mirror" is useful in describing how biofeedback instruments are used. Simply stated, they provide the patient with a view or "reflection" of physiological processes associated with the stress response. This view, unavailable without the instruments, is then used to gain control over the body's response to stress. The patient first learns to control the external signal from the equipment. As the person becomes familiar with subtle internal shifts of posture, thought, breathing, or other experience or sensation associated with change in the external signal, they practice these on their own. Eventually, the equipment is no longer needed.

The training process combines both trial and error learning with exercises designed to encourage relaxation, such as autogenics or progressive muscle relaxation. Autogenics is an exercise in which patients silently repeat phrases aimed at encouraging the relaxation response. These phrases include themes of heaviness, warmth, and calmness. Progressive muscle relaxation (Wolpe, 1973) is among the more commonly used relaxation exercises. In practice, it involves having the patient tense and relax various muscle groups, usually in order beginning with the feet and finishing with those in the head. The patient is encouraged to focus on the difference in sensation between tension and relaxation.

Conceptual Basis and Historical Development

The instruments used in biofeedback were available long before their use in self-regulation of the stress response. Their use began in the 1950s and 1960s, when research in self-regulation suggested individuals could learn to control autonomic functions if provided accurate information or "feedback." From that point forward, the field of biofeedback grew from a convergence of trends in several disciplines. Schwartz and Olson (1995) identified the trends which were most influential in the development of biofeedback. The antecedent fields included:

Instrumental Conditioning of the Autonomic Nervous System

For several decades, learning theorists assumed that the autonomic nervous system could not be controlled through conscious mediation. A series of human and animal studies suggested otherwise (Harris & Brady, 1974). These studies revealed changes in vasomotor responses, blood pressure, salivation, galvanic skin response, and cardiac rhythm could be conditioned or controlled by external stimuli. The assumptions that autonomic nervous system responses could not come under voluntary control were challenged. It was argued that if a person could improve the accuracy of their perceptions of visceral events, then control of vasomotor responses, blood pressure, salivation, galvanic skin response, and cardiac rhythm could be gained. The legitimacy of clinical biofeedback grew as additional research supported the findings of these early studies.

Psychophysiology

Psychophysiology refers to the study of interrelationships of physiological and cognitive processes. In biofeedback, the person utilizes thoughts, images, words, and other cognitive mediated stimuli to gain control of physiological processes. These include muscle activity, blood flow, sweat gland activity, and skin temperature, each of which are associated with the stress response. As the medical community began to recognize and accept the interaction between mind-body processes, biofeedback developed as a legitimate treatment option.

Behavior Therapy and Behavior Medicine

Behavioral medicine refers to the application of principles of behavior and learning to medical disorders and health. Clinicians within behavioral medicine recognize the importance of stress, habits, and environmental variables in the contribution to disease, chronic illness, and health. Intervention occurs within the patient's environment and is aimed at assisting the person in becoming responsible in their health and well-being. Biofeedback is based on many behavioral principles and strongly emphasizes the responsibility the patient has in their health care.

Stress Research

Cannon (1932) and Selye (1974) are credited with two significant advances in stress research. Cannon developed the concept of the "fight-or-flight" response, referring to a person's innate response when confronted with stress. Selye identified the stages of alarm, resistance, and exhaustion when referring to how individuals first experience stressors, become used to them, and then become overwhelmed. Together, their work focused attention on the impact stress had on illness and health. Biofeedback and relaxation were supported as methods of treatment aimed at improving health through stress management.

Biomedical Engineering

Significant advances occurred in the area of biomedical engineering following World War II, allowing for measurement of sweat gland activity, skin temperature, and muscle activity. Heart rate, respiration, and brain waves are additional measures used in biofeedback. Computers allow for multiple channel feedback, storage of data, and improved capabilities of reviewing progress.

Electromyography

Electromyography training is among the more commonly used modalities in biofeedback. The use of instruments to monitor muscle tension extends back to the early part of the century. It was not until the 1960s that electromyography was recognized for its potential value in retraining muscle groups. Electromyography in biofeedback is commonly used to treat chronic pain, headaches, and incontinence (Schwartz, 1995).

Electroencephalographic Training

From the late 1960s into the 1970s, a series of studies revealed an association between alpha-wave activity and relaxed, yet alert, states of consciousness. Clinicians began using alpha-wave training for developing a general relaxed state. Electroencephalographic biofeedback training in the clinical setting has been used in treating seizure disorders and attention-deficit disorder (Schwartz, 1995).

Cybernetics

The field of cybernetics examines how information is processed by systems and how change occurs as a result (Watzlawick, Bavelas, & Jackson, 1967). Cybernetic theory suggests that information travels within a series of "feedback loops" which the system then uses to make changes or regulate itself within its environment. Positive feedback leads to change, whereas negative feedback encourages homeostasis, stability, or equilibrium. Humans, to some degree, may be considered as acting on cybernetic principles. They respond to feedback, either positive or negative, when interacting with the environment.

Biofeedback training provides the person with specific information that, without the instruments, is unavailable. The instruments extend the "feedback loop" from a subjective or reflective "scan" of the body to a more objective, detailed assessment of the physiological process being monitored. From the patient's perspective, extending this feedback loop to include information from the instruments is a challenge in the early stages of treatment and may itself be a source of stress. However, once the process is mastered, the detail provided in using the biofeedback instruments, over that of simply scaling tension from 1 to 10, allows for more successful training and skill development.

Cultural Factors

Schwartz and Olson (1995) identified three cultural factors that have contributed to the development of biofeedback in the past twenty to thirty years. First, Eastern and Western techniques of healing have, to a degree, merged in recent years. Methods of biofeedback are similar to methods of healing in Eastern cultures. Biofeedback encourages the use of consciousness to change physiological processes, not unlike those attained through meditation or yoga. Second, rising health costs have forced a move toward cost-effective management of disease and the limits of pharmacotherapy are being recognized. Finally, the move toward wellness and prevention have supported biofeedback and other methods that encourage self-regulation and personal responsibility for one's own health.

Professional Developments

A professional society and professional certification have encouraged the development of research, standards of practice, and acceptance of biofeedback into mainstream healthcare. Practitioners can obtain certification from the Biofeedback Certification Institute of America (Schwartz, 1995).

Current Applications

In addition to its application in treating tinnitus, biofeedback is used in treating a variety of stress-related disorders, including the following: tension and migraine headaches, incontinence, essential hypertension, Raynaud's disease, insomnia, chronic pain, anxiety, irritable bowel syndrome, bruxism, nausea, and seizures. Biofeedback has demonstrated promising results in treating esophageal spasm, hyperhidrosis, dysmenorrhea, diabetes mellitus, and fibromyalgia (Schwartz, 1995).

Contraindications include treatment of patients diagnosed with severe depression, schizophrenia, mania, severe obsessive-compulsive disorder, delirium, acute medical decompensation, or strong potential for a dissociative reaction or fugue state (Schwartz, 1995). Biofeedback may exacerbate symptoms of these conditions by encouraging an internal focus. Caution must also be used when employing biofeedback with patients with dementia or with seizure disorders. Patients taking medication for conditions such as diabetes mellitus, hypothyroidism, seizures, hypertension, glaucoma, and asthma should inform their physician of their training and the potential need for medication adjustment. In treatment of tinnitus, the clinician should be aware of the potential for depression as a mitigating factor.

INSTRUMENTATION AND TRAINING MODALITIES

Instruments in biofeedback are used to monitor and "feed back" to the patient information which they would otherwise be unable to detect. Muscle tension and peripheral skin temperature are the most commonly used modalities in biofeedback training. Training may also occur using the modalities of electrodermal activity, respiration, electroencephalographic feedback, and plethysmography.

Electromyography

Electromyography measures the electrical activity that results from muscle activity or muscle contractions. As muscles contract, an electrical charge is dispersed in the surrounding tissue. When conducting electromyography or muscle tension training, an alcohol swab is used to prepare the skin at the site where the electrodes will be placed. The swab removes dirt and oil that impede conductivity. Conductive cream is applied to the electrodes to ensure adequate conduction. The electrodes monitor the weakened signal generated by muscle activity that has moved to the skin surface. Measurements are provided in microvolts and are represented in either auditory or visual signals for the patient. The patient uses these signals as a guide to lowering muscle tension.

Temperature Training

Peripheral skin temperature is often used in treating migraines, chronic pain, and hypertension. Skin temperature reflects the degree of vasoconstriction in the arterioles, or blood vessels at the tips of the fingers and toes. When a person encounters stress, the sympathetic nervous system generates a contraction in the smooth muscle of the arterioles, the blood vessels at the tips of the fingers and toes. The function of this contraction is to encourage the blood to carry oxygen to those muscles in need, for example the leg muscles. This enables the body to engage the fight or flight response. As a result of the contraction of, and decreased blood flow in, the arterioles, fingers and toes cool.

During peripheral skin temperature or thermal biofeedback, instruments (thermistors) used to monitor peripheral skin temperature are taped to the patient's index finger. The patient learns over time to control the feedback by warming or cooling their hand. The goal in thermal biofeedback is to consistently warm the hand to a temperature that reflects a state of relaxation or 95.5 degrees Fahrenheit.

Thermal biofeedback is generally less "intuitive" than electromyography or muscle tension training. For instance, most patients are able to reflect their overall level of tension by "scanning" their body's current state and represent this tension on a scale of 1 to 10 in terms of how their body "feels." In everyday conversation, it is not uncommon to hear someone complain about the tension in the back of their neck, shoulders, or forehead. It is less common, and probably quite rare, that a person will report, "I'm feeling tense today. My fingers are cold." It may be due to this less intuitive nature of skin temperature training that many patients are initially confused, then intrigued by this form of training. Inevitably, these patients become quite excited once they begin to develop control.

Electrodermal Activity

Electrodermal activity, sometimes referred to as galvanic skin response, relies on the passage of an external electrical current across the palm between two electrodes. When the stress response is turned on, sweat rises through the glands on the palm of the hand as mediated by the sympathetic nervous system. Resistance between electrodes decreases with an increase in the sweat response and higher values are displayed on the biofeedback instruments. Electrodermal activity is very sensitive to change in the patient's emotional and cognitive processes. Caution should be used in its application, especially early in treatment before the patient has developed a sense of trust in the clinician.

Respiration

While breathing therapies, such as diaphragmatic breathing, mindfulness breathing, or paced respiration, may be taught without the use of instrumentation, advances in biofeedback technology provide for monitoring of both thoracic and diaphragmatic breathing. Two belts filled with fluid are used to monitor breathing, one around the chest cavity and the other around the abdominal region. An electrical current is passed within the fluid. As the person breathes, conductivity within the belts change, reflecting the patient's dominant pattern of breathing. The feedback provides a profile of the patient's thoracic and diaphragmatic movements during respiration. The goal in respiration training is to increase the diaphragmatic movement and slow the breathing to as few as 6 to 8 breaths per minute (Schwartz, 1995).

Electroencephalographic Feedback

In electroencephalographic training, electrodes are placed on the scalp to monitor brainwave activity. Alpha activity has been associated with an alert but relaxed state (Lubar, 1989). Theta waves represent drowsiness. Both alpha- and theta-wave training have been used in clinical settings with disorders such as attention deficit disorder, migraines, and seizures.

Plethysmography

Plethysmography is the measurement of blood flow in extremities, such as fingers or toes. It serves to reflect heart rate and, as with temperature training, vasoconstriction. In photoplethysmography, a light source is passed through the skin of the finger. The plethysmograph measures blood volume or how much blood is underneath the sensor. The information provided by the plethysmograph is sensitive to such variables as time and location of the training. As a result, it is difficult to measure "progress" from session to session using this modality. Training is more likely to focus on developing the ability to influence the change in blood flow within a session.

BIOFEEDBACK AND TINNITUS

Stress, tension, and cognitive factors are considered a potential contributor to the severity of tinnitus and/or level of discomfort experienced as a result of the illness (Grossan, 1976; House, Miller, & House, 1977; Kirsch, Blanchard, & Parnes 1989; Kitajima, 1988; Podoshin, Ben-David, Fradis, Gerstel, & Felner, 1991; Schwartz, 1995; Svihovec & Carmen, 1984). Living with tinnitus, just as living with any chronic illness, can contribute to a person's stress level (Rolland, 1994). The subjective disturbance for tinnitus patients can range from mild irritation to depression and suicidal ideation (see Chapter 2).

As with many chronic illnesses, where stress is potentially both cause and effect, a vicious cycle can develop. The tinnitus contributes to a person's stress level. This increase in the stress response may then lead to an exacerbation of symptoms. For example, Kitajima (1988) found that stress may direct attention to sounds that had previously existed under the threshold of perception. Even persons who may lead a relatively "stress free" lifestyle may be pulled into this cyclic process. There may be no other significant stressor in the patient's life outside the tinnitus.

The interactional nature of stress and chronic illnesses, such as tinnitus, provides for two "windows" of treatment, including (1) surgical or pharmacological methods, and/or (2) methods directed at moderating patient's response to the condition (Tyler & Babin, 1993). Biofeedback training aims to encourage a change in response to the symptoms of tinnitus and other conditions in the environment that contribute to the stress response. Biofeedback may be useful in treating disorders, including tinnitus, which are impacted by stress, which precipitate a stress response, and in cases where symptoms may be triggered or exacerbated by the stress precipitated by the condition itself.

Clinically, it is helpful to encourage an understanding of this "stress-symptom-stress" cycle when engaging patients in biofeedback training. This understanding helps increase motivation and contributes to the recognition of responsibility for treatment necessary in biofeedback.

Schwartz (1995) offers several speculations on how biofeedback works when used in treating tinnitus. These include distraction, habituation effects, cognitive changes, improved sleep, and reduced muscle tension. Distraction occurs as the patient focuses attention on breathing, thoughts, or other internal stimuli. With less attention given to the tinnitus, patients report being less annoyed and improved coping. Habituation, according to Schwartz, refers to the repeated pairing of the tinnitus with the relaxation response. Eventually, the tinnitus no longer carries with it association of stress, tension, and irritation.

Cognitive changes may include hopeful expectations for change and a decrease in helpless patterns of thinking. As the person first experiences relief, hope for change may improve. With continued success in practicing biofeedback strategies, the patient's confidence and sense of self-control is regained. Improved sleep may lead to decreased tension during the day and greater success employing techniques of self-regulation. Finally, decreased muscle tension may also contribute to an overall decrease in stress and arousal.

Research in Biofeedback and Tinnitus

Results from studies examining the efficacy of biofeedback over the past 20 years have been generally supportive of biofeedback as a viable option in the treatment of tinnitus. Early researchers recognized the impact stress or anxiety had on tinnitus (Grossan, 1976; House et al., 1977). These studies were the initial attempts in applying biofeedback to tinnitus. While they suggested that patients with tinnitus may benefit from biofeedback training, much of this early research was plagued by methodological problems. More recently, the research in biofeedback and tinnitus has expanded to include multilevel assessments, more in-depth follow-up, and attempts to differentiate the effective component in biofeedback.

Literature Reviews

Kirsch et al. (1989) provides a critique and summary of studies examining the efficacy of relaxation and biofeedback in the treatment of tinnitus. All studies examined by Kirsch and colleagues utilized biofeedback alone or in combination with relaxation training. The authors reviewed single case, single group, and controlled outcome studies, noting that results from individual studies often varied within each category of design. They concluded that "methodological problems . . . limit confidence" (1989, p. 63), in results which suggested that biofeedback was effective in treating tinnitus. For example, several studies reported that annoyance and intrusiveness decreased and coping increased. However, the authors expressed concern that the global measures used in determining efficacy led to the mixed results among the studies.

Basing their impressions on the current state of the research, the authors suggest that biofeedback is generally helpful in treating tinnitus. However, given the reliance on global outcome measures in the studies, they add that it is difficult to determine its degree of efficacy. In response to the methodological problems of the early research, Kirsch et al. suggest adopting a multidimensional assessment in measuring treatment outcomes.

Anderson, Melin, Hagnebo, Scott, and Lindeberg (1995) reviewed thirty-eight studies on hypnosis, biofeedback, and cognitive behavioral treatment. Their conclusions held less promise for the treatment of tinnitus with biofeedback than those of Kirsch. Results indicated that cognitive behavioral approaches, combined with relaxation training, had been studied more often than either hypnosis or biofeedback. In the single case reports and single group design studies that examined biofeedback, most indicated that biofeedback had a generally positive effect. However, the authors concluded that there was little support among these studies that linked treatment directly to a decrease in tinnitus. Furthermore, among the fifteen controlled group studies examined by the authors, the more controlled the study, the more disappointing the results in support of biofeedback. They held concerns over the mechanism by which biofeedback supposedly worked, questioning whether biofeedback was simply "another way of implementing relaxation training." They concluded that there were too few studies with baseline measures or control groups, appropriate sample sizes, and appropriate follow-up.

Group Studies

Kirsch, Blanchard, and Parnes (1987) conducted a multiple baseline evaluation of the treatment of tinnitus with both relaxation training and biofeedback. In their summary of the literature to date, the authors acknowledged that biofeedback shows promising results in treating tinnitus. However, they expressed concern for the general lack of controls, poor baseline measures, and deficient criteria used in determining efficacy in previous studies. This study sought to improve on these concerns by combining multiple baseline and treatment measures in evaluating relaxation training, electromyography, and thermal training.

Six subjects were randomly assigned to either a two-week or a five-week baseline period. A diary monitoring tinnitus and sleep disturbance was kept during the baseline, treatment, and for one-month following treatment. The pretreatment assessment included a symptom history interview, baseline measures on muscle tension and temperature, an audiological evaluation,

and several psychological tests, including the: MMPI, Beck Depression Inventory (BDI) (Beck et al., 1961), State-Trait Anxiety Inventory (STAI) (Spielberger et al., 1970), and the Psychosomatic Symptom Checklist (PSC) (Cox et al., 1975). Posttreatment assessment included each of the previously mentioned psychological tests, with the exception of the MMPI. Visual analog scales measuring satisfaction with treatment and the impact of treatment on coping, stress, and severity of the tinnitus were completed. During a three-month follow-up, participants completed BDI, STAI, and PSC. The diary was also kept four weeks prior to the three-month follow-up assessment.

Treatment included relaxation and imagery training, two sessions of electromyography biofeedback, and four sessions of thermal training. Subjects were encouraged to use relaxation during their biofeedback training. Following treatment, analysis of the diaries revealed little to no change in sleep or tinnitus disturbance. Change was noted on the global measures of coping, satisfaction with treatment, and stress caused by the tinnitus. Improvements were noted for four subjects in their ability to reduce electromyographical biofeedback. Subjects showed little change in their ability to control temperature.

This study demonstrated that improvements in tinnitus will depend on the measures employed. The daily diaries indicated no change while the global measures suggested improvements occurred. Despite the small number of subjects who participated, the results are promising.

Podoshin et al. (1991) compared electromyography biofeedback with acupuncture and Cinnarizine. Fifty-eight subjects with tinnitus were randomly assigned to various treatment and control groups. The biofeedback patients trained using placements on the frontalis muscles during ten weekly sessions. In the biofeedback control group, participants were connected to the biofeedback instruments, however the sound and visual scales were not connected. Fifty percent of the biofeedback treatment group reported improvements in tinnitus and disturbance. Thirty percent reported improvement in the acupuncture group. Ten percent reported improvement in the Cinnarizine group. No improvements were reported in the control group.

Carmen and Svihovec (1984) studied the effect of relaxation and limited biofeedback training on eleven subjects diagnosed with tinnitus. The subjects completed seven to thirteen sessions of relaxation treatment. In three of these sessions, frontalis electromyography activity was observed. At the eighteenth month follow-up, 90 percent of the subjects attributed a reduction in tinnitus and their negative reaction to tinnitus to the relaxation/biofeedback training.

Walsh and Gerley (1985) combined thermal biofeedback and Jacobsonian relaxation with thirty-two patients diagnosed with tinnitus. The patients received eight weekly sessions of thermal biofeedback training with taped relaxation. Sixty-five percent of the patients reported a reduction in loudness or annoyance. The researchers concluded that there is a significant relationship between increased blood flow, skin temperature, and decrease in the intensity of tinnitus symptoms.

Ireland, Wilson, Tonkin, and Platt-Hepworth (1985) reported on the treatment of thirty patients using relaxation training. Based on their review of the literature, they concluded that biofeedback was effective in reducing tinnitus and the discomfort it produces. Furthermore, they reflected on the possibility that biofeedback and relaxation training may be so similar that the treatment effect may occur with relaxation training alone. They cite several potential benefits in using relaxation training versus biofeedback, including cost-effectiveness (relaxation training can be conducted in a group), and the lack of need for equipment. However, their study revealed little effect on the tinnitus by relaxation training alone, suggesting that comparisons to biofeedback may be misguided. In partial support of

relaxation training, several subjects reported anecdotally that they were less annoyed after treatment. Unfortunately, a measure on annoyance was not included in the study.

Not all research has been supportive of biofeedback. Haralambous et al. (1987) also criticized earlier studies for their poor design, lack of control, and lack of specific measurement devices. In response to Ireland et al. (1985), they attempted also to identify the effective elements of biofeedback. Twenty-six patients were randomly assigned to three groups. In the two treatment groups, training consisted of eight weekly sessions of electromyography biofeedback. An additional component was given to the second treatment group. They were informed not to expect any improvement in the first five sessions, however to expect "dramatic improvement" in their tinnitus and general feelings of well-being after the fifth session. The third group consisted of waiting-list control subjects. Results showed no significant improvements on any of the measures employed, including: tinnitus loudness, frequency, and annoyance; sleep onset difficulty; severity of distress caused by tinnitus; depression and anxiety; and ideological measures.

Single-Subject Studies

Biofeedback has shown mixed results in single-subject designs. Elfner, May, Moore, and Mendelson (1981) demonstrated a reduction in annoyance and frustration, without a reduction in tinnitus level, by employing thermal biofeedback. Follow-up results of one year after biofeedback therapy indicated that the subject was still able to reduce annoyance on a daily basis through his practice.

Borton, Moore, and Clark (1981) conducted a case study demonstrating no reduction in severity or annoyance following electromyography training with placement on the frontalis muscles. These results were obtained even though the patient was able to control and lower electromyography activity.

Studies in which biofeedback was included as part of a comprehensive approach have produced promising results. Duckro, Pollard, Bray, and Scheiter (1984) combined both electromyography and thermal training in the management of complex tinnitus. The researchers approached tinnitus in a similar manner to which chronic pain has been approached conceptually, in treatment, and in the literature. They introduced the application of an integrated, biopsychosocial approach to the management of severe tinnitus. In this study, the patient was trained first using electromyography. After showing control of muscle tension, the researchers introduced thermal training. Treatment also included pain management training, social skills training, assertive training, in vivo exposure to being alone (the patient had a fear of being alone), cognitive treatment of depression, and marital therapy. Improvements were noted on scores on the Beck Depression Inventory, the Willoughby Personality Schedule, and a self-rating of fear of being alone. Tinnitus severity decreased after the sixth day of treatment. Results had been maintained at the three-month follow-up. The authors note that both biomedical treatment and psychotherapy had been ineffective in alleviating symptoms prior to the program. They argue that, only after a comprehensive and integrative, biopsychosocial understanding of and approach to the symptoms had been implemented, did the patients suffering decrease.

Erlandson, Carlsson, and Svensson (1989) used electromyography to enhance the awareness of the importance of emotional factors and increased stress reactivity to tinnitus in a 56-year-old male with disabling tinnitus of a two-year duration. The patient was given fifteen sessions of electromyography training, eleven weekly sessions with the remaining sessions spread over a one-year period. During the training sessions, discussions of the relationship between stress and environmental factors were held. As training continued, the patient became more familiar with what factors in his environment contributed to increased stress. This led to the patient's greater control over risk factors, which contributed to the symptoms and his tension levels. The patient's posttreatment tinnitus ratings decreased, as did his anxiety levels as measured by Taylor's Manifest Anxiety Scale (Taylor, 1953). Qualitatively, a number of positive changes were noted by the patient, including a reduction in tinnitus, an improvement in tolerance, concentration, and emotional stability, and improvements in sleep.

TREATMENT PROTOCOL

Assessment and Intake

During the initial biofeedback session, several areas should be addressed including the history and symptomology of the tinnitus, an introduction to biofeedback concepts and methods, and a discussion of patient responsibilities.

In the process of reviewing the history of the tinnitus, Schwartz (1995) suggests covering possible causes of the tinnitus, its location (right, left, or bilateral), severity, type, quality of sounds, past and present treatments, and current medications. This information will be useful as the clinician decides whether biofeedback is the most appropriate step at this time or whether a referral to the patient's family physician or an audiologist is appropriate. Biofeedback should only be employed after other potential physical causes have been ruled out (such as a tumor). During the process of reviewing the patient's history, a therapeutic relationship begins to develop as the clinician shows interest in the patient's experience.

The clinician should also address the impact tinnitus is having on the patient's life and current methods used to manage both the tinnitus and the reported impact. It is important to recognize that the impact may extend in a number of areas, including work, family interactions, perceptions of self, hopes for the future, and general health.

Providing the person the opportunity to portray how the condition has impacted their living is important in establishing trust, normalizing the patient's experience, and setting the stage for developing alternative coping strategies. In having the patient explore the various areas in which the symptoms have impacted their life, the clinician is also encouraging definition of where improvements are likely to occur.

During the initial session of biofeedback, the patient is introduced to the concepts, instruments, and role of the therapist in biofeedback. Conceptual areas to also cover include the relationship between stress and health, the fight or flight response to stress, and the interactional relationship between stress and chronic illness.

When introducing the patient to the instruments, it may be helpful for the clinician to provide a metaphoric, as well as a formal, definition of biofeedback. The metaphor of a mirror or weight scale can be useful in conveying how the equipment is used in the learning process. For example, when someone attempts to lose weight, his or her first step may be to use a weight scale in determining their starting point. After noting their current weight, the person may then change either diet or exercise patterns. The scale is then used in determining if the current adjustments in diet or exercise have had the desired effect. If the adjustments have resulted in weight loss, the person may choose to continue with what has worked thus far. If not, the person may then alter their approach. Biofeedback instruments are used in this same manner. The information gathered from the instruments is used in deciding what works.

Some patients may have unrealistic expectations regarding how the equipment functions. It may be important to emphasize that the instruments do not *make* a person relax, rather they simply serve to indicate whether or not the body is relaxed, or if it is becoming more relaxed. Another common concern to address is the potential for electric shock by the instruments. Calming these concerns and assisting the person to become comfortable with the equipment is necessary. Providing a brief demonstration during the first session, with electromyography leads connected to the patient's forearm, will assist in developing a sense of comfort and familiarity with the instruments.

Expected outcomes and estimated length of sessions and treatment should be addressed during the initial session. Training may take from twelve to fifteen weeks on the average. If no change is noted in the patient's attempts to control the feedback or in symptomology after six to seven weeks, it may be necessary to refer the patient to another form of treatment.

Informing patients of their responsibility will prepare them for their role in the training. Patients are asked to practice biofeedback and relaxation strategies at least once, sometimes twice per day with the practice session lasting between 10 to 15 minutes. Without regular practice, biofeedback will not have the desired effect. In this respect, the relationship between the patient and clinician can be compared to that of player and coach. The clinician provides the guidance, structure, and support. The patient, not unlike the player, devotes time to practice. The clinician encourages motivation, but ultimately, it is the patient's responsibility for change.

Training Sessions

While the introductory session may last 60 to 90 minutes given the amount of information to cover, the typical training session lasts between 30 minutes to 1 hour. The recommended frequency and structure of sessions varies, from once per week to two sessions per week early in training. Most clinicians will agree that during the initial phase of training, once per week is the minimum.

Electromyography is the most commonly used modality in treating tinnitus. Electrode placement with electromyography for tinnitus treatment is generally one of two locations: the trapezius (neck and shoulders) and the frontalis muscle (forehead) (Svihovec & Carmen, 1984). Placement consists of first, cleaning the skin with an alcohol swab to allow for a proper connection of the electrodes to the skin's surface. Second, a small amount of conductive cream is used on each electrode prior to placement. Third, the actual placement of electrodes. Placement for a reading of frontalis activity is approximately 1½ inches above the eyebrows. (An overview of electrode placements in electromyograpy is provided by Basmajian and Blumenstein, 1989). Finally, throughout the process, discussing and commenting on each step taken during placement of the electrodes can increase the patient's comfort with the instruments, the clinician, and the training process.

In peripheral skin temperature training, also commonly used for tinnitus, placement is on the index finger of either hand. Proper placement involves taping the thermistor to the side of the index finger above the distal interphalyngeal (DIP) joint. The lead, or wire to which the thermistor is attached, is then taped at the base of the finger, as the first 3 inches of the lead can pick up temperature readings. Finally, the lead is taped to the palm of the hand to provide stability if and when the patient moves. Again, it is useful to talk the patient through these components of the session.

When conducting temperature training, several considerations should be given to potential artifacts that may inadvertently impact temperature readings. These include room temperature, moving air, "blanketing" or covering of the thermistor, chill from the patient coming in from outside, and temperature drift in the instrument itself (Peek, 1995).

Goals to consider for the first full training session include increasing the patient's comfort with the instruments, increased awareness of the relationship between tension and readings provided by the equipment, and encouraging the patient's ability to develop a relaxed state. Generally, patients experience and display an inherent interest or fascination in viewing and manipulating the readings. Encouraging a period of "trial and error" learning can enhance the patients'

confidence, while also assisting in identifying constraints in the ability to produce relaxation.

During the initial session and early part of each session, physiological baselines are taken to provide for comparisons during and across session. One-minute resting baselines are commonly used and should be taken following a period of adaptation to the office environment. Upon reviewing baselines at the end of session and comparing these to changes during training, the patient is provided reinforcing feedback and increased confidence to continue in their efforts.

The initial and subsequent training sessions can include instruction in various forms of relaxation procedures, such as autogenic training, imagery, and/or progressive muscle relaxation. Music or soft sounds of nature are also useful on their own or coupled with a more formal relaxation exercise. Given the important role proper breathing plays in developing the relaxation response (Schwartz, 1995), instruction in diaphragmatic breathing is useful early in training, perhaps as early as the first session. Diaphragmatic breathing is a simple procedure that patients can use during their home practice.

As training progresses, the clinician can consider providing the patient time alone to train with the equipment. The clinician's absence should only occur in brief periods and only after the patient has developed a sufficient level of comfort with the equipment. Benefits of the clinician's absence include decreasing the patient's stress due to "performance" anxiety and generalization of training to occasions in the patient's environment when they are alone elsewhere (Schwartz & Gemberling, 1995). Advantages of remaining with the patient include opportunities for providing suggestions during training or changing recommended protocols that do not provide adequate training. Also, the presence of another person (in this case, the clinician) during training helps toward generalizing the "skill" of relaxation to social situations. Finally, being present allows the clinician an opportunity to monitor artifacts or factors that may inadvertently influence feedback. For example, in peripheral skin temperature training, it is important to have the patient avoid trapping the thermistor between the index finger and the arm chair or knee when the hand is at rest. This will inadvertently contribute to increased temperatures.

At the end of the training session, the clinician and patient review physiological changes that have occurred. The use of computers in biofeedback have been quite valuable to this end. Programs are available that analyze and display data from the session, providing both the patient and clinician with a clear format for review. During the review period, the patient and clinician assess which strategies employed have been instrumental in effecting positive change and which have produced increases in tension. The goal is to assist the patient in becoming familiar with the internal cues associated with change in the external cues of the biofeedback instrument.

The final portion of the training session will include a discussion of home practice. The patient is encouraged to develop a home practice structure that includes at least 10 to 15 minutes each day. During these times, the patient is to practice what is learned during the session. The clinician may consider having the patient record a variety of parameters of their home practice for the purpose of increasing compliance and providing reinforcing feedback. These parameters include time and length of practice, exercise used during practice, pre- and postpractice subjective response (thoughts, feelings, and physical sensations), symptom occurrence, and the impact symptoms are having on daily activity. Given the subjective nature of tinnitus, a self-report scale is useful in assessing the severity of symptoms. Svihovec and Carmen (1984) recommend a 9-point scale, where 0 represents no tinnitus and 8 represents extremely loud tinnitus. Eventually, if using peripheral skin temperature training, the patient can be provided an inexpensive hand thermometer to record pre- and postpractice temperatures. Subsequent sessions will include a review of home practice. In addition to encouraging compliance, such reviews reinforce the importance placed on the patient's responsibility in the treatment.

Training Goals

The training goal for electromyography biofeedback for tinnitus is two microvolts maintained for approximately ten minutes. In temperature training, 95.5 degrees reflects a sufficient state of relaxation. Ultimately, the goal of treatment is to impact the severity of tinnitus and the discomfort it adds to the patient's life. Improvements in severity can be monitored using scales allowing for the subjective nature of tinnitus. As previously mentioned, Svihovec and Carmen (1984) recommend a 9-point scale, where 0 represents no tinnitus and 8 represents extremely loud tinnitus. Schwartz (1995) recommends a 6-point scale that separates activity versus rest and sleep conditions.

SUMMARY

Biofeedback can be an effective treatment for many stress-related illnesses, including tinnitus. In the treatment of tinnitus, the goals of biofeedback include: (1) impacting the symptoms through mediation of the stress response, and (2) increasing the patient's capacity to manage the illness by decreasing annoyance and decreasing the impact tinnitus has on daily life. Consequently, training should include counseling to address how cognitive factors impact the condition (see Chapter 11) and how tinnitus is impacting the person's life. Resolution of external stressors will contribute to successful treatment of the illness. As a treatment option, biofeedback training can be combined with other forms of treatment or when other forms of treatment have not produced desired results.

REFERENCES

Andersson, G., Melin, L., Hagnebo, C., Scott, B., & Lindeberg, P. (1995). A review of psychological treatment approaches for patients suffering from tinnitus. *Annals of Behavioral Medicine, 17*(4), 357–366.

Basmajian, J. V. (1989). *Biofeedback: Principles and practice for clinicians.* Baltimore: Williams & Wilkins.

Basmajian, J. V., & Blumenstein, R. (1989). Electrode placement in electromyographic biofeedback. In J. V. Basmajian (Ed.), *Biofeedback: Principles and practice for clinicians* (pp. 369–382). Baltimore: Williams & Wilkins.

Beck, A. T., Ward, C. H., Mendelson, M., Mock, J., & Erbaugh, J. (1961). An inventory for measuring depression. *Archives of General Psychiatry, 5,* 561–571.

Borton, T., Moore, W. H., & Clark, S. R. (1981). Electromyographic feedback treatment for tinnitus aurium. *Journal of Speech and Hearing Disorders,* 39–45.

Cannon, W. B. (1932). *The wisdom of the body.* New York: Norton.

Carmen, R., & Svihovec, D. (1984). Relaxation-biofeedback in the treatment of tinnitus. *The American Journal of Otology, 45*(5), 376–381.

Cox, D. J., Freundlich, A., & Meyer, R. G. (1975). Differential effectiveness of electromyographic feedback, verbal relaxation instructions, and medication placebo with tension headaches. *Journal of Consulting and Clinical Psychology, 43,* 892–898.

Duckro, P. N., Pollard, A., Bray, H. D., & Scheiter, L. (1984). Comprehensive behavioral management of complex tinnitus: A case illustration. *Biofeedback and Self-Regulation, 9*(4), 459–469.

Elfner, L. F., May, J. G., Moore, J., D., & Mendelson, J. M. (1981). Effects of EMG and thermal feedback training on tinnitus: A case study. *Biofeedback and Self-Regulation, 6*(4), 517–521.

Erlandsson, S., Carlsson, S. G., & Svensson, A. (1989). Biofeedback in the treatment of tinnitus: A broadened approach. *Goteborg Psychological Reports, 19,* 1–12.

Friedman, R., Sedler, M., Myers, P., & Benson, H. (1977). Behavioral medicine, complementary medicine, and integrated care: Economic implications (pp. 949–962). In J. L. Randall & L. S. Lazar (Eds.), *Primary care: Complementary and alternative therapies in primary care, 24,* (4). Philadelphia: W. B. Saunders Company.

Grossan, M. (1976). Treatment of subjective tinnitus with biofeedback. *Ear, Nose, and Throat, 55,* 314–318.

Haralambous, G., Wilson, P. H., Platt-Hepworth, S., Tonkin, J. P., Hensley, R., & Kavanagh, D. (1987). EMG biofeedback in the treatment of tinnitus: An experimental evaluation. *Behaviour Research and Therapy, 25*(1), 49–55.

Harris, A. H., & Brady, J. V. (1974). Animal learning: Visceral and autonomic conditioning. *Annual Review of Psychology, 25,* 107–133.

House, H. W. (1978). Treatment of severe tinnitus with biofeedback training. *The Laryngoscope, 88,* 406–412.

House, J. W., Miller, L., & House, P. R. (1977). Severe tinnitus: Treatment with biofeedback. *Transactions of the American Academy of Ophthalmology and Otolaryngology, 84,* 697–703.

Ireland, C. E., Wilson, P. H., Tonkin, J. P., & Platt-Hepworth, S. (1985). An evaluation of relaxation training in the treatment of tinnitus. *Behaviour Research and Therapy, 23,* 423–430.

Kirsch, C. A., Blanchard, E. B., & Parnes, S. M. (1987). A multiple-baseline evaluation of the treatment of subjective tinnitus with relaxation training and biofeedback. *Biofeedback and Self-Regulation, 12*(4), 295–312.

Kirsch, C.A., Blanchard, E. B., & Parnes, S. M. (1989). A review of the efficacy of behavioral techniques in the treatment of subjective tinnitus. *Annals of Behavioral Medicine, 11*(2), 58–65.

Kitajima, K. (1988). Biofeedback training for tinnitus relief. In M. Kitahara (Ed.), *Tinnitus: Pathophysiology and management* (pp. 131–140). Tokyo: Igaku-Shoin.

Olson, R. P. (1995). Definitions of biofeedback and applied psychophysiology. In M. S. Schwartz (Ed.), *Biofeedback: A practitioner's guide* (pp. 27–31). New York: The Guilford Press.

Peek, C. J. (1995). A primer of biofeedback instrumentation. In M. S. Schwartz (Ed.), *Biofeedback: A practitioner's guide* (pp. 45–95). New York: The Guilford Press.

Podoshin, L., Ben-David, Y., Fradis, M., Gerstel, R., & Felner, H. (1991). Idiopathic subjective tinnitus treated by biofeedback, acupuncture, and drug therapy. *Ear, Nose, and Throat Journal, 70*(5), 284–289.

Rolland, J. S. (1994). *Families, illness, and disability: An integrative treatment model.* New York: Basic Books.

Schwartz, M. S. (1995). *Biofeedback: A practitioner's guide.* New York: The Guilford Press.

Schwartz, M. S., & Gemberling, A. L. (1995). Therapist presence or absence. In M. S. Schwartz (Ed.), *Biofeedback: A practitioner's guide* (pp. 176–183). New York: The Guilford Press.

Schwartz, M. S., & Olson, R. P. (1995). A historical perspective on the field of biofeedback and applied psychophysiology. In M. S. Schwartz (Ed.), *Biofeedback: A practitioner's guide* (pp. 3–18). New York: The Guilford Press.

Selye, H. (1974). *Stress without distress.* Philadephia: Lippincott.

Spielberger, C. D., Gorsuch, R. L., & Luschene, R. E. (1970). *STAI Manual for the State-Trait Anxiety Inventory.* Palo Alto: Consulting Psychologists Press.

Svihovec, D., & Carmen, R. (1984). Tinnitus treatment using biofeedback-relaxation techniques. In J. G. Clark & P. Yanick (Eds.), *Tinnitus and its management: A text for audiologists* (pp. 119–135). Springfield, IL: Charles C. Thomas.

Taylor, J. A., (1953). A personality scale of manifest anxiety. *Journal of Abnormal and Social Psychology, 48,* 285–290.

Tyler, R. S., & Babin, R. W. (1993). Tinnitus. In C. W. Cummings (Ed.), *Otolaryngology-Head and Neck Surgery.* Mosby-Year Book, Inc.

Walsh, W. M., & Gerley, P. P. (1985). Thermal biofeedback and the treatment of tinnitus. *Laryngoscope, 95,* 987–989.

Watzlawick, P., Bavelas, & Jackson, D. (1967). *Pragmatics of human communication.* New York: W. W. Norton.

Wolpe, J. (1973). *The practice of behavior therapy.* New York: Pergamon Press.

CHAPTER 13

Cognitive-Behavior Modification

Robert W. Sweetow, Ph.D.

INTRODUCTION

The shared objective of researchers, clinicians and tinnitus sufferers is the elimination of this unwanted auditory intruder. Perusal of the literature on tinnitus management reveals a long list of procedures that were initially heralded but are no longer in use. Clinicians anxious to assist patients suffering from this frustrating malady have been repeatedly buoyed by reports of initial treatment success, only to be disappointed by the lack of follow-up data demonstrating lasting improvement. Unfortunately, even with comprehensive testing (see Chapter 6), there is great difficulty identifying the cause of idiopathic tinnitus. Consequently, efforts have been aimed at controlling the symptom. Strategies cited in the literature include masking with home devices, tinnitus maskers, and hearing aids (see Chapter 14), electrostimulation (see Chapter 16), nutritional counseling (including the use of herbs such as ginkgo biloba), and vitamin supplements such as niacin, zinc, and so on. More recently, the combination of directive educational counseling

with low-intensity, broadband noise generators or hearing aids have been proposed to facilitate habituation. Short-term success with these procedures has been inconsistent, at best. With the exception of hearing aids, the record of long-term success has been even lower.

This frustrating lack of achievement led to the question of why symptom management has been such a dismal failure. Was it because the symptom of tinnitus is so heterogeneous in terms of its underlying cause, its physical manifestations and its psychological implications? After all, individuals interpret tinnitus in a wide variety of ways. Some find it little more than an occasional annoyance, while others report severe disruption of their lives (McFadden, 1982). Patients indicate that the tinnitus may "cause" difficulties in the areas of sleep, concentration, hearing, social relationships, and work. Many report that the tinnitus is responsible for increasing fatigue, stress, anxiety and depression (see Chapter 2). Yet, despite the fervor of the patient's subjective response, there appears to be little correlation between the reported loudness of the tinnitus and the degree to which a person is adversely affected. Thus, it seems reasonable to assume that it is the patient's reaction to the tinnitus, rather than the symptom itself, that separates the individual who simply experiences tinnitus from the individual who may seek ongoing help (Sweetow, 1986). Therefore, another explanation for the failure of adequate management of the tinnitus patient is that attempts at symptom control may be directed at the wrong manifestation of tinnitus. Many therapeutic attempts have been directed toward eliminating or minimizing *the sound*. Conceivably, management attempts would be more successful if they were directed toward a tinnitus-related symptom that is more manageable.

One commonality shared by nearly all uncompensated tinnitus patients is an unhealthy attitude and/or a maladaptive reaction to the symptom. A reaction is a learned behavior. Unlike an internally produced "sound," like tinnitus, all behaviors are subject to modification. Therefore, regardless of the cause of tinnitus, the differentiation of the compensated versus the uncompensated patient is ultimately a function of how the patient reacts to the tinnitus. If a person is not "bothered" by the tinnitus, it ceases to be a problem. This is not to say that attempts should not be made to identify and, if possible, rectify the underlying disease process. But given the reality that most cases of subjective tinnitus are idiopathic in nature, psychological intervention aimed at successfully reducing the stress, distress, and distraction associated with tinnitus can be productive and may produce the most attainable goals (see Chapter 11).

Because there are no universally successful approaches to managing tinnitus or the tinnitus patient, it behooves professionals to explore other disciplines whose efforts toward management of subjective symptoms sharing similarities with tinnitus have met with greater degrees of success. One such discipline is the study of pain control.

A noninvasive approach toward pain management that has proven to be successful is cognitive-behavioral therapy.

DEFINITION OF COGNITIVE-BEHAVIORAL THERAPY

Cognitive-behavioral therapy can be simply defined as the therapeutic effort to modify maladaptive thoughts and behaviors by applying systematic, measurable implementation of strategies designed to alter unproductive actions. There are two main components to this approach, as implied by its name. One is *cognitive restructuring*, or an attempt to reconceptualize the problems presented by the disorder into a form that is amenable to a viable solution. More simply, cognitive restructuring helps patients think differently and adopt a different attitude about their problem. The other component is *behavioral modification*. Identifying factors that contribute to the problem and the subsequent reaction, then finding ways to modify them through behavioral actions comprise this component. The combined approach assists patients to identify and correct maladaptive behaviors, distorted conceptions, and irrational beliefs. Patients can then monitor the role that negative thoughts exert in maintaining their adverse reaction to their unwanted symptoms. An excellent discussion of this approach has been written by Turk, Meichenbaum, and Genest (1983).

HISTORY OF COGNITIVE-BEHAVIORAL THERAPY

The origins of cognitive-behavioral therapy can be traced back to the 1950s when a small group of therapists, dissatisfied with conventional psychotherapy, developed new techniques based on experimental psychology (Wolpe & Lazarus, 1966). In its early forms, cognitive-behavioral therapy was comprised of a conglomerate of therapeutic approaches. A partial list of these approaches include the following:

Systematic desensitization: Wolpe (1958) popularized this form of progressive muscle relaxation utilizing contrasting physical sensations. The precursor of this approach, which was based on a graded anxiety hierarchy (easiest to most difficult), was actually described in seventeenth-century England.

Token economy used operant principals popularized by B. F. Skinner (1953) to provide tangible rewards for subjects. Operant conditioning means that the subject's response is dependent on the presence of a particular stimulus. Just as rats could learn more rapidly to perform certain behaviors when they received reinforcement such as food, so could humans alter behavior when conditioned that a specific behavior following the presence of a particular stimulus would be rewarded. It too, had its early use in the seventeenth century for patients "afflicted" with nail biting and alcoholism.

Aversion therapy (Cautela & Kearney, 1986) involves covert sensitization attained by having patients visualize scenes pairing undesired behavior with a highly unpleasant consequence. This strategy, under the guidance of a therapist, may help reduce unwanted, but persistent behaviors. If the patient recognizes negative consequences of his actions, the actions may cease. It was first described in ancient Rome to treat alcoholism.

Rational-emotive therapy, Ellis (1962), supported the view that it is not events that disturb people, but rather their view of the events. Meichenbaum (1977), reporting on his work with schizophrenics, refined Ellis' theories by adding the importance of self-talk and self-guided speech to guide behavior. When solving problems, patients "talk silently to themselves" and these private self-statements may be part of a chain of actions leading to the solution. This process may be equated with "thinking" and "believing."

Cognitive-restructuring is used to guide patients to recognize and subsequently abandon unhelpful thinking patterns and replace them with constructive cognitions and thoughts. In addition, it is designed to help patients reconceptualize problems into manageable units.

Behavior therapy is based on the tenet that words and concepts are meaningful only when linked to direct experience. But, in addition, there is a systematic application of conditioning principals to the clinical disorder. Many operant approaches focus on behavior and ignore cognition. Meichenbaum (1977) stressed the importance of automatic thought processes on subjective perception and eventual resolution of intractable disorders. Beck (1979) and Burns (1980) have been among the most influential scholars infusing cognition into behavioral therapy. Used alone, either cognitive therapy or behavior therapy is not as effective as when used together (Thorpe & Olson, 1990).

APPLICATIONS OF COGNITIVE-BEHAVIORAL THERAPY

Cognitive-behavioral therapy has been successfully utilized for patients suffering from chronic pain, depression, anxiety, panic disorders, post-traumatic stress, phobias, personality disorders, obsessive-compulsiveness, marital therapy, sexual dysfunctions, eating disorders and addictions. It is one of the most widely used and accepted psychological strategies for coping with intractable disorders. Beck, Rush, Shaw, and Emery (1979) first described the application of cognitive therapy for depression. Much of their work is directly applicable to tinnitus patients because of the frequency with which depression and other emotional disorders are associated with tinnitus. Cognitive intervention consisting of attention diversion, imagery training, and distraction techniques have been used successfully for patients suffering from chronic low back pain (Turk et al., 1983).

SIMILARITIES OF TINNITUS WITH PAIN

Tinnitus shares many similarities with pain. Both are subjective, both are invisible, both are often intractable, and both may be affected by extraneous events. In the following discussion of pain, notice how easily and appropriately the symptom of tinnitus can be substituted for the symptom of pain. The Subcommittee of Taxonomy defines pain as: "An unpleasant sensory and emotional experience associated with actual or potential tissue damage, or described in terms of such damage."

Melzack and Wall (1965) hypothesized that pain perception is governed by means of a gate control. Opening or closing the gates facilitate or inhibit the flow of nerve impulses from the peripheral nerves to the central nervous system. When the amount of information passing into the gate exceeds a certain critical level, the neural areas responsible for the pain experience and response are activated. The opening and closing of the gates is profoundly affected by the efferent descending influences from the brain.

If one gate is flooded with certain sensations, the others close. For example, if a person has a chronic stomach pain, but then accidently stubs his toe, the flood of sensation from the toe close the gate for the stomach pain sensations. The gates essentially keep a person from paying attention to all the sensations a body receives at one time.

Melzack and Wall indicated that the final perception of pain can be described by the following components and treatments:

Component	Treatment
Sensory-discriminative	• Relaxation procedures
Motional-affective	• Attention diversion
	• Somatization
	• Imagery manipulations
Cognitive-evaluative	• Cognitive therapy
	• Preparing and confronting the patient
	• Coping with feelings at critical moments
	• Self-reinforcement for having coped

This classic work was the first cogent description of how psychological factors influence and sustain the pain perception.

Tinnitus patients, like individuals suffering from panic attacks, often make "catastrophic misinterpretations" of the sensation, viewing them as symptoms of a worsening physical ailment, and one that is out of control. As a consequence, fear escalates rapidly with only slight provocation (even a slight increase in the loudness or quality of the tinnitus). Beck (1979) treats these panic disorders with cognitive therapy.

Attempts have been unsuccessful at resolving the question: "Are psychopathological factors in chronic pain patients a consequence of experiencing pain, or do preexisting disorders act as predisposers to the pain becoming 'chronic'?" (Gatchel & Turk, 1996). An analogous question exists for tinnitus patients: "Are the emotional problems experienced by a certain segment of tinnitus patients a consequence of the tinnitus itself, or were these patients more susceptible to emotional problems to begin with, and was the tinnitus merely a trigger?"

Stress and maladaptive coping strategies are manifested in a variety of manners, both physical and psychological. Tinnitus patients are well served by education concerning the undeniable correlation between exacerbation of tinnitus perception and stress.

Pain treatment differs from tinnitus treatment in that the underlying cause of pain is often identifiable and treatable. As a result, well tested drugs can be prescribed whose purpose is to address the anatomical sites responsible for the pain, or the structures in the brain responsible for interpreting the pain. However, many attempts at medication for tinnitus control lack focus regarding specific auditory or central structures. When the cause of pain cannot be pharmaceutically controlled, or when medication cannot be tolerated due to side effects, there are well-tested treatment plans available for altering a patient's reaction to pain.

For example, Meichenbaum and Turk (1976) reviewed a large body of literature indicating that patients' perception of control of pain can result in a higher threshold of pain and/or pain tolerance; however, they point out that when only cognitive techniques are employed, results are equivocal. Thus, they agree with Thorpe and Olson (1990) that cognitive approaches should be combined with behavioral modification.

Subjective pain is overtly expressed as behaviors. As such, these behaviors are vulnerable to the influence of systematic consequences with which they come in contact. Similar to pain, inactivity leads to increased focus and preoccupation with tinnitus and these cognitive/attentional changes increase the likelihood of misinterpreting symptoms. In addition, tinnitus, pain, and depressed patients often share a sense of learned helplessness. Learned helplessness refers to behavioral passivity in the face of uncontrolled stress (Seligman, 1975).

Pain is affected by a large number of variables: excitatory and inhibitory, emotional and biological; which may affect the experience independently of the organic disease entity. Brena and Chapman (1983) called the following five components the 5 "D"s of learned pain syndrome:

1. Dramatization of complaints
2. Dysfunction of conditions (such as sex drive) unrelated to pathology
3. Drug misuse
4. Dependency (helplessness)
5. Disability (paid and otherwise)

Davidson (1976) stated that the behavioral component of pain management may be addressed by an operant approach consisting of the following goals:

1. Reduction of pain behavior such as:
   a. signals to others that tend to elicit reinforcement
   b. the use of unnecessary medication
2. Reduction of excessive health care utilization behaviors including:
   a. continued pursuit of unattainable "cure"
   b. continued pursuit of authentication of the problem
   c. continued pursuit of attention, additional palliative medication, or more prescribed rest

3. Increased activity level
   a. restoration of optimal activity level to make posttreatment target behaviors accessible
4. Rearrangement of contingencies to pain and well behavior by family and significant others
   a. reduction in direct and indirect reinforcement of pain behavior and secondary gain
   b. increase in reinforcement of effective well behavior
5. Establishment and maintainance of well behavior
   a. correction of skill deficits
   b. remediation of problem behaviors from which time-out was sought through pain behaviors
   c. promotion of access to sustaining well behaviors
   d. where indicated, legitimization of retirement and helping the patient and family to carry it out effectively.

Davidson cautions that all of the previously mentioned operant techniques should only be applied if there is evidence of learned behavior to pain and if the target behavior is within the repertoire of the patient. He also advises that this type of therapeutic approach must be sustained by the patient's family or support system.

As stated earlier, it is not difficult to substitute *tinnitus* for *pain* throughout the preceding discussion. For tinnitus, it is quite plausible that a similar sequence of events occur.

- A physical sensation is produced by damage to a peripheral structure. Cognitions alter the threshold or the critical level necessary to evoke the tinnitus perception.
- The patient may engage in catastrophic misinterpretations of the tinnitus, viewing it as a sign of impending deafness or a symptom of a life-threatening ailment.
- The patient may feel that he has no control of the problem.
- Learned helplessness may ensue. The patient might alter his behavior by "giving up the fight," staying home, withdrawing socially, and/or rendering himself incapable of concentrating at work.

- The five "D"s (dramatization of complaints, dysfunction of conditions unrelated to the tinnitus, drug misuse, dependency, and disability) may result.

Cognitive-Behavioral Therapy for Tinnitus Patients

The application of cognitive therapy for emotional disorders and cognitive coping skills therapy with patients suffering from intractable pain led Sweetow (1986) to suggest employing the combined approach of cognitive-behavioral therapy for tinnitus patients.

Changing cognitive patterns and learned behavior requires systematic reconditioning, not simply a determination to do well! Just saying, "you can learn to live with it" is not sufficient. Likewise, it is not advisable to attempt to modify the patient's personality. The patient will reject attempts at treatment, if he perceives the therapist as believing he is unstable or that the problem is "all in his head." Instead, the consequences of the behaviors and thought patterns must be made the central issue. Thus, cognitive-behavioral therapy incorporates a series of testable hypotheses. To arrive at these hypotheses, a thorough assessment of the patient's problem must first be undertaken. Assessment is both diagnostic and therapeutic. It is difficult to separate assessment from process. Organized procedures should be mutually agreed upon to alter maladaptive behaviors and thoughts. Progress should be measurable and monitored regularly and follow-up is essential.

The basic flow of cognitive-behavioral therapy for tinnitus entails the following steps:

I. Define the problem in terms of a framework that allows for amenable solutions

Understanding and assessing a patient's preconceived beliefs about the consequences of his inability to cope with tinnitus is essential in establishing a therapy plan.

The assessment segment of cognitive-behavioral therapy for tinnitus patients is accomplished via written questionnaires, personal interviews, and severity scaling inventories (see Chapter 11). Similar to the evaluation preceding any type of treatment, the questionnaire and interviews should be comprehensive and consider the following:

- onset of the problem
- potential causes and trigger events
- location and nature of the tinnitus
- exacerbating factors
- other medical and otological details
- treatment history

In addition, for purposes of cognitive-behavioral therapy, the nature of how the patient perceives the tinnitus and how it is dealt with cognitively and behaviorally should be established. For example, questions such as "When are you aware of the tinnitus?" and "When does the tinnitus bother you?" may help launch discussions of cognitive distortions, as will be described shortly. Statements made by the patient must be well defined. It is not adequate for a patient to say "I can't fall asleep," or "The tinnitus is driving me crazy." Instead, these remarks must be carefully and operationally defined. Examples of unacceptable versus acceptable operationally defined responses follow.

Inadequate Response	Acceptable Response
The tinnitus keeps me awake.	I fall asleep relatively easily but then I awaken twice each night and then it takes about an hour to fall back asleep.
The tinnitus is driving me crazy.	I am finding it difficult to concentrate when I can't find any quiet time. This makes me angry and I'm losing my temper around my family.

Carefully question the patient in order to determine what specific ways the tinnitus is affecting attitudes and behavior. Does he stay at home when he hears the tinnitus, does the tinnitus depress him, does it make him angry, does it prevent him from working? Problems should be quantified in terms of frequency, duration, and intensity.

- *Frequency* refers to how often the patient thinks about the tinnitus during the course of the day
- *Duration* refers to the length of time these thoughts persist
- *Intensity* refers to the strength of the negative reaction, be it anger, sadness, helplessness, and so on.

2. Identify the behaviors and thoughts affected by the tinnitus

Questionnaires and personal interviews should determine the behaviors affected by the tinnitus and the strategies currently utilized. For example:

- Does the tinnitus interfere with sleep, work, social relationships?
- How does the patient react when the tinnitus is the first thing heard in the morning?
- Is the patient withdrawing from social and family situations?
- How do others react to the patient with regard to the tinnitus?

Also, the therapist should ascertain whether there is a legal case pending concerning the tinnitus. These last two questions may help determine whether there are secondary gains associated. The therapist must assess behavioral contingencies, reinforcers, stimulus pairings in the patient's environment, and the patient's responsiveness to such events.

3. List the maladaptive strategies and cognitive distortions currently employed

Dysfunctional thoughts that are exaggerated, distorted, mistaken, or unrealistic lead to in-comprehensible reactions. The following list describes common cognitive distortions. Patients should be informed that these distortions are made by most people and occur regularly. Usually, they are not particularly harmful, but if they sustain an unacceptable status quo in terms of reactions or behaviors, they are maladaptive and should be modified.

Dichotomous—all or nothing thinking; for example, "Yes, my tinnitus doesn't bother me as much as it used to, but it is still there, so it's unacceptable."

Selective abstraction (mental filter)—one aspect of a complex situation is the focus of attention, while others are ignored; for example, "I was upset this afternoon about my tinnitus, so I'm not getting better."

Mind reading—assuming others thoughts without having evidence; for example, "I know my friends think I'm crazy."

Jumping to conclusions—assuming negative expectations about future events as established facts; for example, "When I wake up in the morning and hear my tinnitus, I know it is going to be a terrible day."

Emotional reasoning—assuming emotional reactions reflect the true situation; for example, "I feel overwhelmed about my tinnitus, therefore it is going to be impossible to overcome."

Labeling—attaching a global label to oneself rather than to specific events or actions; for example, "I'm cursed."

Overgeneralization—an event is characteristic of life in general, as opposed to specific; for example, "I couldn't concentrate on my homework last night because of the tinnitus. I will never graduate and achieve my life's dreams."

Disqualifying the positive—positive experiences that would conflict with negative views are discounted; for example, "The fact that I haven't thought about tinnitus in a few days is just a fluke."

Catastrophizing—negative events are treated as intolerable rather than in perspective; for example, "I couldn't sleep last night, so I did poorly at a job interview. This tinnitus is ruining my life."

Should statements—using should and have to statements to provide motivation or control; for example, "I should be able to ignore this tinnitus."

Personalization—assuming one is the cause of a particular event when in fact other factors are responsible; for example, "I should have never agreed to have that stapedectomy, because it caused my tinnitus."

4. Distinguish between the tinnitus experience and the maladaptive behavior

A patient may assign the blame for certain behaviors on the presence of tinnitus. He may say "the tinnitus is making me depressed," or the "tinnitus is preventing me from working." These statements confer attributes to tinnitus that are unwarranted. The patient must recognize that the tinnitus does not have the power to produce such events. It is the patient's reaction and behaviors that produce these responses. The therapist can help the patient remove tinnitus' status as an entity of its own by encouraging the patient to analyze the reality and logic of his statements.

5. Identify alternate thoughts, behaviors, and strategies

Three main processes are employed to reach the objectives. They are:

1. changing the way one interprets, thinks and feels
2. modifying one's actions for a specific purpose, and
3. removing inappropriate beliefs, anxieties and fears

Burns (1980) lists a variety of charting methods to help patients identify and modify maladaptive thoughts, behaviors, and strategies.

An example is a simple three-column chart, called a Dysfunctional Thoughts Record, in which the patient's task is to record a specific situation he wants to alter in the left column; the negative, maladaptive cognitive distortion in the middle column; and an alternative, rational thought in the right-hand column. For example, the patient may record the following:

Situation	Cognitive Distortion	Rational Thought
I wake up and hear my tinnitus so I know its going to be a bad day.	Jumping to conclusions All or nothing thinking	What I do will determine how my day goes, not the fact that I hear the tinnitus.

Another method is to ask the patient to grade emotions on a 1 to 10 scale. This procedure is very useful in eliminating all or nothing distortions. Alternatively, the therapist can remind the patient of a serious catastrophe, (such as a life-threatening illness of a loved one), have the patient grade it on 1 to 10 scale, and compare that situation to his tinnitus. This approach may reduce catastrophizing.

A technique that may assist the patient recognize his own maladaptive strategies is to have the patient reverse roles with the therapist so that the therapist presents negative views while the patient is asked to challenge those unsubstantiated views. For example, the therapist can detail the hopelessness of the situation, while the patient formulates alternative solutions.

6. Encourage the patient to formulate and prioritize attainable target goals

When mutually developing goals, ensure that the targets are not unrealistic. The patient should establish initial goals that can be relatively easily achieved. For example, the patient who has difficulty falling asleep might record the following objectives, which can be monitored by his significant other.

Behavior	Current Status	Moderate Improvement	Realistic Goal
Falling asleep	Takes 2 hours	1 hour	30 minutes

Note that these objectives are realistic, as opposed to saying, "I want to fall asleep every night within 5 minutes."

7. Collaboratively devise and rehearse strategies that can be measured

As succinctly stated by Beck, Rush, Shaw, and Emery (1979) "cognitive therapy" is "collaborative empiricism." The patient is the chief decision maker, with the therapist serving as a resource. Prior to beginning cognitive-behavioral therapy, the therapist must communicate certain convictions to the patient. First, the patient needs to understand that the therapist takes the problem of tinnitus seriously and that it deserves a comprehensive evaluation before deciding on the proper treatment mode. Next, the therapist should acknowledge that he knows the tinnitus is real, not imagined, and that the patient's reaction to the tinnitus may well be a normal reaction to an abnormal condition. However, the goal of the therapy is to alter reactions and behaviors if they are maladaptively hindering eventual peaceful coexistence with the tinnitus. The therapist also should acknowledge that he has limitations, and no magical cure!

Some cognitive-behavioral therapists use homework assignments. Homework should be collaboratively selected and should be in attainable and measurable units. Ideally the patient will suggest the same homework assignments that the therapist *would* have suggested. Collaborate by saying "so what I understand is that you have agreed to take responsibility for trying to . . ." If a patient "fails" in completing the assignment, it should be viewed as an opportunity to jointly examine the self-thoughts that led to the "failure." Sometimes, the assignments

consist of maintaining a diary, or charting frequency, duration, and intensity as described earlier. When diaries are used, asking the patient's significant other to maintain records may also be useful in joint counseling sessions. It is a realistic concern that focusing attention on the tinnitus for charting purposes during the early stages of therapy could result in its perceived exacerbation, and the patient should be informed of this possibility.

Distraction, rather than focusing may be preferable. However, maintaining distraction indefinitely in the presence of a constant high-intensity stimulus is extremely difficult (McCaul & Malott, 1984). Even so, a variety of distraction methods can be effective. Among the more popular techniques are replacement imagery, cognitive rehearsal, desensitization with flooding imagery, coping imagery (combining cognitive rehearsal with desensitization and flooding), thought stopping, and refocusing. An overview of these procedures is presented in Turk, Meichenbaum, and Genest (1983).

As with other forms of counseling and educational therapy, providing the patient with home reading materials may be useful. In putting together such materials, the therapist should consider the following suggestions (Burns, 1980):

- Organize and present the materials in natural, logical categories such as diagnosis, treatment, expected outcome, and so on.
- Present details in both writing and verbally.
- Tailor the instructions to the language level of the patient.
- Don't overload; gradually present the material over time.
- Emphasize the "how-to" component, not just the "why."
- Assess comprehension and skill by asking the patient to describe what he or she is going to do after the session.
- Give the patient a self-monitoring tool to assess his or her own performance.
- Include the family in the educational process, whenever possible.

8. Regularly assess success or failure of coping strategies

Cognitive-behavioral therapy is built on the premise that the patient's assumptions can be self-tested. For example, a patient can make a list of positive consequences that might occur if he changes his typical pattern of staying home when the tinnitus is apparent first thing in the morning. Then, at the end of the day, he can chart accomplishments that were achieved, compared to simply staying home. As another example, a patient who reports that he is aware of his tinnitus "all the time," can alter this maladaptive thought by being asked to report any times during the day when he was focused on other matters and thus unaware of the tinnitus. Also, a significant other might be recruited to record the amount of time it takes for the patient to fall asleep following implementation of specific strategies such as altering the customary bedtime, or drinking a glass of warm milk before retiring.

Overall progress in coping with tinnitus can be assessed and compared to a pretherapy baseline using subjective inventories. Numerous subjective severity scales are available (see Chapter 11). Formal assessment scales are needed to establish a baseline measure that can be compared to subsequent monitoring. Quantifiable measures are also required because it is difficult to determine whether "I'm feeling kind of bummed out" is an improvement over "I'm not feeling so hot."

Assessment data that are of limited reliability or unknown validity are worthless from a research standpoint, but may be quite useful from a clinical view. For example, if a patient does not complete an answer on a survey, this can serve as a useful counseling issue for clarification purposes. Furthermore, test-retest reliability is irrelevant when dealing with behaviors that are changeable and situation specific. (Nelson, 1983). For example, a tinnitus patient may react quite differently to his tinnitus when he is depressed versus when he is happy.

9. Question and challenge unsubstantiated statements

Challenge statements that contain absolutes ("never, always, everyone, no one"). When a patient states "I'll never be able to do it; It would be too hard for me; I'll just fail," point out that he just made three cognitive distortions in this one defeatist outburst. Challenge the patient, in a non-hostile manner, to provide evidence why the goals cannot be achieved. When a patient indicates that his wife is losing respect for him because he is too weak to fight off the tinnitus, ask him if she has told him as much, or is he "mind reading" and making assumptions without evidence. Challenges should be made in a non-hostile manner; direct confrontation is usually discouraged but can help if the patient is not willing or able to participate actively in the process.

10. Lay a framework for maintenance of positive changes

Bandura's (1977) social learning theory states that environmental factors, behavioral responses, and mediational processes are constantly interacting so it makes no sense to try to locate the beginning of any behavioral sequence. The "expectation" of a bad situation creates anxiety and fear. Also important is the concept of self-efficacy. The patient who wonders "can I handle the problem?" or "what do I need to do to handle the problem?" needs positive encouragement and evidence that the objectives can indeed be achieved.

The time frame for positive change should be realistically discussed with the patient. Cognitive-behavioral therapy should produce success (as defined by the therapist and the patient) within six to eight weeks. If no progress has been made during this period, it is probably not going to be successful. Attainable short-term goals should be attempted initially. Teach the patient to anticipate failures and setbacks in order to short circuit overreaction. Inform the patient that progress will not be constant and that lack of progress and setbacks can be informative. The patient needs to learn to not get too buoyed by the peaks or too discouraged by the valleys on the way to progress.

Cognitive-behavioral therapy lies between directive and client-centered approaches. Guided discovery is preferred over direct confrontation. This style maximizes patient involvement, encourages the patient to take responsibility, and minimizes the feeling that the therapist is imposing his or her own ideas on the patient. In addition, there are a variety of other actions that the cognitive-behavioral therapist should perform. Among them are:

- Continually check with the patient to determine the patient's understanding of the strategies and techniques being employed.
- Use teamwork. Encourage the patient throughout the session to be active in therapy.
- Pace the session so that there is a clear beginning, middle, and end. Avoid peripheral digression.
- Utilize excellent listening and empathic skills. Recognize the patient's internal reality.
- Display high levels of warmth, concern, confidence, and genuineness.
- Be confident, and professional.
- Use guided discovery. Use a questioning format ("then what, what would happen if, what does that mean?") to assist the patient in reaching conclusions.
- Focus on key thoughts and help the patient recognize dysfunctional thinking.
- Manifest a broad repertoire of cognitive techniques and move between them as appropriate.
- Manifest a broad repertoire of behavioral techniques and move between them as appropriate.
- Encourage patients to attribute positive change to themselves, not to the therapist.

MYTHS ABOUT COGNITIVE-BEHAVIORAL THERAPY

The following statements are myths about cognitive-behavioral therapy (the realities are italicized).

1. Cognitive-behavioral therapy is "the power of positive thinking." *In reality it is the power of realistic thinking. It is collaborative planning and testing.*
2. Cognitive-behavioral therapy is simple. *It takes time and careful thought.*
3. Cognitive-behavioral therapy is talking people out of their problems. *Cognitive-behavioral therapy is not debate; it employs guided discovery.*
4. Cognitive-behavioral therapy ignores the past. *Cognitive-behavioral therapy pays only as much attention to the past as is necessary.*
5. Cognitive-behavioral therapy means no medication. *Working in conjunction with a mental health professional is important in assessing whether the simultaneous use of medication might assist in the cognitive-behavioral modification process.*
6. The goal of cognitive-behavioral therapy is to eliminate emotion. *The objective is to bring emotions under control.*
7. Cognitive-behavioral therapy can only be used with bright, intellectual patients. *The therapist must adapt the pace and intensity of therapy to the patient's level.*
8. Cognitive-behavioral therapy cannot be used with seriously disturbed patients. *Professionals untrained in mental health therapy should refer as appropriate.*

PATIENT RESISTANCE

It is not unusual for the therapist to encounter serious patient resistance to a psychological approach to a problem that the patient perceives as a physical malady. Noncompliance with homework or collaboration is a natural consequence of a maladaptive thinking style. Conveying to patients that they are held in high regard as worthwhile persons will help overcome resistance. Remind the patient that even though the initial generator of the tinnitus may have been peripheral (that is, the ear), it is ultimately the brain that perceives and interprets the tinnitus, and it is therefore the brain that can produce changes. The neurophysiological model proposed by Jastreboff and Hazell (1993) used in conjunction with (or in certain cases, subsequent to) cognitive-behavioral therapy can help create a sense of balance between the patient's perception of the therapy being a "simple psychological" intervention and the patient's deeply rooted belief that the tinnitus is a physical problem. The explanation afforded by this model can be very helpful to help deflect the initial feeling of guilt or weakness regarding a perceived inability to cope. It is important to treat the patient with respect and educate him or her regarding the possible causes of tinnitus and why the brain is intricately tied into the perception and the ultimate difficulty in habituating to the symptom. McFadden (1982) stated that "treatment of psychological factors without adequate preparation of the patient often results in confusion and alienation." So it is vital to inform the patient that while the tinnitus is real, the maladaptive response to it is exacerbating its perception and making habituation more difficult. Moreover, cognitive-behavioral therapy, albeit a primarily psychological approach, may have significant physical ramifications as suggested by the principles of neural plasticity and cortical reorganization (Kilgard & Merzenich, 1998). Resistance is often minimized when the patient recognizes that this approach can alter physical function.

POSSIBLE PHYSICAL OUTCOMES

Cognitive interpretations and affective arousal may directly affect physiology by increasing sympathetic nervous system arousal (Bandura et al., 1985) and producing endogenous opioids, (Bandura et al., 1987). Endogenous opioids and neuropeptides (endorphins) activate efferent control systems in the central nervous system that are important in pain suppression and may prove to be relevant to tinnitus perception.

Catecholamines are neurotransmitters involved in regulating heart rate, blood pressure, mobilizing blood glucose, shunting blood from the viscera to brain and muscle, and so forth. Frankenhauser (1980) suggests that psychological factors trigger both the sympathetic-adrenomedullary response and the pituitary-adrenocortical systems, thus influencing secretion of catecholamines. It is possible that modifications of cognition can lead to decreased catecholamines, decreased muscle tension, and increased availability of neurotransmitters such as serotonin and endogenous opioids such as endorphins. So, not unlike anticonvulsant drugs that have been reported to temporarily minimize tinnitus, perhaps cognitive restructuring alters neurotransmitters in a more specific goal-oriented manner than is obtainable by using an unfocused approach from drugs.

RESULTS AND FOLLOW-UP ISSUES

Jakes (1992) reported that the use of cognitive restructuring alone resulted in slight, but not statistically significant improvements in emotional distress when compared to tinnitus maskers, tinnitus maskers plus cognitive therapy, placebo maskers, or waiting list controls. Henry and Wilson (1997) reported similarly uninspiring results using attention-diversion, imagery, and distraction.

There are very few studies of the long-term effect of cognitive-behavioral therapy on tinnitus patients. Sweetow (1986) reported success (as defined by statistically significant improvements on the Tinnitus Severity Scale) (Sweetow & Levy, 1989), but there were no data regarding sustained long-term improvements. Jakes et al. (1986) compared success attained with relaxation training only to attention diversion along with relaxation training. They found no differences between the two treatments. They hypothesized that overall therapeutic impact may have been due to cognitive training (attempts to alter beliefs and attitudes about the tinnitus) presented prior to the relaxation training.

Henry and Wilson (1997) allocated sixty tinnitus subjects with chronic tinnitus to one of three conditions: (1) cognitive coping skills training (attention diversion, imagery training and thought management skills) combined with education, (2) education only, or (3) control (waiting list). The two treatment groups improved significantly over the control group in terms of frequency of use of coping strategies, benefits derived from coping strategies, reduction of irrational beliefs, and knowledge about tinnitus. Subjects receiving cognitive training along with education improved significantly more than the education-only group for greater reductions in distress and handicaps associated with tinnitus. Depression, subjective loudness ratings, noticeability, and bothersome of tinnitus was not different for those two groups. At the twelve-month follow-up, the differential treatment effects had dissipated. Thus, booster sessions were considered essential.

Marlatt and Gordon (1985) address the problem of sustaining progress for the long term and propose the following steps to guard against relapse:

1. make the patient aware of high-risk situations
2. teach the patient to identify early signs of impending relapse, and
3. develop explicit strategies for handling these situations and warning signs.

In order to develop these plans, it is necessary to explore the patient's long-term expectations for future problems and outcomes. Then, once strategic plans are implemented, periodic booster sessions, approximately every three months for the first year, and every six months the second following the initial six to ten sessions should be provided.

WHO SHOULD ADMINISTER COGNITIVE-BEHAVIORAL THERAPY TO TINNITUS PATIENTS?

It is anticipated that most of the readers of this chapter will not be trained as mental health professionals. Therefore, one might question whether they have adequate skills to provide cognitive-behavioral therapy for tinnitus patients. It is this author's contention that cognitive-behavioral therapy has numerous parallels to aural rehabilitation, a process which most audiologists feel relatively comfortable. Aural rehabilitation and cognitive-behavioral therapy can both be employed either in individual or in group therapy modalities (Sweetow, 1984). Both techniques require good listening skills, empathy, and common sense. Like a hearing loss, tinnitus affects the entire family. As with aural rehabilitation, it is helpful to break the problems associated with the tinnitus down into smaller components so that success can be achieved readily. And, similar to aural rehabilitation, cognitive-behavioral therapy can be effectively used in conjunction with, or as a preparation for, many of the other therapeutic approaches detailed in this book. Wilson et al. (1998) address this issue, as well.

The therapist, regardless of his training, must be clearly aware of his professional limitations, however. In addition to, or in lieu of, cognitive-behavioral therapy, direct counseling from a trained psychologist or psychiatrist may be in order. Tinnitus patients have been described as rigid, desperate, obsessive, or neurotic (House, 1981). Many present additional problems contributing to tinnitus distress (such as divorce, money, and occupation). Some have a history of depression. It is difficult to definitively state whether the emotional status of tinnitus patients existed before the onset of tinnitus, or whether it is a result of the tinnitus. The professional must be prepared to recognize when personality disorders, psychiatric and mental disorders dictate that an outside referral to a mental health professional is warranted. For this reason, establishment of a network with a multidisciplinary team is crucial.

CONCLUSIONS

Cognitive-behavioral therapy is an approach that can help patients make a positive adaptation to the presence of tinnitus. It involves a collaborative effort in which the patient, not just the therapist, is responsible for the outcome. Like other therapies for incurable conditions, patients must understand that it is not designed to eliminate the condition, rather to alter the patient's cognitions, attitudes and associated behaviors in a manner such that the tinnitus is no longer perceived to exert a negative impact on the patient's life. Cognitive-behavioral intervention can accomplish these goals and have an overall positive impact on the patient's life providing the patient understands and accepts these objectives, the assessment process is complete, the interpretation of the patient collected data is logical and correct, and the execution of the intervention is sufficient.

REFERENCES

Bandura, A. (1977). Self-efficacy: Toward a unifying theory of behavioral change. *Psychology Review, 84,* 191–215.

Bandura A., O'Leary, A., Taylor, C., Gauthier, J., & Gossard, D. (1987). Perceived self-efficacy and pain control: Opioid and nonopioid mechanisms. *Journal of Personality and Social Psychology, 53,* 563–571.

Bandura, A., Taylor, C. B., Williams, S. L., Mefford, I. N., & Barchas, J. D. (1985). Catecholamine secretion as a function of perceived coping self-efficacy. *Journal of Consulting and Clinical Psychology, 53,* 406–414.

Beck, A. T., Rush, A. J., Shaw, B. F., & Emery, G. (1979). *Cognitive therapy of depression.* New York: Guilford Press.

Brena, S. F., & Chapman, S. L. (1983). *Management of patients with chronic pain.* New York: Spectrum Publications Jamaica.

Burns, D. (1980). *Feeling good: The new mood therapy.* New York: Signet.

Cautela, J., & Kearney, A. (1986). *The covert conditioning handbook.* New York: Springer.

Davidson, P. (1976). *The behavioral management of anxiety, depression and pain.* New York: Brunner/Mazel, 167–177.

Ellis, A. (1962). *Reason and emotion in psychotherapy.* New York: Lyle-Stuart.

Frankenhaeuser, M. (1980). Psychobiological aspects of life stress. In S. Levine & H. Ursin (Eds.), *Coping and health.* New York: Plenum.

Gatchel, R. J., & Turk, D. C. (1996). *Psychological approaches to pain management.* New York: Guilford Press.

Henry, J. L., & Wilson, P. H. (1997). The psychological management of tinnitus: Comparison of a combined cognitive educational program, education alone and a waiting-list control. *International Tinnitus Journal, 2*(1), 9–20.

House, P. (1981). Personality of the tinnitus patient. In *Tinnitus CIBA Foundation Symposium 85.* London: Pitman, 191–203.

Jakes, S. C., Hallam, R. S., McKenna, L., & Hinchcliffe, R. (1992). Group cognitive therapy for medical patients: An application to tinnitus. *Cognitive Therapy and Research, 16,* 67–82.

Jakes, S. C., Hallam, R. S., Rachman, S., & Hinchcliffe, R. (1986). The effects of reassurance, relaxation training and distraction on chronic tinnitus sufferers. *Behavior Research and Therapy, 24,* 497–507.

Jastreboff, P. J., & Hazell, J. W. P. (1993). A neurophysiological approach to tinnitus: Clinical implications. *British Journal of Audiology, 27,* 7–17.

Kilgard, M. P., & Merzenich, M. M. (1998). Cortical map reorganization enabled by nucleus basalis activity. *Science, 279,* 1714–1718.

Marlatt, G. A., & Gordon, J. R. (1985). *Relapse prevention.* New York: Guilford.

McCaul, K., & Malott, J. (1984). Distraction and coping with pain. *Psychol Bulletin, 95*(5), 16–33.

McFadden, D. (1982). *Tinnitus. Facts, theories, and treatments.* Washington, DC: National Academy Press.

Meichenbaum, D. (1977). *Cognitive-behavioral modificaiton: An integrative approach.* New York: Plenum.

Meichenbaum, D. H., & Turk, D. (1976). The cognitive-behavioral management of anxiety, anger, and pain. In *The behavioral management of anxiety, anger, and pain.* Davidson, P. O. (Ed.). New York: Brunner-Mazel.

Melzack, R. & Wall, P. (1965). Pain mechanisms: A new theory. *Science, 150,* 971.

Nelson, R. O. (1983). Behavioral assessment: Past present, and future. *Behavioral Assessment, 5,* 195–206.

Seligman, M. (1975). *Helplessness: On depression, development, and death.* San Francisco: W. H. Freeman.

Skinner, B. F. (1953). *Science and human behavior.* New York: Macmillan.

Sweetow, R. W. (1984). Cognitive-behavioral modification in tinnitus management. *Hearing Instruments, 35,* 14–52.

Sweetow, R. W. (1986). Cognitive aspects of tinnitus patient management. *Ear and Hearing,* 7(6), 390–396.

Sweetow, R. W. (Ed.). (1987). Management of the tinnitus patient. *Seminars in Hearing, 8*(1).

Sweetow, R. W., & Levy, M. C. (1989). Diagnostic and therapeutic tinnitus severity scaling. *Tinnitus Today, 14*(3), 4–8.

Thorpe, G. L., & Olson, S. L. (1990). *Behavior therapy: Concepts, procedures and applications.* Boston: Allyn and Bacon.

Turk, D. C., Meichenbaum, D., & Genest, M. (1983). *Pain and behavioural medicine: A cognitive-behavioral perspective.* New York: Guilford.

Wilson, P. H., Henry, J. L., Andersson, G., Hallam, R. S., & Lindberg, P. (1998). A critical analysis of directive counselling as a component of tinnitus retraining therapy. *British Journal of Audiology, 32,* 273–286.

Wolpe, J. (1958). *Psychotherapy by reciprocal inhibition.* Stanford, CA: Stanford University Press.

Wolpe, J., & Lazarus, A. (1966). *Behavioral therapy techniques.* New York: Pergamon Press.

CHAPTER 14

Tinnitus Masking

Jack A. Vernon, Ph.D.
Mary B. Meikle, Ph.D.

1st Patient: "I don't understand this masking idea—why add another sound when I already have one I don't want to hear?"

2nd Patient: "What they try to do is *substitute* the masking sound for your tinnitus—it's as though the masker has covered up the tinnitus. I can't even tell my tinnitus is there, when I'm wearing my maskers."

1st Patient: "But why is it any better listening to those masking sounds?"

2nd Patient: "Well, all sounds are not alike. For one thing the masking sounds are pretty mild. They're a low-level type of noise that's not annoying like my tinnitus."

1st Patient: "So you think it's OK to listen to noise all the time?"

2nd Patient: "No, masking sounds are very boring so before you know it you "tune them out." I know the masking noise will be there all the time, kind of like the air conditioner noise, so after a while I don't even notice it."

1st Patient: "Is that the main reason you're willing to put up with masking?"

2nd Patient: "There are some other reasons . . . one is that an outside sound can be turned off whenever I want, unlike my tinnitus. That means I get to control when I hear my tinnitus and when I don't."

1st Patient: "So you're saying if I cover my tinnitus using a boring external sound that is not too loud, I'll be able to ignore it and I also won't hear my tinnitus?"

2nd Patient: "That's right—if your tinnitus is maskable. Remember they need to do some testing to see what kind of noise works best for covering up *your* tinnitus."

INTRODUCTION

The conversation reproduced above represents comments we have heard many times in the Oregon Tinnitus Clinic. These comments summarize two important themes: First, most of our knowledge about how tinnitus masking works was gained from patients and their observations concerning their tinnitus. Second, it is the patients, not the clinicians, who determine whether or not masking offers an acceptable form of relief. Our

313

task as clinicians is to understand and apply technical knowledge of masking devices so that, working together with each patient, we can jointly determine the best solution for that individual's particular combination of hearing capabilities and tinnitus.

Goals of this Chapter

Subjective tinnitus is a difficult clinical problem and until the early 1970s it defeated most efforts to provide relief. Lacking effective means for treating it, many hearing specialists tended to dismiss tinnitus as not being within their area of training or expertise. As a result, the entire field of tinnitus research suffered from benign neglect, causing most people to believe that nothing could be done for tinnitus. There still are many health professionals as well as patients who remain unaware of the benefits that can be obtained from a properly conducted masking program. It is our hope that this chapter will help to bring tinnitus masking further into the mainstream of day-to-day clinical practice.

As with any technically complex subject, there are a number of ways to do it wrong, and many fewer ways to do it right. With attention to a few technical details, however, it is relatively easy to add tinnitus masking techniques to the existing array of procedures available in the standard audiology or otolaryngology clinic. This chapter is intended to provide a summary of the methods needed to perform tinnitus masking effectively, as well as an overview of the experience upon which those methods are based.

Tinnitus Masking as a Management Tool for Clinically Significant Tinnitus

By "clinically significant tinnitus" we mean severe, constant, unrelieved tinnitus as opposed to the insignificant or minor tinnitus that occurs in the large majority of individuals who report tinnitus. Tinnitus is "clinically significant" when it is the *primary* complaint and when it causes the patient to

seek treatment. Considerable information exists to show that about 80 percent of those who report tinnitus have it only mildly (Brown, 1990; National Center for Health Statistics, 1968). It is the other 20 percent, who have disturbing tinnitus that interferes with sleep and with normal daily activities, for whom treatment efforts such as masking must be provided.

In the remainder of this chapter, for brevity we will omit the words "clinically significant" when discussing tinnitus that requires treatment. It should be understood in what follows that we are *not* speaking of tinnitus in general, but instead referring to tinnitus that is severe enough to cause the individual to seek treatment.

As is well known there are at present no cures for tinnitus, although there is little doubt that cures eventually will be forthcoming as research continues in this area. Tinnitus masking is certainly not a cure. Instead masking provides a form of relief, making it an important tool for treatment and management of severe tinnitus until a more permanent relief becomes available.

It should be kept in mind that patients differ greatly in regard to the nature of their tinnitus and also in regard to etiological factors. Thus, it is unlikely that any proposed treatment will work equally well for all tinnitus patients. That statement applies to tinnitus masking. As will be discussed, there are a number of cases in which masking has not succeeded in relieving tinnitus, although it has been shown that proper use of masking can benefit a majority of patients with severe tinnitus.

Masking as a form of treatment for tinnitus has only been available since 1976, and wearable masking equipment is still undergoing development and improvement. As with any new technology, it takes a while to learn how best to apply it. Moreover there is still a great deal to be learned about tinnitus, and many aspects of tinnitus masking that are not well understood. Thus, even today, it is usually not possible to predict ahead of time which patients will benefit from masking and which will not. That fact leads to the following important caution for both patient and clinician:

"THOU SHALT NOT PREJUDGE."

We have encountered many tinnitus patients who have been told by health care professionals that masking would not work for them—and then we have found that those statements simply were not true. It is difficult to understand why predictions such as those were made when it is easy to test a patient and make a determination based on fact rather than on guesswork. When dealing with tinnitus patients it is crucial that preconceived judgments not be allowed to interfere with the necessary examination procedures. The *only* way to determine whether or not masking is appropriate for a given patient is by actual test with the various types of masking devices.

BACKGROUND AND HISTORY OF TINNITUS MASKING

Although tinnitus masking differs in a number of ways from conventional masking of one sound by another, nevertheless the concept of tinnitus masking owes its existence to the universal human experience of how sounds can mask each other. Many patients have discovered on their own that the sound of running water, for example while taking a shower, prevents them from hearing their tinnitus. Despite that common observation we have yet to meet a tinnitus patient who has recorded shower sounds in order to relieve tinnitus without having to stay in the shower all day long! In fact, what we do as clinicians is simply to provide something akin to those sounds that many patients have already found are helpful to them.

Specific Attempts to Relieve Tinnitus Using Masking

Prior to the electronic era, attempts to relieve tinnitus using masking sounds were sporadic and awkward. Several interesting examples from 1821 are provided by the famous French physician, Jean Marie Gaspard Itard, who described a number of different noise environments to "cover up the internal noise." His advice to use noise as a treatment for tinnitus ran as follows:

> . . . producing a roaring fire in the grate considerably relieves the disturbance resulting from tinnitus which sounds like the distant murmuring of wind and a river in flood. The same approach can be adopted with whistling tinnitus, by putting green or slightly damp wood on the fire. When the tinnitus is like the sound of bells, as long as it is not too loud, it may be masked by the resonance of a large copper bowl into which falls a trickle of water from a vase of the same capacity, with a tiny hole pierced in its base. (Translated by S. D. G. Stephens, 1987, p. 11).

He added that these types of external noises, rather than preventing sleep, helped to induce more profound sleep. For a patient who reported that her tinnitus was rendered inaudible by the sounds of running water, Itard advised her to take up residence near a water mill. Other masking efforts were made subsequently by V. Urbantschitsch in 1883, using tuning forks (Feldmann, 1987a) and by Spaulding (1903) who attempted to mask his patients' tinnitus by playing them tones on his violin.

The dawn of the electronic age brought with it the necessary tools for providing sustained, controllable sound that could be varied freely in regard to spectral content and intensity. Although interesting attempts were made by several investigators in the decades between 1920–1950 (see review by Feldmann, 1987a), electroacoustic devices were too large and cumbersome to provide a practical means of controlling tinnitus prior to the development of miniaturized circuits and wearable hearing aids.

The First Attempts at Wearable Tinnitus Maskers

In 1972 the era of wearable tinnitus maskers was initiated by the joining together of three necessary components: First, an individual with severe tinnitus who brought his predicament to the attention of the health care community—this was the late Charles Unice, M.D., a general practitioner who had developed severe tinnitus shortly before that, and who was responsible for founding the American Tinnitus Association (see Chapter 18). Second, researchers who were interested and willing to apply sophisticated acoustical and electronic techniques to help solve the problems presented by tinnitus. Third, resources for constructing wearable sound generators, provided initially by one of the major hearing aid manufacturers at that time (Zenith Hearing Instruments, Inc., under the direction of Mr. James Johnson).

All three of the necessary factors for clinical use of tinnitus masking came together in the early 1970s. Among the few researchers at that time who were working on tinnitus, one of the present authors (J. Vernon, of the Department of Otolaryngology, University of Oregon Medical School) was then attempting to develop an animal model for tinnitus in rhesus monkeys. That work came to the attention of Dr. Charles Unice, who came to Portland seeking to involve the Oregon workers in clinical work on tinnitus. In the course of interaction between Drs. Unice and Vernon it was accidentally observed that Dr. Unice could not hear his tinnitus when standing near one of the many fountains that occupy prominent architectural spots in Portland. Thus was born the concept of developing a wearable sound generator that could mimic acceptable noise such as that made by rushing water (DeWeese & Vernon, 1975; Vernon, 1975).

The first two such devices were designed and made by the Zenith Corporation, and they proved to be an immediate success. They provided complete suppression of tinnitus perception in the first two patients who wore them. Subsequently, wearable masking devices were provided for a large number of patients, not only in Oregon but also at other otologic centers in the United States, the United Kingdom, Australia, Germany, Denmark, and many other countries (Agnew & Johnson 1993; Çelikyurt, Bahadirlan, & Gülçür, 1995; Coles, Baskill, & Goodrum, 1987; Fusté, Doménech, & Traserra et al., 1995; Gabriels, 1991, 1996a; Hazell, 1987; Hazell & Wood, 1981; Hazell, Wood, & Cooper et al., 1985; McCormick & Pritchard, 1987; Schleuning, Johnson, & Vernon, 1980; Shulman & Goldstein, 1987; Vernon, 1975, 1977, 1979; Vernon, Schleuning, Odell, & Hughes, 1977; von Wedel, 1987; Walter & Johansen, 1987).

Further Development of Wearable Masking Devices

That first generation of tinnitus maskers consisted of behind-the-ear devices that were relatively crude. They lacked capabilities for shaping the noise band, and the frequency range was lower than what is now known to be optimal. As time went by however other manufacturers took up the challenge of designing maskers that would be more appropriate for the majority of tinnitus sufferers (Vernon, 1975, 1979, 1981; Vernon & Meikle, 1981). It should be recalled that in most cases, tinnitus is relatively high-pitched (Reed, 1960; Vernon, 1978; Meikle & Walsh, 1984; Meikle et al., 1995; also see Chapter 6). Continued investigation revealed that in many cases, tinnitus can be masked at lower intensity levels if the masking noise occupies a higher frequency range than provided by those original maskers (Pritchard & McCormick, 1987; Vernon, 1979). It is now possible to purchase masking devices that can be tuned to different frequency ranges as needed. In addition, a variety of styles are available including behind-the-ear, in-the-ear, and completely in-the-canal devices. (For commercial sources of masking devices, see Section I in the Appendix on page 356.)

In the intervening years a great deal of work on masking devices has taken place. Perhaps the single most important development, after the recognition that the masking sound must usually include a higher-frequency range, is the development of the "Tinnitus Instrument" or combination unit.

The latter device combines both a sound generator and a hearing aid within the same case (each with its own volume control, if performance is to be acceptable). The terms "Tinnitus Masker" and "Tinnitus Instrument" are terms agreed upon by the United States Food & Drug Administration, who have officially classified these devices as *therapeutic devices* (as opposed to prosthetic devices; the distinction is important because most health coverage plans do not compensate for prosthetic devices).

At the Tinnitus Clinic in Portland, Oregon, the Tinnitus Instrument quickly became the primary instrument of choice for patients that have both hearing impairment and tinnitus (70 percent or more of all tinnitus patients, depending on how hearing impairment is defined). Figure 14-1 illustrates the frequency response of several different commercially available tinnitus maskers and tinnitus instruments.

Tinnitus Relief from an Old Standby: Hearing Aids

The development of wearable masking devices led to greater recognition of the importance of the tinnitus patient's sound environment. A high percentage of hearing-impaired individuals have tinnitus, and it has been known for a long time that properly fitted hearing aids can help to provide relief for tinnitus in some patients. When hearing aids reduce or eliminate the wearers' perceptions of their tinnitus, it is probably because the amplification makes it possible for them to hear ambient noise that can then mask the tinnitus (Saltzman & Ersner, 1947; Vernon, 1977). This masking effect is such a welcome result that hearing aid dispensers have been known to inform their clients that the hearing aid is all they will need to relieve their tinnitus. Unfortunately that statement is true for only a small percentage of tinnitus patients. However, for that group of patients the use of hearing aids to relieve tinnitus provides important benefits, to be discussed in more detail later.

Bedside Maskers and Other Nonwearable Devices

Sleep disturbance from tinnitus is prevalent among individuals with severe tinnitus (Tyler & Baker, 1983; Meikle, Johnson, & Vernon, 1984; George & Kemp, 1991; Gabriels, 1996b; also see Chapter 3). In a recent report describing 1,618 consecutive tinnitus patients, nearly 70 percent reported problems sleeping (45 percent "sometimes"; 25 percent "often") (Meikle, Johnson, & Griest et al., 1995). Although wearable masking devices include in-the-ear models that some patients wear to help them sleep, many individuals prefer to use bedside maskers. These devices are now commercially available in various configurations. (For more detailed information, see Section II in the Appendix on page 356.)

A number of patients have found that static from a mistuned FM radio can provide an adequate masking background for sleeping. That type of sound source, however, does not offer adjustability of the frequency band, thus it may be generally less effective for those who need a specific frequency range of masking sounds.

Other sources of selectable noisebands suitable for use as bedside maskers are available in the form of cassette tapes and CDs (Vernon, 1988; 1992). These need to be played on a tape player or CD player with good high-frequency performance and that provides continuous repetition of the same track. (Information on sources for masking tapes and CDs is provided in Section III of the Appendix on page 356.)

Once the patient has identified a masking sound that is both effective and pleasant, it may take several nights to become accustomed to sleeping in the constant presence of the background noise. The background noise provides some additional benefits beyond that of tinnitus masking—the bedside masker tends to set up an acoustical "shield" that can screen out other, unwanted night-time sounds that tend to disrupt sleep. For patients with severe tinnitus, anything that promotes a more soothing sleep environment is worth pursuing.

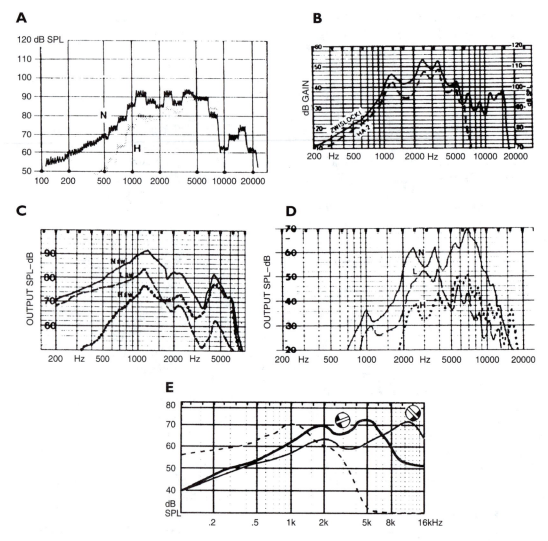

FIGURE 14-1. Frequency ranges of commercially-available tinnitus masking devices. In all graphs, x-axis represents test frequencies and y-axis represents dB SPL; in A, C, and D, letter symbols represent various selectable masking bands (N = normal or default value; H = higher-frequency; L = lower frequency). Note scales differ slightly between graphs. All devices were tested using Zwislocki coupler except where noted otherwise.

A. Starkey AM/Ti (formerly Viennatone AM/Ti)—The instrument used for studies reported by Hazell et al. (1985), still available and in use at some tinnitus clinics; note that sound energy peaks in the approximate range 1 to 4 kHz. (Measured in 2 cc coupler.)

B. Audiotone TA-641—An instrument used by many United States patients in the 1980s, now no longer made; note the improved high-frequency output with significant energy extending through 15 kHz (solid line, data with Zwislocki coupler; dashed line, 2cc coupler).

C. Starkey TM-3—A currently-available masker with adjustable frequency spectrum; with normal "N" setting the peak energy is in range 1 to 5 kHz, while the "L" setting cuts out most energy above about 1.5 kHz.

D. Starkey TM-5—A currently-available masker with adjustable high-frequency output; with normal "N" setting the rolloff is more gradual toward low frequencies and falls off steeply above about 7 kHz; in "H" mode the low-frequency rolloff is steeper and there is additional energy up to about 17 kHz.

E. Starkey TM/TML/TMC—A currently-available device available either as a masker only or as a Tinnitus Instrument (masker plus hearing aid), with optional User Tunable Masking Filter. The filter provides adjustable frequency spectrum for the masking noise as indicated by the three different user-selectable curves, whose center frequencies can be tuned to different frequencies in the range 1 to 15 kHz .

DEVELOPMENT OF MODERN TECHNIQUES FOR MASKING TINNITUS

The ability of noise to reduce or eliminate our perception of other external sounds is well-known and is experienced by all of us in the presence of noisy environments such as when a vacuum cleaner is running, when near a noisy engine, or when running water in the bath or shower. In recent times, considerable effort has been devoted to identifying those sounds that are most effective for "covering up" or masking tinnitus.

Initial Studies of Tinnitus masking

Among the first systematic studies of tinnitus masking stimuli were those performed by Feldmann (1971). From that work he learned that tinnitus masking does not follow the same rules as the masking of one external sound by another. There proved to be great individual differences in regard to the nature of sounds that effectively masked tinnitus: In 34 percent of his patients, it was necessary for the frequency of the masking sound to be close to that matching the pitch of the person's tinnitus. In another 32 percent, the frequency content of the masking sound did not matter as nearly *any* sound appeared to be capable of effectively masking the tinnitus; and in 20 percent, masking could be achieved but only at high sound levels. In some unfortunate cases (11 percent), no sound could be found that would effectively suppress or eliminate the perception of tinnitus. Very similar results were later obtained in several different clinics (Mitchell, 1983; Tyler & Conrad-Armes, 1984; Mitchell, Vernon, & Creedon, 1993), despite using very different techniques for presenting the stimuli and recording patients' responses.

Feldmann also discovered the important phenomenon subsequently named "residual inhibition" (Vernon & Schleuning, 1978). He described an "inhibitory effect" in which the individual's perception of tinnitus was partially or completely suppressed for a period of time *after* the masking stimulus was turned off (1971). He reported, "Prolonged stimulation may in some cases stop the tinnitus for quite a considerable period of time." That discovery carries important implications for tinnitus therapy using masking stimuli, as will be shown in a later section. In sum, although Feldmann himself did not apply his discoveries to any form of tinnitus therapy, his work established a firm foundation for the use of tinnitus masking as a useful clinical procedure.

After the clinical advances made in the 1970s, interest in tinnitus masking as a research topic began to grow. As will be seen in the following sections, a number of important contributions have been made to the body of knowledge concerning clinical use of masking for relief of tinnitus.

Development of Clinical Procedures for Masking

Soon after the advent of the first wearable maskers, techniques for testing tinnitus according to a standardized protocol began to be applied in a large series of patients with the primary complaint of tinnitus (Vernon & Schleuning, 1978, 1980; Vernon & Meikle, 1981). These efforts to develop a standard test battery received considerable discussion in the burgeoning tinnitus literature at that time (see, for example, the 1981 CIBA Symposium on Tinnitus) (Evered & Lawrenson, 1981). The standard protocol that emerged consisted of four main elements that have been employed widely since the early 1980s:

1. Tinnitus pitch matching, using external comparison tones
2. Tinnitus loudness matching using external tones at the pitch of the tinnitus (the method pioneered by Fowler in 1942 and 1943)
3. Determining the Minimum Masking Level (MML) in dB, typically using a broad band of noise
4. Testing for the occurrence and duration of residual inhibition following one minute of masking using a standard stimulus (typically, the same noiseband as in the previous item 3)

The frequency range of the noiseband used for Tests 3 and 4 deserves some comment: In view of the high prevalence of high-pitched tinnitus (to be discussed later), it is usually desirable to limit the low-frequency content of the noiseband since tinnitus is sometimes temporarily exacerbated by exposure to low-frequency noise. (For that reason, 2k to 12k Hz bands of noise have been used commonly for testing patients in the Oregon Tinnitus Clinic.)

With regard to the dB level of the noise used for Test 4 above, several clinics have experimented with different dB levels, usually within the range 0 to 20 dB re MML (Terry, Jones, Davis, & Slater, 1983; Tyler, Babin, & Niebuhr, 1984). The noise level appears to exert a significant influence on the duration of residual inhibition, although the choice of noise levels may vary between clinics. In the Oregon Tinnitus Clinic it is customary to set the level at 10 dB above MML for testing residual inhibition, a setting based on comparative data obtained in the early days of the clinic (J. Vernon, unpublished observations). If the patient finds that level uncomfortable, the Residual Inhibition test is performed at the patient's maximum comfortable level for the ear in question.

Additional details describing use of these four tests can be found in a number of publications (Vernon & Meikle, 1981; Hazell, 1987; Vernon, 1987; Meikle, Johnson, & Press et al., 1995; see also Chapter 6). These four tests can to some extent be accomplished using an audiometer if it has flexible control of tone frequencies and can adjust sound levels in 1 dB steps. The tests are, however, more easily performed using special equipment that is designed specifically for presenting appropriate acoustic stimulation. Use of a specially-designed tinnitus testing system is helpful for generating a wide range of different tones, as well as noisebands with different center frequencies, thus making it easier to match the characteristics of the patient's tinnitus.

In the early years of the Tinnitus Clinic, we assembled a collection of the necessary bench equipment to provide a dedicated tinnitus-testing system (including high-quality sound sources for pure tones and noise; adjustable low-pass and high-pass filters; dB attenuators; mixer circuitry and amplifier; and earphones with good high-frequency response.) Similar efforts have also been reported by other clinics (Terry et al., 1983; van den Abbeele & Frachet, 1991). A simpler solution, but one that is unfortunately no longer available, was provided by several commercially produced tinnitus synthesizers (the Starkey Tinnitus Research Audiometer and the Norwest Tinnitus Synthesizer, neither of which is currently marketed). It is our hope that future tinnitus research will soon be able to take advantage of digital tinnitus testing systems, controlled by small desktop computers currently under development (Henry, Fausti, Flick, Helt, & Mitchell, 1996; Lay & Nunley, 1996).

Figure 14-2 summarizes measurements of pitch, loudness matches, and Minimum Masking Levels (MMLs) obtained in a large sample of patients at the Oregon Tinnitus Clinic (Meikle, Johnson, & Press et al., 1995). Figure 14-2a documents the fact that tinnitus pitch matches are quite high in frequency—at or above 4 kHz in the majority of cases. Figure 14-2b illustrates the now-classic finding, first reported by Fowler (1942, 1943) that tinnitus loudness matches tend to be low—the median loudness match for tinnitus clinic patients is 4 dB, and 88 percent are at or below 10 dB. Figure 14-2c shows that similar generalizations apply to Minimum Masking Levels (median of 6 dB, 80 percent at or below 15 dB).

Figure 14-3 shows the residual inhibition measures in the same group of patients. Most commonly, residual inhibition following one minute of masking is of short duration, but in a few patients the duration may exceed ten minutes or more.

Importance of Tinnitus Pitch and Loudness Measures

There are several reasons why it is important to document the pitch and loudness of tinnitus for each patient: First, to provide

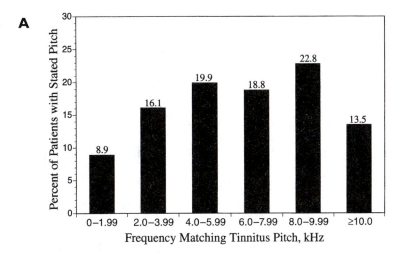

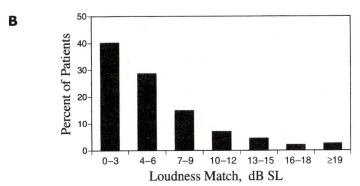

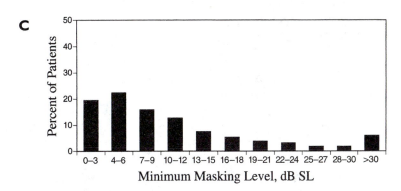

FIGURE 14-2. Psychoacoustic measures of tinnitus in 1,630 patients at the Oregon Tinnitus Clinic. All measures were obtained using the Norwest SG-1 Tinnitus Synthesizer equipped with earphones having excellent high-frequency response. (Not all patients were able to complete all tests, mainly because of poor high-frequency hearing and corresponding limitations of the test equipment.)

A. Tinnitus Pitch Matches (N = 1514)
   All tests were performed at a loudness level matched to that of the patient's tinnitus and all included a test for octave confusion. If a patient had more than one tinnitus sound, then only the pitch of the most troublesome sound was included here.
B. Tinnitus Loudness Matches (N = 1422)
   Tests employed a loudness balance method to adjust an external tone (with frequency matching the pitch of the tinnitus) so as to be equal in loudness to the tinnitus.
C. Minimum Masking Levels (MMLs) (N = 1383)
   A band of noise (2 to 12 kHz) was presented at threshold and then increased in small (1 to 2 dB) steps just until it "covered" the tinnitus; patients whose tinnitus could not be masked or with hearing loss too severe to permit testing are excluded.

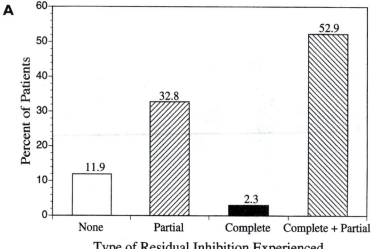

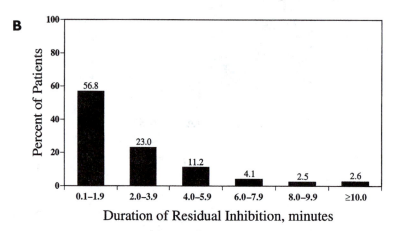

FIGURE 14-3. Measures of Residual Inhibition in 1,630 patients at the Oregon Tinnitus Clinic. Test conditions as described in Figure 14-2; residual inhibition (RI) was measured following 1 minute of masking using a band of noise (2 to 12 kHz) at MML + 10 dB.

A. RI scored at noise-offset as follows: None = Tinnitus at usual loudness; Partial = Tinnitus loudness reduced; Complete = Tinnitus completely inaudible; Partial + Complete = Tinnitus first inaudible then heard at reduced loudness until fully recovered

B. The time required for recovery of the tinnitus to its normal, premasking level was recorded using a stopwatch; total RI duration was recorded as the sum of Partial + Complete. (Patients with no RI were not included in this figure.)

baseline information. Just as in clinical management of chronic pain and other aversive symptoms, quantification of the perceptual dimensions of the patient's problem is the first step in documenting the nature and severity of the problem at a specific point in time. Second, to facilitate *acoustical therapy.* Knowledge concerning the pitch and loudness of tinnitus is likely to be important in considering how best to achieve effective masking. Third, for *evaluating treatment effects.* Both the pitch and the loudness of tinnitus may be altered by ongoing treatment. In order to detect and quantify such treatment effects, it is necessary to know what the tinnitus was like before any treatment began. Precise measures of the loudness match may also be important for patients involved in litigation or compensation review. Although it is beyond the scope of this chapter, careful documentation of patients' reliability in matching their tinnitus to external sounds can be used as evidence to rule out allegations of malingering (Vernon, 1996; also see Chapter 6 and Chapter 17).

Tinnitus Pitch

As Feldmann and others have shown, in about a third of tinnitus patients the effectiveness of masking stimuli is greatest (that is, less-intense masking sounds are required) when the frequency of the masking sound is closely matched to the pitch of the tinnitus (Feldmann, 1971; Mitchell, 1983; Vernon & Meikle, 1981). From these observations it is easy to see that for about one-third of the patient population, the most effective masking band will include the frequency range corresponding to the pitch of their tinnitus. Such patients can be described as requiring "frequency-specific masking."

Because the tinnitus is high-pitched in the majority of cases (Figure 14-2a) it is not surprising that development of wearable maskers capable of generating higher-frequency noisebands has been an important design goal in order to provide frequency-specific masking for those who require it. Controlled studies in which the frequency range of masking noise was varied in relation to the pitch of tinnitus have confirmed the importance of that approach (Pritchard & McCormick, 1987).

Tinnitus Loudness Match

As indicated earlier, the loudness matches for a given individual can be used as legal evidence to support the person's statement that he or she actually has tinnitus (Vernon, 1996). The standard approach involves presentation of an external tone matched to the pitch of the tinnitus. After determining threshold, the tone is raised in 1 dB steps until the person indicates that the tone is equal in loudness to the tinnitus. The same loudness matching procedure is then repeated five or six times in one session, interspersed with other distracting activities (such as discussing the individual's audiometric evaluation or their questionnaire results). If the different loudness measures all fall within a 2 dB range, that is taken as evidence that tinnitus is actually present. The rationale is that loudness matches cannot be reproduced with such high reliability unless there actually is an internally-perceived sound (i.e., the tinnitus) to serve as a reference for all the matching attempts.

Comparison between Tinnitus Loudness Match and the Minimum Masking Level

It seems self-evident that wearable tinnitus maskers should not be so loud as to interfere with speech communication or other hearing needs. To be successful, the masking noise should be as low in intensity as possible in order for it to be nonintrusive and easily ignored.

Research has indicated that the dB difference between the loudness match for the tinnitus and the Minimum Masking Level (MML) may be useful as a predictor of the acceptability of masking sounds (Vernon, Griest, & Press, 1990). If the MML is much higher than the tinnitus loudness match, the patient is unlikely to consider the masking sound an acceptable substitute for the tinnitus. On the other hand if the MML is equal to or lower than the tinnitus loudness match, acceptance of the masking sound is likely.

The Importance of Residual Inhibition Tests

The importance of measuring residual inhibition is twofold: First, it gives many patients a feeling of renewed hope that their tinnitus is not so intractable after all. Particularly when they have had constant, nonvarying tinnitus for a long time, it is a dramatic demonstration that their tinnitus *is* in fact capable of being modified, even if only briefly. Secondly, it introduces patients to the idea that they may be able to use and manipulate external sounds in order to obtain significant tinnitus relief.

The prevalence of residual inhibition is extremely high: Nearly 90 percent of all Tinnitus Clinic patients have been reported to exhibit either partial or complete residual inhibition following one minute of masking by a broad band of noise at 10 dB above their Minimum Masking Level (Vernon & Meikle, 1988; Meikle, Johnson, Griest et al., 1995). In addition, residual inhibition may accumulate and become more prolonged over time if masking stimuli are presented on a long-term basis. Some patients begin to notice, after weeks or months of using tinnitus masking, that they can induce residual inhibition by wearing their masking devices for only a short time, after which they can remove the masking sound and continue to experience a tinnitus-free interval for an extended period. In some cases residual inhibition tends to accumulate, with tinnitus-free intervals becoming longer and longer over time as masking is continued. In a few cases what appears to be permanent or sustained relief of tinnitus has eventually resulted.

Once patients are able to recognize the phenomenon of residual inhibition they are often able to identify it when it occurs in response to some external sound in their environment such as the shower, a radio or television program just before bed, or the noise audible within an airplane during flight. (Noise during air travel sometimes creates an unexpected problem for the Tinnitus Clinic. Some of the patients who have flown to the clinic have discovered upon arrival that their tinnitus is suppressed or even absent for a day or so, thus delaying testing.)

The high prevalence of residual inhibition suggests that it is a phenomenon of fundamental importance for understanding neural mechanisms responsible for tinnitus. When objective methods for studying the presence or absence of tinnitus become more widely available (such as the various types of brain imaging currently under active development, such as Cacace et al., 1996; Lockwood & Salvi et al., 1998), it is to be hoped that future efforts will be devoted to elucidating the neural mechanisms responsible for residual inhibition induced by masking. At this time, very little is known about the neural basis for either tinnitus masking or residual inhibition. It is interesting that in a recent volume devoted to discussion of possible neural mechanisms for tinnitus, there was no speculation concerning possible neural mechanisms for tinnitus masking and residual inhibition.

HOW TINNITUS MASKING DIFFERS FROM CONVENTIONAL MASKING

The term "masking" has a long history of use in audiology (Davis & Silverman, 1947). Masking can be defined as the reduction or elimination of the perception of one sound by the presentation of other sound(s). Most of us use the term "masking" without considering that it originated as a metaphor; that is, the term was used originally in visual contexts where masks were used to cover or conceal something (such as masks used to cover the face at Halloween, or the painter's use of masking to cover and conceal areas to be left unpainted). One dictionary definition of "masking" is "the concealment or screening of one sensory process by another" (Morris, 1969).

It is important to emphasize that the term "masking" does *not* necessarily imply that the masking sound must completely cover or totally suppress the sound we wish to mask—despite the fact that in standard audiological practice, masking of the nontested ear is designed to completely obscure the hearing in that ear. By contrast, in auditory research designed to investigate the masking of one external sound by another, the extent of masking is commonly measured as a continuum of possible masking effects, ranging from very little to complete. A similar approach must be applied to tinnitus masking, where the masking effects can be partial or complete.

Many workers have demonstrated that tinnitus masking does not behave like conventional sound-on-sound masking (Feldmann, 1987b; Johnson & Mitchell, 1984; Vernon, 1991; Vernon, Johnson, Schleuning, & Mitchell, 1980).

The major differences can be summarized as follows:

1. In conventional masking, it is difficult for a tone to mask a band of noise. In contrast, an external pure tone can often mask tinnitus that sounds like a broad band of noise. Even with tinnitus that is perceptually very intense, it may take an external tone of no more than a few dB above threshold to "cover" or eliminate the perception of tinnitus, regardless of whether the tinnitus sounds like a tone or like a band of noise.

2. In conventional masking, of one sound by another, there is an orderly frequency relationship such that a given masking sound tends to mask higher-frequency sounds more easily than it masks those that are below it in frequency (Wegel & Lane, 1924). That relationship does not apply to tinnitus masking; instead, individuals vary greatly in regard to the frequencies and intensities that are effective for masking their tinnitus.

3. In conventional masking, there is a "critical band" surrounding the tone to be masked, within which masking tones are effective and outside of which they are not (Fletcher & Munson, 1937; Greenwood, 1961). In contrast, there does not seem to be a critical band for tinnitus masking in most individuals (Shailer, Tyler, & Coles, 1981; Johnson & Mitchell, 1984). In some patients the tinnitus can be masked easily by nearly any frequency; in a few, no masking is obtainable at any frequency; and in a substantial percentage, the most effective masking sounds are those whose predominant frequency is close to the pitch of the tinnitus.

4. In monaural tone-on-tone masking, it is easy to produce the sensation of "beats" when two tones of equal loudness are close, but not identical, in regard to frequency and phase. In the case of tinnitus that is perceived as a single pure tone, it is very uncommon to obtain "beats," despite many efforts using masking tones that are systematically varied in the effort to approximate the frequency, phase, and perceived loudness of the tinnitus (but see Chapter 8).

5. In conventional masking, it is difficult for one external sound to mask another sound if the two sounds are presented to opposite ears. With tinnitus masking, it has sometimes been easily possible to reduce or eliminate the perception of tinnitus in one ear by presenting a moderate or low level sound to the opposite ear (Tyler, Babin, & Niebuhr, 1984).

6. Upon termination of conventional masking, the sound that is being masked is normally perceived as being at its original, premasking level (unless the masker was intense enough to cause auditory fatigue). Upon termination of tinnitus masking, the tinnitus typically undergoes a temporary reduction or even absence known as "residual inhibition." The tinnitus then gradually recovers to its original level, with large individual differences between patients in regard to the length of the recovery period.

These differences in the behavior of tinnitus masking were unexpected because tinnitus sensations bear such a strong resemblance to external sounds that it was natural to suppose that tinnitus would behave like external sounds in other ways. In fact, many tinnitus patients have described their sense of bewilderment when they first discovered that their tinnitus sounds were *not* in fact coming from the outside world, and their surprise when no one else could hear them. Those readers who experience high-pitched, ringing tinnitus may recall how difficult it is to distinguish between their own tinnitus and some of the high-frequency test tones generated during audiometric testing.

Lack of Possible Neural Explanations for Tinnitus Masking

The strong resemblances between tinnitus and external sounds might lead auditory physiologists to expect that tinnitus masking involves neural mechanisms similar to those that are thought to underlie conventional masking. However, from the very outset of research on tinnitus masking, it has been clear that the neural phenomena responsible for tinnitus masking must be very different (Feldmann, 1971; Vernon, 1991; also see Discussion, pp. 287–290 in Evered & Lawrenson, 1981).

Considerable attention has been paid to the neural mechanisms responsible for conventional types of masking in which external sounds are presented so as to mask or interfere with each other. A number of hypotheses concerning underlying neural processes have been advanced, ranging from a simple "line-busy" phenomenon (where the two sounds compete for the same sensory elements at the periphery) to more complex synaptic interactions usually involving the central nervous system. Many questions remain concerning the neural basis of conventional sound-on-sound masking, and efforts are still underway to explain complex masking phenomena such as "masking level differences" (Jeffress, Blodgett, & Deatherage, et al., 1952), forward and backward masking (Jeffress, 1970), and "central masking" (Zwislocki et al., 1968; Zwislocki, 1971). Tinnitus masking, however, does not appear to obey the same perceptual laws as those that govern the masking phenomena described earlier. That fact suggests that tinnitus masking probably involves quite different, as yet unknown, neural phenomena.

Attempts to account for neural mechanisms underlying both tinnitus and the phenomena of tinnitus masking must also take into account the fact that approximately 40 percent of tinnitus patients report multiple tinnitus sounds (Meikle & Griest, 1991; Meikle, Johnson, & Griest, et al., 1995). Such patients may report that a given masking stimulus has covered only one of their tinnitus sounds, leaving their other tinnitus sounds in the same frequency range unaffected. That situation requires that the clinician make further efforts to identify a masking sound that can effectively cover all of the individual's tinnitus (or if not all, at least the most objectionable portion). It also suggests that neural investigations will need to consider the possibility that neural generators for tinnitus, wherever they may be located, may well involve multiple neuroanatomic locations and/or a variety of different underlying neural mechanisms.

EFFECTIVE CLINICAL USE OF TINNITUS MASKING

There are three major categories of wearable tinnitus masking equipment: (1) tinnitus maskers, (2) hearing aids, and (3) Tinnitus Instruments (combination units containing both a masker and a hearing aid within the same case). The versatility offered by these three types of devices is a key element in a successful masking program. To take advantage of that versatility, the examiner's role is to test each patient carefully to discover which of the available types of devices functions best for that particular patient.

As yet there is no way to define one standardized testing routine that will work for every patient—there is too much unpredictability caused by the individualistic and variable way in which different patients' tinnitus responds to masking. For example, some patients will need a Tinnitus Instrument on one ear and a hearing aid or a tinnitus masker on the other; other patients may need to have the same type of device on both ears.

It is also difficult to predict whether one or two wearable devices will be required. It is true that most patients with bilateral tinnitus require wearable devices on *both* ears to cover the tinnitus, yet other patients with seemingly identical tinnitus need to wear only one device to accomplish the same effect. Even more puzzling, some patients with unilateral tinnitus require masking devices on both ears. Experience demonstrates that trial-and-error testing with different types and combinations of wearable devices is the only way to obtain a successful fitting of masking devices (Johnson & Hughes, 1991; Tyler & Stouffer, 1991).

For a clinician to be effective in fitting wearable devices for masking of tinnitus, it is desirable during the testing procedure to have available a collection of both in-the-ear (ITE) and behind-the-ear (BTE) devices. The available selection of devices should also include the three major categories of tinnitus masking equipment: (1) tinnitus maskers, (2) hearing aids, and (3) Tinnitus Instruments (combination units).

Patients most commonly have bilateral tinnitus. Therefore, it is often necessary to have two of each unit. However, in some patients the tinnitus behaves differently in the two ears, and thus masking therapy is complicated by the need to treat each ear separately. Bearing in mind that patients may have asymmetrical hearing loss, the stock of devices that the examiner needs for testing patients becomes quite large. Just as with hearing aid fitting, there is an equipment investment that is important for any clinician who wishes to provide truly effective tinnitus masking.

In what follows it is assumed that a given ear is evaluated first by itself, to establish the effectiveness of the various types of devices when fitted to that ear. Having determined what works best for each ear separately, in any given patient, it is then essential to check what happens when the devices for the two ears are activated at the same time. In some patients, adding masking to the second ear may reduce the effectiveness of the device applied to the first ear. The clinician's task is to work out the best possible combination, which may in some patients require trying a number of different equipment configurations.

Guidelines for Successful Tinnitus Masking

The examiner needs to pay close attention to what patients say during trials of the various masking devices. For example the patient might say, "Your sound is too high" or "Your sound is too far above my sound." The examiner should be aware that most patients are not fluent in attempting to describe what they hear, and such statements might mean either that the masking sound is too loud or that it is too high-pitched. With careful adjustments the examiner can determine what sort of change is actually required to make the masking sound more effective for the individual in question. There is one cardinal rule: Just as in determining the right eyeglass prescription, the final decision must be made by the patient, not the examiner. The clinician's role is to offer the widest possible range of choices.

The major guidelines in setting up a successful masking program are as follows:

1. It is important to create an environment in which patients feel free to ask questions and volunteer comments.
2. The clinician's role is to provide the patient with opportunities to experience a variety of different types of masking devices.
3. The patient is the one who determines the acceptability and effectiveness of masking.

Category 1: Patients with Significant Hearing Impairment

Based on the audiometric examination and the patient's report, the examiner knows whether the patient being tested is one of the 70 to 80 percent of tinnitus patients who have significant hearing difficulties. If so, the approach to treatment always begins with tests of hearing aids to see whether the tinnitus may be masked simply by amplifying the patient's listening environment.

In what follows, testing and evaluation of hearing-impaired patients using hearing aids is described first, followed by testing and evaluation using tinnitus instruments.

Use of Hearing Aids for Relief of Tinnitus

We always try hearing aids first because, if the aids are successful in masking the tinnitus, the patient is likely to receive a double benefit—that is, better speech communication as well as tinnitus relief. When we speak of the use of hearing aids for masking of tinnitus, we refer to the fact that hearing aids can by themselves cause tinnitus to become inaudible or substantially reduced in loudness. When hearing aids do succeed in eliminating or reducing tinnitus it is probably because they restore the wearer's ability to hear background noise, which can act as a masking stimulus by creating an unobtrusive form of interference that effectively "covers" or reduces the level of the tinnitus.

Testing routine. Note that the test should not be done in a soundproof room. For the hearing aid to pick up and amplify ambient noise (the basis for masking of tinnitus using hearing aids), testing must be done in a normal sound environment that is *not* unusually quiet.

To evaluate the ability of a hearing aid to relieve tinnitus one should first adjust the aid so that it is functioning optimally for that person's hearing loss. Adequate attention should be paid to establishing the proper amplification through the usual adjustment procedures (manipulating the volume control while presenting speech stimuli, asking the patient to speak, and so on). One then asks the patient "Tell me about your tinnitus—how does it sound right now?" For patients whose tinnitus can easily be masked by any frequency, the amplification of ambient noise often succeeds amazingly well in "covering" the tinnitus.

If there is no change in the tinnitus when the hearing aid is on, it may help if the aid's frequency response can be adjusted. Since many patients have high-frequency hearing loss as well as tinnitus with pitch above 6 kHz, it is likely that the hearing aid will need to be adjusted to provide optimum amplification for those higher frequencies. The exact nature of the change cannot be specified ahead of time, and the rule of thumb is to keep trying alternative adjustments if masking is not achieved.

A positive masking result with use of hearing aid(s) may be to produce either "Partial masking" or "Complete masking," and the result should be so recorded. The result is recorded as "No masking" if there is no change in the tinnitus despite efforts to adjust the frequency response of the aid.

Relation of tinnitus pitch to masking produced by hearing aids. If the patient's tinnitus is relatively low-pitched (below about 4 kHz), especially if the hearing loss involves that same frequency range, a well-fitted hearing aid can often be quite effective in covering the tinnitus. Figure 14-4 shows an example of a typical patient whose tinnitus could be masked successfully using a hearing aid.

If a patient has high-pitched tinnitus (above about 4 to 5 kHz), it is possible that the background environmental noise will not contain sufficient high frequencies to cover the tinnitus. However it is always worth trying the hearing aid regardless of the tinnitus pitch because some patients can experience effective tinnitus masking by *any* sound regardless of frequency. The hearing aid is a simple solution for such cases so it is clearly an efficient and cost-effective way to obtain tinnitus relief while also providing hearing help.

Patients with severe hearing loss. In certain cases the patient's hearing loss is so great that hearing aids are unable to enhance speech communication. That fact does not necessarily preclude the use of hearing aids for obtaining tinnitus relief. The example illustrated in Figure 14-5 is a patient for whom hearing aids provided no improvement in speech intelligibility. Nevertheless,

Patient H. H. (36 yrs. – Male)

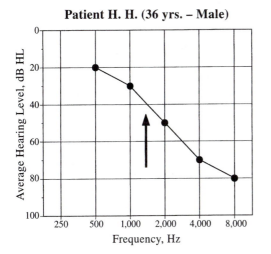

Patient D. P. (63 yrs. – Female)

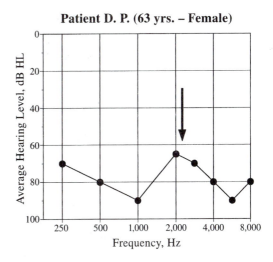

FIGURE 14-4. Use of hearing aids to relieve low-pitched tinnitus. In this and the following figures, arrows indicate the frequency of tones matching the predominant pitch of the tinnitus. Right ear: 0, Left ear: X. Data for the right ear are shown for this patient. He had worked sixteen years in a sawmill without using hearing protection, and was unaware of his hearing loss but reported bilateral tinnitus, worse on the left. Bilateral hearing aids (with open molds to preserve acuity for speech frequencies) provided immediate relief for the tinnitus, so long as there was a slight level of background noise.

FIGURE 14-5. Use of a hearing aid relieves tinnitus even in an ear with "no usable hearing." (Please see Figure 14-4 for explanation of symbols.) This 63-year-old patient reported severe tinnitus in one ear only, resulting from Ménière's disease twenty years earlier. A hearing aid with flat frequency response and occluded molds provided effective masking, although the aid did not improve hearing for speech or other environmental sounds.

a hearing aid provided very significant relief for her (unilateral) tinnitus. She was quite emphatic in stating her desire to obtain a hearing aid despite its negligible benefit for speech communication. This example makes it clear why we have the unbreakable rule: "If the patient has hearing impairment, *always* try hearing aids first regardless of the nature and extent of the hearing loss."

Overall success rate using hearing aids to provide masking. In the past, some hearing aid dispensers have advised all tinnitus patients that they could obtain tinnitus relief through the use of hearing aids. However, a review of the actual results obtained in patients attending the Oregon Tinnitus Clinic who had been so advised contradicts that generalization. A total of 192 patients were identified within our computer data base who had been told previously that their tinnitus could be relieved simply by using hearing aids. The testing at the Tinnitus Clinic, which included a very thorough evaluation using a wide variety of equipment, revealed that only 7 percent of this group actually succeeded in obtaining tinnitus relief using hearing aids. Of the remaining 93 percent, 53 percent required other types of equipment (either maskers or Tinnitus Instruments) to achieve successful relief of tinnitus, and 40 percent proved to be unmaskable by any of the equipment tried. Had this group of 192 patients been governed by the advice of their hearing aid dispensers, it is clear that only a small fraction would have succeeded in obtaining tinnitus relief.

The low success rate when attempting to mask tinnitus using hearing aids probably reflects the fact that the majority of tinnitus patients have high-pitched tinnitus, as discussed in the next section.

When Hearing Aids Are Not Enough: Use of Tinnitus Instruments

The Tinnitus Instrument was developed for patients who need to have hearing amplification combined with tinnitus masking. We have found that the majority of tinnitus patients have their maximal hearing loss above 4 kHz, and perhaps not surprisingly, 75 percent of them match their tinnitus pitch at or above that same frequency (Meikle, Johnson, & Griest, et al., 1995). As Figure 14-2a shows, in approximately 55 percent, the tinnitus is above 6 kHz. It is for patients such as these that the Tinnitus Instrument was developed. As was illustrated in Figure 14-1, successive development of these devices has yielded progressively higher-frequency masking bands.

For patients with high-frequency hearing loss, hearing aids are not usually sufficient to cover the tinnitus because normal environmental sound typically is limited to frequencies predominantly *below* about 4 kHz. Therefore, the Tinnitus Instrument was designed to supply the higher-frequency bands that so often are needed to cover higher-pitched tinnitus. Even for patients whose high-pitched tinnitus can be masked by considerably lower-frequency bands, it is often desirable to use a high-frequency band in order to minimize interference with the speech frequency range. As Figure 14-1 shows, the Tinnitus Instruments offer selectable frequency bands so that the masker frequency can be adjusted to obtain the optimal masking effect for a given patient.

Testing routine. Experience has shown that there must be separate volume controls for the hearing aid portion and the masker portion of the Tinnitus Instrument. Further, it is extremely important for the examiner to adjust the hearing-aid portion of the Tinnitus Instrument first, *before* turning on the masking sound. The idea is to set the hearing aid to be as effective as possible and then "add in" only the amount of masking sound that is needed to cover the tinnitus.

Instructions to patients. Patients who are candidates for Tinnitus Instruments need to receive careful instructions: they risk complete failure if they turn the masker on first, before they turn the hearing aid on. If they attempt to set the masker level first, it is likely their hearing loss will require a high level of masking sound in order for it to be heard adequately. That means that when they turn on the hearing aid portion of the unit, the added amplification will make the preexisting masking noise uncomfortably intense.

Patients also need to be reminded that they should always set the masker at the *lowest* level that covers their tinnitus (or, in some cases, the level that succeeds in reducing it to an acceptable level). It is understandable that some patients might try to use masking at a greater intensity than is necessary, following the mistaken idea "If a little is good, a lot must be better." It is important to discourage such tendencies because, if carried too far, they could cause the masking sound to interfere with speech perception, or conceivably lead to temporary exacerbation of the tinnitus. The following is an example of patient instructions such as we provide:

> When you adjust your Tinnitus Instrument to obtain the best possible tinnitus relief, you should *first* turn on the amplification (hearing-aid portion of the instrument). Adjust the hearing-aid portion so that external sounds and your own voice sound as normal as possible. After that you should turn on the tinnitus masking sound, but only to a very low intensity level. If you are still able to hear your tinnitus, you may increase the level of the masking sound by very small steps until it "covers" your tinnitus or until the loudness of your tinnitus is reduced.
> *Never increase the masking sound to an uncomfortably loud level*—the masking sound should always be comfortable to listen to. After you have been wearing the Tinnitus Instrument for a while you may find that you wish to adjust the masking sound slightly, either increasing or decreasing its intensity level as needed to get the most comfortable tinnitus masking effect.

The final instructions to patients concern battery life. When the batteries in wearable equipment are nearing the end of their useful life, the high frequencies begin to be degraded first. That effect has caused some patients to complain that although their maskers are still producing sound, the sound no longer seems to mask their tinnitus. Patients need to be cautioned that they should replace the batteries if the masking sound appears to have lost some of its effectiveness.

The first Tinnitus Instrument. Dr. G. is one of the most unusual and most interesting cases that we have encountered. We were very fortunate to have him as a patient in the early days of the Tinnitus Clinic. His audiogram is illustrated in Figure 14-6. At the time we first saw him he was 57 years old, a dentist who had been

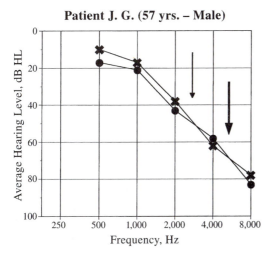

Patient J. G. (57 yrs. – Male)

FIGURE 14-6. Use of Tinnitus Instruments to relieve bilateral tinnitus. (Please see Figure 14-4 for explanation of symbols.) Initial tests indicated a pitch match around 2,800 Hz (thin arrow). Hearing aids were tried first, but they did not provide tinnitus relief although the amplification provided significant help for the patient's hearing. After the "octave confusion" test was initiated, it was found that his tinnitus pitch actually was an octave higher, at 5,600 Hz. Tinnitus Instruments (combining amplification plus masking noise) were then obtained for him and he experienced complete relief from his tinnitus.

using the high-speed dental drill for more than 20 years. He had considerable hearing loss which was probably due to his work experience. His tinnitus was bilateral, with pitch matched to approximately 3 kHz and a loudness match of 8 dB SL. Inasmuch as he had both tinnitus and hearing loss at 3 kHz, we fitted him with bilateral hearing aids. He responded well to amplification, indicating that he could now hear birds, appreciate music, and even attend social gatherings and understand speech. However, the hearing aids did not relieve his tinnitus in the slightest. We were surprised as we expected that his tinnitus (which apparently matched a tone very close to 3 kHz) would be easily masked when he wore hearing aids.

Through a long, drawn-out series of testing sessions, several things were revealed. First, Dr. G.'s initial visit to our clinic had predated the recognition of the "octave confusion" that often occurs when tinnitus patients attempt to match their tinnitus pitch. When we rechecked his tinnitus pitch match using the test for octave confusion, we discovered that his tinnitus actually matched a tone closer to 6 kHz, where we obtained a loudness match of 6 dB SL. Next and even more important, it was Dr. G.'s idea to borrow a pair of tinnitus maskers that he then attached to his hearing aids (using rubber bands!). This patient actually invented the concept of the Tinnitus Instrument, totally relieving his tinnitus in the process.

Unilateral Tinnitus Instruments. A different clinical example is provided by the patient shown in Figure 14-7, who reported severe tinnitus in the left ear only and whose audiogram indicated substantial high-frequency hearing loss. This patient was an excellent candidate for a Tinnitus Instrument, having significant high-frequency hearing loss in addition to high-frequency tinnitus (matched to a 10 kHz tone). As we hoped, he could be easily masked. Use of a Tinnitus Instrument to provide high-frequency masking in his left ear

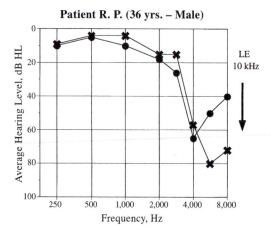

Patient R. P. (36 yrs. – Male)

FIGURE 14-7. Unilateral high-frequency tinnitus relieved by a Tinnitus Instrument. (Please see Figure 14-4 for explanation of symbols.) This case exemplifies the multiple benefits obtainable from use of Tinnitus Instruments: The patient achieved complete tinnitus suppression during the day, significant hearing help, and improved ability to sleep.

completely relieved his tinnitus and provided significant improvement in speech intelligibility. In addition, by wearing his instrument to bed at night he obtained the help he needed for sleeping.

Bilateral versus unilateral masking. If the tinnitus is bilateral or "in the head," two units will probably be needed. The pitch of the tinnitus may differ between the two ears and there may be other spectral differences as well. Therefore, each ear should be tested first by itself to determine the most effective frequency range for masking sounds applied to that ear. During testing, the patient should be instructed to attend only to the tinnitus in the ear with the masker, and to try to disregard any other tinnitus sounds. This is a more complicated testing situation than when there is unilateral tinnitus, and the patient may require some practice in attending to each ear separately. Further, the examiner needs to question the patient carefully to be sure it is clear which tinnitus sounds or locations are affected by the masker. Most commonly, the masking effects are limited to the stimulated ear but some-

times a single masker can produce coverage for tinnitus in both ears.

If the tinnitus is worse on one side than the other, the ear with the most disturbing tinnitus should be tested first. If that ear is successfully masked, it is often the case that the patient will sigh with relief and say that no further masking efforts are needed. The patient may volunteer that the less intense tinnitus on the other side is not a significant problem. In such cases the examiner should be prepared for the fact that the patient is likely to call back after a few days and report that now the tinnitus on the less intense side has become more bothersome. It is unlikely that the tinnitus has actually increased on that side; instead, it is probable that the patient finds it more difficult to ignore the milder tinnitus after the more intense tinnitus on the first side has been rendered inaudible.

After recording the masking effect for each ear when tested separately (either "Complete masking," "Partial masking," or "No masking"), it is important to repeat the test with both maskers operating simultaneously. The examiner needs to pay close attention to the sound level, adjusting the first unit to be just loud enough to cover the tinnitus and then turning on the second unit on the other side. Its loudness should be increased gradually until it just covers the tinnitus on that side. When both maskers are operating at the same time it is likely that both can be set at lower levels than when operating *solo*. However, in some cases there is a rather surprising interaction between the two maskers, necessitating higher sound levels when they operate together than when they operate separately (Vernon, Press, Griest, & Storter, 1991). In passing, it should be noted that such effects probably indicate the complexity of the underlying neural mechanisms responsible for masking-induced changes of tinnitus.

Tinnitus Instruments for tinnitus relief during sleep. There are instances in which we recommend the use of the Tinnitus Instrument even though a hearing aid alone may achieve effective coverage of the tinnitus. If the patient has tinnitus that interferes with sleeping, the advantage of the Tinnitus Instrument is that the hearing aid portion of the device can be turned off at night, and the unit can then be worn as a masker in order to generate noise that can reduce or eliminate the tinnitus. Although the same benefit can be obtained using a bedside masker, a wearable device may be more convenient for some people, particularly those who travel frequently or those who find it inconvenient to set up a bedside masker.

Category 2: Patients with Normal or Nearly-normal Hearing

Testing and evaluation techniques using maskers in normally hearing patients are outlined in the first section that follows, with a subsequent discussion of the use of Tinnitus Instruments in such patients.

Tinnitus Maskers for Relief of Tinnitus in Normally-hearing Ears

The percentage of tinnitus patients who are without significant hearing impairment is small. Depending on the criterion used to define normal hearing, the figure for the Oregon Tinnitus Clinic ranges from 7 to 8 percent (those with all thresholds through 8 kHz ≤ 20 dB) to about 25 to 30 percent (those with average threshold at 1, 2, 4, 6 kHz ≤ 25 dB). The normally-hearing group tends to be younger, on average, than the general tinnitus population and also includes a relatively high percentage of individuals with sudden-onset tinnitus, often caused by accidents involving head trauma. This is the group for whom tinnitus creates substantial interference with their work life, and for whom stress, fatigue, and loss of sleep produce especially disabling effects. Recent data reveal the unexpected finding that normally hearing tinnitus patients tend to be significantly *more* disabled than those who also have hearing impairment (Meikle, Griest, & Press et al., 1997). Thus, this group is especially in need of tinnitus relief.

Testing routine. The first device to be tried with such patients is always the tinnitus masker. Because the pitch of tinnitus is commonly very high in normally-hearing individuals, the most effective masking is usually obtained with a high-frequency noiseband, ideally with its peak output close to the frequency matched to the patient's tinnitus pitch. But because of the unpredictability of tinnitus masking effects, it is good to have adjustable-frequency maskers available in case the high-frequency band is not an effective masker. In such cases it is always worth a try to see if a lower frequency band might provide some degree of masking.

In normally-hearing ears, the coupling of the masker to the ear should be accomplished with as little interference as possible with ambient sound. For that purpose, either a tube fitting (for behind-the-ear maskers) or a vented mold (for in-the-ear maskers) should be used. Again, patients should be instructed how to adjust the masking level by increasing the masking sound by small steps until it just covers the tinnitus. They should also be reminded to replace the battery if at some point the masking sound seems to alter or become less effective.

Figure 14-8 illustrates a typical case in which a tinnitus masker provided effective relief. Note that the patient's hearing levels were normal or nearly so. This patient, Mr. R. W., had tinnitus consisting of a hissing sound which was matched to a noiseband centered at about 3 kHz, with a loudness match of 4 dB SL. He judged that his tinnitus was identical to the masking sound produced by the wearable tinnitus masker. For most patients the noiseband produced by a tinnitus masker is much preferred over the typical high-pitched, tonal tinnitus sound. But in this case the tinnitus and the masking sound were the same. When R. W. requested that he be fitted with a tinnitus masker we responded, "You already have that sound — of what value is it for you to wear a device that generates that same sound?"

It took some time for this patient to explain all the reasons why he welcomed

Patient R. W. (46 yrs. – Male)

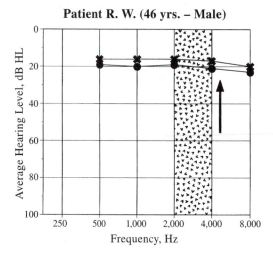

FIGURE 14-8. Use of a Tinnitus Masker in an individual with normal hearing. (Please see Figure 14-4 for explanation of symbols.) A relatively low frequency band of noise succeeded in completely covering this individual's tinnitus. The tinnitus was present in the right ear only and resembled a "hissing" sound (shaded area) plus a tone at 4,500 Hz. In addition to wearing the masker all day, the patient used the masker at night in order to achieve uninterrupted sleep.

the imposition of the masking sound, but in the end his responses taught us a great deal about the masking of tinnitus. First, he pointed out that the masking sound was an "outside" sound and therefore carried no negative implications for his health or hearing status. Second, he reported that the external masking sound did not seem very loud and as a result he could easily ignore it. Third, R. W. said that with masking he could determine when he would and when he would not hear his tinnitus. That he could be in control, he felt, was much better than having the tinnitus exerting control over him. Finally, as he continued to use masking over an extended time period, he began to experience cumulative residual inhibition. After using masking for about three years, the tinnitus completely disappeared.

Residual inhibition as extensive as that is most unusual and not an effect most patients can realistically anticipate. When treating patients using masking techniques, it is im-

portant to emphasize that the production of residual inhibition is *not* the purpose of the masking sound. Residual inhibition is an excellent and hoped-for "bonus" that occurs in some cases, but the main purpose of masking is to provide immediate relief from the noxiousness of the tinnitus sound.

A different type of tinnitus that benefited from use of a tinnitus masker is that of Ms. K. F., shown in Figure 14-9. She reported having tinnitus in her left ear only, and it proved to have an unusually low pitch (matched to 750 Hz). A low-frequency masking band easily masked her tinnitus, and she was able to use her masker throughout the day without any noticeable interference with speech comprehension.

Still another type of masking situation is represented by Ms. B. L., shown in Figure 14-10. Her tinnitus started after an automobile accident in which she received severe head trauma. Although her hearing loss was present before the accident, the tinnitus did not start until several days afterward. The tinnitus was in her right ear only and was matched to a narrow band of noise centered at 3,150 Hz. Our first attempt to provide masking was unsuccessful as she required a masking level (54 dB SL) that was 44 dB higher than the loudness match for her tinnitus. Fortunately we then tried masking *both* ears at the same time, even though only one ear had the tinnitus. With bilateral masking, the masking levels were only 14 dB SL in each ear—only 4 dB above her tinnitus loudness match. She found the bilateral masking very helpful and readily accepted devices for both ears. With this patient we learned the importance of evaluating ipsilateral, contralateral, and bilateral masking before determining the final masking recommendation.

Tinnitus Instruments for Relief of Tinnitus in Nearly-normal Ears

Although it may seem illogical, it is sometimes the case that patients with fairly normal hearing obtain better results with Tinnitus Instruments than with tinnitus

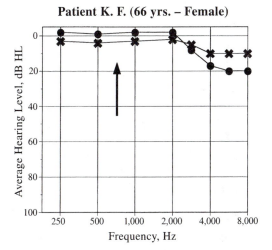

FIGURE 14-9. Use of a Tinnitus Masker for low-frequency tinnitus. (Please see Figure 14-4 for explanation of symbols.) This patient had tinnitus in the left ear only which was completely suppressed by use of a low-frequency masker (supplying a noiseband with major energy in the range 0.5 to 3 kHz).

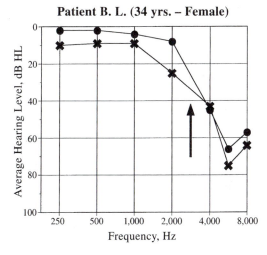

FIGURE 14-10. Use of bilateral Tinnitus Maskers for unilateral tinnitus resistant to masking. This patient described her tinnitus as a band of noise, in the right ear only, which she matched to a one-third octave band centered at 3,150 Hz, at 10 dB SL. With unilateral masking it was necessary to raise the masker level to 54 dB SL to achieve "coverage" of the tinnitus, and the patient understandably found that masking level unacceptable. When bilateral Tinnitus Maskers were provided, she obtained complete tinnitus relief at a masking level of only 14 dB SL in each ear.

maskers. The reason may be related to observations that the majority of normally-hearing tinnitus patients have very high-pitched tinnitus (Meikle, Griest, & Press, et al., 1997). Patients in that category usually state that they do not need hearing help in order to understand speech. However, such patients often need to have masking sounds that are at or above 8 kHz, where their thresholds are likely to be elevated even though they are not aware of any hearing loss. To obtain maximum benefit from masking, such patients need amplification at higher frequencies as provided by use of Tinnitus Instruments.

It is important for normally-hearing patients to actually experience what the Tinnitus Instrument sounds like. Without that experience, the patient cannot make an informed decision regarding what type of masking device is most effective and most acceptable to listen to.

Difference between Effectiveness Versus Acceptability of Masking

From the preceding sections it should by now be clear that there is a difference between the *effectiveness* of masking and its *acceptability*. "Effectiveness" refers to the ability of the masking device to provide adequate coverage of the tinnitus so that the individual can no longer hear it, or hears it at reduced loudness. "Acceptability" refers to the tolerability, or better yet, the *comfort* with which the patient can listen to the masking sound and accept it as a substitute for the tinnitus. Clearly, the masking sound should never be loud enough to be annoying or to disrupt the wearer's attempt to hear other external sounds.

There are often masking sounds that are effective in covering up tinnitus, but which the patient does not find acceptable to listen to. The careful clinician will not stop after testing one or two masking possibilities. Instead, the effort should be made to try the many possible alternatives—in-the-ear, behind-the-ear, unilateral, bilateral, with different frequency bands, and so forth. It is up to the clinician not only to offer patients the widest possible opportunities for evaluating different masking alternatives, but also to provide the necessary guidance in fitting and adjusting the devices.

Complicated Cases

Audiologists are used to the fact that patients differ greatly in regard to the ease and rapidity with which their hearing can be tested. The same is true for the ease with which different patients' tinnitus can be tested. Some individuals' reactions to the various wearable devices can be tested fairly rapidly, particularly if they have unilateral tinnitus that can easily be masked. The tests of wearable devices become more time-consuming when patients have bilateral tinnitus, tinnitus consisting of multiple sounds, variable tinnitus, or tinnitus that is difficult to mask. A few patients have *all* of these complicating factors. Although these complexities prolong the testing session, in the interest of establishing an accurate clinical picture of the individual in question, they are important to document.

Multiple Tinnitus Sounds

Dealing with such complications can present difficult challenges to the clinician. For example, approximately 27 percent of tinnitus patients hear a number of different tinnitus sounds in different localizations (Meikle & Griest, 1991). There are great individual differences, and the combinations can be very complex—perhaps a high-pitched ringing in the left ear, a roaring noise in the right ear, and a sound like "crickets" described as being "in the head." Each of these sounds may require a different frequency range of masking noise in order to be covered.

In general, the examiner can approach this task by determining which sound(s) it is necessary to "cover" in order for the patient to experience adequate tinnitus relief. Very often, patients with complex tinnitus are satisfied if the most intrusive of the tinnitus sounds are effectively masked, and are willing to ignore other weaker sounds so long as they do not cause sleep disturbance or other significant problems. During this evaluation, the examiner must work closely with the patient to determine which particular combination of masking devices is most acceptable in terms of masking effectiveness, in addition to providing hearing help if amplification is needed.

Localization Shifted by Masking

Occasionally patients whose tinnitus is perceived as unilateral will report that the masking sound has "pushed the tinnitus over into the other ear." Experience suggests that such patients probably have bilateral tinnitus, with one side stronger or more audible (Johnson & Hughes, 1991). They are typically unaware of weaker tinnitus on the second side until the stronger side is either masked or put into residual inhibition. In such cases the patients often believe that they do not need masking for the weaker tinnitus that has not previously bothered them. The clinician should be prepared for the fact that such patients may later decide, often after only a few days, that they do in fact need masking for both ears.

Another complicated situation can arise in patients whose tinnitus is localized "in the ears." In a few of these patients the masking sound appears to push the tinnitus centrally so that it is perceived "in the head" as long as masking is presented. It is difficult to imagine what neurological process underlies such a perceived shift in localization of tinnitus, nevertheless it is a real phenomenon that is reported by some patients. If masking in these cases succeeds only in moving the tinnitus to a new location, without reducing or eliminating the tinnitus, masking probably cannot be used effectively for such patients.

When Tinnitus Masking Does Not Work

It is always distressing to the clinician as well as the patient when nothing can be found to provide relief for a given patient. This situation occurred more frequently in the early days of tinnitus masking, before the current range of devices was available, but it still is the case that a certain percentage of individuals will not be able to benefit from masking. Patients need to be told that this can occur right from the outset, in the same way that surgeons explain to their patients that a proposed surgical procedure may or may not achieve the desired effect. Unlike the situation with surgery, efforts to identify effective masking devices are noninvasive. The patient has nothing to lose and a great deal to gain from trying masking.

If the masking trials are all unsuccessful, and no effective masking device(s) can be identified, the clinician's responsibilities are not yet ended. If the patient's tinnitus is severe, it is essential to offer other forms of treatment such as a trial with drug therapy, relaxation training, stress-reduction counseling, or other treatment alternatives.

HOW SUCCESSFUL IS TINNITUS MASKING?

There are many different ways to evaluate the success with which masking is achieved, and there is still no widespread agreement on the best measure to use. From the psychoacoustic point of view, effective masking of tinnitus is achieved when masking renders the patient's tinnitus inaudible or else greatly reduced in loudness. Psychoacoustic data on the efficacy of masking stimuli are important for several purposes, as discussed in the next section. However, they do not tell the whole story: Patients may not find the masking stimuli to their liking even though they succeed in covering the tinnitus. There are dimensions in judging the overall success of masking that have little to do with the effectiveness of the masking stimulus.

In what follows we first describe testing to determine the maskability of tinnitus in each patient. We will show that all but a

small percentage of patients can be either completely or partially masked using a broad band of noise generated by bench equipment and presented under earphones. That procedure can demonstrate to the patient that masking provides relief, but it does not guarantee that the patient will accept masking as a therapy.

The second part of the masking tests involves testing each patient with a variety of different wearable devices in order to determine both the *effectiveness* and the *acceptability* of ear-level masking devices. We will show that a sizable percentage of patients experience effective masking with these devices, when properly fitted and adjusted, although not all patients find the masking sounds acceptable.

Our discussion of the success of tinnitus masking ends by summarizing data from patients who used masking as a long-term therapeutic procedure. Analyses involving follow-up observations are essential because the long-term results of masking cannot always be predicted based on the initial evaluation session. We will summarize results from a number of different clinics showing that masking as a therapy for tinnitus can be successful in a large percentage of patients for whom it is recommended.

Masking Efficacy: Psychoacoustical Aspects

Effective masking of tinnitus is a psychoacoustic phenomenon that occurs when a sound is identified that can "cover" or suppress an individual's perception of tinnitus; that is, the tinnitus is either not perceived or is greatly reduced during the time that the masking sound is present. As described in the following sections, the efficacy of masking stimuli is measured in two different ways: First, using either bench equipment or a Tinnitus Synthesizer to yield precise documentation of the loudness of tinnitus in dB relative to patients' hearing thresholds; and second, using wearable ear-level devices.

Measuring the Efficacy of Masking Using Electroacoustic Equipment

Testing (either with a Tinnitus Synthesizer or with bench equipment) is done under circumaural earphones specially selected to have good high-frequency response (such as the Koss Pro 4A). The test procedure involves generating a broad band of noise (2k to 12 kHz is typical in the Oregon Tinnitus Clinic) and determining the threshold for that noise. The level of the noise is then raised in small steps (typically 1 to 2 dB) and each time the patient is asked to report whether or not the tinnitus is still audible. In most cases the broadband noise succeeds in covering the tinnitus (rendering it completely inaudible) at a fairly low level, usually on the order of 10 dB SL or less. That result is recorded as "Complete masking," and the lowest level at which the noise completely covers the tinnitus is recorded as the Minimum Masking Level (MML). In a few cases, the noise level reaches the patients' loudness discomfort level or the limits of the equipment before complete masking is

achieved. In such cases, if the loudness of the tinnitus undergoes partial reduction, the occurrence of "Partial masking" is recorded at the lowest level at which it was observed. The MML cannot be measured in such cases. In about 5 percent of the patients we have tested, there is no reduction of the tinnitus and in these cases, "No masking" is recorded.

Figure 14-11 summarizes the results obtained from a sample of 1,395 patients at the Oregon Tinnitus Clinic who were tested using a Tinnitus Synthesizer. It is clear that a very high percentage of patients experienced masking effects—92 percent exhibited complete masking in at least one ear, 4.5 percent exhibited partial masking, and only 3.5 percent experienced no masking effects. These results are all the more impressive when we recall that Minimum Masking Levels are generally very low. As Figure 14-2b shows, 50 percent of patients were completely masked by a noise level no greater than 6 dB above threshold, and 80 percent were completely masked by a level no greater than 15 dB. The fact that the masking noise usually covers the tinnitus at

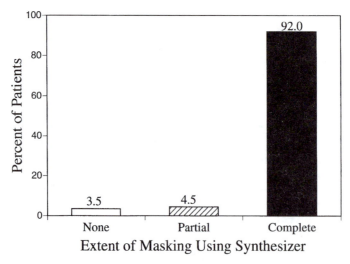

FIGURE 14-11. Effectiveness of masking achieved using the Tinnitus Synthesizer. The extent of masking was evaluated by asking patients to report how their tinnitus sounded while the masking sound was turned on. If tinnitus was completely inaudible, the masking effect was scored as "complete." If the tinnitus was reduced in loudness, masking was scored as "partial."

relatively low sensation levels undoubtedly contributes to the successful use of masking for long-term therapy.

Although partial masking is not as desirable an end result as complete masking, nevertheless the value of partial masking should not be underestimated. Many individuals have benefited significantly from provision of partial masking, some of them wearing their maskers both night and day. These patients report that they are able to tolerate their tinnitus when its level is sufficiently reduced to permit them to sleep and to go about their daily routine without interference.

Masking Efficacy Using Wearable Devices

Ear-level masking devices, like hearing aids, require careful work to achieve a proper fitting. First, the fitting of masking equipment requires attention to the localization of tinnitus—it does no good to provide effective masking for only one ear if there is severe tinnitus in other sites that is left untreated. Second, as we noted earlier, the frequency range of masking is important in many cases. Although some patients can be effectively masked by nearly any sound, for many patients it is critical to adjust the masking band to provide a frequency range corresponding to the pitch of the individual's tinnitus.

Early tinnitus maskers did not provide adjustable frequency bands such as those now available (refer again to Figure 14-1). The development of masking devices capable of generating different frequency bands now makes it possible to obtain a better fit between the masking sound and the patient's tinnitus. For example, patients with very high-pitched tinnitus were often difficult to fit with the original maskers that generated noisebands in the range of about 1k to 4 kHz, as the masker level needed to be set at a relatively high intensity level in order to cover tinnitus at 8 kHz and above. However, setting the masker at a high intensity level was then likely to interfere with speech perception. When higher-frequency

noisebands were provided (for example, Figure 14-1d or 14-1e), significantly less sound energy was required to cover the tinnitus, thus the masker volume control could be set low enough that there was little or no interference in the speech frequency range.

The ability of a masking device to generate either "partial" or "complete" masking is established by the patient's report as the examiner adjusts the volume control to obtain the best possible masking effect. Because wearable devices do not have volume controls that provide precision dB adjustments, their effectiveness is typically measured using a relatively gross scale. If the tinnitus proves to be maskable, the examiner notes whether the observed effect was obtained at a volume setting that was "low," "moderate," or "high."

Figure 14-12 summarizes the results obtained when wearable masking devices were tested in the same sample of 1,395 patients shown in Figure 14-11 (note that the masking effects of hearing aids are included in this summary). Comparing Figure 14-12 with Figure 14-11 reveals that masking by wearable devices is somewhat less effective than the masking provided by the Tinnitus Synthesizer. With wearable devices the percentage of patients experiencing complete masking (70.5 percent) was lower, and the percentage experiencing partial masking (19.6 percent) was higher, than with the synthesizer. Also, there were more patients who experienced no masking effects (9.9 percent) when using ear level devices. These differences may be attributed to several technical differences between the synthesizer versus wearable equipment. First, the transducers (speakers) in the wearable devices are not as effective for high-frequency reproduction as the transducers in the earphones. Second, the synthesizer is more powerful than the wearable equipment. Third, placement of the wearable devices is subject to greater variability than for the circumaural earphones used with the synthesizer. Fourth, the noise stimuli generated by the synthesizer are correlated (that is, generated by a single source that supplies identical signals to the

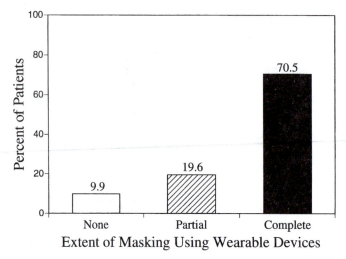

FIGURE 14-12. Effectiveness of masking achieved using wearable masking devices. Scoring of the extent of masking was done as described for Figure 14-11.

two earphones) whereas for an individual wearing two masking devices, the noise stimuli that are generated are independent of each other. The presentation of correlated noise to the two ears may conceivably provide more effective suppression at the level of neurological process(es) underlying tinnitus (Johnson & Hughes, 1991).

There are, however, a few patients who experience *better* masking with wearable equipment than with the synthesizer. That fact suggests that ear canal resonances or other features of the acoustical coupling between the ear and the masking device may have a sizable impact on the effectiveness of masking. There is preliminary evidence to support that suggestion (Vernon, 1987c). In addition, a patient using two wearable devices is hearing two independent noise sources, which are uncorrelated. There may be some sort of "masking level difference" phenomenon (Jeffress et al., 1952; see also Johnson & Fenwick, 1984) that affects responses to binaural tinnitus masking in certain patients.

Subjectively, comments by tinnitus patients indicate that they do actually feel as though their tinnitus is being "covered up" by the masking noises produced during testing in the clinic—either completely covered, or only partly covered, as the case

may be. The demonstration of masking is often a very dramatic occurrence for individuals who have been experiencing severe, unrelieved tinnitus for a long time.

Acceptability of Wearable Masking Devices

After testing the effectiveness of wearable masking devices, the clinician must then determine whether or not the patient finds the masking devices acceptable; that is, does the patient consider the masking sound an acceptable substitute for his tinnitus? This is a highly individual and subjective matter, and it is not possible to predict which sounds will in fact be acceptable to a given patient. While it appears that many patients feel bands of noise are more acceptable to listen to than the high-pitched "ringing" tinnitus so often complained about, not all patients agree. Occasionally there are individuals who indicate they would prefer to listen to a masking sound consisting of a high-pitched tone. In a few such cases we have been able to provide special masking devices that generate a tone instead of noise. In these instances the tonal masking was used not as a constant form of acoustic stimulation, but rather as a series of relatively brief acoustic exposures (lasting perhaps 15 to 30 minutes) that provided tinnitus relief in the form of residual inhibition after the masking sound was removed.

In addition to the acceptability of the masking sound itself, there is also the question of the acceptability of wearing an ear-level device. There are many reasons why individuals may choose not to wear a tinnitus masking device. If the tinnitus is a relatively minor irritation for the patient there is little motivation to accept the costs, inconvenience, and potential intrusiveness of a wearable masking device. In contrast, when tinnitus is very intense, patients will go to great lengths to obtain and use effective masking devices, disregarding questions of vanity, convenience, and cost.

We ask tinnitus patients to rate the perceived loudness of their tinnitus using a Visual Analog Scale from "0" (no tinnitus) to "10" (extremely loud) (Meikle, 1991; Meikle & Griest, 1991). There is a direct relationship between the patients' loudness ratings and their interest in a masking program. Those with ratings below about "5" are seldom interested in pursuing any type of treatment, and are usually satisfied merely to learn that their condition is not life-threatening, that they are not "going deaf" nor "going crazy," and that help is available should they later decide they need it. (We also counsel such patients on the importance of avoiding loud sounds that could make their tinnitus worse.)

Patients with loudness ratings at "7" or above are those that are definitely interested in obtaining treatment, while those with intermediate ratings, in the range of about "5" to "6," are sometimes interested, sometimes not. It should be emphasized that patients with loudness ratings of "10" are those that are most apt to be suicidal, and demonstrating the effectiveness of masking can be a dramatic and important occurrence for patients in this group. (It is extremely important not to let such patients become discouraged if masking does not work. In that case, some alternative form(s) of therapy must be tried in order to prevent such patients from losing all hope and acting rashly.)

The *acceptability* of wearable devices (maskers, Tinnitus Instruments, and/or hearing aids) can be gauged by reviewing the extent to which patients who can be effectively masked agree to obtain equipment. At the Oregon Tinnitus Clinic, approximately 15 percent of those who can be masked indicate they do not wish to obtain wearable devices. Table 14-1 lists the reasons why those individuals declined the recommended treatment. The largest percentage (4 percent of those who could be masked) refrained because they felt their tinnitus was not severe enough to warrant the expense and inconvenience. The table also lists other reasons, such as that effective masking required a higher stimulus intensity than some patients wished to accept (2.7 percent) or that some patients felt their tinnitus was preferable to the masking sound (3.3 percent).

Long-term Clinical Effectiveness of Wearable Masking Devices

The use of tinnitus masking devices for extended time periods provides convincing evidence that these devices are truly helpful to patients. By now there have been many different clinics involved in efforts to provide masking for tinnitus patients. These efforts have varied widely, not only in regard to the procedures and equipment employed, but also in regard to the methods used for evaluating treatment outcomes. Because a detailed comparison of the strengths

Table 14-1. Reasons why patients declined wearable devices

Reason for Declining	Percent of Patients*
Tinnitus not severe enough	4.1 %
Prefers tinnitus to masker	3.3
Masker intensity too high	2.7
Masker increases tinnitus	1.3
Patient not ready to purchase	0.7
Other reasons	3.0
	15.1

*Based on a total sample of 1,019 patients for whom ear-level masking was effective

and weaknesses of many small studies is beyond the scope of the present discussion, we have chosen to emphasize a statistical approach in reviewing the ultimate clinical success of masking. In this section we focus on large-scale studies where the large number of subjects helps to compensate for the inherent variability in tinnitus patients' responses to treatment.

The largest and therefore most useful sets of data concerning the efficacy of masking have come primarily from five otologic centers. Three are located in the United Kingdom: The Tinnitus Clinic of the University College Hospital, and the Royal National Throat, Nose, and Ear Hospital (both in London); and the Institute for Hearing Research General Hospital in Nottingham. Two of the centers are in the United States: The Tinnitus Center of the State University of New York Health Science Center at Brooklyn, New York, and the Tinnitus Clinic of the Oregon Health Sciences University in Portland, Oregon. (Unfortunately, results from a large study of tinnitus masking conducted in Germany could not be included in this comparison because, although many of the subjects had significant hearing impairment, no effort was made to provide units involving both masking and hearing amplification; see von Wedel, 1987.)

The various investigations of tinnitus masking efficacy in the United States and in the United Kingdom differed in a number of details, primarily in regard to the nature of the specific masking devices available; the proportion of binaural fittings; and the criteria used to determine success. It seems self-evident that masking efficacy is very much dependent on the adequacy of the available equipment. For example, hearing-impaired patients usually do not do as well with tinnitus maskers as with Tinnitus Instruments because they need help for their hearing, in addition to needing tinnitus therapy. Failure to include Tinnitus Instruments was probably the main reason that the German study cited earlier did not generate as high a success rate as in the British and United States studies.

The following is a summary of the efficacy of tinnitus masking as reported by the five British and American clinics:

Tinnitus Masking Programs in the United Kingdom

Results from London and Nottingham were obtained in a jointly-conducted study and were reported together (Hazell, Wood, & Cooper et al., 1985). Data on masking effectiveness were obtained from a total of 368 patients in London and Nottingham. The masking equipment was provided without charge to the patients. Of the 368 patients receiving tinnitus masking devices, 57 percent received a masker, 22 percent received a Tinnitus Instrument, 18 percent received a hearing aid, and 4 percent received two different devices (one for each ear).

The effectiveness of the devices was evaluated using a questionnaire administered a minimum of six months following the initiation of masking. Patients were asked (among many other questions), "Whilst wearing the instrument, did it help you to mask the tinnitus?" and were instructed to check one of five different response categories ("All the time, three-quarters of the time, half the time, one-quarter of the time, never"). To simplify comparisons we collapsed the first three of those response levels to derive a new category, "Substantially helped"; and likewise collapsed the last two levels (one-quarter of the time, or never) to derive the category "Not substantially helped."

For the present review we used data summarized in Table 19 (page 85) of the study performed by Hazell, Wood, & Cooper et al. There were 239 patients who were "Substantially helped" and 129 who were "Not substantially helped," yielding a success rate of 69 percent.

Comment on United Kingdom masking trials. Conduct of these trials was hampered by several problems reported by the authors, including a high rate of repairs needed for the Tinnitus Instruments, and the fact that many patients had difficulty adjusting the volume controls. In addition, all of the masking devices provided bands of noise in a lower frequency range than that now considered desirable for most patients. Further, most of the binaural devices were supplied for patients at only one of the centers despite the high prevalence (61 percent) of patients with binaural tinnitus at all the centers. In view of these less-than-optimal conditions, the 69 percent success rate seems quite remarkable. Despite the various difficulties, the authors commented "One of the most rewarding consequences of successful masking therapy is that many patients no longer need to take sleeping pills" (Hazell, Wood, & Cooper et al., 1985, p. 84). A further comment concerned the presumed mechanisms of masking effects, which they said ". . . can make a great deal of difference to how noticeable the tinnitus is. Probably, this is partly the effect of tinnitus suppression by the masking and partly the result of the assistance it gives to the process of habituation" (Ibid., p. 93).

Tinnitus Masking Programs in the United States

In what follows we will evaluate the success rates in several large masking trials in the United States. Our task is complicated by the fact that a number of different measures of masking success have been used in those studies, making it difficult to compare their results. The United States results are also somewhat difficult to compare to the British results as none of the United States studies provided the type of long-term follow-up used in the United Kingdom, which were performed after six months of masking.

Despite those limitations it is possible to base the United States evaluations on data that reflect patients' actual experience with masking, by using data obtained following the standard thirty-day trial period that is allowed each person who wishes to try a masking device. As the measure of masking success, we used patients' decisions to purchase the masking devices they had tried, based on the rationale that patients would not purchase the devices unless they had found them helpful during the thirty-day trial period.

The Tinnitus Center of the State University of New York Health Sciences Center in Brooklyn.

Four large patient samples were evaluated consecutively, starting in 1977 and ending in 1994 (Goldstein & Shulman, 1991, 1996; Shulman & Goldstein, 1987). Several different methods for calculating the success of masking were used in those studies, resulting in reported success rates that varied from 85 percent to 19 percent. The large variations in regard to masking success may also have resulted from procedural differences, but that is difficult to determine because the reports provide relatively little information concerning the masking procedures employed (for example, there was no information on the number of binaural versus monaural fittings).

In order to calculate an overall success rate for masking, we combined the results from all four samples, thus obtaining a total of 799 patients who were advised to purchase masking devices. Of the 799 patients who received recommendations to purchase devices, 356 patients actually did so (42 percent purchased maskers, 19 percent Tinnitus Instruments, 22 percent hearing aids, and 17 percent purchased two different devices, one for each ear). Expressing the number who purchased masking devices (N = 356) as a percentage of the overall group who received recomendations to purchase devices (N = 799) yields a masking success rate of 45 percent.

The Tinnitus Clinic of the Oregon Health Sciences University.

Determinations of masking success have been made for three successive, nonoverlapping samples. Sample 1 consisted of 493 patients seen in 1976 to 1978 and Sample 2 consisted of 105 patients seen in 1979 (Schleuning, Johnson, & Vernon, 1980). Sample 3 consisted of 638 patients seen in 1984 to 1989. (Johnson, Griest,

& Press et al., 1989). Combining all three patient samples, data from a total number of 1,236 patients were available, of whom 828 received recommendations to purchase wearable devices (37 percent maskers, 36 percent Tinnitus Instruments, 24 percent hearing aids, and 3 percent were advised to purchase different devices for each ear). Of those who received recommendations to purchase masking equipment, a total of 506 actually purchased the recommended devices after the trial period ended. Expressing the number who purchased masking devices (N = 506) as a percentage of the group who received recommendations to purchase devices (N = 828) yields a masking success rate of 61 percent.

Comment on United States masking trials. There is a substantial difference between the percentage purchasing devices in New York (45 percent) versus the percentage purchasing devices in Oregon (61 percent). One factor that might account for such a difference is the relatively low percentage of Tinnitus Instruments recommended to the patients in New York (19 percent) compared to the Oregon group where, since the early 1980s, a consistent finding is that approximately 60 percent of those receiving equipment recommendations are best helped by Tinnitus Instruments.

Comparisons of Masking Success in the United Kingdom Versus the United States

It seems to be more difficult to obtain long-term follow-up data in the United States than in the United Kingdom, probably because distances are generally much greater in the United States, and patients' contacts with the health care system tend to be less frequent because of the higher costs of health care in this country. To date, no prospective study of tinnitus masking has been conducted in the United States using measurement techniques strictly comparable to those used in the United Kingdom for the large-scale, prospective trial described earlier.

Despite that lack a small amount of data are available from a retrospective sample of patients seen at the Oregon Tinnitus Clinic during 1990 to 1991, in which a total of 151 patients (59 percent) reported they purchased the recommended masking equipment (Vernon, Griest, & Press, 1992). The last 77 patients in that survey were also questioned using an item resembling that used in the United Kingdom study. The 1992 study in Oregon included the question, "Did your tinnitus masking device provide relief of your tinnitus?" A total of 59 patients responded "Yes," amounting to 77 percent of the subjects who were asked that question. These observations illustrate the fact that the manner in which subjects are questioned about their results has a significant effect on the resulting estimates of treatment success. The results also suggest that a higher percentage of people found the devices helpful than were willing to pay for the devices.

In all the follow-up surveys conducted so far, whether in the United Kingdom or the United States, it is always found that some patients stop using their masking devices because they have developed prolonged residual inhibition, and no longer are in need of tinnitus masking. Thus one may not conclude that stopping use of masking indicates a masking failure, and likewise it is not valid to use the number of patients continuing to use masking over the long term as an indicator of the success of masking. It is also quite common for patients to state they wish to keep their masking equipment even if they no longer use it. (In instances where the tinnitus appears to have "settled down" to a lower level over time, patients may wish to keep their masking equipment in case the tinnitus later reverts to its original aversive condition.) For these reasons, it appears that one cannot obtain a valid measure of the success of masking simply by determining how many people are still using it after some lengthy period such as a year or two.

Differences between the 69 percent success rate in the United Kingdom versus the

45 to 77 percent rates in the United States may reflect several factors: The patients in the United Kingdom received their masking devices free of charge, thus eliminating the cost that undoubtedly acts to reduce the percentage of purchasers in the United States. Another factor may be the differences in criteria for determining success. Recall that in the United Kingdom, successful masking was based on patient's ratings of the treatment effects at a six-month follow-up examination. For evaluating the success of masking in the United States, however, most of our conclusions regarding masking efficacy have been based on patients' decisions to purchase equipment after the thirty-day trial period, because most of the United States studies did not provide six-month follow-up data or other long-term observations such as those available in the United Kingdom study.

Given the many differences between the various clinics in regard to masking equipment, treatment protocols, and measurement techniques, it is not surprising that differences have been found between the effectiveness of masking at the various treatment centers in the United Kingdom and the United States. These observations underline the need for widespread standardization of methods for evaluating tinnitus treatments.

TINNITUS AND HYPERACUSIS: TREATMENT RELATED TO MASKING

In recent times it has become apparent that tinnitus can be complicated by another hearing problem that is sometimes even more severe than the tinnitus. That problem is *hyperacusis*, which can be described as a collapse of loudness tolerance (Vernon & Press, 1998). Patients with hyperacusis find that almost all sounds are uncomfortably loud (excepting their own voice), and they get the idea that their hearing is "too sensitive." Abnormally sensitive thresholds are *not* the problem, in fact the majority of

hyperacusis patients have some form of hearing loss (Vernon, 1987b; Sood & Coles, 1988; Brandy & Lynn, 1995).

The term "hyperacusis" is currently used differently by different audiologists and tinnitus clinics, and there is as yet no consistent definition to guide diagnostic use of this term. It is widely acknowledged that "hyperacusis" involves a greatly reduced loudness tolerance for part or all of the frequency range, manifested in a small dynamic range (the absolute difference between an individual's threshold for a given stimulus and the Loudness Discomfort Level, or LDL, for the same stimulus) (Hazell & Sheldrake, 1992). However there is little agreement concerning where the line could or should be drawn between ordinary loudness recruitment and the severe pathological condition that renders the individual dysfunctional in all but the most quiet sound environments.

Despite the lack of a consistent definition for "hyperacusis," there is some information concerning its prevalence. A survey conducted recently by the American Tinnitus Association indicated that of approximately 35,000 individuals who received the survey, 112 (0.32 percent) returned questionnaires that indicated they suffered from hyperacusis. If all of those who actually had hyperacusis responded, and if that same percentage applies to the 10 million-plus individuals with severe tinnitus in the United States (Brown, 1991), it would appear that approximately 32,000 individuals in the United States have both tinnitus and hyperacusis. Thus it appears that hyperacusis as a complication of tinnitus is fairly rare; however, it can be an exceedingly bad problem and one that requires careful professional attention.

The survey conducted by the American Tinnitus Association provided some interesting information about hyperacusis. When asked which was worse, hyperacusis or tinnitus, 53 percent indicated that hyperacusis was worse while 19 percent indicated that the two were equal. Hyperacusis was present in both ears for 89 percent of the patients. Males constituted 69 percent of the cases while females constituted 37 percent, almost a two-to-one ratio. That distribution suggests that a major cause of hyperacusis may be exposure to damaging levels of sound (a situation affecting many more men than women). When asked whether the tinnitus or the hyperacusis started first, 53 percent responded that the tinnitus started first. In the remaining 47 percent of cases, about half indicated that hyperacusis started first, the remainer indicating that both conditions started simultaneously.

When loudness tolerance is measured in hyperacusis patients it is usually found to be most abnormal in the higher frequencies (Vernon, 1992). A typical example of the results obtained in a hyperacusis patient, using pure tones to measure Loudness Discomfort Levels has been measured as follows: LDLs of about 25 dB above threshold at 250 Hz, 20 dB at 500 Hz, and perhaps 10 to 15 dB up through 2 to 3 kHz; then LDLs of no more than 3 to 5 dB (or even less!) at frequencies above 4 kHz. Such LDLs can be measured reliably, suggesting that there is a genuine neurological basis for the abnormally low loudness tolerance.

Hyperacusic patients experience a problem with loudness intolerance that is much greater than that experienced by individuals with simple loudness recruitment, such as often accompanies hearing loss. Patients with hyperacusis cannot tolerate even moderate levels of sound. As a result, these unfortunate people tend to move through life wearing earplugs and/or earmuffs at all times (Gabriels, 1996b). They find unexpected sounds such as truck noises or sirens to be nerve-shattering experiences and consequently tend to become socially isolated, staying home and indoors nearly all the time.

The treatment we use for hyperacusis is effective but necessarily quite slow. Thus it is important to encourage patients to follow the program very faithfully, and not become discouraged and give up. The program consists of two parts: (1) Systematic desensitization using structured acoustic stimuli, and (2) avoiding overdependence on earplugs or other ear protection (Vernon, 1987b).

Desensitization to Re-establish Normal Loudness Tolerance

This is done by having patients spend a portion of each day listening to a specially-constructed noiseband, at their maximum comfort level. Originally we had patients listen to white noise but, over time, we found that "pink noise" is a more effective desensitizing stimulus, perhaps because white noise contains high frequencies at which the individual's dynamic range is inordinately small, thus creating irritation and aggravation rather than leading to acclimatization. Since the environmental sounds to which daily life exposes us normally contain very little sound energy above about 4,000 Hz, we reasoned that the use of "pink noise" (which is lacking in the high frequencies) might improve the desensitization process by avoiding the high frequencies that are so aversive to hyperacusis patients. To provide an appropriate listening experience that can be used easily by patients, we developed special listening materials, available either on cassette tapes or CDs (for details, see Section III in the Appendix on page 356). These materials are listened to under earphones in order to provide maximum consistency and control of the sound level.

Each time a patient dons the earphones and listens to the pink noise it is important that a proper, individualized listening level be established. To do so, the patient is instructed to begin each listening session by increasing the loudness of the pink noise very gradually above threshold in order to determine the level at which the noise is just starting to be uncomfortable, and then reducing the noise level only slightly. The patient then uses that loudness level for the duration of the listening session, assuming that it remains comfortable. The patient is also instructed that the goal is gradually to increase the listening level for the noise over time, by raising each day's listening level slightly relative to the preceding day. In this way, the procedure takes advantage of increasing loudness tolerance as it starts to develop. As a general rule we tell hyperacusis patients to expect to take about two years to recover normal loudness tolerance, although they may well experience noticeable improvement within a few months.

Listening to pink noise for a total of two or more hours per day is recommended as a minimum, but the listening period can be divided into shorter intervals if necessary so long as the listening level is carefully reestablished at the start of each and every listening period. Since listening to pink noise is boring, we recommend that patients provide themselves with some other activity, such as reading, sewing, or other activities that are compatible with the wearing of earphones.

In a few cases we have found that what started out to be a satisfactory loudness level became objectionable as the listening period continued. In such cases we recommend immediate cessation of the current desensitization schedule, followed by a day of rest, and then cautious reinstatement of the desensitization program using shorter listening periods. We also instruct such individuals to call us immediately if they again experience objectionable effects from listening to the pink noise. In at least one case, the patient was not able to continue use of the desensitization CD as her tinnitus increased whenever she listened to the CD (regardless of how low the sound level was set). Although the noise levels used for desensitization are not damaging, it is not yet known what sort of neurological processes underlie either hyperacusis or its desensitization, therefore it is important to act conservatively in order to avoid undue hazard owing to unknown pathological processes.

Avoiding Overuse of Ear Protection

It is very important to instruct hyperacusic patients *not to overprotect their ears!* Such individuals tend to wear earplugs all the time and frequently complain that earplugs do not adequately screen out objectionable noises and thus do not provide adequate protection for them. They should be counseled, however, that by screening out lower-level environmental sounds, constant wearing of earplugs tends to make hyperacusis become progressively worse. Hyperacusis patients who persist in wearing earplugs all the time actually cause their problem to become aggravated. As a result, hyperacusis is most severe in those who have had it longest, and it takes longer to obtain successful recovery in such patients.

At the beginning of therapy we counsel hyperacusis patients to avoid truly loud sounds, while at the same time avoiding overprotecting their ears. Since all sounds appear uncomfortably loud to them, they are in a dilemma to know when to protect and when not to protect. To resolve that dilemma we rcommend that they obtain an inexpensive sound level meter (obtainable for under $40 at electronic equipment stores) and measure the sound pressure levels of the sounds to which they are usually exposed. We recommend that they begin their desensitization program by setting 65 dB SPL as the cutoff level above which they will wear ear protection. At first, sound levels below 65 dB may produce some discomfort, but the patient needs to understand that there must be an effort on his or her part to accept some sounds that are moderately uncomfortable in order to begin the desensitization process. As therapy progresses, the cutoff level can and should be raised gradually until finally the patient wears ear protection only when there is a real need for it (for example, at sound levels $\geq$ 85 dB SPL).

Hyperacusis patients typically complain that they cannot go out because, when they leave the protection of their home, they can be devastated by unexpected sounds such as a truck passing, an automobile backfiring or sounding its horn at close range, and so forth. Since it is important that these patients lead as normal a life as possible, some form of controlled protection is needed for them. Fortunately there is a device available which attempts to meet the special needs of the hyperacusis patient. It is the *Refuge©* hearing aid (produced by Micro-Tech, Plymouth, MN) that looks like an ordinary in-the-ear hearing aid. The device functions like an earplug in that it blocks the ear canal, thus attenuating incoming sound. In addition, the electronic circuitry in the Refuge provides compression amplification that reduces or eliminates the amplification of higher-level sounds. For low-level sounds, the device provides carefully controlled amplification so that the wearer maintains a normal sound environment. The aim is to maintain normal exposure to acceptable sound levels, thus avoiding overprotection of the ears with consequent worsening of hyperacusis.

It is likely that the prevalence of hyperacusis is greater than generally supposed. Thus it is imperative that a definition of the condition be established that is agreed upon by all health care professionals. Moreover it is also important that a standardized test for hyperacusis be established, most likely one involving measurement of Loudness Discomfort Levels and determining whether or not a standard criterion is met. We would suggest that such tests include measurement of LDLs over a wide range of test frequencies (such as octave steps over the range 1k to 8k Hz), because the hyperacusic patients we have seen and tested exhibited an inverse relationship between the test frequency and loudness tolerance—the higher the test frequency, the less the individual's loudness tolerance at that frequency.

FUTURE DIRECTIONS FOR TINNITUS RESEARCH AND DEVELOPMENT

There are many opportunities for future research that will yield important and influential information to guide treatment decisions. The following suggestions are offered as a very tentative and incomplete outline of several potentially useful research directions:

Acoustical Modifications of Masking Techniques

Several different lines of investigation have involved modifications of tinnitus masking stimuli in order to see if there are ways to render them more effective for particular subsets of patients. First, preliminary work on residual inhibition has suggested that various types of tonal maskers might be more effective than noisebands for producing long-lasting residual effects (Vernon, Press, Griest, & Storter, 1991). The suggested masking stimuli were evaluated in a group of thirteen patients and included pairs of tones centered around the frequency of the tinnitus, as well as single tones placed at various frequency separations relative to the tinnitus frequency. Although the small number of observations renders the results inconclusive, it is clear that certain individuals exhibited unusually prolonged residual inhibition under one or more of the various test conditions. It is thus possible that specially-designed masking stimuli could be more effective for certain categories of patients, for example those with tonal tinnitus, those with different tinnitus tones in the two ears, and so on. These preliminary findings need to be extended to a larger group of subjects.

Further work on the spectral content of noisebands used for tinnitus masking would be desirable. It is a consistent observation that masking produced in the clinic, using the Tinnitus Synthesizer, is more effective than that produced by wearable maskers (refer again to Figures 14-8 and 14-9). This difference might be due in part to the synthesizer's wider bandwidth or greater sound power, thus providing more effective stimulation for those who have significant hearing loss; however, it might also be due to the fact that the Tinnitus Synthesizer generates steeper "skirts" for its masking noiseband; that is, wearable devices generate noisebands whose frequency spectra show a more gradual rolloff, both at the high-frequency and the low-frequency ends. Past experience with wearable maskers suggests that these gradual slopes tend to work against effective masking, especially on the low-frequency side where the resulting loudness becomes objectionable to the wearer. Research to evaluate that idea would be helpful, in order to quantify the effectiveness of wearable devices with noisebands having steeper high-frequency and low-frequency rolloff. Current digital techniques would seem well able to solve the technical problems of shaping such bands.

Another potentially useful research direction involves use of bone-conducted sound for masking. Until now, all wearable tinnitus maskers have utilized airborne stimuli. It seems reasonable to assume that there may be advantages for bone-conducted masking in some cases. For example, bilateral tinnitus may require only one bone conduction device as compared to the dual fitting usually required for air conduction units. Another possible advantage might occur in cases where the tinnitus is perceived as being located within the head rather than at the ears—conceivably, bone-conducted masking might provide a masking sensation whose localization is more similar to that of the tinnitus in such cases (see Chapter 6).

In the past, bone conduction transducers were not capable of producing audible stimulation much above about 4,000 Hz, a limitation rendering them inappropriate for many tinnitus patients since at least 75 percent of patients match their tinnitus pitch above 6,000 Hz. Present day bone conduction transducers greatly surpass that restriction, some even being capable of transmitting ultrasonic frequencies that are well above the frequencies needed for tinnitus masking (Corso, 1963; Lenhardt et al., 1991). Recent research has also shown that presentation of ultrasonic stimulation via bone conduction can achieve partial or complete tinnitus masking in a large percentage of cases (Meikle, Edlefsen, & Lay, 1999).

Combining Acoustical Masking with Other Therapies

Pharmacological Techniques Combined with Masking

It has been established that the drug Xanax (alprazolam) can provide effective relief of tinnitus in many cases (Johnson, Brummett, & Schleuning, 1993). A related possibility is that Xanax and masking might work synergistically to provide more effective relief than either treatment alone. The rationale is that different agents that are capable of reducing the loudness of tinnitus might exert their beneficial effects via some of the same elements within the central nervous system. Combinations of different therapies are therefore important to test, especially in those tinnitus patients for whom either therapy by itself is only partially effective. Similarly, the possible potentiation of masking by other types of drug therapy should be investigated using drugs that may be found to have beneficial effects on tinnitus.

Another possibility that deserves further research effort involves the effects of aspirin on tinnitus. It has been observed that aspirin-induced tinnitus is very easily masked and that almost any sound puts it into residual inhibition (McFadden, 1982). If that observation can be reproduced reliably in a larger sample of individuals, it might suggest that administering aspirin to individuals with tinnitus due to other causes might conceivably render the resulting "compound tinnitus" more amenable to masking. Although tinnitus patients are usually advised to avoid aspirin as it is likely to exacerbate their existing tinnitus, to date no one has yet determined whether aspirin might in fact make preexisting tinnitus more easily maskable. Patients who are found to be nonmaskable, using current ear-level equipment, might possibly find that they can use aspirin as an adjunctive treatment to improve the maskability of their tinnitus.

Electrical Stimulation and Masking

There has been confusion as to the exact nature of tinnitus relief produced by electrical stimulation (see Chapter 16). Some claim that electrical stimulation simply produces a sound that acts as a masker. If that is true then a combination of electrical stimuli and masking sounds might interact in beneficial ways, possibly achieving more effective masking results. Efforts to produce relatively noninvasive electrical stimulators (for example, using transcutaneous application of electrical currents, see Staller, 1997) might well be extended to exploring such possibilities. If the two modalities of stimulation can be used to potentiate each other's effects, combinations of acoustical plus electrical stimulation might offer a wider range of spectral or intensity configurations (and thus, possibly, more optimal masking conditions) than can be achieved with either modality by itself.

Use of Tinnitus Masking for Improving Diagnostic Understanding

To date there has been little effort to analyze differences between patients in regard to the ways in which masking stimulation interacts with the perceived characteristics of their tinnitus. We know, for example, that some patients are masked more effectively using dichotic presentations, while others achieve better masking effects when the masking sounds are presented diotically under earphones (Johnson & Hughes, 1991; Tyler & Stouffer, 1991). Although such observations may indicate important individual differences in regard to the neurological substrates for tinnitus, so far there have been few attempts to correlate such differences with concurrent recordings of subjects' auditory brain stem responses, otoacoustic emissions, or functional MRI (magnetic resonance imaging). The recent work evaluating tinnitus alterations using Positron Emission Tomography (PET) is, however, extremely encouraging (Lockwood & Salvi, 1998; also see Chapter 5). As research into tinnitus continues to progress, over time it is likely that cor-relating masking-induced changes in tinnitus with brain changes that are observed using various types of imaging techniques will generate much valuable information.

The use of masking to produce residual inhibition would be another valuable technique, in order to evaluate brain activity in one and the same subject with and without the presence of tinnitus. Further work may confirm that such techniques provide valid indicators of the "site of lesion" for the tinnitus and thus provide valuable information concerning underlying neural mechanisms.

Longitudinal Studies of Tinnitus

Prospective studies, employing longitudinal evaluation of neurological changes in tinnitus patients who are just beginning a program of masking therapy, would constitute an important area for future research. Currently there is little knowledge concerning neural alterations in individuals who experience reduction of tinnitus associated with extended use of masking (over weeks and months). It would be instructive to look for trends in measurable neurological activity in individuals employing long-term masking, using state-of-the art imaging techniques, electrophysiological measures, or other objective methods. Although objective indicators for tinnitus have so far remained elusive, it is possible that longitudinal studies using objective techniques coupled with a well-designed masking protocol could lead to effective methods for documenting the presence and nature of tinnitus.

As an example, imaging studies might show progressive brain alterations in patients who experience increasing durations of residual inhibition resulting from continued use of wearable tinnitus masking devices. In some cases, residual inhibition gradually accumulates to the point where the tinnitus is no longer audible at any time. A well-designed longitudinal study of such cases to evaluate brain activity before masking is begun, and repeated from time to time as residual inhibition begins to last for longer and longer intervals, could provide unique opportunities for examining the various objective indicators for tinnitus. In this way it may be possible to determine which types of objective measurements (auditory brain stem responses, longer-latency responses in the auditory nervous system, various types of brain imaging, and so on) might serve best as sensitive and reliable indicators of tinnitus.

REFERENCES

Agnew, J., & Johnson, R. M. (1993). New tinnitus masking devices allow patient, clinician tuning. *Hearing Instruments, 44,* 25–26.

Arnold, W., Bartenstein, P., Oestreicher, E., Römer, W., & Schwaiger, M. (1996). Focal metabolic activation in the predominant left auditory cortex in patients suffering from tinnitus: A PET study with [¹⁸F]Deoxyglucose. *ORL, 58,* 195–199.

Brandy, W. T., & Lynn, J. M. (1995). Audiologic findings in hyperacusic and nonhyperacusic subjects. *American Journal of Audiology, 44,* 46–51.

Brown, S. C. (1990). Older Americans and tinnitus: A demographic study and chartbook. *GRI Monograph Series A, No. 2.* Washington, DC: Gallaudet Research Institute.

Brummett, R. E. (1997). Are there any safe and effective drugs available to treat my tinnitus? In J. A. Vernon (Ed.), *Tinnitus treatment and relief* (pp. 34–42). Boston: Allyn & Bacon.

Cacace, A. T., Cousins, J. P., Moonen, C. T. W., Van Gelderen, P., Miller, D., Parnes, S. M., & Lovely, T. J. (1996). In-vivo localization of phantom auditory perceptions during functional magnetic resonance imaging of the human brain. In G. E. Reich & J. A. Vernon (Eds.), *Proceedings of the Fifth International Tinnitus Seminar* (pp. 397–401). Portland, OR: American Tinnitus Association. New York: Kugler Publications.

Çelikyurt, C., Bahadirlar, Y., & Gülçür, H. O. (1996). A PC–based system for management of tinnitus using masking. In G. E. Reich & J. A. Vernon (Eds.), *Proceedings of the Fifth International Tinnitus Seminar* (pp. 303–304). Portland, OR: American Tinnitus Association. New York: Kugler Publications.

Coles, R. R. A., Baskill, J., & Goodrum, K. (1987). A comparative trial of ear-canal and behind-the-ear tinnitus maskers. In H. Feldmann (Ed.), *Proceedings of the Third International Tinnitus Seminar* (pp. 265–269). Karlsruhe: Harsch Verlag.

Corso, J. F. (1963). Bone-conduction thresholds for sonic and ultrasonic frequencies. *The Journal of the Acoustical Society of America, 35,* 1738–1743.

Davis, H., & Silverman, S. R. (1960). *Hearing and deafness* (revised ed.). New York: Holt-Rinehart.

DeWeese, D., & Vernon, J. (1975). The American Tinnitus Association. *Hearing Instruments: (December),* pp. 19, 38.

Evered, D., & Lawrenson, G. (Eds.) (1981). *Tinnitus. CIBA Foundation Symposium 85.* London: Pitman Press.

Feldmann, H. (1971). Homolateral and contralateral masking of tinnitus by noisebands and by pure tones. *Audiology, 10,* 138–144.

Feldmann, H. (1983). Time patterns and related parameters in masking of tinnitus. *Acta Otolaryngologica, 95,* 594–598.

Feldmann, H. (1987a). Masking of tinnitus—Historical remarks. In H. Feldmann (Ed.), *Proceedings of the Third International Tinnitus Seminar Münster* (pp. 210–213). Karlsruhe: Harsch Verlag.

Feldmann, H. (1987b). Masking phenomena in tinnitus. In H. Feldmann (Ed.). *Proceedings of the Third International Tinnitus Seminar Münster* (pp. 224–228). Karlsruhe: Harsch Verlag.

Fletcher, H., & Munson, W. (1937). Relation between loudness and masking. *Journal of the Acoustical Society of America, 9,* 1–10.

Fowler, E. P. (1942). The "illusion of loudness" of tinnitus—Its etiology and treatment. *Laryngoscope, 52,* 275–285.

Fowler, E. P. (1943). Control of head noises. Their illusions of loudness and timbre. *Archives of Otolaryngology, 37,* 391–398.

Fusté, J., Doménech, J., Traserra, J., Traserra-Coderch, J., & Cuchi, A. (1996). Masking in the management of tinnitus unresponsive to drug therapy. In G. E. Reich & J. A. Vernon (Eds.), *Proceedings of the Fifth International Tinnitus Seminar* (pp. 310–311). Portland, OR: American Tinnitus Association.

Gabriels, P. (1991). Fitting protocol for the tinnitus patient. *Tinnitus Assessment and Rehabilitation. Papers presented at the Third Bi-Annual Workshop, Australian Association of Audiologists in Private Practice.* Melbourne: Australian Association of Audiologists in Private Practice (pp. 38–45).

Gabriels, P. (1996a). Children with tinnitus. In G. E. Reich & J. A. Vernon (Eds.), *Proceedings of the Fifth International Tinnitus Seminar* (pp. 270–274). Portland, OR: American Tinnitus Association.

Gabriels, P. (1996b). Tinnitus and hyperacusis. In G. E. Reich & J. A. Vernon (Eds.), *Proceedings of the Fifth International Tinnitus Seminar* (pp. 46–50). Portland, OR: American Tinnitus Association.

George, R. N., & Kemp, S. (1991). A survey of New Zealanders with tinnitus. *British Journal of Audiology, 25,* 331–336.

Goldstein, B. A., & Shulman, A. (1991). Tinnitus masking. A longitudinal study of efficacy/ diagnosis 1977–1990. In J. M. Aran & R. Dauman (Eds.), *Tinnitus 91. Proceedings of the Fourth International Tinnitus Seminar* (pp. 375–380). New York: Kugler Publications.

Goldstein, B. A., & Shulman, A. (1996). Tinnitus masking—A longitudinal study of efficacy/ diagnosis 1977–1994. In G. E. Reich & J. A. Vernon (Eds.), *Proceedings of the Fifth International Tinnitus Seminar* (pp. 315–321). Portland, OR: American Tinnitus Association.

Greenwood, D. D. (1961). Auditory masking and the critical band. *Journal of the Acoustical Society, 33,* 484–501.

Hazell, J. W. P. (1987). Tinnitus masking therapy. In J. W. P. Hazell (Ed.), *Tinnitus* (pp. 96–117). London: Churchill Livingstone.

Hazell, J. W. P., & Sheldrake, J. B. (1992). Hyperacusis and tinnitus. In J. M. Aran & R. Dauman (Eds.), *Tinnitus 91. Proceedings of the Fourth International Tinnitus Seminar* (pp. 245–253). New York: Kugler Publications.

Hazell, J. W. P., & Wood, S. M. (1981). Tinnitus masking—A significant contribution to tinnitus management. *British Journal of Audiology, 15,* 223–230.

Hazell, J. W. P., Wood, S. M., Cooper, H. R., Stephens, S. D. G., Corcoran, A. L., Coles, R. R. A., Baskill, J. L., & Sheldrake, J. B. (1985). A clinical study of tinnitus maskers. *British Journal of Audiology, 19,* 65–146.

Henry, J. A., Fausti, S. A., Flick, C. L., Helt, W. J., & Mitchell, C. R. An automated technique for tinnitus evaluation. In G. E. Reich & J. A. Vernon (Eds.), *Proceedings of the Fifth International Tinnitus Seminar.* Portland, OR: American Tinnitus Association. (pp. 325–326). New York: Kugler Publications.

Jeffress, L. A. (1970). Masking. In J. V. Tobias (Ed.), *Foundations of Modern Auditory Theory Vol. 1* (pp. 85–114). New York: Academic Press.

Jeffress, L. A., Blodgett, H. C., & Deatherage, B. H. (1952). Masking of pure tones by white noise as a function of the interaural phase of both components. *The Journal of the Acoustical Society of America, 34,* 1124–1126.

Johnson, R. M. (1998). The masking of tinnitus. In J. A. Vernon (Ed.), *Tinnitus treatments and relief* (pp. 164–186). Boston: Allyn & Bacon.

Johnson, R. M., Brummett, R., & Schleuning, A. (1993). Use of alprazolam for relief of tinnitus. *Archives of Otolaryngology—Head & Neck Surgery, 119,* 842–845.

Johnson, R. M., & Fenwick, J. (1984). Masking levels (Minimum Masking Levels) and tinnitus frequency. In *Proceedings of the Second International Tinnitus Seminar, New York 1983. The Journal of Laryngology and Otology, Suppl. 9* (pp. 63–66). Ashford, Kent, U.K.: Invicta Press.

Johnson, R., Griest, S., Press, L., Storter, K., & Lentz, B. (1989). A tinnitus masking program: Efficacy and safety. *The Hearing Journal, 42,* 18–25.

Johnson, R. M., & Hughes, F. M. (1991). Diotic versus dichotic masking of tinnitus. In J.-M. Aran & R. Dauman (Eds.), *Tinnitus 91. Proceedings of the Fourth International Tinnitus Seminar* (pp. 387–390). New York: Kugler Publications.

Johnson, R. M., & Mitchell, C. R. (1984). Critical bandwidth-masking bands. In *Proceedings of the Second International Tinnitus Seminar, New York 1983. The Journal of Laryngology and Otology, Suppl. 9* (pp. 69–73). Ashford, Kent, U.K.: Invicta Press.

Lay, J., & Nunley, J. (1996). Tinnitus evaluation system based on computerized auditory research laboratory. In G. E. Reich & J. A. Vernon (Eds.), *Proceedings of the Fifth International Tinnitus Seminar* (pp. 327–328). Portland, OR: American Tinnitus Association.

Lenhardt, M. L., Skellett, R., Wang, P., & Clarke, A. M. (1991). Human ultrasonic speech perception. *Science, 253,* 82–84.

Lockwood, A. H., Salvi, R. J., Coad, B. A., Towsley, M. L., Wack, D. S., & Murphy, B. W. (1998). The functional neuroanatomy of tinnitus. Evidence for limbic system links and neural plasticity. *Neurology, 50,* 114–120.

McCormick, M. S., & Pritchard, J. (1987). Do tinnitus maskers reduce tinnitus levels: A two-year review of tinnitus matching and masking. In H. Feldmann (Ed.), *Proceedings of the Third International Tinnitus Seminar* (pp. 299–300). Karlsruhe: Harsch Verlag.

McFadden, D. (1982). *Tinnitus: Facts, theories, and treatments.* Washington, DC: National Academy Press.

Meikle, M., & Walsh, E. T. (1984). Characteristics of tinnitus and related observations in over 1800 tinnitus clinic patients. In *Proceedings of the Second International Tinnitus Seminar, New York 1983. The Journal of Laryngology and Otol-*

ogy , Suppl. 9 (pp. 17–21). Ashford, Kent, U.K.: Invicta Press.

Meikle, M. B. (1991). Methods for evaluation of tinnitus relief procedures. In J.-M. Aran & R. Dauman (Eds.) *Tinnitus 91. Proceedings of the Fourth International Tinnitus Seminar* (pp. 555–562). New York: Kugler Publications.

Meikle, M. B., Edlefsen, L. L., & Lay, J. L. (1999). Suppression of tinnitus by bone conduction of ultrasound. *Abstracts of the Association for Research in Otolaryngology,* 223.

Meikle, M. B., & Griest, S. E. (1991). Computer data analysis: Tinnitus Data Registry. In A. Shulman (Ed.), *Tinnitus. Diagnosis/treatment* (pp. 416–430). Philadelphia: Lea & Febiger.

Meikle, M. B., Griest, S. E., Press, L. E., McLaughlin, T. L., & Perrin, N. A. (1997). Disability caused by tinnitus with and without hearing impairment. *Abstracts of the Association for Research in Otolaryngology,* 66.

Meikle, M. B., Johnson, R. M., Griest, S. E., Press, L. S., & Charnell, M. G. (1995). Oregon Tinnitus Data Archive 95–01. *World Wide Web*: <http://www.ohsu.edu/ohrc–otda/>, 1995.

Mitchell, C. (1983). The masking of tinnitus with pure tones. *Audiology, 22,* 73–87.

Mitchell, C. R., Vernon, J. A., & Creedon, T. A. (1993). Measuring tinnitus parameters: Loudness, pitch, maskability. *Journal of the American Academy of Audiology, 4,* 139–151.

Morris, W. (Ed.). (1969). *The American Heritage Dictionary of the English Language.* New York: American Heritage Publishing and Houghton-Mifflin.

National Center for Health Statistics. (November 1968). Hearing status and ear examination: Findings among adults, United States, 1960–1962. *Vital and Health Statistics, Series 11, No. 32.* Washington, DC: U.S. Department of Health, Education and Welfare.

Nunley, J. (1995). New prostheses to aid patients. In G. E. Reich & J. A. Vernon (Eds.), *Proceedings of the Fifth International Tinnitus Seminar* (pp. 335–340). Portland, OR: American Tinnitus Association.

Preves, D., Millier, R., Yanz, J., Anderson, B., & Hagen, L. (1998). A combination custom active hearing protector/hearing aid. *The Hearing Journal, 51,* 34–43.

Pritchard, J., & McCormick, M. S. (1987). Are high frequency tinnitus maskers effective? In H. Feldmann (Ed.), *Proceedings of the Third International Tinnitus Seminar Münster.* (pp. 303). Karlsruhe: Harsch Verlag.

Reed, G. F. (1960). An audiometric study of two hundred cases of subjective tinnitus. *Archives of Otolaryngology, 71,* 94–104.

Reich, G. E., & Griest, S. E. (1991). A survey of hyperacusis patients. In J. M. Aran & R. Dauman (Eds.), *Tinnitus 91. Proceedings of the Fourth International Tinnitus Seminar* (pp. 249–253). New York: Kugler Publications.

Saltzman, M., & Ersner, M. S. (1947). A hearing aid for relief of tinnitus aurium. *Laryngoscope, 57,* 358–366.

Schleuning, A. J., Johnson, R. M, & Vernon, J. A. (1980). Evaluation of a tinnitus masking program: A follow-up study of 598 patients. *Ear & Hearing, 1,* 71–74.

Shailer, M. J., Tyler, R. S., & Coles, R. R. A. (1981). Critical masking bands for sensorineural tinnitus. *Scandinavian Audiology, 10,* 157–162.

Shulman, A., & Goldstein, B. (1987). Tinnitus masking—A longitudinal study of efficacy-diagnosis: Treatment 1977–1986. In H. Feldmann (Ed.), *Proceedings of the Third International Tinnitus Seminar Münster.* (pp. 251–256). Karlsruhe: Harsch Verlag.

Sood, S. K., & Coles, R. R. A. (1988). Hyperacusis and phonophobia in tinnitus patients. *British Journal of Audiology, 22,* 228.

Spaulding, A. J. (1903). Tinnitus, with a plea for its more accurate musical notation. *Annals of Otology, 32,* 263–272.

Staller, S. J. (1997). Suppression of tinnitus with electrical stimulation. In J. Vernon (Ed.), *Tinnitus Treatment and Relief* (pp. 77–90). Boston: Allyn & Bacon.

Stephens, S. D. G. (1987). Historical aspects of tinnitus. In J. W. P. Hazell (Ed.), *Tinnitus.* London: Churchill Livingstone.

Terry, A. M. P., Jones, D. M., Davis, B. R., & Slater R. (1983). Parametric studies of tinnitus masking and residual inhibition. *British Journal of Audiology, 17,* 245–256.

Tyler, R. S. (1991). The psychophysical measurement of tinnitus. In J.-M. Aran & R. Dauman (Eds.), *Tinnitus 91. Proceedings of the Fourth International Tinnitus Seminar* (pp. 17–26). New York: Kugler Publications.

Tyler, R. S., Babin, R. N., & Niebuhr, D. P. (1984). Some observations on the masking and post-masking effects of tinnitus. In *Proceedings of the Second International Tinnitus Seminar, New York 1983. The Journal of Laryngology and Otology, Suppl. 9* (pp.150–156). Ashford, Kent, U.K.: Invicta Press.

Tyler, R. S., & Baker, L. J. (1983). Difficulties experienced by tinnitus sufferers. *Journal of Speech and Hearing Disorders, 48*, 150–154.

Tyler, R. S., & Conrad-Armes, D. (1984). Masking of tinnitus compared to masking of pure tones. *Journal of Speech and Hearing Research, 27*, 106–111.

Tyler, R. S., Kuk, F. K., & Mims, L. A. (1987). Ipsilateral and contralateral postmasking recovery of tinnitus. In H. Feldmann (Ed.), *Proceedings of the Third International Tinnitus Seminar* (pp. 275–279). Karlsruhe: Harsch Verlag.

Tyler, R. S., & Stouffer, J. L. (1991). Binaural tinnitus masking with a noise centered on the tinnitus. In J.-M. Aran & R. Dauman (Eds.), *Tinnitus 91. Proceedings of the Fourth International Tinnitus Seminar* (pp. 391–394). New York: Kugler Publications.

van den Abbeele, T., & Frachet, B. (1992). Tinnitus matching. Technological features. In J.-M. Aran & R. Dauman (Eds.), *Tinnitus 91. Proceedings of the Fourth International Tinnitus Seminar* (pp. 57–59). New York: Kugler Publications.

Vernon, J. (1975). Tinnitus. *Hearing Aid Journal, Nov., 13*; 82–83.

Vernon, J. (1977). Attempts to relieve tinnitus. *Journal of the American Audiology Society, 2*, 124–131.

Vernon, J. (1978). Information from U.O.H.S.C. tinnitus clinic. *American Tinnitus Association Newsletter, 3*, 1–4.

Vernon, J. (1979). The use of masking for relief of tinnitus. In H. Silverstein & H. Norell (Eds.), *Neurological surgery of the ear.* Birmingham, AL: Aesculapius.

Vernon, J. (1981). The history of masking as applied to tinnitus. In *Tinnitus. Proceedings of the First International Tinnitus Seminar, New York 1979. The Journal of Laryngology and Otology* (Suppl. 4, pp. 76–79). Ashford, Kent, U.K.: Invicta Press.

Vernon, J. (1982). Relief of tinnitus by masking treatment. (1982). In G. M. English (Ed.), *Otolaryngology.* Philadelphia: Harper & Row (Chapter 53; pp. 1–21).

Vernon, J. (1987a). Assessment of the tinnitus patient. In J. W. P. Hazell (Ed.), *Tinnitus.* (pp. 71–87). London: Churchill Livingstone.

Vernon, J., Griest, S., & Press, L. (1990). Attributes of tinnitus and the acceptance of masking. *American Journal of Otolaryngology, 11*, 44–50.

Vernon, J., Griest, S., & Press, L. (1992). Plight of unreturned questionnaires. *British Journal of Audiology, 26*, 137–138.

Vernon, J., Johnson, R., Schleuning, A., & Mitchell, C. (1980). Masking and tinnitus. *Audiology and Hearing Education, 6*, 5–9.

Vernon, J., & Schleuning, A. (1978). Tinnitus: A new management. *Laryngoscope, 88*, 413–419.

Vernon, J., Schleuning, A., Odell, L., & Hughes, F. (1977). A tinnitus clinic. *Ear Nose & Throat Journal, 56*, 181–189.

Vernon, J. A. (1987b). Pathophysiology of tinnitus: A special case—Hyperacusis and a proposed treatment. *The American Journal of Otolaryngology, 8*, 201–202.

Vernon, J. A. (1987c). Real-ear evaluation of tinnitus maskers. In H. Feldmann (Ed.), *Proceedings of the Third International Tinnitus Seminar* (pp. 363–369). Karlsruhe: Harsch Verlag.

Vernon, J. A. (1988). Current use of masking for the relief of tinnitus. In M. Kitahara (Ed.), *Tinnitus pathophysiology and management* (pp. 96–106). Tokyo: Igaku-Shoin.

Vernon, J. A. (1992). Tinnitus: Causes, evaluation, and treatment. In G. M. English (Ed.). *Otolaryngology, Revised edition* (Chapter 53). Philadelphia: Lippincott.

Vernon, J. A., (Ed.). (1998). *Tinnitus treatment and relief.* Boston: Allyn & Bacon.

Vernon, J. A., & Meikle, M. B. (1981). Tinnitus masking: Unresolved problems. In D. Evered & G. Lawrenson (Eds.), *Tinnitus. CIBA Foundation Symposium 85* (pp. 239–256). London: Pitman Press.

Vernon, J. A., & Meikle, M. B. (1988). Measurement of tinnitus: An update. In M. Kitahara (Ed.), *Tinnitus pathophysiology and management* (pp. 36–52). Tokyo: Igaku-Shoin.

Vernon, J. A., & Press, L. (1998). Treatment for hyperacusis. In J. A. Vernon (Ed.), *Tinnitus treatment and relief* (pp. 223–227). Boston: Allyn & Bacon.

Vernon, J. A., Press, L. S., Griest, S. E., & Storter, K.V. (1991). Acoustic stimulation and tinnitus. In J. M. Aran & R. Dauman (Eds.), *Tinnitus 91. Proceedings of the Fourth International Tinnitus Seminar* (pp. 363–369). New York: Kugler Publications.

Vernon, J. A., & Schleuning , A. J. (1980). Tinnitus: Its care and treatment. *American Academy of Otolaryngology 1980 Instruction Series* (Course 576). American Academy of Otolaryngology.

von Wedel, H. (1987). A longitudinal study in tinnitus-therapy with tinnitus-maskers and hearing aids. In H. Feldmann (Ed.), *Proceedings of the Third International Tinnitus Seminar* (pp. 257–260). Karlsruhe: Harsch Verlag.

Walter, B., & Johansen, P. A. (1987). Effect of tinnitus masker. 5 years follow-up. In H. Feldmann (Ed.), *Proceedings of the Third International Tinnitus Seminar* (pp. 301–302). Karlsruhe: Harsch Verlag.

Wegel, R. L., & Lane, C. E. (1924). The auditory masking of one pure tone by another and its probable relation to the dynamics of the ear. *Physiological Review, 23,* 266–285.

Zwislocki, J. J., (1971). Central masking and neural activity in the cochlear nucleus. *Audiology, 10,* 48–59.

Zwislocki, J., Buining, E., & Glantz, J. (1968). Frequency distribution of central masking. *Journal of the Acoustical Society of America, 43,* 1267–1271.

Appendix

SECTION I.
SOURCES OF MASKING DEVICES

At this writing there are two commercial sources for tinnitus masking devices located in the United States:

Starkey Labs, Inc.,
P.O. Box 9457, Minneapolis, MN 55344
Telephone: 1-800-328-8602 (in the
            United States)
Web Site: <http://www.starkey.com>

General Hearing Instruments, Inc.,
P.O. Box 23748, New Orleans, LA 70183
Telephone: 1-800-824-3021 (in the United
            States and Canada)
Web Site:
<http://www.generalhearing.com>

SECTION II.
BEDSIDE MASKING DEVICES

There are many bedside masking devices available commercially. A particularly versatile array of devices, suitable for tinnitus masking, is manufactured by:

Marpac Corporation,
P.O. Box 3098, Wilmington, N.C. 28406
Telephone: 1-800-999-6962 (in the United
            States and Canada)
Web Site: <http://www.marpac.com>

A masking pillow (sound is broadcast from microstereo speakers located inside the pillow) is available as the "Sound Pillow" from:

Phoenix Productions,
2935 Thousand Oaks, Suite 6-269,
San Antonio, TX 78247
Telephone: 1-877-846-6488

SECTION III.
MASKING TAPES AND CDS

While some individuals may choose to record their own masking bands or other form of constant, easily-ignored noise, those who lack the resources to do so may obtain masking tapes and CDs designed to mask tinnitus:

1. An analog CD with selectable noise-bands is available at nominal charge from the following:

Oregon Tinnitus Clinic,
NRC 04, 3181 S.W. Sam Jackson Park Rd.,
Portland, OR 97201
Telephone: (503) 494-7954
Web Site:
<http://www.ohsu.edu/ohrc/tinnitusclinic/

Each of the different bands on the CD contains a noiseband covering a different frequency range so that the user may select the band that provides most effective tinnitus masking. The CD also provides a band of "pink noise" for use in the Hyperacusis Desensitization Program (refer to pages 346–347). The Tinnitus Clinic also has masking tapes available for those who do not wish to use a CD player.

2. A set of masking CDs with uniquely shaped noise is available as the "Dynamic Tinnitus Mitigation" system from:

Petroff Audio Technologies,
23507 Balmoral Lane, West Hills, CA 91307
Telephone: (818) 716-6166
Web Site: <http://www.tinnitushelp.com>

The system consists of a set of four audio CDs that provide a wide array of different types of noise, plus miniature headphones and a user's manual containing suggestions for successful management of tinnitus.

CHAPTER 15

Tinnitus Habituation Therapy (THT) and Tinnitus Retraining Therapy (TRT)

Pawel J. Jastreboff

INTRODUCTION

In the 1980s several key observations instilled doubt as to whether the mechanisms of tinnitus are confined to the auditory system, typically to the cochlea and the auditory nerve. The study of clinical and research data indicated the involvement of other systems within the brain in clinically-relevant tinnitus. From these observations, a neurophysiological model of tinnitus was created, and based on this model a treatment aimed at the habituation of tinnitus, Tinnitus Habituation Therapy (THT) was proposed. THT can be achieved by various methods. One method, Tinnitus Retraining Therapy (TRT), involves counseling and sound therapy to habituate tinnitus. To comprehend THT and TRT, it is important to understand the neurophysiological model of tinnitus, and therefore this chapter first provides an outline of the model.

Development of the Concept of Tinnitus Habituation: Clinical Observations Contradict Dominant Role of the Auditory System in Tinnitus

The first observation that contradicted the belief that the mechanisms of tinnitus are contained within the auditory system was that while approximately 10 to 20 percent of the general population experience tinnitus, only about a quarter of this population suffer from it (Coles, 1996; Davis, 1996; Coles, 1996; McFadden, 1982). Second, the psychoacoustical characterization of tinnitus in the group that simply experienced tinnitus did not show any difference when compared to the group that suffered from tinnitus, and furthermore, the severity of tinnitus and its impact on life was not correlated with these measurements (Hazell et al., 1985). Third, the average audiogram for people with tinnitus is practically identical and statistically undistinguishable from the average audiogram obtained from the general population (Hazell, 1996). Finally, the psychoacoustical characterization of tinnitus (that is, pitch, loudness, and maskability) did not offer any predicted value for assessing treatment outcome (Jastreboff et al., 1994). Disregarding whether the loudness of tinnitus was high or low, or whether it was easy or difficult, or even impossible to suppress it, the probability of improvement was the same.

These observations strongly suggested that since the psychoacoustical description of tinnitus does not seem to be related to its severity and has no bearing on the probability of recovery, then the auditory system is not the dominant factor in clinically significant tinnitus. Tinnitus is referred to as "clinically significant" when it creates problems and the individual seeks treatment. Other systems within the brain have to be included in understanding when and why tinnitus causes suffering.

Notably, the finding that the average audiogram is practically the same for people with tinnitus and the general population disposes of the opinion that tinnitus is directly related to hearing loss. This is further supported by the observation that many tinnitus patients have normal hearing (Hazell et al., 1985; Hazell, 1996) (and unpublished results from the University of Maryland Tinnitus and Hyperacusis Center) and about 30 percent of the people who are totally deaf do not have tinnitus (Hazell et al., 1995a; McFadden, 1982a). This postulate is contradictive to other theories and models of tinnitus that focus on the auditory system, typically limiting the mechanisms of tinnitus to the auditory periphery; for example, the cochlea and the auditory nerve (Kiang et al., 1970; Zenner & Ernst, 1993; Moller et al., 1993; Moller, 1984; McFadden, 1982).

Functions of the Limbic and Autonomic Nervous Systems

If not the auditory system, then what other systems need to be included in the model of tinnitus? The observation of tinnitus patients provided the answer (Jastreboff, 1990; Newman et al., 1995; Kuk et al., 1990; Stouffer et al., 1991; Stouffer & Tyler, 1990). The patients for whom tinnitus is clinically significant exhibit a strong emotional reaction to it, a high level of anxiety, and a number of psychosomatic problems. This indicates the involvement of two systems within the brain—the emotional, limbic, and the autonomic nervous systems.

The limbic system is a heterogenous array of brain structures at or near the edge (limbus) of the medial wall of the cerebral hemisphere, includes the following cortical structures: the olfactory cortex, hippocampal formation, cingulate gyrus, and subcallosal gyrus; and the following subcortical regions: the amygdala, septum, hypothalamus, epithalamus (habenula), anterior thalamic nuclei, and parts of basal ganglia. The limbic system exerts an important influence upon the endocrine and autonomic motor systems. The limbic system influence directly neuroendocrine, autonomic, and controls multifaceted behavior, including emotional expression, seizure activity, memory storage and recall, and the motivational and mood states (Swanson, 1987).

The autonomic nervous system, one of the two main divisions of the nervous system, provides the motor innervation of smooth muscle, cardiac muscle, and gland cells. The autonomic system controls the action of the glands; the functions of the respiratory, circulatory, digestive, and urogenital systems; and the involuntary muscles in these systems and in the skin. The system also has a reciprocal effect on the internal secretions, being controlled to some degree by the hormones and exercising some control, in turn, on hormone production. The autonomic nervous system consists of two physiologically and anatomically distinct, mutually antagonistic components: the sympathetic (thoracicolumbar), and parasympathetic (craniosacral). The sympathetic division stimulates the heart, dilates the bronchi, contracts the arteries, inhibits the digestive system, and prepares the organism for physical action. The parasympathetic division has the opposite effect, it prepares the organism for feeding, digestion, and rest (Brooks, 1987).

For both divisions the pathway of innervation consists of a synaptic sequence of two motor neurons, one of which lies in the spinal cord or brain stem as the preganglionic neuron, the thin but myelinated axon (preganglionic or B fiber) emerges with an outgoing spinal or cranial nerve and synapses with one or more of the postganglionic neurons composing the autonomic ganglia; the unmyelinated postganglionic fibers in turn innervate the smooth muscle, cardiac muscle, or gland cells. The preganglionic neurons of the sympathetic part lie in the intermediolateral cell column of the thoracic and upper two lumbar segments of the spinal gray matter; those of the parasympathetic part compose the visceral motor (visceral efferent) nuclei of the brain stem, and with the cranial nerves, especially the vagus and accessory nerves, pass to ganglia and plexuses within the various organs. The lower part of the body is innervated by fibers arising from the lateral column of the second to fourth sacral segments of the spinal cord. Impulse transmission from preganglionic to postganglionic neuron is mediated by acetylcholine in both the sympathetic and parasympathetic parts; transmission from the postganglionic fiber to the visceral effector tissues is classically said to be by acetylcholine in the parasympathetic part and by noradrenaline in the sympathetic part. Recent evidence suggests the existence of further noncholinergic, nonadrenergic classes of postganglionic fibers (Brooks, 1987).

From the point of view of tinnitus, it is important that the limbic system is involved in all aspects of life involving motivation, mood, and emotions, and that it activates the endocrine and autonomic nervous systems. A highly activated limbic system results in mood swings, a person being controlled by emotions, potential changes in hormone levels (with all its consequences), and through activating the autonomic ner-

vous system, can influence all body functions. Typically patients exhibit syndromes indicating a dominance of sympathetic division of the autonomic nervous system, which stimulates the heart, inhibits the digestive system, and in general prepares the body for physical action. This in turn leads to problems with sleep, which is very common (Coles, 1996). Abnormally high activation of these systems results in stress, anxiety, and loss of well-being. These patients are extremely annoyed by their tinnitus, which as it is argued in this chapter, due to the feedback loop connecting the auditory, limbic, autonomic nervous systems, continues to get worse.

Please note that the high level of activation of the limbic and autonomic nervous systems by any factor, even without tinnitus present, will result in the same syndromes as described by tinnitus patients, and that only sleep deprivation can account for many behavioral and psychological changes reported by patients (such as inability to concentrate, mood swings, problems with logical decision, rapid illogical reactions to encounter problems; see Chapter 2). The difference is that when the external factors go away (stress induced by necessity of extreme amount of work, personal relationship ends, and so forth) activation of the limbic and autonomic nervous systems decreases to the normal level. But with tinnitus cases, tinnitus remains present. Once the conditioned reflex arcs are established, the activation of both systems increases to the level where the physical defenses of the body force the individual to sleep, abandon stressful activities (resigning from work or social contacts), and a plateau is reached.

Another crucial issue reflects the physiological fact that a high level of activation of the sympathetic part of the autonomic nervous system, because of any reason, activates the fight or flight reaction, and suppresses or even eliminates positive emotions, resulting in the inability to enjoy life. In cases of severe tinnitus, it is frequently observed these patients no longer enjoy activities previously pleasant to them, and life ceases to offer joy. This in turn yields depression.

Typical complaints, such as problem with sleep, anxiety, depression, and a variety of emotions attached to tinnitus including fear and tension, strongly indicate that the tinnitus signal activates both the limbic and autonomic nervous systems in the brain, and that this activation is sustained. Accordingly, the basic postulate of the neurophysiological model of tinnitus is that the auditory system, including the cochlea, plays only a secondary role in the emergence of clinically significant tinnitus. The auditory system provides the initial signal, but the problems with tinnitus arise from the improper activation of the limbic and autonomic nervous systems. The activation occurs by means of both subcortical and cortical loops, acting through association developed in the manner of conditioned reflexes. The interaction of signals among these structures is presented schematically in Figure 15-1A.

An Outline of the Neurophysiological Model of Tinnitus

When a new auditory signal is presented for the first time, the sound is transduced in the cochlea and detected at subcortical centers, which activate the cortical area and it is perceived and evaluated. The pattern of the signal is compared to other patterns stored in memory and its relevance is assessed as being either neutral, positive, or negative. As a new signal, it evokes a slight activation of the limbic and autonomic nervous systems. On the behavioral level this can be described as attracting attention to the new signal, and putting the brain and body in the state of alertness. If the signal is evaluated as neutral and does not carry significant information (for example, sounds of a refrigerator in our house), a repetitive presentation of the same stimulus will not activate the limbic and autonomic nervous systems. It will not attract our attention and we will not be aware of its presence. The signal has been habituated.

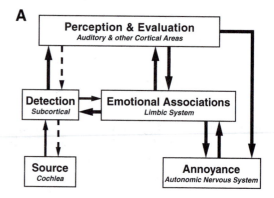

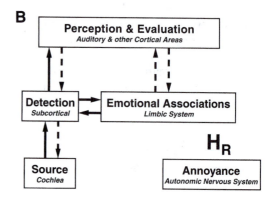

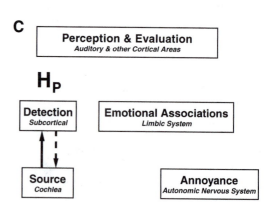

FIGURE 15-1. Block diagram outlining systems involved in clinically relevant tinnitus and changes occurring as a result of tinnitus habituation. Thickness of the arrows indicates the significance of a given connection. **A**—before treatment; **B**—habituation of reactions to tinnitus; **C**—habituation of tinnitus perception.

It is important to realize that two types of habituation can occur. The first type is the *habituation of the reaction* to the signal, that is, activation of the autonomic nervous system (which yields the fight or flight reaction and annoyance) is habituated. This reaction is extinguished, and consequently even when we perceive this specific signal, the reflex reactions to this signal disappear. The second type of habituation is the *habituation of the perception* of the signal, that is, the signal is detected in the subcortical centers, but does not reach the level of our awareness and consequently we are not "hearing" it, except when we focus our attention on it; again, an example would be the sound of a refrigerator.

The habituation of reactions occurs when the neuronal activity representing the sound of the refrigerator, while present in the auditory system, is blocked and does not reach the autonomic nervous system (Figure 15-1B). This neuronal activity still mildly activates the limbic system, a condition needed to sustain perception of the signal.

The situation is totally different if, during the initial evaluation, the new sound acquires a negative association, such as something unpleasant, annoying, or even dangerous. Then neuronal activity corresponding to this sound will activate the limbic system, inducing fear or irritation, and activate the autonomic nervous system providing the "fight or flight" reaction. Activation of these systems will reinforce the conditioned reflex loop, and consequently repetition of this sound will enhance the activation of the limbic and autonomic nervous systems. Then, without the need for full awareness and recognition, this specific sound will induce a very quick and strong reaction of our autonomic nervous system (lower loop from the cochlea to the autonomic nervous system in Figure 15-1A). The creation and enhancement of these conditioned reflexes can be described as a "vicious circle." The presence of the sound evokes annoyance and strong emotions, which enhances the awareness to the signal, which further enhances annoyance and emotions, which further enhances the awareness, and so on. The reactions to the sound serve as a negative reinforcement, and the repetitive presentation of the signal results in strengthening the reflex loop, which results in self-enhancement of the reactions.

The brain reacts to tinnitus as if it is an external sound. If the initial perception of tinnitus is not associated with anything negative, and it does not induce strong annoyance, then both the reaction to, and the perception of, tinnitus are habituated. Consequently these people experience, but do not suffer from, tinnitus. Fortunately this occurs for about 75 percent of the people who have tinnitus (McFadden, 1982).

However, if the initial association of tinnitus is negative; for example, the person is told there is no hope, the tinnitus can get worse, there might be a brain tumor, or tinnitus is associated with progressive hearing loss, then the initial negative relationship is created and the perception of tinnitus strongly activates both the limbic and autonomic nervous systems. Once this "negative counseling" occurs, and tinnitus is labeled as something wrong, then the brain starts to automatically monitor the presence of, and changes in, tinnitus, which in turn increases the annoyance induced by tinnitus. The conditioned reflex loop is even more enhanced, because it is impossible to run away from tinnitus, or attack and destroy it, and the continuous presence of tinnitus yields the continuous activation of the autonomic nervous system resulting in increased annoyance.

The situation is particularly significant because of a specific limitation of the brain. Although we are able to detect very weak, but significant, signals and enhance them, even distinguish them against background noise, our brain can only perform one task requiring our full attention at a time. For example, we cannot read a book and write a letter at the same time. However, in everyday life we are emerged in a huge number of simultaneous stimuli surrounding us, and if we had to consciously select which stimuli we should pay attention to, we would not be able to do anything else.

Two mechanisms provide a solution to this problem. Based on previous experience, the subcortical centers subconsciously select and filter out unimportant signals so that we are only aware of the signals that are significant, particularly signals that indicate something unpleasant or dangerous. Habituation of perception of the insignificant signals occurs and we are not aware of all the sounds that surround us. The second mechanism involves a subconscious creation of a list of tasks to be performed based on their importance, and one task is performed at a time, with the most important task placed at the top of the list. While we have some control over which task we do first, our control is seriously limited in cases of stimuli that are associated with something negative or dangerous. If the stimulus has a strong negative connotation we lose our control over monitoring this signal altogether and automatically our attention focuses on this specific stimulus. A classical example would be to attempt to listen to a someone speaking when a tiger is in the same room, or trying to sleep with a loose and dangerous snake in the bedroom.

Once tinnitus achieves a strong negative connotation, which is enhanced through the vicious circle, a strong conditioned reflex with negative reinforcement is established. Consequently, the people lose the ability to focus their attention on other signals and perform other tasks, as their attention is continuously focused on tinnitus. People experience the inability to concentrate on one subject, which has a profound impact on their ability to work and follow conversation. This in turn frequently creates the false impression that tinnitus is masking the conversation, and that because of tinnitus, the ability to hear and understand speech decreases. Indeed, tinnitus disturbs the ability to understand conversation, not because it is physically masking the sound but because it disrupts our concentration and attention that is needed to follow a conversation.

Continuous activation of the autonomic nervous system has an impact on the person's life by interfering with their sleep. When the autonomic nervous system has a high level of activation, then the person experiences difficulty falling asleep, sleep is shallow and does not provide enough of the Rapid Eye Movement phase (which is essential for restoration of the brain), causing sleep deprivation. For many people the symptoms that they assume are a consequence of tinnitus actually result from their sleep deprivation (see Chapter 3). The people who experience sleep deprivation without tinnitus have problems concentrating, thinking, are unstable emotionally, and have problems with emotional control. Consequently, they have a tendency to overreact to small problems, and the quality of their work deteriorates. Finally if the period of sleep deprivation is prolonged, the cumulative effect of all these symptoms may cause depression.

The issue of depression, which is so prevalent among tinnitus patients, results from another, even more pronounced mechanism. A highly activated sympathetic part of the autonomic nervous system, together with a negative emotion, such as fear, annoyance, or discomfort, can suppress or even eliminate positive emotions, resulting in the inability to enjoy life. In everyday life this translates to a situation when the person is unable to enjoy life and activities that were previously enjoyed. A clear example of this, which is actually used in a behavioral conditioning suppression technique (Estes & Skinner, 1941), and in an animal model of tinnitus (Jastreboff et al., 1988), is counteracting alimentary motivation (hunger, thirst) with fear. In everyday life this occurs when somebody is waiting in the dentist's office knowing that in a few minutes he/she is going to be asked to come inside to have a dental procedure performed. If at this time the person is offered a nice dinner, most probably he will not be able to eat at all, and even if he forces himself to eat, he might have a problem with his gastrointestinal tract and would not be able to enjoy the meal.

Patients who experience continuously high activation of the limbic and autonomic nervous systems consequently lose their ability to enjoy life. This is a common complaint. If prolonged, this may cause severe depression, which the patient correctly associates with tinnitus, which in turn further enhances the negative association of tinnitus and its vicious circle.

Notably, the activation of limbic and autonomic nervous systems induced by tinnitus occurs via two pathways: the upper loop (cortical) which involves verbalization and conscious thinking, and the lower subconscious (subcortical) (Figure 15-1A). The cortical loop is involved in verbalized beliefs such as "I am going deaf, I am going crazy, I have a brain tumor." Activation of the subcortical loop does not require any conscious belief or strong emotion related to tinnitus. The situation is similar to being forced to listen to a neighbor playing the same song over and over for 16 hours a day. While we fully realize the sound of the song is not causing damage to our ear and is not related to any medical problem, it can be extremely annoying and disruptive and cause a high level of anxiety and discomfort.

The neurophysiological model provides an explanation why the psychoacoustical characterization of tinnitus has no correlation with tinnitus severity and treatment outcome. In this model, the clinically significant problems the patient experiences are associated with the level of activation of the autonomic nervous system, and through this annoyance is induced. Notably, the level of annoyance does not depend on the strength of the tinnitus-related activity within the auditory pathways, but on the strength of the connection between the auditory system and the limbic and autonomic nervous systems, which is reflected in the level of activation of these systems. Consequently, patients who suffer from tinnitus have a stronger connection between the auditory and the limbic and autonomic nervous systems as compared with people who do not suffer but just experience tinnitus.

This postulate is based on the observation that the strength of a reaction to any stimulus, once the stimulus is detected, is not controlled by the strength of the stimulus, but rather by the strength of the conditioning to a given stimulus. For example, it is possible to induce a very strong reaction to a weak stimulus providing that the negative reinforcement is strong. On the other hand, even loud sound can induce a weak reaction if the reinforcement is weak. In the case of tinnitus, the reinforcement is the strength of the reaction of the autonomic nervous system, which is being self-enhanced via the vicious circle, and does not depend on the initial strength of the tinnitus signal. This explains why patients who have soft tinnitus might experience a high level of annoyance, while patients who have relatively loud tinnitus are able to habituate it.

Theory of Discordant Damage (Dysfunction)

Throughout the text, data has been quoted to support the postulate that there is only an indirect relationship between tinnitus and hearing loss. At the same time, the epidemiological data indicate that the prevalence of tinnitus is higher in people with hearing loss. Furthermore it has been documented that exposure to loud sound can create temporary or permanent tinnitus. This issue is important because many patients are afraid that tinnitus indicates oncoming hearing loss, and through this belief tinnitus achieves a negative connotation. As part of the demystification of tinnitus, during the counseling process the lack of relationship between tinnitus and hearing loss should be presented, which can be explained by the discordant damage theory (Jastreboff, 1995; Jastreboff, 1990). This theory proposes that the source of tinnitus is related to the area of the basilar membrane where there is the largest difference between functional inner hair cells and dysfunctional outer hair cells.

This theory provides solutions for several puzzling aspects of tinnitus. First, the largest difference would occur at the bottom of the slope of the audiogram, because this is the area where we should still have relatively functional inner hair cells and maximal damage to the outer hair cells. Clinical observation has confirmed this prediction showing that this is the frequency range where typically the pitch of tinnitus occurs (Jastreboff, 1996). Second, this theory could also explain why about 30 percent of tinnitus patients have normal hearing (Hazell,

1996; Hazell et al., 1985). It is important to recognize that damage to outer hair cells, up to 30 percent, if it is relatively homogenous, might not be detected in the audiogram (Clark et al., 1984). Consequently a limited area of dysfunctional outer hair cells may not be detected on the audiogram. Therefore, even in cases of normal hearing there are still areas of damaged outer hair cells with intact inner hair cells, resulting in unbalanced activity between Type I and Type II fibers. This, in turn, causes unbalanced activity probably at the level of the dorsal cochlear nucleus, which is further enhanced in the auditory pathways and finally perceived as tinnitus. Notably, recordings from single units from the external nucleus of the inferior colliculus in rats with experimentally induced tinnitus indicate the emergence of abnormal, epileptic-like activity which might be related to tinnitus, with an indication of disinhibition, probably mediated by GABA, as a potential mechanism creating this activity (Jastreboff, 1995; Chen and Jastreboff, 1995).

Finally this theory may explain why about 30 percent of totally deaf people do not experience tinnitus (Hazell, 1996; Hazell et al., 1995). If both systems are equally damaged and there is no difference in the activation of the Type I and Type II auditory nerve fibers, then there is no imbalance and tinnitus might occur only as a result of a normal increase of the gain within the auditory pathways, which however can be compensated by the filtering property of the subcortical centers.

Consequently, since hearing loss reflects the combined function of inner and outer hair cells, and since partial damage of outer hair cells can be compensated by the remaining outer hair cells and plastic modifications of the connection in the auditory pathways, it is possible to have tinnitus without hearing loss, while damage to the cochlea predominantly affecting outer hair cells might cause both hearing loss and tinnitus. In this respect the emphasis is put on damage of the outer hair cells system while inner hair cells are preserved, and on contrasting the difference between the damaged outer hair cells and inner hair cells, rather than on a sum of the damage of both systems, which is reflected in hearing loss.

Hypersensitivity of the Auditory Pathways

Tinnitus is a complex phenomenon and its emergence can result from a number of various mechanisms. Indeed, in the same patient several mechanisms may coexist and contribute to various extents to tinnitus. One of those mechanisms is the increase of the gain within the auditory system. This increase can occur both at the level of the cochlea and within the subcortical auditory pathways, and it is typically evoked by decrease of auditory input. Two lines of evidence support the postulate that the auditory system undergoes continuous dynamic changes in sensitivity, and that in the situation of decreased signals from the periphery, the signals within the auditory pathways are enhanced and abnormal sensitivity occurs. The first comes from an experiment performed on humans. Eighty subjects with normal hearing and no tinnitus were put into an anechoic chamber and asked to describe any sensations they had. They experienced a significant increase in their perception of sounds that appeared to be loud, and notably within a few minutes 94 percent of them developed temporary tinnitus (Heller & Bergman, 1953).

Results of electrophysiological investigations of the auditory pathways may provide an explanation of this phenomenon. Single unit recordings revealed a high level of spontaneous activity occurring within the auditory pathways without any sound stimulation. When the sound level is very low, the individual neurons of the auditory pathway become more sensitive (Boettcher & Salvi, 1993), the sensitivity of neuronal networks processing these signals increases as well resulting in increased detection of small signals. Consequently, the subcortical centers, which were previously able to filter out this spontaneous activity will start to pick up small modifications in the spontaneous activity, which would be perceived as tinnitus. This explanation has been further supported by recordings from animals.

In animals with permanent or temporary hearing loss or damage to the cochlea, about a quarter of the neurons in the cochlear nuclei complex and in the inferior colliculi exhibited increased sensitivity to any kind of stimulation (Boettcher & Salvi, 1993), and an abnormal increase in the evoked potential recorded from the auditory pathways was observed (Gerken, 1992; Gerken et al., 1985; Gerken, 1979). Electrophysiological and psychoacoustical evidence strongly supports the postulate that signals are continuously filtered, and when auditory input decreases significantly, or the cochlea is damaged, the subcortical systems are unable to compensate this change and the perception of tinnitus emerges.

It has to be stressed that the perception of tinnitus does not mean the emergence of clinically significant tinnitus. A person can perceive tinnitus, but may not necessarily suffer from it. The clinical problem arises from the activation of other systems in the brain, and the auditory system only provides the first initial signal on which the conditioned response of the limbic and the autonomic nervous systems occurs.

Hypersensitivity to Sound—Hyperacusis and Phonophobia

A prediction arising from the neurophysiological model of tinnitus was that if abnormal enhancement within the auditory system might yield tinnitus, then the presence of tinnitus might be accompanied by this abnormal increase of gain, which on a psychoacoustical level would be reflected as hypersensitivity to sound. On the behavioral level, hypersensitivity to sound results in decreased tolerance to external sound, measured audiometrically as decreased loudness discomfort levels. This phenomenon can result from several mechanisms. The first class of mechanisms encompasses the abnormal functioning of the auditory system, which can involve the peripheral part (most probably dysfunction of the outer hair cells system) and the central part (increased sensitivity of neurons in auditory pathways resulting from sound deprivation, such as hearing loss, or changes in neurotransmitter and neuromodulators). As in this case hypersensitivity is based solely on the auditory system, it is labeled hyperacusis. The second class of mechanisms reflects the abnormal excitation of the limbic and autonomic nervous systems while the auditory system is functioning normally. Since it typically involves fear of sound, it is labeled phonophobia.

According to the author, recruitment, which is typically linked to sound hypersensitivity, is not related at all. Recruitment reflects the inevitable increase of the slope of loudness growth function due to hearing loss. It may coexist with hyperacusis or phonophobia, but both phenomena can emerge without any recruitment. Sometimes recruitment might contribute to sound hypersensitivity but typically it does not, and while patients with hearing loss have recruitment only a portion exhibit sound hypersensitivity.

Note that for TRT, it is irrelevant to large extent whether this hypersensitivity to sound results from the increased peripheral gain, for example in the outer hair cells system, or is more central, or both. The neurophysiological model predicts that in a significant number of cases this abnormal increase of gain should be present and that people who have only hypersensitivity without tinnitus are more likely to experience tinnitus in the future. Thus, hypersensitivity may be considered a pre-tinnitus state (Jastreboff et al., 1998; Jastreboff, 1990).

In the 1980s, when the neurophysiological model was created (Jastreboff, 1990), the above prediction was contrary to the data presented in the literature. It was reported by Vernon that hypersensitivity to sound is uncommon and occurs in 0.1 percent of the population of tinnitus patients (Vernon, 1987). In a recent chapter they increased this number to 0.3 percent (Vernon & Press,

1998). Tyler and Conrad-Armes noted decreased loudness discomfort levels in some tinnitus patients they studied (Tyler & Conrad-Armes, 1983). However, after we systematically measured the loudness discomfort levels in our patients, the results showed that about 40 percent of tinnitus patients have increased sensitivity to sound, as evident by their average LDLs below 100 dB HL and their subjective perception. Considering that clinically significant tinnitus affects approximately 4 to 5 percent of the general population, and considering that 40 percent of the tinnitus patients have hyperacusis (Jastreboff et al., 1996b; Coles, 1996b; Jastreboff et al., 1996b), at least 2 percent of the general population experience hyperacusis to various degrees. This would translate to approximately 5 million people in the United States. Furthermore, in our practice we have a number of patients who exhibit hyperacusis only, which indicates that this estimation is actually too low.

The wide prevalence of hyperacusis and its coexistence with tinnitus has a profound implication. If increased gain in the auditory pathway can result in tinnitus, then hyperacusis without tinnitus can be regarded as potential pre-tinnitus state. As discussed later, the use of sound (sound therapy) is one of two components of TRT. The presence of hyperacusis prevents using sound levels that would be recommended otherwise, as it could yield increased discomfort, result in establishing phonophobia, and failure of the treatment. Accordingly, the presence, extent and subtype of hyperacusis is one of the main criteria in determining the TRT protocol.

Tinnitus Habituation Therapy

The neurophysiological model provides not only solutions to a number of puzzling aspects of tinnitus, but what is more important from the clinical perspective is that it has resulted in a new method for helping tinnitus patients, Tinnitus Habituation Therapy (THT) (Jastreboff, 1998; Jastreboff et al., 1998; Jastreboff, 1990). At the moment there is no method that can be used successfully to attenuate tinnitus source for a significant number of patients without profound side effects. However two features of the brain can be utilized to achieve control over tinnitus—brain plasticity and its ability to habituate a variety of stimuli. One essential feature of the brain is its enormous plasticity. We are able to learn, and that means change the synaptic connections between neurons throughout our life. And while this plasticity is different at different stages of our life, still it is significant throughout all our life. We can use this feature to achieve the habituation of tinnitus; that means, the auditory system and the connection of the auditory system with the limbic and autonomic systems can be retrained. By proper retraining procedures, the tinnitus signals can be blocked, thereby preventing the activation of these systems. Thus, neurophysiology provides us with both a model allowing for better understanding tinnitus and for showing us the direction through which we can achieve control of tinnitus.

If we block the activation of the limbic and the autonomic nervous systems, then even if tinnitus is perceived it will not induce any reaction, and consequently there would be no annoyance (Figure 15-1B). An example of this would be the patient who perceives tinnitus, but the sound holds as much meaning as the sound of a refrigerator. The sound is easily ignored and the patient's attention can be shifted to other tasks. As a result, tinnitus ceases to be an issue for the patient. This corresponds to the classical definition of habituation, as disappearance of a reaction induced by a stimulus, denoted in Figure 15-1B as H_R. As evident from this figure, habituation of reactions occurs when tinnitus-related neuronal activity, present in the auditory pathways, is prevented from reaching the limbic and autonomic nervous systems. The neuronal networks composing the central nervous system have the ability to selectively enhance or suppress a specific pattern of neuronal activity (Pribram, 1987). Consequently, it is possible for such a network to selectively block, filter-out, tinnitus related activity while not changing the processing of other patterns of activity. Specifically, the networks providing the limbic system with auditory information (connections between the medial geniculate body and the amygdala) are involved.

Achieving only habituation of reactions would be sufficient for allowing the patient to return to normal life. However it is possible to gain even more relief. If it is possible to block the tinnitus-related neuronal activity and prevent it from activating the cortical area by filtering out the tinnitus signal at the subconscious level (presumably within subcortical centers), then the subject would not even be aware of the presence of tinnitus, and consequently would also achieve the habituation of the perception of tinnitus (Figure 15-1C—H_p). In this case, neuronal networks belonging totally to the auditory pathways are involved. As a result, in the ideal case tinnitus is not perceived, except when attention is focused on it. While some people achieve this stage of habituation of perception, in practice patients still perceive tinnitus a small percentage of the time, but because the habituation of tinnitus reaction has also occurred, patients are not annoyed by tinnitus even when they are aware of its presence. On the other hand, in about 20 percent of patients undergoing TRT for over two years, habituation of perception reaches such a level, that they experience episodes (on the average 10.5 days) when they are unable to perceive their tinnitus even when they focus on it (Sheldrake et al., 1996). The clinical goal is to achieve both types of habituation by reaching the state where patients are hardly ever aware of the presence of tinnitus (< 10 percent of the time), and when they are aware, it will not bother them.

Notably, the habituation approach can be used in theory for other sensory systems (achieving habituation of phantom limb and phantom pain) and for removing any type of phobias, such as a fear of spiders, heights, claustrophobia, and so forth. Indeed, we are

using successfully a specific protocol for patients with phonophobia.

It is important to realize that Tinnitus Habituation Therapy is not a cure for tinnitus—when perceived the tinnitus will have the same loudness and pitch as before the treatment. However the habituation of tinnitus is achieved by filtering out and blocking tinnitus related neuronal activity from reaching the brain area responsible for consciously perceiving this activity, so it does not cause awareness of tinnitus and does not activate the autonomic nervous system. The habituation of tinnitus can be achieved using various methods. The simplest one consists of two components, counseling and sound therapy, which is known as Tinnitus Retraining Therapy—TRT.

Tinnitus Retraining Therapy

There are other methods of achieving habituation of tinnitus. All include specific counseling, but sound therapy can be omitted or replaced by other methods. A version of this approach is used for patients who have a relatively weak connection between the auditory and limbic system (Category 0), when a less intensive version of sound therapy is used, and in some cases even this is not implemented by patients. It can be replaced by hypnosis and/or self-hypnosis aimed at detaching tinnitus with any negative association and creating associations with pleasant phenomena. Once medications are available that would attenuate tinnitus-related neuronal activity, then habituation could be achieved by combining counseling and medications. Notably, although it is possible to omit sound therapy, it is not advisable even when other methods are available. The use of sound is easy, intuitive, and patients respond well to the idea of using low-level sound. Other methods are recommended as supplementary therapies, which can be used in conjunction with TRT.

Since sound therapy is not necessary to achieve tinnitus habituation, and even when TRT is used, the sound and not any particular device is important: sound generators are not an essential part of TRT. In theory, except cases with severe hyperacusis, TRT can be performed with only counseling and enriched background sound in about 80 percent of cases. This, however, is not practical as it is much easier to conduct sound therapy and better achieve patient compliance with the protocol, with the use of sound generators. In cases of significant hearing loss, amplification of enriched background sound by hearing aids is used successfully. In this situation two goals are achieved: sound needed for TRT is provided, and the patient's hearing problem is helped.

Counseling

The first part of TRT involves retraining counseling; that is, teaching the patient about the mechanisms of tinnitus and how habituation can be achieved. The following main points are discussed: (1) tinnitus/hyperacusis results from compensation by the auditory system of otherwise irrelevant damage or dysfunction within the auditory pathways; (2) tinnitus as a problem arises due to enhanced activation of emotional and autonomic centers in the brain; (3) it is possible to utilize normal functions of the brain to attenuate these abnormal activations and to achieve control over tinnitus by habituating reactions induced by tinnitus and by habituating its perception. On the basis of neuroscience, mechanisms of specific strategies are explained so patients understand why it is important to avoid silence and furthermore increase the level of the background sound, why masking prevents habituation, and why stress can worsen tinnitus. While counseling, the interaction with the patient should be open, frequently treating the patient as a partner. It is necessary to allow sufficient time for answering all questions. It is essential that the patient accepts that the concepts "make sense" and relate to his situation.

The important part of the counseling process is the demystification of tinnitus. The patient is given sufficient information regarding the mechanisms of tinnitus emergence and its affect on life, and through this the negative associations of tinnitus are gradually removed. It is crucial to realize that the habituation of tinnitus can occur only if tinnitus does not have a strong negative association. Once tinnitus becomes neutral, its habituation will occur naturally without the need of any special help. Indeed, depending on the patient population for a center, for 10 to 30 percent of patients all that has to be done to help the patient control his tinnitus is to provide counseling and instruct him to avoid silence and increase the level of auditory background.

Demystifying tinnitus decreases the activation from the cortical area to the limbic and autonomic nervous systems and through this, the activation of the autonomic nervous system is decreased. Consequently, if this activation is smaller, tinnitus will become less important, which in turn will cause the next activation to be even smaller, and so on. In other words, the vicious circle will go in the reverse direction. As the importance of tinnitus is decreased, the reaction induced by tinnitus is also decreased, this in turn decreases the level of annoyance and the amount of attention directed to it.

Although in theory inducing habituation by retraining counseling may be sufficient, adding the additional component of sound therapy is very helpful in the majority of cases. The therapy utilizes a basic property of perception: We do not perceive an absolute value of a stimulus, but rather the difference between the stimulus and the background. A classical example would be the perception of the brightness of a small candle in a dark room compared to its brightness in the full sun. While the physical intensity of the candle light would be exactly the same under both conditions, in the dark the brightness of the light would appear to be very high, while in the sun it would appear weak. Since we cannot eliminate the tinnitus signal, at least at the moment, the sound therapy helps to decrease the difference between the tinnitus signal and the background neuronal activity by increasing this background activity.

Sound Therapy

Introducing sound creates a reversal situation to the one when people were put into an extremely quiet environment which resulted in tinnitus emergence (Heller & Bergman, 1953). The patients are provided with constant, low-level sound. Indeed the statement "avoid silence" is one of the important messages that the patient takes home from the counseling session. Once the tinnitus-related neural activity is decreased, then consequently the strength of neuronal activation going to the limbic system, autonomic nervous system, and to cortical areas is also decreased. This results in decreased tinnitus annoyance, which in turn further decreases awareness of the tinnitus signal. This is another mechanism through which the vicious circle is reversed. The strength of the tinnitus gradually decreases, allowing the brain to habituate to the tinnitus-related neuronal activity in a more efficient way.

Masking

Note, that if we suppress ("mask") the tinnitus signal, so that it is not perceived, then habituation of the tinnitus signal cannot occur by definition. Habituation involves retraining and therefore necessitates the detection of the tinnitus-related neuronal activity. If the tinnitus signal is suppressed and cannot be detected, relearning and consequently habituation cannot occur. Thus, suppression of tinnitus ("masking") is counterproductive to habituation.

Clinical observation fully supports this statement. A group of patients were selected, who for a long period of time, up to fifteen years, were utilizing "masking" of their tinnitus. Although they experienced relief while "masking," as soon as they switched off the masking sound the tinnitus was as intrusive as previously. These patients were switched to a habituation protocol and within one year it was possible to achieve habituation of their tinnitus, while in the previous fifteen years no change was observed (Hazell & Sheldrake, personal communication).

In addition, even "partial masking" is not recommended as the retraining of tinnitus will occur not on the original tinnitus signal, but on a modified tinnitus signal. Even if habituation of this modified tinnitus signal is achieved, when the "partial masking" sound is stopped, the original unchanged tinnitus signal will reappear. Some habituation of the original signal will be observed, however the effectiveness of habituation would be lessened. In Figure 15-2 the effectiveness of habituation is plotted in relationship to the physical intensity of the sound used.

Once sound increases above the threshold of hearing it will cause a gradual decrease in the difference between the tinnitus signal and background neuronal activity, and the effectiveness of the therapy should increase. When we reach the level of "partial masking," however, which occurs when the sound intensity goes beyond the point of mixing with tinnitus and external sound, the effectiveness of habituation would begin to decrease. Finally, when total suppression of tinnitus is reached, the effectiveness of habituation would be zero.

Notably, it is sound that is important and not the particular device that provides the sound. It is possible to use environmental sound by instructing the patient to play the TV, radio, nature tapes, and a variety of other

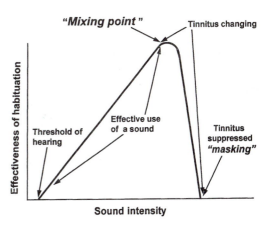

FIGURE 15-2. Dependence of habituation effectiveness on the intensity of the sound used for the sound therapy.

sounds. For patients with hearing loss it is advisable to use environmental sounds enhanced by hearing aids. It is important to recognize that in these cases, the purpose of the hearing aids is to act as an amplifier of the external sounds, and consequently without external sound, they do not offer any benefit for tinnitus. Furthermore, as the hearing aids are used for tinnitus and not for enhancing communication ability, they should be worn all the time. To allow perception of low frequency environmental sounds and bearing in mind that the majority of patients typically have normal low frequency hearing, the fitting of the hearing aids should be as open as possible. The use of in-the-canal hearing aids is strongly discouraged, except when patients have severe hearing loss for frequencies below 500 Hz.

For the majority of tinnitus patients, however, the optimal approach involves the use of broad band noise generators that are worn behind the ear with an open fitting. These devices offer several advantages. First, they provide sound that evokes relatively random neuronal activity that resembles spontaneous activity. In this way we are increasing the spontaneous activity that the brain can easily filter and habituate. Indeed the majority of our patients quickly habituate to the sound generated by the devices, and they are not aware they are wearing them, particularly because low sound levels are used.

The second advantage of the sound generators is that the sound level can be well controlled and the sound is stable, both in frequency and time domains. As such, it is again easy to habituate while achieving a reasonably stable level of increased background neuronal activity. Third, the sound from the generators share with tinnitus the feature of being attached to the head. Consequently, when the patient moves their head the sound from the generators moves also, which further facilitates the habituation of tinnitus. Fourth, it is easier for the patient to comply with the sound protocol because it is much easier for the patient to put the generators on in the morning, set them, and wear them throughout the day

without thinking about them, than it is to maintain enriched sound background, in which case they would need to have a radio, tape recorder, or CD player around all the time, and they would need to keep the sound at a reasonably stable level throughout the day. Therefore, about 70 percent of our patients are fit with binaural sound generators.

If hearing of patients allows, two sound generators are always used. There are several reasons for it. Two sound generators, set at the same subjective loudness, assure symmetrical stimulation of the central auditory pathways. The symmetrical stimulation prevents development of abnormal receptive fields, which could result in impairment of central auditory processing. Additionally, use of only one noise generator can result in a shift of unilateral tinnitus to the opposite ear.

This combination of counseling and sound therapy, known as TRT, can be performed with or without instrumentation, and is just one method of achieving tinnitus habituation. TRT should not be associated with use of sound generators or hearing aids, since *the sound is important and not the specific, technical method of its delivery.* Moreover, use of sound generators without proper counseling will not result in habituation of tinnitus and is not TRT.

Notably, it is possible to achieve habituation and perform THT without using additional external sound, for example by combining counseling and biofeedback, or even utilizing counseling alone, but this approach is not optimal. In all cases it is advisable to tell the patient to at least avoid silence. On the other hand, even TRT patients can be advised to use other therapies that promote the habituation of tinnitus, particularly any kind of approach that would decrease the activation of the autonomic nervous system, stress level, and anxiety. In this respect therapies like biofeedback, hypnosis, and stress management might be helpful. Once we have a medication that could interfere with tinnitus neuronal activity, it would become a useful component of THT and might replace the need for sound generators.

Sleep Problems

In one specific situation the use of sound is particularly advisable; namely, when patients experience tinnitus-related sleeping problems (see Chapter 3). An increased level of anxiety might be responsible for difficulty in falling asleep and for waking up during the night. Normal sleep occurs in approximately 90-minute cycles, during which we go through different stages of sleep, including periods of time when we wake up or sleep is shallow. Under normal conditions we can fall back to sleep, when sleep is shallow (due for example to anxiety), and the patient awakes in a quiet environment, the tinnitus sound will appear to be very loud and intrusive and might prevent them from falling back to sleep. The simple and effective solution is to advise patients to have some sound around them during the night. Then, when they wake up, they will still hear sound and the tinnitus will not be as intrusive. Consequently they would be able to fall back to sleep much easier. For many patients the use of sound during the night is extremely beneficial.

An important parameter of the sound therapy is that the sound level should not induce annoyance or irritate the patient. Therefore, the patient should be instructed to keep the sound level lower than this irritating level. Otherwise patients with tinnitus, but without hyperacusis, are instructed to set the level of the sound generators or environmental sounds close to, but not above, the mixing point. For patients with hyperacusis the use of low-level sound, close to threshold, can be an effective method for desensitizing the auditory system, and indeed many of our patients have benefited from this therapy.

Categories of the Patients

Based on the neurophysiological model it is possible to place the patient into one of five general categories, with substantial differences in the treatment for each category (Table 15-1) (Jastreboff, 1998). Each category can be further divided into several subcategories, but for simplicity only the main division is presented here. .There are four characteristic features that are used for this

Table 15-1. Categories of patients

Category	Hyperacusis	Prolonged sound-induced exacerbation	Subjective hearing loss	Impact on life	Treatment (in addition to counseling and enrichment of background sound)
0	—	—	—	low	common only
1	—	—	—	high	sound generators set at mixing point
2	—	—	present	high	hearing aid with stress on enrichment of the auditory background
3	present	—	not relevant	high	sound generators set above threshold of hearing
4	present	present	not relevant	high	sound generators set at the threshold; very slow increase of sound level

Abbreviations: Hyperacusis—significant sensitivity to environmental sounds typically associated with LDLs below 100 dB HL; Prolonged sound-induced exacerbation of tinnitus/hyperacusis when the effects persists to the following day; Subjective hearing loss—perceived subjectively by a patient as having a significant impact on patient's life; Impact on life—the extent of impact of tinnitus on patient's life; Treatment for each category involves counseling and the use of enriched auditory background.

classification. One is the impact of tinnitus on the patient's life. This reflects the strength of the connection between the auditory system and the limbic and autonomic nervous systems. The second feature is the subjective perception of hearing loss by the patient. The important point is the subjectivity of this perception. If a patient shows a small hearing loss on the audiogram, but whose hearing is of crucial importance (for example, he may have a job in which he has to understand every single word, or he may be a professional musician and any distortion affects his performance), then a hearing aid might be recommended to achieve both help for tinnitus and to provide the patient with better hearing. On the other hand, someone who has tinnitus and moderate to significant hearing loss on audiogram, but the hearing loss does not present a problem, would be a better candidate for sound generators rather than hearing aids. The third component is the presence or absence of hyperacusis. If hyperacusis is present with the threshold of significant hyperacusis defined as the average LDL of 100 dB HL, then the protocol will involve desensitization first, and the next step will depend on whether hearing loss is present and the extent of tinnitus. It is necessary to assess the relative contribution of hyperacusis and phonophobia, since LDLs are reflecting the sum of both phenomena.

The fourth characteristic is the presence of prolonged worsening of hyperacusis and/or tinnitus after exposure to moderate or loud sound. This "kindling" or "winding up" effect is of particular significance and it is a significant feature of patients with hyperacusis resulting from disease. Forty-eight percent of the patients with Lyme disease have hyperacusis, which exhibits kindling as a result of exposure to moderate or even very low sound levels (Fallon et al., 1992). A number of patients without Lyme disease can also exhibit a similar effect.

A number of patients report worsening of their tinnitus or hyperacusis as a result of exposure to sound. In most cases this worsening lasts only a few minutes or hours.

In some cases it can last for days or weeks. To sort out the patients who exhibit this effect a criterium is used that is labeled the "morning after" effect. That is, if the patient experiences worsening of their tinnitus and/or hyperacusis the next morning after sound exposure from the previous day, then the patient is classified as having prolonged impact of noise exposure. The resulting categories from this classification are presented in Table 15-1.

Category 0 consists of patients who do not have hyperacusis, do not have significant hearing loss, and whose tinnitus has little impact on their life. For these patients, the directive counseling session, including the advice to avoid silence and to enrich their sound environment, is usually sufficient and there is no need for any instrumentation. Patients with recent onset of tinnitus, no more than a couple months, and who have not received any "negative counseling" (Jastreboff & Hazell, 1993) belongs to this category as well. Negative counseling is referred to when patients are told that nothing can be done, they will have to learn to live with it, have a brain scan to exclude brain tumor, and so on. Depending on the population of patients at a given center this group may pertain to between 10 percent and 30 percent of the patient population.

Category 1 consists of patients who have significant tinnitus, but no hyperacusis and no subjective hearing loss. For these patients the most effective approach is the use of sound generators set at the level close to the "mixing point." The majority of patients belong to this category, and they exhibit a high level of success in controlling their tinnitus.

Category 2 consists of patients like Category 1, but who have significant subjective hearing loss. For these patients to achieve improvement both in tinnitus and hearing, we recommend hearing aids, typically programmable. We instruct the patient to wear them all the time while enriching their sound environment. It is stressed to the patient that the sound is important for the treatment and not the hearing aids. The main purpose of the hearing aids is to amplify and improve the level of sound, and providing better communication is secondary.

Category 3 consists of patients with significant hyperacusis, which is not enhanced for a prolonged period of time as a result of sound exposure. Tinnitus may, or may not, be present. Sound generators are necessary to help desensitize the hyperacusis. The desensitization procedure begins with the sound level set close to, but clearly above, the threshold of hearing. This level is increased during the treatment to the level appropriate to their tinnitus (if present). Indeed, these patients tend to recover faster than patients with tinnitus only.

Category 4 consists of patients who have tinnitus and/or hyperacusis and exhibit prolonged worsening of their symptoms as a result of sound exposure. This is the most difficult category to treat and the success rate is lower, below 50 percent. In this case we set the sound generators at the threshold. For cases when there is general hypersensitivity of perception, the patients are advised to wear the devices for a week without turning them on to desensitize the perception of the touch of the devices. These patients require continuous monitoring. During the progress of the treatment, the sound level is increased very slowly.

Effectiveness of TRT

At the moment we have seen over 1,000 patients, who typically present serious tinnitus and hyperacusis. Our patient population tends to be more severe compared to the average population of tinnitus patients going to otolaryngology clinics as most of our patients have already seen several otolaryngologists; some have Lyme disease, Ménière's disease, or extreme hyperacusis; and occasionally we have suicidal cases. We do not use any preselection criteria for patients. Anyone who wants to be seen is accepted and treated at our clinic. This is possible because habituation occurs at a higher level within the brain than the potential source of tinnitus and affects the interaction of the auditory system with other

systems in the brain. Consequently, the source of tinnitus is irrelevant.

The effectiveness of the treatment has been assessed by evaluating patients' status before, during and at the completion of the treatment using prepared questionnaires. The questionnaires were designed to assess three main aspects: impact on life, annoyance level, and awareness of tinnitus. The dominant feature of the impact of tinnitus on the patient's life was evaluated by using a scale from 0 to 10 during the first visit and all subsequent follow up visits or telephone interviews. Furthermore patients were asked to list all the activities that were affected by tinnitus and/or hyperacusis during each visit. In addition they were asked to respond to a specific list of activities and report whether these activities were affected by their tinnitus and hyperacusis. Since this is considered as the most important criterium for patients to qualify as showing improvement, it was necessary for patients to show at least a 20 percent change on the scale of impact on life, and at the same time show at least one activity which was previously affected by tinnitus and hyperacusis to be performed normally, or improvement in all activities previously affected, to be classified as showing improvement in impact of tinnitus on their life.

A second set of questions were aimed at assessing the habituation of the reaction of tinnitus, and patients were asked to rate the annoyance induced by tinnitus on a scale from 0 to 10. The third set of questions were aimed at assessing the habituation of the perception. The patients were asked on a scale of 0 to 100 to judge the percentage of time when they were aware of their tinnitus during the last couple of weeks.

To qualify the patient as showing significant improvement it is necessary that more than one of these categories show improvement, in addition to at least a 20 percent improvement in the impact of life. If the patient showed improvement in only one dimension, but did not exhibit improvement in others, or if improvement was smaller than the required 20 percent, the patient was qualified as showing nonsignificant improvement and put into the category of no improvement. All the questions presented to patients included the possibility of tinnitus getting worse.

Out of over 1,000 patients, 194 random cases were evaluated on the basis of the initial interview, follow-up visits, or telephone interviews, if patients were not contacting the center (Jastreboff et al., 1996a). These patients underwent treatment with the approach decided exclusively by the patient category. All patients received initial counseling, included advice about avoiding silence, and need for enrichment of background sound. Seventy-nine percent of patients received behind-the-ear sound generators (Viennatone Am/Ti), 9 percent were fitted with various kinds of hearing aids according to their need, with appropriate counseling. The remaining 11 percent received an initial session of counseling but decided not to continue with the protocol.

The group with sound generators and hearing aids had a similar proportion of patients showing significant improvement, 81.8 percent and 83.3 percent respectively, with the average of 82.0 percent. Fourteen point five percent reported no change or the improvement was not sufficient according to our criteria. Three point five percent reported worsening of their problem. In the group which received only one session of counseling, only 22.7 percent of patients showed significant improvement, with 59.1 percent without significant change and 18.2 percent reporting worsening of their problems. Comparison of the effectiveness of the full treatment versus the single counseling session was statistically significant ($p < 0.001$; $X^2 = 37.04$, df = 2 using better, the same, and worse groups).

The values of measures used in assessing the treatment outcome, were statistically indistinguishable at the beginning of the treatment between the "Better" and "Same" categories of patients (Effect on life 6.567 ± 0.667 vs. 6.881 ± 0.300; Awareness 89.556 ± 4.745 vs. 76.013 ± 3.147; Annoyance 7.733 ± 0.605 vs. 6.805 ± 0.320, for "Same" and "Better" groups). Assessment of the changes was performed by calculating for each variable, the difference (after—before), which was expressed as a percentage of the initial value. Those values were averaged separately for improving and not improving groups. Since results obtained with the use of sound generators and hearing aids were practically identical, these data were combined. In this group patients classified as showing significant improvement had an average decrease of effect on life by 54.90 percent, awareness by 42.60 percent, and annoyance by 57.71 percent. The changes were clearly less in groups classified as "Same" (10.72 percent of effect on life, 12.20 percent awareness, and 11.47 percent annoyance). A shift in the direction of improvement for all the measures observed in the "Same" group reflect the fact that patients who actually showed some improvement (but not significant according to our criteria) were categorized as showing no improvement. Evaluation of tinnitus patients who did not undergo treatment showed that these parameters tend to be stable or have a tendency to worsen (Sheldrake et al., 1996). The proportion of patients showing at least some improvement was 88 percent.

Several observations argue against the possibility of a placebo effect. All the interviews and evaluations were performed between six months and three years after beginning treatment, while the placebo effect would appear only for a few months. Nearly all patients, and particularly all cases showing improvement, were checked and interviewed more than once. Furthermore, we followed a number of patients for a period up to six years, and in this population of patients we have not observed a relapse back to their previous level of tinnitus. We are certain that we will observe such a relapse, but it seems that the ratio is so low that it is seen only in patients who later developed new significant medical problems (such as cancer).

CONCLUSION

In conclusion, it seems that the neurophysiological model of tinnitus offers both an explanation to some puzzles regarding the mechanisms of tinnitus and offers an acceptable method to achieve control of tinnitus, Tinnitus Habituation Therapy. Furthermore, Tinnitus Retraining Therapy, the simplest form of Tinnitus Habituation Therapy, seems to be effective for about 80 percent of the general tinnitus population and while it requires about eighteen months to achieve a stable level of control of tinnitus, positive results are typically observed within the first six months. Finally, given that Tinnitus Habituation Therapy and Tinnitus Retraining Therapy are harmless and can not in any way hurt the patient, it is proposed that these are effective and safe methods for treating tinnitus patients.

REFERENCES

Boettcher, F. A., & Salvi, R. J. (1993). Functional changes in the ventral cochlear nucleus following acute acoustic overstimulation. *Journal of the Acoustical Society of America, 94,* 2123–2134.

Brooks, C. M. (1987). Autonomic Nervous System, nature and functional role. In G. Adelman (Ed.), *Encyclopedia of neuroscience* (pp. 96–98). Boston: Birkhauser.

Chen, G. D., & Jastreboff, P. J. (1995). Salicylate-induced abnormal activity in the inferior colliculus of rats. *Hearing Research, 82,* 158–178.

Clark, W. W., Kim, D. O., Zurek, P. M., & Bohne, B. A. (1984). Spontaneous otoacoustic emissions in chinchilla ear canals: Correlation with histopathology and suppression by external tones. *Hearing Research, 16,* 299–314.

Coles, R. R. A. (1996). Epidemiology, aetiology and classification. In J. A. Vernon & G. Reich (Eds.), *Proceedings of the Fifth International Tinnitus Seminar, 1995* (pp. 25–30). Portland, OR: American Tinnitus Association.

Davis, A. (1996). The aetiology of tinnitus: Risk factors for tinnitus in the UK population—A possible role for conductive pathologies? In J. A. Vernon & G. Reich (Eds.), *Proceedings of the Fifth International Tinnitus Seminar, 1995* (pp. 38–45). Portland, OR: American Tinnitus Association.

Estes, W. K., & Skinner, B. F. (1941). Some quantitative properties of anxiety. *Journal of Experimental Psychology, 29,* 390–400.

Fallon, B. A., Nields, J. A., Burrascano, J. J., Liegner, K., DelBene, D., & Liebowitz, M. R. (1992). The neuropsychiatric manifestation of Lyme borreliosis. *Psychiatric Quarterly 63,* 95–117.

Gerken, G. M. (1979). Central denervation hypersensitivity in the auditory system of the cat. *Journal of the Acoustical Society of America, 66,* 721–727.

Gerken, G. M. (1992). Central auditory temporal processing: Alterations produced by factors involving the cochlea. In A. Dancer, D. Henderson, R. Salvi, & R. Hamernik (Eds.), *Effect of noise on the auditory system* (pp. 146–155). Philadelphia: Mosby.

Gerken, G. M., Saunders, S. S., Simhadri-Sumithra, R., & Bhat, K. H. V. (1985). Behavioral thresholds for electrical stimulation applied to auditory brain stem nuclei in cats are altered by injurious and noninjurious sound. *Hearing Research, 20,* 221–231.

Hazell, J. W., Wood, S. M., Cooper, H. R., Stephens, S. D., Corcoran, A. L., Coles, R. R., Baskill, J. L., & Sheldrake, J. B. (1985). A clinical study of tinnitus maskers. *British Journal of Audiology, 19,* 65–146.

Hazell, J. W. P. (1996). Support for a neurophysiological model of tinnitus. In J. A. Vernon & G. Reich (Eds.), *Proceedings of the Fifth International Tinnitus Seminar, 1995* (pp. 51–57). Portland, OR: American Tinnitus Association.

Hazell, J. W. P., McKinney, C. J., & Aleksey, W. (1995a). Mechanisms of tinnitus in profound deafness. *Proceedings of the Fifth International Conference on Cochlear Implants,* Melbourne, Australia, October 24–28th, 1995 (In Press).

Hazell, J. W. P., McKinney, C. J., & Aleksy, W. (1995b). Mechanisms of tinnitus in profound deafness. *Annals of Otolology, Rhinology, and Laryngology, 166*(Suppl.) 418–420.

Heller, M. F., & Bergman, M. (1953). Tinnitus in normally hearing persons. *Annals of Otology, 62,* 73–93.

Jastreboff, P. J. (1990). Phantom auditory perception (tinnitus): Mechanisms of generation and perception. *Neuroscience Research, 8,* 221–254.

Jastreboff, P. J. (1995). Tinnitus as a phantom perception: Theories and clinical implications. In J. Vernon & A. R. Moller (Eds.), *Mechanisms of Tinnitus* (pp. 73–94). Boston, London: Allyn & Bacon.

Jastreboff, P. J. (1996). Usefulness of the psychoacoustical characterization of tinnitus. In J. A. Vernon & G. Reich (Eds.), *Proceedings of the Fifth International Tinnitus Seminar, 1995* (pp. 158–166). Portland, OR: American Tinnitus Association.

Jastreboff, P. J. (1998). Tinnitus; the method of. In G. A. Gates (Ed.), *Current Therapy in Otolaryngology Head and Neck Surgery* (pp. 90–95). St. Louis, Baltimore, Boston: Mosby.

Jastreboff, P. J., Brennan, J. F., Coleman, J. K., & Sasaki, C. T. (1988). Phantom auditory sensation in rats: An animal model for tinnitus. *Behavioral Neuroscience, 102,* 811–822.

Jastreboff, P. J., Hazell, J. W. P., & Graham, R. L. (1994). Neurophysiological model of tinnitus: Dependence of the minimal masking level on treatment outcome. *Hearing Research 80,* 216–232.

Jastreboff, P. J., Gray, W. C., & Gold, S. L. (1996a). Neurophysiological approach to tinnitus patients. *American Journal of Otology, 17,* 236–240.

Jastreboff, P. J., Gray, W. C., & Mattox, D. E. (1998). Tinnitus and Hyperacusis. In C. W. Cummings, J. M. Fredrickson, L. A. Harker, C. J. Krause, M. A. Richardson, & D. E. Schuller (Eds.), *Otolaryngology head & neck surgery* (pp. 3198–3222). St. Louis, Baltimore, Boston: Mosby.

Jastreboff, P. J., & Hazell, J. W. P. (1993). A neurophysiological approach to tinnitus: Clinical implications. *British Journal of Audiology, 27,* 1–11.

Jastreboff, P. J., Jastreboff, M. M., & Sheldrake, J. B. (1996b). Utilization of Loudness Discomfort Levels in the treatment of hyperacusis, tinnitus, and hearing loss. *Association for Research in Otolaryngology, 19,* 44.

Kiang, N. Y. S., Moxon, E. C., & Levine, R. A. (1970). Auditory-nerve activity in cats with normal and abnormal cochleas. In G. E. W. Wolstenholme & J. Knight (Eds.), *CIBA Foundation Symposium on Sensorineural Hearing Loss* (pp. 241–273), London: Churchill.

Kuk, F. K., Tyler, R. S., Russell, D., & Jordan, H. (1990). The psychometric properties of a tinnitus handicap questionnaire. *Ear Hearing, 11,* 434–445.

McFadden, D. (1982). Tinnitus: Facts, theories, and treatments. *National Academy Press,* Washington, DC.

Moller, A. R. (1984). Pathophysiology of tinnitus. *Annals of Otology, Rhinology, and Laryngology, 93,* 39–44.

Moller, M. B., Moller, A. R., Jannetta, P .J., & Jho, H. D. (1993). Vascular decompression surgery for severe tinnitus: Selection criteria and results. *Laryngoscope, 103,* 421–427.

Newman, C. W., Wharton, J. A., & Jacobson, G. P. (1995). Retest stability of the tinnitus handicap questionnaire. *Annals of Otology, Rhinology, and Laryngology, 104,* 718–723.

Pribram, K. H. (1987). Holography and brain function. In G. Adelman (Ed.), *Encyclopedia of neuroscience* (pp. 499–500). Boston: Birkhauser.

Sheldrake, J. B., Jastreboff, P. J., & Hazell, J. W. P. (1996). Perspectives for total elimination of tinnitus perception. In J. A. Vernon & G. Reich (Eds.), *Proceedings of the Fifth International Tinnitus Seminar, 1995* (pp. 531–536). Portland, OR: American Tinnitus Association.

Stouffer, J. L., & Tyler, R. S. (1990). Characterization of tinnitus by tinnitus patients. *Journal of Speech and Hearing Disorders, 55,* 439–453.

Stouffer, J. L., Tyler, R. S., Kileny, P. R., & Dalzell, L. E. (1991). Tinnitus as a function of duration and etiology: Counselling implications. *American Journal of Otology, 12,* 188–194.

Swanson, L. W. (1987). Limbic system. In G. Adelman (Ed.), *Encyclopedia of neuroscience* (pp. 589–591). Boston: Birkhauser.

Tyler, R. S., & Conrad-Armes, D. (1983). The determination of tinnitus loudness considering the effects of recruitment. *Journal of Speech and Hearing Research, 26,* 59–72.

Vernon, J., & Press, L. (1998). Treatment for hyperacusis. In J. A. Vernon (Ed.), *Tinnitus treatment and relief* (pp. 223–227). Boston: Allyn and Bacon.

Vernon, J. A. (1987). Pathophysiology of tinnitus: A special case—hyperacusis and a proposed treatment. *American Journal of Otology, 8,* 201–202.

Zenner, H. P., & Ernst, A. (1993). Cochlear-motor, transduction and signal-transfer tinnitus: Models for three types of cochlear tinnitus. *Eur. Arch. Otorhinolaryngol. 249,* 447–454.

CHAPTER 16

Electrical Stimulation for Tinnitus Suppression

René Dauman

INTRODUCTION

As all senses, hearing is based on the cortical perception of *biological electricity*. In the cochlea acoustical vibrations are converted into action potentials. Although the precise underlying process in tinnitus is yet unknown (see Chapter 4), one can assume that tinnitus perception is related with the brain processing of an abnormal biological electrical activity. The proposal to utilize *artificial electricity* in the attempt to relieve tinnitus sufferers appears thus logical from a physiological point of view.

The Two Forms of External Electricity

To appreciate the electrical potentials in the auditory system and the stimuli used to reduce tinnitus, it is important to distinguish between *direct current* (DC) and *alternating current* (AC). DC stimulation is known to damage neighboring tissues. For instance in long bones, low levels of DC current induce new bone formation, which has been attributed to the irritant nature of electro-chemical products released from the electrode during the stimulation (Yasuda, 1974).

Some Characteristics of Biological Electricity

DC Potentials in the Cochlea

Three categories of DC potentials are produced in the cochlea. The *receptor potential* which is a negative voltage (–65 mV) recorded between the inside of a viable outer or inner hair cell and the extracellular fluid (Russell & Sellick, 1978). The *endocochlear* or *endolymphatic potential* is a resting potential measured between the endolymph and perilymph. This positive (+80 mV) potential is due to an active mechanism inside the stria vascularis, maintaining a high concentration of potassium and a low concentration of sodium within the scala media against their gradients of concentration. Those two potentials of opposite polarity, endolymphatic potential and intracellular receptor potential, result in a large gradient across the apical surface of the hair cells, which plays an important role in the transduction process (Davis, 1965). The third DC potential is the *summating potential*, which is recorded between electrodes placed on each side of the organ of Corti. It is a stimulus-related voltage that closely follows the stimulus waveform envelope. In contrast with the first two DC potentials, the summating potential can be recorded in humans using electrocochleography and tone bursts of various frequencies as stimuli (Dauman, Aran, & Portmann, 1986).

AC Potentials in the Cochlea

Two types of AC potentials are produced within the cochlea. The *cochlear microphonic* is recorded between two electrodes located on both side of the organ of Corti, similar to the summating potential. It is a stimulus-related potential and reflects the alternating current generated by the hair cells. The second AC voltage is the *action potential*, measured between a microelectrode placed in an auditory nerve fiber and an extracellular electrode. Unlike the summating potential and the cochlear microphonic, the action potential is a postsynaptic response since it arises from the auditory nerve fibers. Action potential reflects the excitation of the afferent neurons by the neurotransmitter released by the inner hair cells. Due to its postsynaptic origin, action potential is a transient, electrical event. It is the major component of the electrocochleographic response obtained in humans or animals. In experimental measurements, two types of action potentials are recorded from individual neurons, spontaneous and sound-induced, which differ mainly by the spike rate and synchronization, both enhanced by sound.

Brain Electrical Potentials

Brain electrical evoked potentials can be recorded differentially between two scalp electrodes, for example one at the vertex and the other at the ipsilateral mastoid. To be detected far from their sources (Sohmer & Feinmesser, 1967) and distinguished from electrical background noise, they must undergo synchronous averaging.

Within the 8 ms following a brief stimuli (Jewett, Romano, & Williston, 1970) there are a series of five waves, separated by approximately 1 ms, which are attributed to the activation of the auditory nerve, the cochlear nucleus, and the lateral lemniscus, successively. Therefore, they are referred as *brain stem electrical potentials*. According to three-dimensional measurements (Grandori, 1986), these potentials are essentially due to changes in the orientation of neural currents within the mentioned nuclei of the brain stem.

Other potentials include *middle latency responses* and *event-related potentials*, that utilize the ability to discriminate between frequent and rare stimuli (Picton, 1995).

FIRST ATTEMPTS TO ALLEVIATE TINNITUS WITH FLOW OF ELECTRIC CHARGES

Only one year after the discovery of electricity by Volta, a German physician named Grappengeiser (cited by Feldmann, 1984) connected deaf patients with tinnitus to a DC battery. He found that, in order to suppress tinnitus, current had to flow with the positive terminal (electrode delivering the current) close to the ear. If the current was reversed, the patients reported hearing a rushing sound and, occasionally, an increase in their tinnitus. Grappengeiser also noted that changes in tinnitus happened only while the electric current was turned on. In 1855, Duchenne de Boulogne used Faraday's AC induction coil to deliver current to the ear through an electrode immersed in water in the external ear canal. Eight of the ten patients treated were said to have been cured of their tinnitus, although little information is available. Interestingly, some of the characteristics of electrical tinnitus suppression described in the nineteenth century were replicated later in controlled experiments.

UNEXPECTED TINNITUS SUPPRESSION WITH ELECTRICITY USED FOR OTHER PURPOSES

In 1960 Hatton, Erulkar, and Rosenberg were exploring the physiology of the vestibular system using electrical stimulation. They were surprised that almost half of their deaf patients (fifteen out of thirty-three) reported a reduction in their tinnitus during stimulation. They found that *positive* (anodal) *pulses of DC* delivered on the side of tinnitus, near the cheek, were more effective than other locations or negative DC. This was particularly true when the patients had severe hearing loss. They also noticed that tinnitus was suppressed only during current flow, and that tinnitus could be entirely suppressed when the current was presented just above the patient's ability to detect it. In spite of these positive findings, Hatton et al. (1960) concluded that electrical tinnitus therapy was not viable because of the damaging effects of DC on tissues and because of the need to stimulate the patients constantly.

The interest in electrical tinnitus suppression reappeared in the late 1970s, with the first attempts to restore *hearing* in the *profoundly deaf*. These studies, which will be reviewed in next sections, were carried out either with extra-cochlear current, using a stimulating electrode located at the promontory or in the round window niche, or with intra-cochlear current. The effects on tinnitus were rather unexpected and confered additional interest to the electrical stimulation of the cochlea in hearing-impaired subjects.

TINNITUS SUPPRESSION ACCORDING TO THE SITE OF ELECTRICAL STIMULATION

General Comments

A great variety of routes have been investigated in the utilization of electricity for achieving tinnitus relief. Since the underlying process in tinnitus is yet unknown, it is not surprising that the mechanism by which electrical stimulation might influence tinnitus is still unclear. This lack of knowledge did not hamper the continuation of using electrical stimulation in tinnitus sufferers. Consistent improvements in the delivery of current to the auditory nerve occurred with the increasing use of cochlear implants in hearing-impaired subjects. The closer to the auditory system is the source of electrical current, the easier it is to analyze how electricity might influence tinnitus (Coles, 1996). Therefore, the external sites of stimulation will be discussed first, even though this does not respect the chronology of the reported studies.

Many parameters are important in the study of electrical suppression of tinnitus, including the characteristics of electricity used, the types of subjects investigated, and the experimenters' definition of a successful outcome. For instance, some studies assessed profoundly or severely hearing-impaired subjects, whereas others used patients with moderate hearing impairment. Experiments also differed in how much, and for how long, loudness change in tinnitus was required to be considered successful. In addition, whether tinnitus reduction continued after the current was turned off, and whether the electrical stimulus could be heard by patients differed from one study to another.

Another difficulty results from the contribution of the placebo effect. Behind the simplicity and banality of the term "placebo effect," a multifactorial phenomenon is hidden. Placebo effect depends upon the treated individual, but is also influenced by the clinician who is in charge of the patient, and the interaction between the two. Furthermore, with regards to the evaluation of placebo effect on tinnitus, a supplementary difficulty is caused by the use of a device, whether it is a hearing aid, a noise generator, or a system delivering electrical current. In drug therapy for tinnitus, it is relatively easy to eliminate, or to take into consideration, the placebo effect by using a double-blind procedure (for example, Dauman,

Frachet, & Tyler, 1996; Murai, Tyler, Harker, & Stouffer, 1992). On the contrary, with a device or a system involving auditory perception to be effective, the distinction between placebo effect and a true therapeutic effect is harder to establish (Dauman, 1997).

Extracochlear Stimulation with Transcutaneous Electrodes

Transcutaneous stimulation was initially investigated to avoid the constraints of transtympanic or round window electrode. Chouard, Meyer, and Maridat (1981) found that 30 of 64 patients (47 percent) experienced tinnitus relief after sessions of 20 minutes using various currents at different stimulus locations (especially tragus and behind the earlobe). Some patients reported relief for days and even weeks after stimulation. As had been noted by other investigators, Chouard et al. found that positive (anodal) DC current produced the geatest benefit. However, in contrast with a study utilizing transtympanic technique (Cazals, Negrevergne, & Aran, 1978), Chouard et al. reported that the chances for a positive outcome were smaller with high frequency hearing loss.

Morgon et al. (1984) investigated the efficiency of electrical stimulation combined with low frequency (144 Hz) acoustical stimuli. The addition of an acoustic stimulation was attempted to improve the efficiency of electrical stimulation, but this choice was purely empirical. Using a commercial device called Tinnitop, patients underwent six sessions of 45 minutes, one every ten days, using pulsed electrical AC (sine wave) in combination with the low-frequency sound. Unlike previous studies, the criterion for success was a sustained reduction in tinnitus loudness for a period of one week. Twenty-seven of the fifty patients (54 percent) reported reductions in their tinnitus loudness after one or more sessions. In spite of initial success, the investigators published no further work on this device, as tinnitus relief rapidly showed to be inconsistent and highly dependent upon

experimental conditions (Morgon, 1944, personal communication). See Table 16-1.

Other studies explored electrical stimulation combined with drug therapy. Local lidocaine in combination with low-level DC in the ear canal (iontophoresis), has been advocated to anesthetize the eardrum. In 1985, Brusis and Loennecken used iontophoresis to build up an electric field, enabling lidocaine to penetrate through the tympanic membrane. Fifty patients received this therapy on a daily basis, up to ten consecutive treatments. Tinnitus was reduced completely or partially in thirty-one patients (62 percent) after repeated application to one or both ears. Ten patients (20 percent) experienced complete suppression, in some of these subjects tinnitus did not return and in others it returned at a lower level than before the treatment. In contrast to intravenous application, lidocaine did not induce side effects when applied by iontophoresis. However, it is unclear whether the reduction in tinnitus loudness was due to lidocaine, DC current, or the combination of the two, and also why intratympanic lidocaine should affect the cochlea.

Shulman (1985) reported on the Audimax Theraband, which was a wearable device that delivered undetectable, low-level AC between each mastoid. Electrodes were maintained with a headband. The signal was amplitude modulated to penetrate the skin and swept from low (200 Hz) to high frequency (20,000 Hz). Patients began wearing the device for 1 hour on the first day and progressively increased their use to 5 hours per day. The device was worn at home and tinnitus loudness was reported in a daily journal. Shulman studied three groups of patients and found that seven of the first thirteen patients (54 percent) experienced a tinnitus decrease, and that one patient (8 percent) got worse. A second group of eight patients was tested and none of them experienced any tinnitus relief. This was attributed to a hardware problem and a third group of twelve patients was studied. Six of these patients had been included in one of the two previous studies and there was no

Table 16-1. Extracochlear stimulation: Transcutaneous electrodes

Authors	Stimulation site	Patient #	Stimulus	Definition of success	Results
Grappengeiser (1981)	close to ear	10 deaf	DC+	suppression	temporary
Duchenne (1855)	EAC[1] (water)	10	AC	"cure"	8
Hatton et al. (1960)	near cheeks	33 deaf	pulsed DC+	reduction	15/temporary
Chouard et al. (1981)	tragus, BTE[2]	64 (HL[3])	DC+	relief	30/temporary
Morgon et al. (1984)	Tinnitop	50	AC & LFS[4]	week red.[5]	27/temporary
Brusis & Loennecken (1985)	EAC iontoph.	50	Lidoc. + DC	partial relief	31
Shulman (1985)	Theraband	13/8/12	modul.AC[6]	daily j.[7]	7/0/8
Thedinger et al. (1987)	Theraband	30	single blind	improvement	5 (on/off)[8]
Dobie et al. (1986)	Theraband	20	double blind	relief	5 (on/off)[9]
Vernon (1987)	Theraband	16	single blind	relief	0
Cazals et al. (1986)	Theraband	21	open trial	relief	0
Engelberg & Bauer (1985)	around ear	10	LF pulses[10]	relief or fr.[11]	6
Engelberg & Bauer (1985)	around ear	20	single blind	relief or fr.[11]	9/1[12]
Vernon & Fenwick (1985)	around ear	23	AC	40% reduction	5/temporary

[1] External Ear Canal (EAC)
[2] Behind the Ear (BTE) lobe
[3] various degrees of Hearing Loss (HL)
[4] Low Frequency Sound (LFS)
[5] one week reduction
[6] amplitude modulated AC

[7] decrease on daily journal
[8] device on (#2) or off (#3)
[9] device on (#2) or off (#3)
[10] Low-Frequency pulses (LF)
[11] Loudness reduction or decrease in tinnitus frequency
[12] improvement in treated (#9) and placebo (#1) groups

control group. Eight of the twelve patients (67 percent) experienced tinnitus relief with three subjects showing complete suppression and residual inhibition.

Because patients are unable to detect the Theraband stimulus, subsequent researchers used controlled experiments to determine the true effectiveness of the device. The Theraband was worn at times turned on and at times turned off. Patients were asked to rate the loudness of their tinnitus on a daily basis without knowing whether they were receiving electrical stimulation. Thedinger, Karlsen, and Schack (1987) studied thirty patients receiving actual or placebo stimulation over a period of two weeks in a single-blind crossover fashion. Five patients experienced improvement. Two patients improved with the device turned on and three improved with the device turned off. Two other controlled studies were performed with the Theraband, one by Dobie, Hoberg, and Reeves (1986) and one by Vernon (1987). Both found limited benefit.

Dobie et al. studied twenty patients: two experienced benefit with the device turned on and three reported benefit with the device turned off. Vernon reported that none of his sixteen patients experienced any tinnitus relief with the device. Similarly disappointing results were found by Cazals, Bourdin, Negrevergne, and Dauman (1986). In twenty-one subjects with the Theraband device, no relief was observed in any subject. The general trend from these reports on the Theraband device is that they contrasted greatly with the optimism of the first investigator (Shulman, 1985).

More traditional forms of electrical stimulation were assessed in the 1980s and 1990s. The outcomes of these studies were mixed. Engelberg and Bauer (1985) stimulated ten patients with a handheld probe at thirteen specific locations on the auricle of the ear with tinnitus. The sites were selected for their increased electrical conductivity as measured by low electrical resistance. The stimulus was a low-intensity, low-frequency variable square wave. Each location was stimulated for up to 2 minutes, and patients needed treatments up to three times per week for up to seventeen sessions. Although the investigators did not precisely define what they considered to be an improvement in tinnitus, they reported that six of the ten subjects (60 percent) reported "improvements" in their tinnitus lasting from a few hours to several months. In some cases, patients reported a decrease in tinnitus frequency and in some cases the effect was a reduction in tinnitus loudness. In a second more-controlled part of their study, Engelberg and Bauer (1985) investigated twenty subjects divided into two groups with one group receiving treatment and the other group receiving a placebo in a single-blind protocol. Nine of the ten subjects (90 percent) receiving treatment reported improvements in their tinnitus, while only one of the subjects in the placebo group experienced an improvement. This remarkably high success rate may relate to the investigators' criterion for success, which included decrease in tinnitus pitch as well as loudness reduction.

A number of other studies were performed during this period with varying degrees of success. Investigators continued to be frustrated by the effectiveness of DC stimulation, which has long been known to cause damage. The use of safer AC current in various configurations, stimulations sites, and waveforms continued to be inconsistently successful. In 1985, Vernon and Fenwick repeated many of the earlier experiments by Chouard et al. They used a variety of waveforms and stimulated in front and behind the ear. Using a more rigorous criterion for success (a 40 percent reduction in tinnitus loudness after treatment), these investigators achieved little success with only five of their twenty-three subjects (22 percent) reporting benefit. Unlike Engelberg and Bauer, none of these subjects experienced any change in tinnitus pitch during or after stimulation. Of the few patients who experienced tinnitus suppression during stimulation, typically only one waveform was effective for a given patient. In addition, tinnitus relief after the stimulation was interrupted; that is, residual inhibition, did not exceed a few hours.

In conclusion, the effectiveness of transcutaneous electrical stimulation is unclear. Most of the studies showed either unsubstantial or short-term results. The analysis of the controlled experiments suggests that it is hard to eliminate a placebo effect in the claimed success. Furthermore, the mechanism of action of the trancutaneously-applied current is uncertain, even though excitation of the auditory nerve is plausible for some investigators.

Extracochlear Stimulation with Alternating Current (AC) Applied at the Eardrum

Like the transcutaneous approach, stimulation with a noninvasive eardrum electrode was attempted to overcome the inconvenience of transtympanic as well as round window electrode. This method was investigated by Kuk et al. (1989), who assumed that electrical stimulus could be transmitted more efficiently through the ossicles to the inner ear than by surface electrodes on the external ear or neck. AC stimulation from 62 to 8,000 Hz was used, with various stimulus waveforms (sine, triangular, and square waves). The effectiveness of electrical stimulation was evaluated from psychophysical measurements (loudness rating, annoyance rating, contralateral broadband noise masking level) made at the various stages of the procedure (pre-, during, and posttreatment).

Ten patients reporting relatively constant, nonfluctuating tinnitus, in at least one ear were investigated. Most of these patients reported that their tinnitus had low- and high-pitched components. During the course of electrical stimulation five subjects reported no change in their tinnitus; in all these nonresponders, no auditory sensation could be elicited in spite of maximum current level ranging between 335 and 2,000 μA. Five patients reported a change in tinnitus; that is, they experienced a lowering of tinnitus loudness or annoyance by at least 33 percent (difference between the ratings before and during the treatment, divided by the rating obtained before the treatment and multiplied by 100). Three of the responders reported nonauditory sensations (tingling, warmth) similar to those described by the nonresponders. It was therefore not possible to predict the effect on tinnitus from the existence and the quality of the auditory sensation during stimulation.

In general, patients who experienced tinnitus reduction reported a reduction in the low-pitch component of their tinnitus; this occurred for all stimulus frequencies that were effective in tinnitus reduction, and at current level lower than that required to reduce the high-pitch tinnitus component. Stimulus frequencies that were effective in tinnitus reduction varied across individuals and did not appear to be related to the patients' audiograms or dominant tinnitus pitch-match frequency.

In all five responders, the contralateral noise level required to mask the tinnitus decreased during the 10-minute electrical stimulation. Square and triangular waves were more effective than sine waves in reducing tinnitus. The duration of tinnitus reduction following the 10-minute stimulation varied from 40 seconds to about 4 hours.

The responsive and the nonresponsive groups showed some psychophysical differences before electrical stimulation was started. In the nonresponsive group all patients reported bilateral tinnitus of equal severity in both ears, whereas in the responsive group all subjects reported a predominance of their tinnitus on one side. All patients in the responsive group showed acoustic postmasking effect (tinnitus reduction followed by gradual return to its premask level, or tinnitus reduction followed by an abrupt return), while only two subjects in the nonresponsive group exhibited similar masking recovery pattern. Minimum masking level in the contralateral ear was greater than 40 dB sensation level in the nonresponsive group, whereas most responders to electrical stimulation required less than 40 dB sensation level.

The design of the experiment did not allow for the measurement of potential placebo effects because the AC stimuli could be either heard or felt at suprathreshold level, and the trials consisted of increasing the level until some form of sensation was produced. Without a control for placebo effect on all patients, it may be overly optimistic to conclude that AC can effectively reduce tinnitus. However, several observations on the patients' response patterns suggest that influence of placebo effect is unlikely. First, the responsive patients reported maximum tinnitus reduction at a certain stimulus intensity level; higher or lower levels reduced the effectiveness. Second, some stimulus frequencies were more effective than others in tinnitus reduction. Third, the patients' subjective reports to different frequencies of stimulation varied. Last, triangular and square waves were more effective than sine wave in tinnitus reduction in all responsive patients.

From these results, Kuk et al. concluded that stimulating the eardrum with AC can be effective in reducing tinnitus in that ear for some patients. It eliminates the potential tissue damage of DC stimulation. Tinnitus reduction can occur without the electrical stimuli being audible. Another advantage of this technique of electrical stimulation is the long poststimulation reduction period, which lasted 4 hours in two patients, after only 10 minutes of stimulation. Kuk et al. considered that AC stimulation can be effective in tinnitus reduction with various degrees of hearing loss, and not only in profoundly deaf individuals as Hatton et al. (1960) suggested with DC. But to be successful, electrical stimulation must be performed with carefully-selected stimulus characteristics and, perhaps, preferably used in patients where tinnitus can be masked with low-level acoustic stimuli. See Table 16-2.

Extracochlear Stimulation at the Promontory or the Round Window

A systematic analysis of tinnitus reduction with these two sites of stimulation was performed in several reports from the group in Bordeaux. In the original report (Cazals et al., 1978), sensations induced by electrical stimulation of the cochlea through a trans-tympanic electrode placed at the promontory or a round window electrode were studied in sixteen subjects with a profound or severe hearing loss. A current generator with a DC-coupled output allowed separate or combined stimulations with positive and negative polarities. Input signal parameters (width and frequency of the pulses) were monitored in addition to the output control of intensity. The most important result was that suppression of tinnitus during stimulation by *positive* (anodal) *DC pulses* was observed in six patients, always on the side of electrical stimulation. When these DC positive pulses were interrupted, tinnitus reappeared immediately, which was confirmed in another report (Portmann, Cazals, Negrevergne, & Aran, 1979).

Inverting the current polarity (from positive to negative) was ineffective on tinnitus perception and induced hearing systematically. Therefore, Cazals et al. suggested that positive DC pulses were able to inhibit a pathological activity within the auditory system. The level at which such an inhibition might occur was unclear, but a peripheral effect on the auditory nerve was assumed due to the strict unilaterality of tinnitus suppression on the side of stimulation.

Table 16-2. Extracochlear stimulation: Electrodes placed temporarily close or within the middle ear

Authors	Stimulation site	Patient #	Stimulus	Definition of success	Results
Kuk et al. (1989)	eardrum	10[1]	AC[2]	33% change[3]	5/temporary
Cazals et al. (1978)	P or RW[4]	16[5]	pulsed DC+	suppression	6/temporary
Cazals et al. (1984a)	promontory	70	pulsed DC+[6]	suppression	46/temporary
Graham & Hazell (1977)	promontory	13[7]	AC[8]	suppression	2/temporary[9]
Hazell et al. (1993)	RW	9[10]	AC[11]	suppression	7/temporary

[1] various degrees of Hearing Loss (HL)

[2] various frequencies (62 to 8,000 Hz)

[3] on psychophysical measurements (loudness and annoyance ratings, contralateral noise masking level)

[4] Promontory or Round Window

[5] severe or profound hearing loss

[6] using control of the voltage produced at the electrode level

[7] totally deaf patients

[8] low-frequency sine waves (10 to 30 Hz)

[9] one patient relieved for 4 hours

[10] patients with unilateral deafness

[11] low-frequency sine waves (20 to 100 Hz)

In a later study (Cazals, Negrevergne, Aran, & Portmann, 1984a), seventy tinnitus sufferers were examined during transtympanic electrocochleography. Two difficulties were encountered, which were at that time somewhat disconcerting but are now better known.

First, several subjects who had initially reported a very annoying tinnitus declared on the day of and prior to electrical stimulation that their tinnitus was reduced. Spontaneous change of annoyance over time makes the evaluation of any treatment for tinnitus more challenging. Second, auditory sensation and tinnitus suppression induced by electrical stimulation of promontory were often intermingled with undesirable tactile feelings, certainly due to excitation of middle ear tissues.

In the study published in 1984, a control of the voltage at the patient's electrode was measured, resulting in an important technical improvement in comparison with the report of 1978. When applying a positive train of pulses a *DC shift* was produced within a few seconds, and this DC current was the effective parameter in tinnitus reduction. Another observation also instructive was the fact that after an abrupt offset of the DC positive pulses an *exponential decay of voltage* could be observed at the electrode, whereas such rises in impedance were never observed with negative DC. This finding brought Cazals et al. (1984a) to compare the cochlea excited with DC positive pulses to a capacitor which would charge under stimulation. Their report confirmed that promontory electrode was less effective in tinnitus reduction than the round window (Aran & Cazals, 1981), and showed that a positive DC shift of 1 to 5 V was necessary to suppress tinnitus (66 percent of responsive patients).

Another report warned of the danger for sensory receptors of the cochlea with this type of current (Aran, Wu, Charlet de Sauvage, Cazals, & Portmann, 1983), and therefore Cazals et al. (1984a) recommended to restrict the use of this technique to totally deaf persons. Since tinnitus sufferers in their vast majority do not show a profound or severe hearing loss, one could retrospectively regret that this work was not continued with less dangerous forms of current, such as charge balanced biphasic current pulses (Sheperd, Clark, & Black, 1983). One explanation for this discontinuity that there was a new emphasis on extracochlear implant for profoundly deaf patients (Cazals, Rouanet, Negrevergne, & Lagourgue, 1984b). Adverse effects of chronic intracochlear electrical stimulation using DC was documented a few years later by an experiment in implanted guinea pigs, showing extensive new bone formation in the three scalae and marked spiral ganglion cell loss (Sheperd, Matsushima, Millard, & Clark, 1991).

A group in London investigated the effect of *AC at the promontory and/or the round window.* Graham and Hazell (1977) using transtympanic electrode in totally deaf patients reported that in two out of thirteen subjects (15 percent) a temporary tinnitus suppression was achieved with sinusoidal currents (sine waves) of 10 to 30 Hz, one patient showing a four-hour period of continued tinnitus relief after interruption of current. This was the first reported case of residual inhibition due to electrical stimulation.

A more recent study (Hazell, Jastreboff, Meerton, & Conway, 1993) reported on acute sinusoidal AC stimulating the cochlea through a round window electrode in nine patients with unilateral deafness and severe tinnitus. They observed total suppression of tinnitus in seven individuals and confirmed the greater effectiveness in tinnitus reduction when using low frequencies, especially between 20 and 50 Hz. Frequencies below 100 Hz also resulted in better hearing thresholds and wider dynamic ranges (difference between hearing threshold and auditory discomfort level). This optimal sensitivity for low frequencies was found helpful because tinnitus suppression was never observed for subthreshold stimulation. Hazell et al. (1993) also assessed the loudness growth of auditory perception with increasing levels of current at different frequencies. They observed that the slopes varied considerably with the frequency of electrical stimulation and inferred from this variability an interpretation for the mechanism of electrical suppression of tinnitus. Feldmann's masking experiments have shown that the minimal masking level usually does not vary a lot from one frequency to another (Feldmann, 1971), even though it does in some patients (Tyler & Conrad-Armes, 1984). If electrical suppression of tinnitus was achieved through auditory masking, Hazell and his colleagues (1993) considered that similar loudness growths for hearing across frequencies were to be expected. These investigators therefore concluded that this frequency-dependence for hearing sensations was hardly compatible with a tinnitus suppression through auditory masking.

Experiments with intracochlear implants, which will be detailed subsequently, suggest on the contrary a link between the hearing sensation induced by electrical stimulation and the amount of simultaneous tinnitus reduction (Dauman & Tyler, 1993).

Extracochlear Implants

Tinnitus suppression achieved with acute electrical stimulation usually disappears rapidly after the current is interrupted. Therefore, several investigators have attempted to use chronic stimulation with an extracochlear implant.

Positive DC pulses were used by Fraysse and Lazorthes (1983) in five patients who were specifically implanted for tinnitus suppression by placing an electrode on the round window membrane. Unlike the group in London, these investigators found that low-frequency stimulation (below 150 Hz) induced annoying vibrotactile sensations. Using frequencies varying continuously from 150 to 1,500 Hz, they reported a total tinnitus suppression during stimulation in three patients, a tinnitus reduction in one subject, and a deterioration in tinnitus for the last individual. Two patients experienced total reduction for one month and eighteen months, respectively.

In the study by Cazals et al. (1984b), one out of the four profoundly deaf individuals implanted at the round window had severe preoperative tinnitus and was therefore fitted with a special signal-processing strategy based on positive DC current. At the first fitting, a level of 2 V started to reduce tinnitus and 5 V were necessary to suppress entirely tinnitus. For reasons of safety, the patient received initially a DC stimulator with an output limited to 3 V. After two months the patient reported having used the stimulator almost every day for several minutes with some relief while it was on. Then the maximum output was adjusted to 5 V, but after a period of one month the subject reported that he had tried the stimulation several times and quickly stopped it because it produced unpleasant effect in the head. See Table 16-3.

Low-frequency AC sinusoidal current was used by Hazell et al. (1993) in two cochlear implant patients. These individuals with unilateral deafness, on the side of implantation, had been responsive to tinnitus suppression at the round window and needed chronic stimulation. Therefore, they received the extracochlear device designed in London (Conway & Boyle, 1989). Using the strategy implemented by this group to enable speech perception, good results in tinnitus suppression were attained for three and one-half years, although the low-frequency cutoff frequency was intended to favor transmission of speech. Nevertheless, modification of the device was felt necessary to enhance further its ability to transmit low frequencies (20 Hz or even lower) and therefore allow for a better tinnitus reduction. Eventually, there was no evidence of alteration in the contralateral (better hearing) ear. This concern was of importance as experiments carried out in the guinea pig with a single middle ear electrode placed at the round window and extracochlear AC stimulation showed outer hair cells efferent endings to become dense and vacuolated on transmission electron microscopy (Dodson, Walliker, Bannister, Douek, & Fourcin, 1987).

Table 16-3. Extracochlear stimulation: Chronic implantation at the round window

Authors	Stimulation site	Patient #	Stimulus	Definition of success	Results
Fraysse & Lazorthes (1983)	RW	5	pulsed DC+	suppression	3[1]
Cazals et al. (1984b)	RW	1	DC+	suppression	1[2]
Hazell et al. (1993)	RW	2[3]	AC	suppression	2
Matsushima et al. (1996)	middle ear	3[4]	AC	reduction[5]	3/temporary[6]

[1] two patients showing tinnitus suppression for more than one month
[2] strategy abandoned after three months
[3] patients with complete unilateral hearing loss
[4] severe-to-profound hearing loss in two individuals, mild hearing loss in one subject
[5] tinnitus reduction was accompanied by sleep improvement
[6] need to use repeatedly the device (twice a day)

Better effectiveness of low frequencies (10 Hz) was also reported by Matsushima, Sakai, Takeichi, Miyoshi, Sakajiri, Uemi, and Ifukube (1996). They used an AC device (with a 10 kHz carrier) implanted in the middle ear of three patients. Preoperative hearing loss was severe-to-profound in two of the implanted ears (profound deafness in the contralateral ear in one subject, normal hearing in the contralateral ear of the second patient). In the third subject, the preoperative hearing loss in the implanted ear was mild. Prior to surgery, the three patients showed sleep disturbances (difficulty in falling to sleep and repeated waking up). After only 2 to 3 minutes of stimulation, all three patients fell asleep and this was evidenced by electroencephologram in one of them. Tinnitus suppression was obtained in one individual with a use of 30 minutes of stimulation twice per day. Tinnitus reduction was achieved in another patient, despite the same rate of use as the former one. The last subject experienced tinnitus reduction all day long after 1 hour of stimulation, twice or three times a day. Later, she became highly dependent on the device and used the system several hours per day. This last patient, after a breakdown of the device due to an excessive pressure she exerted on the coil to improve the contact with the skin, showed again severe sleep disturbance and tinnitus worsening. After repairing of the device, tinnitus reduction and sleep improvement were again attained.

For these *extracochlear sites of stimulation* (transcutaneous, ear canal, eardrum, promontory, round window) two mechanisms for tinnitus relief can be hypothetized. Although auditory neural responses to electrical stimulation likely arise from a mechanism that bypasses the hair cells, an interference of electrical stimulation with presynaptic biological potentials cannot be ruled out in the achievement of tinnitus relief. This presynaptic effect could be especially involved with DC pulses, this type of current being presumably capable to modify the DC potentials produced within the cochlea, for instance the endolymphatic potential. Physiological experiments performed by Moxon (1971) using monophasic pulses of current have identified two types of responses differing in their latency. The first component, characterized by a short latency, was attributed to a direct stimulation of auditory nerve fibers. Another series of peaks, termed the "electrophonic component," showed a longer latency and was thought to originate from the mechanical excitation of the basilar membrane and the action of the outer hair cells (Abbas, 1993). The electrophonic response is seen only in ears with functioning hair cells and is probably not important in stimulation of ears with no functional hearing (van der Honert & Stypulkowski, 1984). But electrophonic response has possibly a role in DC-induced tinnitus suppression in patients with well-preserved hearing.

The other mechanism through which electrical stimulation is assumed to modify tinnitus is direct stimulation of the auditory nerve fibers, resulting either in the suppression of a peripheral source of tinnitus or, more likely, in a change in the spontaneous action potential firing rate and thus a masking-like effect. Postsynaptic contribution could be predominantly implicated in experiments using AC.

The relationship between auditory sensation and tinnitus relief during electrical stimulation will be discussed in the next section on intracochlear implants. In this situation the source of electrical stimulation is closer to the auditory nerve fibers, resulting potentially in a more precise analysis of the two phenomena, sound-induced perception and tinnitus suppression.

Intracochlear Stimulation

Although the vast majority of tinnitus sufferers do not have a profound deafness (Coles, 1996; Dauman, 1997; Hazell, 1995; see also Chapter 1), cochlear implants made a large impact on electrical tinnitus suppression over the last ten years, as they did on the entire hearing health care profession (Tyler, 1991). Several factors have contributed to an increasing interest in tinnitus management through cochlear implants. First, in the large population of profoundly hearing-impaired people who were not receiving adequate benefit from hearing aids, there was obviously a proportion of patients who suffered from tinnitus in addition to their communication problems. An estimate of this proportion can be derived from the study by Tyler and Kelsay (1990) indicating that forty-two out of fifty-two

(81 percent) cochlear-implant users reported having tinnitus before they received their implant. Second, the word-recognition benefit received by many profoundly deaf subjects from their cochlear implant (Dorman, 1993) was an encouragement to extend the selection criteria for cochlear implantation to less profound hearing loss. Initially the selection criteria were that the patients obtain less than 10 percent correct word recognition for monosyllables with hearing aids (Tyler, 1991). In 1995, the NIH consensus conference gave its approval to extend the use of cochlear implants to severe hearing loss with insufficient speech recognition (NIH, 1995). This gave another group of tinnitus patients access to cochlear implants. Third, as stress can be reduced by improved communication, cochlear implants can reduce tinnitus by improving communication. Last, cochlear implants have provided a means for studying more precisely the parameters of intracochlear stimulation (Dauman & Tyler, 1993).

Single-Channel Intracochlear Implants

Originally, tinnitus reduction by cochlear implants was reported with single-channel intracochlear devices. When a single-channel (3M/House) electrode was passed 20 mm into the scala tympani, William House observed an unexpected tinnitus relief in twenty-three out of twenty-nine (79 percent) profoundly hearing-impaired patients (reported by House & Brackmann, 1981). The levels of tinnitus could be compared preoperatively and after use of the implant. Eight patients (27 percent) reported that the tinnitus was absent, fifteen (52 percent) said it was reduced, and six (21 percent) felt that it was the same. None of the patients reported tinnitus to be worse after use of the implant.

Thedinger, House, and Edgerton (1985) implanted a group of five hearing patients for tinnitus relief with the 3M/House device. The results were disappointing with regard to hearing conservation and tinnitus reduction, as only one subject reported a tinnitus reduction while listening to speech through his cochlear implant. Hearing deteriorated in these patients although the electrode was placed 6 mm only into scala tympani (House, 1984).

In a more recent follow-up on sixty-five profoundly deaf patients implanted with the 3M/House device, (Berliner, Cunningham, House, & House, 1987), thirty-four patients (53 percent) reported that their tinnitus was improved and seven patients (11 percent) reported that their tinnitus was worse.

Sininger, Mobley, House, and Nielsen (1987) measured tinnitus reduction in one hearing patient implanted with the 3M/House device. This patient had normal low-frequency hearing and a moderate-to-severe high-frequency hearing loss. Sinusoids between 400 and 16,000 Hz were ineffective in reducing tinnitus, but a biphasic pulse train was effective in six of fifteen conditions tested. Sininger et al. suggested that the current may have been insufficient to reduce tinnitus in most conditions because of loudness intolerance induced by bone conduction or electrophonic hearing. Also noteworthy is the observation that the short (6 mm) intracochlear electrode resulted in little change in the residual hearing of this patient. This suggests that intracochlear electrodes may eventually be designed for tinnitus suppression in mildly to moderately hearing-impaired patients (Tyler, 1995).

Hazell, Meerton, and Conway (1989) tested six totally deaf patients who received a single-channel intracochlear implant. They were able to reduce the tinnitus in all six patients using a 100-Hz sinusoid.

Multichannel Cochlear Implants

Most of the studies carried out over the last years on tinnitus reduction by cochlear implants have been performed with multichannel devices.

In their study of some of the better cochlear implant performers (using different multichannel devices, but also a single-channel implant), Tyler and Kelsay (1990) found that out of the forty-two subjects who reported preimplant tinnitus, tinnitus was partially eliminated in nineteen individuals (45 percent) and completely eliminated in fifteen patients (36 percent); seven patients (17 percent) reported that the cochlear implant had no effect on their tinnitus, and only one subject (2 percent) that the implant made his tinnitus worse. A limitation in this study was that only successful cochlear-implant users were chosen as subjects and this report may have overestimated the actual success in tinnitus suppression. It might well be that in implantees less successful in speech recognition, the electrical stimulation of the auditory-nerve fibers would have been less efficient and the effect on tinnitus therefore less positive. It thus appeared useful to evaluate tinnitus pre- and postoperatively in a more general population of cochlear-implant users.

This was investigated by Tyler (1995). Patients selected were eighty-two profoundly deaf male adults implanted in seven hospitals working under a common protocol that was sponsored by a Department of Veterans Affairs Cooperative Studies program. Prior to implantation all candidates were asked whether they had bothersome tinnitus. If they answered affirmatively, they were administered the Tinnitus Handicap Questionnaire (Kuk, Tyler, Russell, & Jordan, 1990). The Tinnitus Handicap Questionnaire was also administered at the first stimulation, three and twelve months poststimulation, and at yearly intervals thereafter. All patients, whether they initially reported bothersome tinnitus or not, were asked to rate their tinnitus on a five-label scale (absent, mild, moderate, severe, intolerable) at their first stimulation and at three, twelve, twenty-four, and thirty-six months postimplantation. Prior to implantation, twenty-two of the individuals (27 percent) reported bothersome tinnitus. Preoperatively, the overall score of the Tinnitus Handicap Questionnaire averaged 33.2 percent (SD = 24.7). The factor 1 (consequences of tinnitus) score averaged 27.8 percent (SD = 27.9), the factor 2 (tinnitus and hearing ability) score averaged 34 percent (SD = 34.7 percent), and the factor 3 (patient's view of tinnitus) score averaged 50.6 percent (SD = 20.6). The degree of tinnitus handicap in this population could not be predicted by biographical, audiological, or communication efficacy variables. Furthermore, Tyler compared the twenty-two individuals who had tinnitus with the sixty profoundly deaf patients who had no tinnitus, and found no significant differences between the two groups before implantation on measures of quality of life, intelligence, depression, or hearing handicap. Of interest, the group with tinnitus obtained somewhat higher speech perception scores than the group without tinnitus.

Of those twenty-two patients with preoperative bothersome tinnitus, three patients received the 3M/Vienna device, ten received the Ineraid device, eight received the Nucleus twenty-two-channel device, and one received an extracochlear single-channel Nucleus device (this patient had a fibrous round window that prevented the introduction of the electrode into scala tympani).

Two of the twenty-two patients (9 percent) showed an increase in their tinnitus after twenty-four months of cochlear implant use. Nine patients (41 percent) showed a clear (greater than 10 percent) decrease in their tinnitus handicap. Three patients who did not report their tinnitus as bothersome preoperatively later reported a severe tinnitus postoperatively (24 months after surgery). Unfortunately, preoperatively these patients were not asked to rate their tinnitus on the none-mild-moderate-severe-intolerable scale; they were only asked if they experienced troublesome tinnitus or not. If their preoperative, nontroublesome tinnitus, is considered to be equivalent to mild or moderate, then the cochlear implant precipitated a marked increase in tinnitus in all three individuals. Although this figure appears small with respect to the total number of investigated individuals (eighty-two), cochlear implant candidates should be informed that there is a 3 to 5 percent chance that their tinnitus may be increased after implantation.

In Tyler's 1995 report, 27 percent (twenty-two of eighty-two) of the profoundly-hearing impaired patients reported bothersome tinnitus before receiving a cochlear implant. This number is considerably lower than that reported by other studies of cochlear implant patients. Preoperative tinnitus was observed in 85 percent (forty-four of fifty-two) by Gibson (1992), 86 percent (eighteen of twenty-one) by Bredberg, Walden, and Lindström (1992), and 85 percent (twenty-eight of thirty-three) by Zwolan, Kileny, Souliere, and Keminck (1992). This apparent discrepancy is likely a result of Tyler's stipulation of bothersome tinnitus. His 27 percent estimate of bothersome tinnitus compares with an incidence of about 8 percent of the general population reporting a moderately or severely annoying tinnitus (Coles, 1996; see also Chapter 1). Axelsson and Ringdahl in 1989 found that about 14 percent of the general population reported that they suffered from tinnitus "often or always," and that this number increased to about 25 percent when only men between fifty and fifty-nine years of age were considered. Brown (1990) estimated about 21 percent of the general population of men between 55 and 64 years old to have tinnitus "every few days" or that "bothers them quite a bit." Thus, it appears that the profoundly hearing-impaired population in Tyler's study has an incidence of tinnitus much larger than that of the general population, but not substantially larger than that of other men of similar ages with severe hearing loss. Furthermore, Tinnitus Handicap Questionnaire scores reported by Kuk et al. (1990) on 275 patients with mild to severe hearing loss, and those reported by Tyler (1995) on implanted individuals (overall score and separate factor scores) did not differ significantly.

Gibson (1992) evaluated tinnitus with a postoperative questionnaire in seventy adults who had received the Nucleus intracochlear implant device. Out of the fifty-two patients who replied, only eight (15 percent) reported no preoperative tinnitus, and analysis of tinnitus was possible in forty-two individuals. Surprisingly a large number of these patients believed that their tinnitus had been lessened by the surgery, fourteen of the forty-two subjects (33 percent) reporting that tinnitus was better and two subjects (5 percent) that it had gone entirely. Tinnitus was judged unaltered by surgery by twenty-two of the forty-two patients (52 percent) and worsened by four patients (10 percent). Of those patients who still had tinnitus after the surgery, one patient developed tinnitus with the surgery, and one patient developed tinnitus from a head trauma several months after surgery. These forty-two patients were asked to rate the relief obtained by switching on the cochlear implant. Six of the forty-two patients (14 percent) reported tinnitus suppression, ninteen of the forty-two subjects (45 percent) reported tinnitus reduction and sixteen subjects (38 percent) reported that tinnitus was unchanged.

When comparing the patients reporting good tinnitus suppression using the cochlear implant and the patients reporting no change in tinnitus using the cochlear implant, Gibson found no prognostic value in preoperative electric testing at the promontory, nor in age, length of total deafness, preoperative use of hearing aid, or etiology. The only difference between the two groups was that the group who benefited had a higher proportion of unilateral tinnitus (36 percent) than the other group (11 percent). The better result on unilateral tinnitus was in agreement with data collected at the promontory or round window (Aran & Cazals, 1981; Cazals et al., 1978; Cazals et al., 1984a).

The lack of prognostic factor observed by Gibson (1992) in tinnitus suppression with cochlear implants is in some disagreement with another study by Zwolan et al. (1992) who administered a questionnaire to thirty-three postlingually deafened patients implanted with the Nucleus device. Questions were designed to assess the effect of cochlear implantation on tinnitus perception and was derived from a tinnitus questionnaire designed by Stouffer and Tyler (1990). The questionnaire was administered pre- and postoperatively. In an effort to quantify tinnitus change after implantation, the variables of tinnitus loudness, duration, and annoyance were evaluated on a 1 to 10 scale. Prior to data collection, it was determined that a change in tinnitus loudness or annoyance would be considered significant if the respondent indicated a change of three or more units. Questions regarding change in location of tinnitus and the presence of residual inhibition (reduction in tinnitus level after the implant was turned off) were also included in the questionnaire. Out of the twenty-eight individuals who reported preoperative tinnitus, tinnitus loudness was decreased in 54 percent (fifteen patients), unchanged in 43 percent (twelve patients), and increased in 3 percent (one patient) following cochlear implantation. Tinnitus annoyance was decreased in 43 percent (twelve subjects), unchanged in 50 percent (fourteen subjects), and increased in 7 percent (two subjects). In those patients reporting a tinnitus decrease, 77 percent reported that tinnitus was decreased or abolished in the implanted ear and 42 percent reported that tinnitus was decreased or abolished in the contralateral ear also. No patient reported decreased tinnitus in the contralateral ear alone. On the basis of contralateral residual inhibition and tinnitus suppression (42 percent of patients), Zwolan et al. suggested that the residual inhibition achieved with cochlear implants was more a centrally mediated effect than a peripheral process.

Ito and Sakakihara (1994) reported on twenty patients who received a cochlear implant for a severe or profound hearing impairment. Preoperatively, five patients (25 percent) reported marked tinnitus, thirteen patients (65 percent) had slight tinnitus, and only two patients (10 percent) reported no tinnitus at all. During promontory stimulation, tinnitus was abolished in four patients (22 percent), reduced in nine patients (50 percent) and unchanged in five patients (28 percent). After surgery, tinnitus was abolished in eight subjects (44 percent), reduced in seven subjects (39 percent), unchanged in two subjects (11 percent), and aggravated in one patient (6 percent). Thus, the investigators reported that intracochlear electrical stimulation was effective in relieving tinnitus in 83 percent of patients who underwent cochlear implant surgery. The analysis of individual results during preoperative promontory stimulation and after cochlear implantation shows comparable effects of electrical stimulation in fourteen subjects, in particular for the five patients with marked preoperative tinnitus. However, a discrepancy appears in four individuals: tinnitus was suppressed or abolished postoperatively in three patients although promontory stimulation was uneffective, and tinnitus was aggravated postoperatively in one patient even though it had been reduced during promontory stimulation. The findings in these four patients confirm that electrical stimulation may have different effects on tinnitus according to the site of stimulation, and that intracochlear stimulation appears more effective to suppress tinnitus than promontory stimulation, at least in profoundly deaf individuals.

Ito and Sakakihara conclude their report by discussing the mechanism of tinnitus suppression in subjects with a cochlear implant. According to Vernon (1977), the presumable mechanism of masking effect induced by environmental sounds in non-implanted tinnitus patients is that basilar membrane vibrates and suppresses the abnormal activity in the hair cells in the inner ear that produces tinnitus, thus suppressing tinnitus. In cochlear implant patients the cochlea is functionally destroyed, the basilar membrane is no longer vibrating, and the hair cells are no longer activated. Therefore, another mechanism of tinnitus suppression in cochlear implant patients must be involved.

One explanation suggested by Ito and Sakakihara is that the electrical stimulation from the implanted electrodes alter the activities of the cochlear nerve, which is in this hypothesis postulated to be the main cause of the tinnitus. In another explanation, the electrical stimulation from the

implant is thought to be transmitted to the cochlear nucleus and superior olive nucleus, and to inhibit the hair cells of the inner ear via the cochlear efferent fibers. However, because hair cells are no longer functionally activated in cochlear implant patients, this hypothesis is unlikely.

Beside these questionnaire-based studies, other reports have attempted to analyze the effects of multichannel cochlear implants during laboratory experiments. McKerrow, Schreiner, Snyder, Merzenich, and Toner (1991) investigated six patients fitted with the UCSF/Storz four-channel implant device. The time course of tinnitus loudness (judged on arbitrary magnitude scale from 0, undetectable, to 10, very loud) was evaluated every 5 minutes in four conditions. In the first one, the patient was not wearing the device. Then the device was switched on for 30 minutes with the only carrier wave (2 to 6 MHz, depending on the channel) delivered to the device. In this control condition, no patient reported audible sound associated with the implant. Afterwards, for another 30 minutes, white noise was introduced at a comfortable listening level, set by the patient to match the normal mean level of operation of his device (in general around 50 dBA). The device was then switched off and removed from the head. In five patients there was a marked tinnitus reduction in the implanted ear with the device in use with noise, and in four of these there was a tinnitus reduction, usually of smaller magnitude, with the device on but no audible sound input (control condition). Five of the six patients showed some poststimulation reduction of tinnitus when the device was switched off. The duration of this residual inhibition, defined as the time needed for the tinnitus to return to the initial level, ranged from 5 to 15 minutes and the return could be either gradual or abrupt. When the comfortable listening level of noise was used, four of the five patients who reported a tinnitus suppression stated that this effect was markedly bilateral. Two other findings are of interest in the report by McKerrow et al. (1991). First, five of the six patients had already noted prior to the study that their tinnitus was improved by the use of the implant. Although the study does not indicate which patient differed from the five others, the hypothesis that experimental data could parallel the subjective estimate of patients would be helpful for the clinical validation of the experiment. Second, one of the two patients who were tested with isolated channels showed a channel-specific tinnitus reduction; that is, the most effective suppressor channel also produced the closest pitch match for the tinnitus. This suggests that the physiologic correlate of this particular tinnitus sensation was spatially restricted along the central or peripheral cochleotopic axis. As already mentioned in the section on extracochlear implants, some frequency specificity of tinnitus suppression had been shown in the study by Kuk et al. (1989), but in that case the frequency selectivity may not have been related to the cochleotopic organization of the auditory system since the stimulation site was constant (eardrum).

Another experiment was performed with two patients who had received the Nucleus device (Dauman & Tyler, 1993). The main difference with the former study was that the speech processor was driven electrically and not acoustically with a white noise. It was thus possible to change the parameters of the electrical stimulation and to evaluate the consequences of these changes on the perception of both stimulus and tinnitus. Stimuli were charge-balanced trains of various repetition rates (frequencies) and inter-electrode distances. A range of electrodes was chosen in each subject, including basal, medial and apical electrodes. For each condition, different current levels were selected between the hearing threshold and the uncomfortable loudness level, and presented randomly, usually with three replications. For each level, the patient was asked to rate on a 0 to 100 scale the loudness of the stimulus and the loudness of the tinnitus. As seen in Figure 16-1, the stimulus

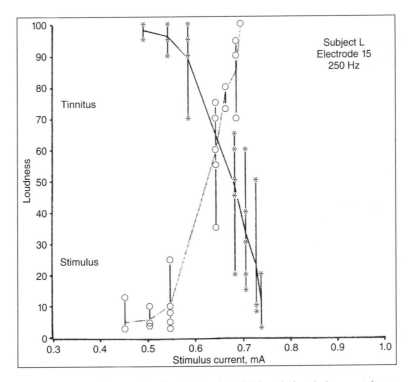

FIGURE 16-1. Loudness ratings for tinnitus (asterisks) and electrical current (open circles) as a function of the stimulus current for one patient using a Nucleus cochlear implant (electrode 15 at 250 Hz). The two curves show opposite slopes with a crossover point around 0.65 mA.

loudness curve and the tinnitus loudness curve show opposite slopes and a crossover point can be defined, where the two curves cross, in this case around 0.65 mA (using bipolar stimulation of electrode 15 at a repetition rate of 250 Hz). Variability of tinnitus loudness was rather large, as opposed to that of stimulus loudness. To compare the effects of varying the stimulus condition (electrode location, frequency of stimulation, inter-electrode distance) two levels were determined, the crossover point and the preferred loudness level for tinnitus reduction. All the parameters influenced these two levels. First, the 125 Hz pulse rate appeared to be the best (that is, requiring the lowest current level) with respect to both crossover point and preferred loudness level for tinnitus reduction. The current level necessary to sufficiently reduce tinnitus without inducing a too loud sound was lower at 125 Hz than at 250 or 80 Hz, which was the lowest frequency evaluated due to the coding strategy. Second, electrode location greatly influenced psychometric functions but in a nonpredictable way, such that a range of electrodes (basal, medial, apical) was not systematically the most effective in reducing the most annoying tinnitus in both patients. Third, the use of different inter-electrode distances showed that the larger the distance, the less current was needed to reduce tinnitus; for example, the bipolar + 3 stimulation being more effective than the bipolar + 1 condition. These data suggest that the optimal parameters for tinnitus reduction should be tailored in each patient. Eventually, a prolonged stimulation (5 minutes at the preferred level for the optimal combination) resulted in a stable tinnitus reduction during stimulation and was followed by a progressive return to the original tinnitus level within about 15 minutes. In conclusion to these experiments, it is expected that with the availability of different programs in the speech processor of a given implanted patient, it will be easier to set up an optimal electrical stimulation for reducing tinnitus, independently from the strategies selected to achieve the best speech understanding. This option might show applicability in patients reporting difficulties in coping with their tinnitus as soon as the device is switched off. See Table 16-4.

CONCLUSION

Electrical stimulation for tinnitus relief has raised a lot of interest among investigators. A wide range of procedures have been described, driving electrical current either through temporary electrodes located at various places or by means of devices implanted in the midlle or inner ear. The benefit of positive DC pulses in reducing momentarily tinnitus was recognized early, but the clinical use of this type of electricity was rapidly restricted to limited periods of time due to its harmfulness in the long term.

Extracochlear stimulation with AC delivered by transcutaneous electrodes did not show consistent results in controlled studies. Spontaneous variability of tinnitus annoyance over time complicates the assessment of effectiveness. Auditory awareness of stimulation makes nonstimulus controls difficult. The lack of standardization in electrical parameters, criteria used to define success, and assessment of tinnitus in the poststimulation period make comparisons across studies and generalization difficult. However, these experiments have indicated that electrical current presented to the peripheral auditory system is capable of reducing tinnitus perception. More research is needed to consider implantable devices for a prolonged stimulation of the cochlea.

Chronic stimulation of the auditory system with electrical implantable prostheses in tinnitus patients has, so far, been limited by the concern of hearing preservation. Early findings on tinnitus suppression were achieved by extracochlear stimulation with an electrode implanted at the round window. The potential of electrical suppression of tinnitus has been considerably extended by the increasing use of multichannel cochlear implants for severe and profound

Table 16-4. Intracochlear stimulation.

Authors	Type of implant	Patient #	Stimulus	Definition of success	Results
House et al. (1981)	3M/House[1]	29[2]	speech	relief	23
Thedinger et al. (1985)	3M/House[3]	5[4]	speech	reduction	1
Berliner et al. (1987)	3M/House[3]	65[5]	speech	improvement	34
Sininger et al. (1987)	3M/House[3]	1[6]	biph. pulse	reduction	1
Hazell et al. (1989)	single UCL	6[7]	100-Hz sin.	reduction	6
Tyler & Kelsay (1990)	multichannel	42[8]	speech	reduction	23
Tyler (1995)	various[9]	22[10]	speech	THQ dec.[11]	9
Gibson (1992)	Nucleus	42[12]	speech	reduction	25
Zwolan et al. (1992)	Nucleus	28	speech	scale ch.[13]	15
Ito & Sakakihara (1994)	multichannel	18	speech	reduction	15
McKerrow et al. (1991)	UCSF/Storz	6	white noise[14]	reduction	5
Dauman & Tyler (1993)	Nucleus	2	comp.contr.15	ratings	2

[1] 20 mm into scala tympani

[2] profoundly deaf patients

[3] 6 mm into scala tympani

[4] hearing subjects

[5] profoundly deaf patients

[6] moderate-to-severe high frequency hearing loss

[7] totally deaf patients

[8] some of the better cochlear implant performers

[9] 3M/Vienna (#3), Ineraid (#10), Nucleus-22 (#8), Nucleus single-channel (#1)

[10] twenty-two patients with bothersome tinnitus (out of eighty-two subjects implanted for profound deafness)

[11] 10 percent decrease in Tinnitus Handicap Questionnaire score

[12] forty-two individuals reporting post-operatively that they had tinnitus prior to implantation

[13] reduction of 3 units on a 1 to 10 loudness-annoyance-scale

[14] control with device on using carrier wave only

[15] computer control of channels, repetition rates, and interelectrode distances

hearing loss. Suppression of tinnitus perception has been reported in many cochlear implant users who had been operated on for a profound hearing loss. Experiments on tinnitus in cochlear implant users have contributed to a better knowledge of the parameters susceptible to improve the effectiveness of electrical stimulation upon tinnitus in hearing patients. Further research is requested to make these advances applicable for tinnitus sufferers with moderate hearing loss (Tyler, 1997).

The mechanism by which these effects occur also require further investigation. Insight into the mechanism of electrical tinnitus reduction could be useful in pharmacological or other treatments. Electrically-induced activation of auditory nerve fibers could be responsible for changing the functional state of auditory nuclei and, therefore, interfere with a potential source of tinnitus in the brain stem (Dauman, 1997). Chronic stimulation of the auditory system by external electricity therefore appears as promising in the achievement of the reduction process to tinnitus annoyance.

ACKNOWLEDGMENT

The help of Jonathan Hazell in reviewing the manuscript was highly appreciated. The author is also grateful to Yves Cazals for his comments on an early version of the manuscript.

REFERENCES

Abbas, P. J. (1993). Electrophysiology. In R. S. Tyler (Ed.), *Cochlear implants: Audiological foundations* (pp. 317–355). San Diego: Singular Publishing Group, Inc.

Aran, J. M., & Cazals, Y. (1981). Electrical suppression of tinnitus. In D. Evered (Ed.), *Tinnitus: CIBA Foundation Symposium 85* (pp. 217–224). London: Pitman Books.

Aran, J. M., Wu, Z. Y., Charlet de Sauvage, R., Cazals, Y., & Portmann, M. (1983). Electrical stimulation of the ear: Experimental studies. *Annals of Otology, Rhinology, and Laryngology, 92*, 614–620.

Axelsson, A., & Ringdahl, A. (1989). Tinnitus—A study of its prevalence and characteristics. *British Journal of Audiology, 23*, 53–62.

Berliner, K. I., Cunningham, J. K., House, W. F., & House, J. W. (1987). Effect of the cochlear implant on tinnitus in profoundly deaf patients. In H. Feldmann (Ed.), *Proceedings of the Third International Tinnitus Seminar 1987*, Munster (pp. 451–453). Karlsruhe: Harsch Verlag.

Bredberg, G., Walden, J., & Lindström B. (1992). Tinnitus after cochlear implantation. In J. M. Aran & R. Dauman (Eds.), *Proceedings of the Fourth International Tinnitus Seminar*, Bordeaux, 1991 (pp. 417–422). Amsterdam/New York: Kugler.

Brown, S. C. (1990). Older Americans and tinnitus: A demographic study and chartbook. *Monograph Series A. No.2.* Washington DC: Gallaudet Research Institute, Gallaudet University.

Brusis, T., & Loennecken, I. (1985). Treatment of tinnitus with iontophoresis and local anesthesia. *Laryngology, Rhinology, Otology (Stuttgart), 64*, 355–358.

Cazals, Y., Bourdin, M., Negrevergne, M., & Dauman, R. (1986). Stimulation électrique transcutanée dans le traitement des acouphènes. *Revue de Laryngologie, 107*, 433–436.

Cazals, Y., Negrevergne, M., & Aran, J. M. (1978). Electrical stimulation of the cochlea in man: Hearing induction and tinnitus suppression. *Journal of the American Audiology Society, 3*, 209–213.

Cazals, Y., Negrevergne, M., Aran, J. M., & Portmann, M. (1984a). Activation and inhibition of hearing with electrical stimulation of the ear. *Advances in Audiology* (Vol. 2, pp. 30–35). Basel: Karger.

Cazals, Y., Rouanet, J. F., Negrevergne, M., & Lagourgue, P. (1984b). First results of chronic electrical suppression with a round-window electrode in totally deaf patients. *Archives of Otorhinolaryngology, 239*, 191–196.

Chouard, C. H., Meyer, B., & Maridat, D. (1981). Transcutaneous electrotherapy for severe tinnitus. *Acta Otolaryngologica (Stockholm), 91*, 415–422.

Coles, R. R. A. (1996). Tinnitus. In A. G. Kerr & S. D. G. Stephens (Eds.), *Scott-Brown's Otolaryngology*, (Chapter 18, Vol. 2, 6th ed.). Oxford: Butterworth-Heinemann.

Conway, M. J., & Boyle, P. (1989). Design of the UCH/RNID cochlear implant prothesis. *Journal of Laryngology* (Suppl. 18), 4–10.

Dauman, R. (1997). Acouphènes: Mécanismes et approche clinique. Encyclopédie Médico-Chirurgicale (Elsevier, Paris), *Oto-rhino-laryngologie*, 20–180–A–10, 7p.

Dauman, R., Aran, J. M., & Portmann, M. (1986). Summating potential and water balance in Ménière's Disease. *Annals of Otology, Rhinology, and Laryngology, 95*, 389–395.

Dauman, R., Frachet, B., & Tyler, R. S. (1996). Almitrine-raubasine and tinnitus: A double-blind placebo-controlled randomized crossover study. In G. E. Reich & J. A. Vernon (Eds.), *Proceedings of the Fifth International Tinnitus Seminar 1995* (pp. 216–224). Portland, OR: American Tinnitus Association.

Dauman, R., & Tyler, R. S. (1993). Tinnitus suppression in cochlear implant users. *Advances in Oto-Rhino-Laryngology, 48*, 168–173.

Davis, H. (1965). A model for transducer action in the cochlea. *Cold Spring Harbor Symp. Quant. Biol., 30*, 181–189.

Dobie, R. A. (1999). A review of randomized clinical trials in tinitus. *Laryngoscope, 109*, 1202–1211.

Dobie, R. A., Hoberg, K. E., & Rees, T. (1986). Electrical tinnitus suppression: A double-blind crossover study. *Otolaryngology—Head and Neck Surgery, 95*, 319–323.

Dodson, H. C., Walliker, J. R., Bannister, L. H., Douek, E., & Fourcin. (1987). Structural effects of short-term and chronic extracochlear electrical stimulation on the guinea pig spiral organ. *Hearing Research, 31*, 65–78.

Dorman, M. F. (1993). Speech perception in adults. In R. S. Tyler (Ed.), *Cochlear implants: Audiological foundations* (pp. 145–190). San Diego: Singular Publishing Group, Inc.

Engelberg, M., & Bauer, W. (1985). Transcutaneous electrical stimulation for tinnitus. *Laryngoscope, 95,* 1167–1173.

Feldmann, H. (1971). Homolateral and contralateral masking of tinnitus by noisebands and by pure-tones. *Audiology, 10,* 138–144.

Feldmann, H. (1984). Suppression of tinnitus by electrical stimulation: A contribution to the history of medicine. In A. Schulman & J. Ballantyne (Eds.), *Proceedings of the Second International Tinnitus Seminar,* New York 1983, *Journal of Laryngology and Otology,* Suppl. 9, 123–124.

Fraysse, B., & Lazorthes, Y. (1983). Implantation chronique d'une électrode au contact de la fenêtre ronde dans le traitement des acouphènes. *Journal Français d'Otorhinolaryngologie, 32,* 307–310.

Gibson, W. P. R. (1992). The effect of electrical stimulation and cochlear implantation on tinnitus. In J. M. Aran & R. Dauman (Eds.), *Proceedings of the Fourth International Tinnitus Seminar, Bordeaux, 1991* (pp. 403–408). Amsterdam/New York: Kugler.

Graham, J. M., & Hazell, J. W. P. (1977). Electrical stimulation of the human cochlea using a transtympanic electrode. *British Journal of Audiology, 11,* 59–62.

Grandori, F. (1986). Field analysis of auditory evoked brain stem potentials. *Hearing Research, 21,* 51–58.

Grapengiesser, C. J. C. (1801). *Versuche den Galvinismus zur Heilung einiger Krankheiten anzuwenden.* Berlin: Myliussischen Buchhandlung.

Hatton, D. S., Erulkar, S. D., & Rosenberg, P. E. (1960). Some preliminary observations on the effect of galvanic current on tinnitus aurium. *Laryngoscope, 70,* 123–130.

Hazell, J. W. P. (1995). Models of tinnitus: Generation, perception, clinical implications. In J. A. Vernon & A. R. Moller (Eds.), *Mechanisms of tinnitus* (pp. 57–72). Boston: Allyn & Bacon.

Hazell, J. W. P., Jastreboff, P. W., Meerton, L. E., & Conway, M. J. (1993). Electrical tinnitus suppression: Frequency dependence of effects. *Audiology, 32,* 68–77.

Hazell, J. W. P., Meerton, L. J., & Conway, M. J. (1989). Electrical tinnitus suppression (ETS) with a single channel cochlear implant. *Journal of Laryngology and Otology* (Suppl. 18), 39–44.

House, J. W. (1984). Effects of electrical stimulation on tinnitus. In A. Schulman & J. Ballantyne (Eds.), *Proceedings of the Second International Tinnitus Seminar,* New York 1983, *Journal of Laryngology and Otology* (Suppl. 9), 139–140.

House, J. W., & Brackmann, D. E. (1981). Tinnitus: Surgical treatment. In D. Evered (Ed.), *Tinnitus: CIBA Foundation Symposium 85* (pp. 204–212). London: Pitman Books.

House, W. F. (1976). Cochlear implants. *Annals of Otology, Rhinology, and Laryngology, 85*(Suppl. 27).

Ito, J., & Sakakihara, J. (1994). Suppression of tinnitus by cochlear implantation. *American Journal of Otolaryngology, 15,* 145–148.

Jewett, D. L., Romano, M. L., & Williston, J. S. (1970). Human auditory evoked potentials: Possible brain stem components recorded on the scalp. *Science, 167,* 1517–1518.

Kuk, F. K., Tyler, R. S., Russell, D., & Jordan, H. (1990). The psychometric properties of a tinnitus handicap questionnaire. *Ear & Hearing, 11,* 434–442.

Kuk, F. K., Tyler, R. S., Rustad, N., Harker, L. A., & Tye-Murray, N. (1989). Alternating current at the eardrum for tinnitus reduction. *Journal of Speech and Hearing Research, 32,* 393–400.

Matsushima, J., Sakai, N., Takeichi, N., Miyoshi, S., Sakajiri, M., Uemi, N., & Ifukube, T. (1996). Implanted electrical tinnitus suppressor. In G. E. Reich & J. A. Vernon (Eds.), *Proceedings of the Fifth International Tinnitus Seminar 1995* (pp. 329–334). Portland, OR: American Tinnitus Association.

McKerrow, W. S., Schreiner, C. E., Snyder, R. L., Merzenich, M. M., & Toner J. G. (1991). Tinnitus suppression by cochlear implants. *Annals of Otology, Rhinology and Laryngology, 100,* 552–558.

Morgon, A., Dubreuil, C., Disant, F., & Chanal, J. M. (1984). New approaches in the treatment of tinnitus by electrostimulation. *Journal Français d'Oto-Rhino-Laryngologie, 33,* 343–351.

Moxon, E. C. (1971). *Neural and mechanical responses to electrical stimulation of the cat's inner ear.* Unpublished doctoral dissertation, Massachusetts Institute of Technology, Cambridge, MA.

Murai, K., Tyler, R. S., Harker, L. A., & Stouffer, J. L. (1992). Review of pharmacological treatment of tinnitus. *The American Journal of Otology, 13,* 454–464.

NIH Consensus Conference. 1995. Cochlear implants.

Picton, T. W. (1995). The neurophysiological evaluation of auditory discrimination. *Ear & Hearing, 16,* 1–5.

Portmann, M., Cazals, Y., Negrevergne, M., & Aran, J. M. (1979). Temporary tinnitus suppression in man through electrical stimulation of the cochlea. *Acta Otolaryngologica (Stockholm), 87,* 294–299.

Russell, I. J., & Sellick, P. M. Intracellular studies of hair cells in the mammalian cochlea. *Journal of Physiology, 284,* 261–290.

Sheperd, R. K., Clark, G. M., & Black, R. C. (1983). Chronic electrical stimulation of the auditory nerve in cats: Physiological and histopathological results. *Acta Otolaryngologica (Stockholm)* (Suppl. 399), 19–31.

Sheperd, R. K., Matsushima, J., Millard, R. E., & Clark, G. M. (1991). Cochlear pathology following chronic electrical stimulation using non charge balanced stimuli. *Acta Otolaryngologica (Stockholm), 111,* 848–860.

Shulman, A. (1985). External electrical stimulation in tinnitus control. *The American Journal of Otology, 6,* 110–115.

Sininger, Y. S., Mobley, J. P., House, W., & Nielsen, D. (1987). Intra-cochlear electrical stimulation for tinnitus suppression in a patient with near-normal hearing. In H. Feldmann (Ed.), *Proceedings of the Third International Tinnitus Seminar 1987, Munster* (pp. 454–457). Karlsruhe: Harsch Verlag.

Sohmer, H., & Feinmesser, M. (1967). Cochlear action potentials recorded from the external ear in man. *Annals of Otology, Rhinology, and Laryngology, 76,* 427–435.

Stouffer, J. L., & Tyler, R. S. (1990). Characterization of tinnitus by tinnitus patients. *Journal of Speech and Hearing Disorders, 55,* 439–453.

Thedinger, B., House, W. F., & Edgerton, B. J. (1985). Cochlear implant for tinnitus. Case reports. *Annals of Otology, Rhinology, and Laryngology, 94,* 10–13.

Thedinger, B. S., Karlsen, E., & Schack, S. H. (1987). Treatment of tinnitus with electrical stimulation: An evaluation of the Audimax Theraband. *Laryngoscope, 97,* 33–37.

Tyler, R. S. (1981). Final general discussion on source of tinnitus (peripheral or central?). In *CIBA Foundation Symposium 85. Tinnitus* (pp. 279–294), London: Pitman Books Ltd.

Tyler, R. S. (1991). What can we learn about hearing aids from cochlear implants? *Ear and Hearing* (Vol. 12, Suppl.), 177S–186S.

Tyler, R. S. (1995). Tinnitus in the profoundly hearing-impaired and the effects of cochlear implants. *Annals of Otology, Rhinology, and Laryngology, 104,* 25–30.

Tyler, R. S. (1997). Perspectives on tinnitus. *British Journal of Audiology, 31,* 381–386.

Tyler, R. S., Aran, J. M., & Dauman, R. (1992). Recent advances in tinnitus. *American Journal of Audiology, 1,* 36–44.

Tyler, R. S., & Conrad-Armes, D. (1984). Masking of tinnitus compared to the masking of pure tones. *Journal of Speech and Hearing Research, 27,* 106–111.

Tyler, R. S., & Kelsay, D. (1990). Advantages and disadvantages reported by some of the better cochlear-implant patients. *The American Journal of Otology, 11,* 282–289.

van der Honert, C., & Stypulkowski, P. H. (1984). Physiological properties of the electrically stimulated auditory nerve. II. Single fiber recordings. *Hearing Research, 14,* 225–243.

Vernon, J. A. (1987). Use of electricity to suppress tinnitus. *Seminars in Hearing,* Vol. 8, No 1.

Vernon, J. A., & Fenwick, J. A. (1985). Attempts to suppress tinnitus with transcutaneous electrical stimulation. *Otolaryngology—Head and Neck Surgery, 93,* 385–389.

Yasuda, I. (1974). Mechanical and electrical callus. *Annals New York Academy of Science, 238,* 457–465.

Zwolan, T. A., Kileny, P. R., Souliere, C. R. Jr., & Keminck J. L. (1992). Tinnitus suppression following cochlear implantation. In J. M. Aran & R. Dauman (Eds.), *Proceedings of the Fourth International Tinnitus Seminar, Bordeaux, 1991* (pp. 423–426). Amsterdam/New York: Kugler.

CHAPTER 17

Medicolegal Issues

Ross Coles

INTRODUCTION

With an increasing public awareness and knowledge about bodily illnesses or disorders that can arise directly or indirectly from some action or lack of action by another person, claims for financial recompense soon follow. This has certainly applied to tinnitus. Initially, tinnitus tended to be a subsidiary item of claim additional to that for hearing loss, usually of the noise-induced kind. More recently though, tinnitus has sometimes been the principal or only complaint. Further, in those cases where tinnitus has devastating effects on lifestyle and ability to work, it usually attracts higher levels of compensation than hearing loss.

TYPES OF INJURY LEADING TO COMPENSATION CLAIMS FOR TINNITUS

Recurrent Noise Exposure

Tinnitus often comes on gradually at some time during or after unprotected exposure to noise (Axelsson & Barrenäs, 1992) of sufficiently high level and duration to cause

noise-induced hearing loss (NIHL). Sometimes it seems to grow out of repeated experiences of temporary tinnitus of ever-increasing duration following each day's noise exposure until eventually the tinnitus is always there, even after a quiet vacation.

Acoustic Trauma

Permanent hearing loss of measurable degree only rarely results from a single noise exposure, unless extremely intense such as from a nearby explosion or gunshot, when it is described as an acoustic trauma. On the other hand recurrent acoustic traumas, such as from weapon firing, frequently cause hearing loss. In those cases tinnitus is common, perhaps with a 60 to 80 percent prevalence (Man & Naggan, 1981) as compared with about 50 percent in association with ordinary NIHL (Coles et al., 1990). This might be something to do with the nature of the incident waveform, and consequent pattern of cochlear damage, since impact noise also seems to cause rather more tinnitus than steady-state types of noise (Alberti, 1987).

The rate of damage to or deterioration of cochlear function is also likely to be important in determining whether or not tinnitus occurs. Note how sudden deafness is almost always accompanied by tinnitus, and that the tinnitus often disappears if the hearing recovers. With the slow development of NIHL or presbyacusis, the brain has a chance to habituate to the gradual developing abnormality in the ongoing auditory neuronal activity (see Chapter 5), which otherwise would be interpreted as a sound, such as tinnitus. But with a relatively rapid onset or increase in degree of cochlear disorder, habituation cannot occur fast enough and tinnitus is more likely to result.

There is another group of people whose tinnitus clearly dates from a sudden loud sound, but which was of insufficient intensity and/or duration to cause measurable hearing loss. The noise may however have caused enough further damage, and consequent change in patterns of neuronal activity, to trigger the onset of tinnitus. Such noises are often unexpected and frightening, and in some of these cases the triggering may have a central neurophysiological rather than cochlear mechanism.

Head or Ear Injury

Tinnitus may result from a minor head or ear injury, even a quite minor one unlikely to cause measurable hearing loss. The mechanisms of tinnitus generation, including triggering of onset, are probably much the same as for acoustic trauma, the most likely in this case being some concussional or direct mechanical damage to the organ of Corti.

In addition, if the injury involves the tympanic membrane or ossicular chain this may cause a conductive hearing loss. Such a hearing loss, due to its attenuation of the tinnitus-masking effect of ambient noise, could have the effect of revealing or exacerbating an underlying tinnitus—either a coincidental one, perhaps associated with presbyacusis, or one consequent on some damage to the internal ear by the same injury.

More severe injuries may cause tinnitus as a result of intracochlear hemorrhage, gross structural damage to the temporal bone, or concussional damage to the auditory nerve or central auditory system.

Ear Syringing

Quite often ear syringing seems to result in onset of tinnitus. If something obviously goes wrong, such as the nozzle coming off the syringe body and violently striking the tympanic membrane, then the direct mechanical injury is evident and the onset of tinnitus is readily understandable. But tinnitus sometimes results from an apparently normal syringing. Possible causes of this have been investigated in some depth by Jayarajan et al. (1995), who found little evidence for an otological mechanism of tinnitus generation. However, in most cases there is also some hearing loss, almost certainly preexisting, and the syringing seems simply to have been a trigger for onset of tinnitus in an ear already somewhat predisposed towards generation of tinnitus. The mechanism of triggering by ear syringing would seem most likely to be either direct from mechanical or acoustical stimulation of the ear, or psychological, from the discomfort, fear, or anxiety it sometimes causes. As Erlandsson discusses in Chapter 2, stress in and of itself can sometimes cause tinnitus. The perception or experience of a stressful event can have subsequent physiological consequences.

These patients are often angry about what they perceive to be an injury. They feel that it should not have happened or a safer method of wax removal should have been used. A compensation claim can then arise, but is usually unsuccessful following a normal ear syringing. (In contrast, when there has been a major error of technique, claims are usually successful). The major hurdle for the complainant is that ear syringing is a traditional and largely safe method of wax removal, and that tinnitus is a sufficiently uncommon complication that the giving of a warning of this particular risk would be regarded by most doctors as unnecessary and perhaps even undesirable. Failure to give such warning would therefore probably not be judged as negligent. The use of pumps giving jets of water at precisely controlled pressures and temperatures helps to avoid gross accidents. Even when no accident occurs, water pumps may also reduce the incidence of tinnitus from syringing, because they are less likely to cause discomfort or giddiness. But cases of tinnitus can arise even with use of a pump, as also they can with instrumental removal of wax under direct vision or by suction. There is still liable to be discomfort, pain, noise, pressure on the eardrum and, importantly, apprehension or fear.

Thus, provided there is no gross mishap, it is difficult for the claimant to prove negligence. One rare exception was a recent case in which the ear syringing was alleged to have been unnecessary in the first place. That was probably correct in fact, but in the end it was too difficult to prove. This leads to the preventive message: it is better to leave healthy wax alone, unless it is causing deafness by completely occluding the ear canal or threatening to do so. Too many things can go wrong in wax removal (Sharp et al., 1990) that it should not be undertaken unless strictly necessary.

Neck Trauma

The association of vertigo and/or imbalance with "whiplash" injuries of the neck has been recognized for decades, but tinnitus is also quite a common symptom (Claussen & Constantinescu, 1995). Typically, whiplash results from a rear-end vehicle collision, where one vehicle is stopped and another runs into the back of it. The stopped vehicle is then jerked forwards, but the inertia of the occupant's head results in violent hyperextension of the neck. Sideways collisions, and front-end ones causing rapid deceleration and forward flexion of the neck, cause whiplash-type injuries too, but of lesser degree for a given force of collision (Toglia, 1976), at least up to the time of introduction of extension-restricting cushions behind the head of the driver and passengers. Many other forms of neck injury, including those secondary to a more obvious blow to the head, can also produce whiplash-type symptoms.

The possible mechanisms by which neck injuries can result in tinnitus (Coles, 1996) include psychological triggering with a preexisting cochlear disorder, labyrinthine concussion with a preexisting cochlear disorder, labyrinthine concussion causing a temporary tinnitus which then persists due to excessive psychological response, and the noise of the impact acting as an acoustic trigger of tinnitus onset. It is apt to point out that with so many possible mechanisms of cervical tinnitus and a latency of onset of tinnitus ranging from zero to up to about four weeks, the causation, symptomatology and diagnosis are considerably uncertain. Nevertheless, compensation claims for tinnitus arising from neck injuries are not uncommon and are often successful—particularly those where there was immediate onset of tinnitus or only a short latent period, where of course the circumstantial evidence is strong.

Psychological Trauma

Acute psychological stresses and strains, and also chronic stress, have for long (Fowler 1943; Fowler & Fowler, 1948) figured in descriptions of factors which may trigger the onset of tinnitus. More recent research (Hallam et al., 1984; Hazell, 1996) continues along this theme, and also attempts to explain the mechanisms of psychological triggering. Consequently, at least in theory, cases of tinnitus triggered by the shock of some blameworthy happening would be compensable, the tinnitus sometimes even being regarded as an atypical form of post-traumatic stress disorder (see Chapter 2).

Pharmacological Injury

Cases of permanent tinnitus caused by drugs are probably rare, and even more rare as the cause of a compensation claim. While temporary tinnitus is an occasional side effect of many drugs, it occurs quite frequently with alcohol, aspirin, quinine, or other anti-malarial medications. On the other hand, a high risk of permanent ototoxic damage and associated symptoms seems largely to be limited to the cytotoxic drugs and amino-glycoside antibiotics (Miller, 1985), used respectively for treatment of cancer or life-threatening infections. Then their use is likely to be more or less essential, and any side-effects have to be accepted as a lesser evil, provided the risk of them is explained and audiological monitoring procedures are carried out where possible.

Surgical Injury

Gross negligence in selection for or performance of surgery seems to be rare nowadays, at any rate with procedures potentially leading to onset or increase of tinnitus. However, there is an unfortunate tendency in the more economically advanced countries for people to forget the possibility of misadventure or bad luck, and automatically to believe that someone must be to blame if something goes wrong with an operation, treatment, or investigation. This leads to more compensation claims than can truly be justified; and even these could have been avoided if the risks of failure, or of side effects such as tinnitus, had been more carefully explained beforehand.

The Missed Acoustic Neuroma

A considerable proportion of acoustic neuromata have as their first symptom a unilateral tinnitus. For instance, in a series of 473 cases of unilateral neuroma, Moffat et al. (1998) reported the presence of tinnitus in 73 percent and tinnitus as the principal presenting symptom in 11 percent. Failure to investigate unexplained unilateral tinnitus with such procedures as magnetic resonance imaging (MRI) may lead to delayed diagnosis and increased morbidity or even mortality, and thence to claims for compensation. It seems that almost the only really effective means of preventing this is the practice of defensive medicine.

However, this tendency may be going too far. For a start, tinnitus is a relatively uncommon form of presentation for this condition which itself is uncommon. Moreover, MRI is quite often of limited availability. This has to be contrasted with the high proportion of people in whom tinnitus is wholly or mostly unilateral, for example, 76 percent in 472 tinnitus-clinic patients (Hazell et al., 1985) and 52 percent of 1,578 people with persistent spontaneous tinnitus in an epidemiological study of the United Kingdom population (Coles, 1984).

In spite of this, few otologists faced with a case of unexplained unilateral tinnitus would dare to rely on their clinical judgment alone. Most would reach for the MRI request form. This might be to avoid possible litigation for not having immediately requested the investigation, but there is also a good clinical reason for it. While there are epidemiological data and other considerations that argue for delaying removal of small intracanalicular tumors (Cox, 1993), a policy of watchful waiting itself entails repeated MRIs, and of course you need a baseline examination against which to compare the later ones.

Triggers of Tinnitus Onset

As already mentioned here and many times in the literature (Fowler, 1943; Fowler & Fowler, 1948; Hallam et al., 1984; Hazell, 1996; Coles, 1997), the actual onset of tinnitus seems to be triggered by some event not itself likely to cause substantial structural damage in the auditory system. Examples include a quite moderate noise exposure, such as from a fairly close gunshot or firework explosion, a warning signal or a telephone malfunction. Other examples are a minor head injury, a whiplash or other neck injury, an ear syringing, or an apparently unrelated event such as emotional strain or trauma. There is usually evidence of an underlying hearing disorder, probably pre-existing such as caused by age-related disorder or noise damage, and it is probably this rather than the triggering event which is the actual cause of the tinnitus. The underlying hearing loss itself may or may not constitute ground for a compensation claim. The triggering event can additionally or alternatively be a reason for a compensation claim if it occurs in circumstances of negligence or of blameworthy injury.

A legal argument often used here is that the underlying hearing disorder, whatever its etiology, would have a low statistical probability, say 25 to 50 percent, of leading to tinnitus at some time later in life, perhaps much later. Thus, the trigger has resulted in actual tinnitus and now, rather than as a mere possibility and at some time in the future. In such statistical arguments, epidemiological data (see Chapter 1; also Coles et al., 1990) can be used to estimate the probabilities of occurrence of tinnitus in various degrees of severity that might be associated with the particular degree of underlying conductive or sensorineural hearing disorder.

Other Causes of Compensable Tinnitus

The previous list of factors leading to tinnitus that might be subject to compensation claim is unlikely to be complete and should not be regarded as such. Indeed, any form of culpable injury, or failure to apply reasonable preventive measures, that directly or indirectly leads to causation of tinnitus or triggering of its onset has the potentiality for a compensation claim.

Tinnitus Onset After End of Period of Noise Exposure

Noise-induced tinnitus can probably arise years after the period of unprotected noise exposure has ceased. The argument is as follows. Epidemiological evidence (Coles et al., 1990; Davis et al., 1992; Chapter 1) indicates that what matters most in the prevalence of troublesome or persistent tinnitus is the amount of hearing disorder, as measured by the hearing threshold levels at the higher frequencies, rather than the actual cause of the disorder such as aging or noise expo-

sure. Those causes lose their significance as determinants of tinnitus prevalence, once account is taken of the high-tone hearing loss. This supports the long-standing clinical dictum that: "Whatever caused the hearing loss, most probably caused the tinnitus too." Most probably, but not certainly: but sufficiently probable that the onus on the diagnostician is to prove the exception rather than the rule. Thus, if the cause of the hearing loss is a cumulation of noise-induced and age-related disorders, then it is probable that a tinnitus coming on years after a period of noise exposure has ceased is due to that cumulated disorder, that is, noise damage as well as the age-related degeneration.

This of course is parallel to the situation where some NIHL may lead to little practical hearing difficulty at the time of its causation, but with added age-related hearing loss may lead to considerable hearing problems later in life. A defendant (potential compensation payer) may argue that the hearing difficulty or tinnitus cannot be due to noise because its onset occurred after the noise exposures ceased. The plaintiff (or claimant) would have to agree that the later onset must be due, at least in part, to addition of hearing loss of other causation, most commonly age-related hearing loss. On the other hand, the defendant would find it difficult to deny that the hearing difficulty would be less severe, and in some cases nonexistent, if there was not the component of noise damage.

Coming back to tinnitus, take as an example a man aged 25 years with a considerable degree of NIHL, whose hearing thresholds at 4 kHz are 45 dB HL. He then moves to quiet work. At age 40 years, he gradually develops a troublesome high-pitched ringing tinnitus. Investigation reveals that his hearing loss has increased by 5 dB, to 50 dB —what might be expected from aging increments. It seems wholly unreasonable and biologically unlikely to postulate that the cause of tinnitus is associated solely with just the 5 dB of age-related hearing loss and has nothing to do with the underlying noise damage sufficient to cause 45 dB of the 50 dB hearing loss. If that were to be maintained, it would mean that the 5 dB "age-effect" on its own would have been associated with onset of tinnitus. That would be difficult to explain if 45 dB of NIHL was not so associated.

Alternatively, this question can be looked at statistically. According to data from the United Kingdom National Study of Hearing, shown here as Figure 17-1, the prevalence of moderately or severely annoying tinnitus can be predicted from the hearing levels at 4 kHz. Let us say that at age 40 this man's likely age-related hearing loss on its own is 5 dB HL, the NIHL is 45 dB HL, and the combined loss 50 dB HL. The expected prevalences of this degree of tinnitus in persons having these hearing losses would be about 1 percent, 10 percent, and 12 percent respectively. That is about twelve times more likely with that degree of NIHL than without it.

ROUTES FOR COMPENSATION CLAIMS

There are wide differences between countries in the provision, availability, and methods for compensation for injuries and bodily illnesses, and tinnitus is no exception. On the other hand there are certain principles that apply in whole or part in many countries and it will be helpful to outline these. They are in fact well illustrated by the various routes to compensation which apply in the United Kingdom and which have been comprehensively reviewed with respect to hearing loss and tinnitus by Hinchcliffe and King (1992).

There are two main routes to compensation—statutory law and common law. Often, the two systems are mutually exclusive: either one system operates throughout the country or state, or the other does. In the United Kingdom though, a worker can have "two bites at the same cherry"—a

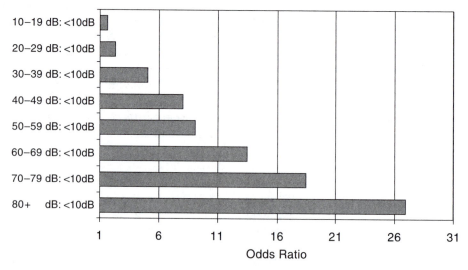

FIGURE 17-1. Relationship between hearing thresholds and prevalence of moderately or severely annoying tinnitus

(Tier B data from United Kingdom National Study of Hearing; Phases 1, 2, and 3 combined; n = 2,522 subjects). (Note: The prevalence in those with HTLs at 4 kHz of less than 10 dB was 1.3 percent).

second bite if the first is not large enough. This may seem curious, but it is actually much fairer for those who are not covered, or are dealt with rather harshly, by the statutory system.

Statutory Law

Statutory law refers to the laws and regulations laid down by the government of the country, state, or province. Typically in the present context, they would refer to health and safety, industrial injuries and diseases, and worker's compensation. They might also include military servicemen's disability pensions, and compensation for criminal or terrorist injuries. They may be administered by government departments or through work-related insurance schemes. While diagnosis and quantitative assessment for compensation is the major interest here, the laws and governmental regulations, codes, and guidance documents aimed at prevention of occupational disease or injury, such as NIHL, are sometimes relevant as well. This is in common-law compensation where negligence by the employer or some other person has also to be proven.

In most cases, the statutory law covering compensation for hearing loss, and sometimes tinnitus in addition, sets out fairly rigid scales. These relate impairment, as usually measured by pure-tone audiometry, either directly to some monetary scale or indirectly via an assessment of percentage hearing or whole-body disability. There is usually much argument as to whether in general the monetary figure is adequate and whether the starting level for payment, the "low fence," is reasonable. But when it comes to individuals, it has to be accepted that such scales can only provide rough justice. For instance, two individuals with the same audiogram may have very different degrees of hearing disability and handicap. Moreover, any such scale usually relates to an average of hearing thresholds over a particular set of audiometric frequencies, for example, 1, 2, and 3 kHz. Two individuals having the same average hearing loss over those assessment frequencies may have very different degrees of hearing loss at other frequencies and hence of hearing disability.

In a few countries an additional sum is payable if there is also a troublesome degree of tinnitus, but often this is conditional on having sufficient hearing loss to qualify for compensation for the hearing loss. Cases of severe tinnitus associated with minor degrees of hearing loss are usually not eligible for compensation under statutory regulations.

On the other hand, injuries sustained as a result of an accident or other form of acute injury are in some countries dealt with by regulations of a more generous and flexible nature. Tinnitus may then be more fairly assessed and compensated.

Common Law

Action under common law is where one person sues another (or others) for compensation for some injury or ill health that had resulted, in a reasonably foreseeable and preventable way, from the act or omission of that other person. Such legal action is open to virtually everyone in the case of nonoccupational injuries, but suing an account of occupational injury or disease is excluded in many countries where worker's compensation regulations apply.

There are important differences between compensation claims under common law and those under statutory regulations (Table 17-1). For instance, in common law, not only does cause and effect have to be proven, usually on a criterion of "balance of probabilities" or "more likely than not," but also a significant part of the injury has to be shown to have arisen out of the negligence of the defendant. Account is also taken of the effect of the hearing impairment and/or tinnitus on the particular claimant's hearing ability, lifestyle, and employability and on his/her family, that is, its disabling and handicapping effects in current WHO

Table 17-1. Comparison of statutory and common law (in cases of noise-induced hearing disorder)

Issue	Statutory Law	Common Law
Specified occupations or amounts of noise exposure	Often	No
Proof of negligence	Not required	Required
Compensation scale	Rigid, specified frequencies	Flexible, often based on case law
Low fence of HTL	Usual, more than minimal	None or minimal
Extra compensation		
• for loss of earnings	No	Yes
• for cost of treatment	No, but hearing aids may be provided	Often
• for greater than average disability or handicap	Rarely	Yes
• for troublesome tinnitus	In some systems	Yes
• for troublesome hyperacusis	No	Yes

terminology (World Health Organization, 1980), or its limitation in activity and restriction in participation effects to use the draft new terminology (WHO, 1997).

Set scales relating impairment to compensation usually do not apply at all, or at least can be forcefully argued against as not strictly applicable to the particular claimant. The result is that quite small degrees of NIHL, such as 5 or 10 dB, may be compensated. Likewise, hearing losses largely or entirely outside the assessment frequencies usual for that country are compensable if considered to be noise-induced and associated with hearing disability. In the same way, tinnitus is more realistically evaluated and compensated, even when there is little associated hearing loss. Hyperacusis which so often accompanies tinnitus (Tyler & Conrad-Armes, 1983a; Coles & Sood, 1988; Hazell & Sheldrake, 1992), can also receive the compensation it may well deserve. The effects of tinnitus and/or hyperacusis sometimes result in large awards on grounds of actual and potential loss of earnings. Special

damages, covering costs of ongoing medical treatment, may also be awarded.

Such court actions are, of course, of adversarial nature and therefore involve large legal costs—often very much larger than the damages awarded. These are usually recovered by the successful plaintiff. Nevertheless, because of the high costs and considerable delays involved in preparing cases every one of which has the potentiality of coming to court, the uncertainty of result in court and the understandable apprehension of most claimants at the prospect of having to go to court, the vast majority of cases are settled by prior negotiation between the legal representatives of claimant and defendant, often between the trade union and the insurance company in fact. In this way, the advantages of flexibility and fairness are combined with relative speed and ease of administration, but often with a slight discount in quantum of damages. Alternatively, settlement schemes may be used to speed things still further, as described in the next section.

Contract Law

Where there are large numbers of common-law claimants against one employer or against several employers using the same insurance company, and the claimants' trade unions are anxious to minimize costs and delay, they may enter into a contract with the employers or insurance company. They then agree to a settlement scheme which avoids the costs and personal anxieties involved in proving noise exposure and negligence. As such, it is a variant on common law but has most of the features of statutory law.

Further advantages to the claimants come from the much increased speed of the process, but these are usually at the price of a considerably reduced scale of monetary award and loss of flexibility in dealing with individual circumstances. The trade unions involved may also have to agree that they will not support a member's claim made outside the contracted scheme. Usually such schemes will cover tinnitus of moderately or severely troublesome nature, but simply by means of an additional lump sum payment and taking no account of the sometimes devastating effects of tinnitus.

DIAGNOSIS OF NOISE-INDUCED TINNITUS

Criterion of Proof

For virtually every compensation purpose, the criterion of proof is that described as "on the balance of probabilities" or "more likely than not." The onus of proof however is on the plaintiff or claimant, and so a diagnostic odds of 50:50 is insufficient. Mathematically, it could be put as requiring a 51 percent or greater probability. This in fact is a great help in arriving at a diagnosis for legal purposes and the question "Is it more likely than not that the noise exposure was at least partly the cause of the tinnitus?" should always be kept in mind.

Evidence of Damaged Hearing

Usually a diagnosis of noise-induced tinnitus cannot be made in absence of a diagnosis of NIHL. An exception to this generalization might be where there was no identifiable NIHL, but the person had noticed prominent tinnitus following daily noise exposures and the duration of this tinnitus gradually lengthened, perhaps after a while only disappearing after a weekend's quiet, and then only after a whole week or two on vacation, and finally becoming permanent. Another possible exception is where there has been a single severe noise exposure or explosion that did not cause an identifiable permanent hearing loss, but nevertheless caused an immediate tinnitus which then persisted. This could arise by several possible mechanisms: (1) a small amount of cochlear damage or additional damage sufficient to cause a change in ongoing auditory neuronal activity, or (2) the tinnitus-exacerbating and perpetuating effect of excessive anxiety about the postexposure tinnitus, or (3) a triggering off of onset of tinnitus in a predisposed ear, as already discussed.

Onset of Tinnitus

Most commonly the noise-induced tinnitus gradually builds up from something barely noticeable at first, until it eventually gets to a point where it can no longer be ignored. Sometimes the tinnitus appears to come on suddenly, but in many such instances it seems more likely that it has been gradually developing and has been suddenly noticed. Because of that possibility, a tinnitus appearing to have come on suddenly should not automatically be attributed to something other than noise damage.

It is sometimes said that a noise-induced tinnitus nearly always comes on early in a period of noise exposure and then usually recedes either of itself or due to habituation processes (Hinchcliffe & King, 1992). However, other authors (Sacher, 1927; McShane et al., 1988; Axelsson & Barrenäs, 1992) indicate that the tinnitus frequently comes on considerably later. Tinnitus is often first noticed at the same time as the first awareness of hearing difficulties, possibly being the factor drawing attention to them. Sometimes its onset is not until well after the hearing loss has been noticed. Further, as argued elsewhere (Coles et al., 1990; Coles, 1997) and earlier in this chapter, the tinnitus may come on some years after noise exposure has ceased and yet still be attributable in part to the underlying noise damage.

Since the majority of claims for compensation for tinnitus relate to chronic noise-induced tinnitus, this section and subsequent ones will relate primarily to that condition. However, many of the features of diagnosis, severity, prognosis, and detection of feigned or exaggerated tinnitus apply also to other causations of tinnitus for which compensation claims may be made.

Character of Tinnitus

Usually the tinnitus is of a continuous type. But it may be intermittent at first. Quite often a person will describe his tinnitus as intermittent, but on further questioning it is found that the intermittency relates to periods when the tinnitus is not heard due to masking by ambient noise or to the person being asleep or it is not noticed due to distraction by other activities. Using questionnaire data from tinnitus patients, Stouffer and Tyler (1990) found that only 68 percent of their 528 respondents recorded their tinnitus as present for over 80 percent of their time while awake. But this may have been more a reflection on their degree of conscious awareness of the tinnitus, as distinct from its actual presence or absence. Indeed, Jastreboff (1998) recommends using the percentage of time that the patient is aware of the tinnitus as a principal metric of outcome of treatment. As an example of this, Sheldrake et al. (1996) reported reductions of awareness time of 58 percent in 130 treated patients, although it is notable that in those not reporting improvement the awareness percentage remained at just over 80 percent. It is suspected that in most of these cases the tinnitus would have been present whenever they were awake, if in fact they were reminded to listen for it.

Often the tinnitus is at a constant level, but sometimes it increases for a while either spontaneously or in relation to stress, tiredness, or exposure to noise. The general tendency is for the patient to habituate to the tinnitus such that it gradually becomes less troublesome, and it may indeed also become less loud. Nevertheless, the natural history of tinnitus is that in occasional cases it increases, often for no apparent reason.

Most commonly the person with noise-induced tinnitus will describe his tinnitus in words suggesting a high-pitched type of sound. Such descriptors as singing, whistling, hissing, ringing, shrieking, piercing, a high-pitched buzz or hum, or even "like cicadas" may be used (Stouffer & Tyler, 1990). The description of the sound may help slightly in diagnosis (Douek & Reid, 1981), for instance to separate out the usual low-frequency descriptors arising from somatosounds (Anon, 1981) and Ménière's disorder. However, the evidence from such descriptions must be used with great caution. Even within a diagnostic category or a particular audiometric configuration, tinnitus sounds seem to vary widely from one person to another and often defy description. Moreover, there may be several sounds constantly present, or intermittent addition of other sounds which may be as short as clicking or ticking sounds. Further, as with any ongoing tinnitus, it may be modulated by the pulse causing an additional throbbing or pulsing element, most commonly when the person is lying down at night. Careful questioning will reveal whether it is merely a pulsatile modulation of an ongoing tinnitus such as noise-induced tinnitus, or a purely pulsing sound which of course would have a different etiology altogether (see Chapter 9).

Pitch Matching

Most commonly, the tinnitus associated with NIHL is pitched close to the frequency of maximum hearing loss (Axelsson & Sandh, 1985). But quite frequently it is at frequencies below or above that, and sometimes at an octave below the last normal-hearing frequency. Occasionally it appears to be present even at low frequencies (Axelsson & Sandh, 1985), but whether that is truly so or whether such findings are the result of the inherent difficulties for the patient in matching his tinnitus is uncertain. I well remember an individual case who saw me one day and I measured his tinnitus pitch at 8 kHz, and he was seen by another expert witness the next day and he measured it at 250 Hz; and that in spite of the patient saying that the tinnitus had not changed! It is evident therefore that not much diagnostic reliance should be placed on either the results of pitch-matching tests (see Chapter 6) or their diagnostic interpretation. Nevertheless, it remains a factor to take into account when assessing the diagnosis in a case of alleged noise-induced tinnitus.

Loudness Matching

It might be thought that the severity of tinnitus depended principally on its loudness, but in fact research studies (Fowler, 1943; Hallam et al., 1984; Meikle et al., 1984; Jakes et al., 1986) have repeatedly shown that although there is a positive correlation between severity and loudness measurements expressed in HL on SL units, it is usually rather poor. Better correlations have been found with subjective loudness scaling or if the person's individual loudness scale is also measured (Hinchcliffe & Chambers, 1983), but the procedures for the latter are relatively complicated and time-consuming and are probably not worthwhile for the present purposes. For loudness matching (Chapter 6) use of an ordinary clinical audiometer is simpler and quicker. Some idea of the likely true loudness can then be obtained by conversion of the results into "effective loudness level," using the method of Matsuhira et al. (1992) or of Tyler et al. (1992).

Minimal Masking Level Measurements

Minimal masking levels of tinnitus can also be measured (Chapter 6) but, as with loudness matching (Coles & Baskill, 1996), there are many procedural uncertainties with both tests. Moreover, the phenomenon of masking decay (Penner et al., 1981) with a continuous masking sound may mean that the results of masking tests relate poorly to degree of tinnitus intrusiveness in everyday life. Of much greater practical help is a carefully taken history of what levels and kinds of everyday sounds render the tinnitus inaudible to the patient. Even in clinical work, it is noteworthy that loudness match and minimal masking levels have been found to have no correlation with tinnitus-related distress (Jastreboff, 1996; Dineen et al., 1997) and too weak a relation with decreasing tinnitus awareness (Jastreboff et al., 1994) to be useful for monitoring treatment (Jastreboff, 1996).

Clinical Examination

As usual, a lookout has to be kept for any substantial diagnostic competitor. This may be revealed from the description of the tinnitus and hearing loss, from the past and present medical history, from the presence of vestibular symptoms, signs and test results, and from other audiological or medical tests.

Tinnitus quite often occurs in people with normal hearing. Stouffer and Tyler (1990) quote three studies of tinnitus patients in whom 20 to 22 percent had subjectively normal hearing. In a large epidemiological study (Coles et al., 1990) just under 10 percent of over 23,000 subjects reported having experienced prolonged spontaneous tinnitus, and of these 56 percent reported no hearing difficulty.

In their own study however, Stouffer and Tyler (1990) found that 18 percent of their 528 tinnitus patients had hearing thresholds at 1 and 4 kHz not exceeding 25 dB HL. They felt it likely that many of these patients had high-frequency hearing losses, and suspected that the percentage of tinnitus patients with normal hearing has been overestimated. Hazell (1996) on the other hand reported a much higher percentage with normal hearing: in 48 percent of 100 tinnitus clinic patients, when normality was defined as hearing thresholds not exceeding 20 dB up to 4 kHz or 30 dB at 6 and 8 kHz. To which ear or ears this applied is not stated, but even if it referred to the better ear only the percentage is remarkably high.

At the other end of the scale, and more in keeping with Stouffer and Tyler's ideas, is a study by Baskill and Coles (1996). Calculations from their reported data suggest that about 15 percent of the ears in 354 tinnitus clinic patients would have had normal hearing, defined by thresholds not exceeding 20 dB at any of eight test frequencies in the range 0.25 to 8 kHz. From the original data, it has been calculated that this proportion drops to only 11 percent if the nontinnitus ears of patients with unilateral tinnitus are excluded. Nevertheless, it is evident that tinnitus does indeed occur with audiometrically normal hearing.

There is also increasing evidence that considerable damage can be done to the internal ear before there is any effect on the threshold of hearing. For instance, Bohne and Clarke (1982) reported noise-induced losses of outer hair cells in the chinchilla of up to 30 percent before permanent threshold shift resulted. Presumably this was due to an inherent redundancy in the number of outer hair cells with respect to threshold of hearing. In man, such hair cell loss may however be responsible for the various other dysfunctions such as disturbances of frequency resolution or abnormalities of otoacoustic emissions (Sallustio et al., 1998), or generation of tinnitus, that sometimes occur without any evident abnormality in the ordinary clinical audiogram. Of particu-

lar relevance in this context is the study of hearing in young people by Smith et al. (1998). Out of 346 randomly selected young adults, 19 percent reported social noise exposure exceeding a criterion amount. They did not have significantly worse hearing than the 81 percent with lesser exposure, but 20 percent of them reported prolonged spontaneous tinnitus as compared with only 7 percent in the less exposed group.

Likewise, tinnitus sometimes occurs where there is no evident abnormality of hearing whatsoever. Perhaps some of these cases are due to hearing what might be called physiological tinnitus, as shown in the classical experiment by Heller and Bergman (1953). In this, they put eighty normally hearing subjects in a soundproof room, one at a time, for up to 5 minutes, and asked them to make notes on the sounds they could detect. Seventy-five of them reported a total of twenty-three descriptions of sounds heard, the most frequent of which were humming, buzzing, and ringing. From their descriptions, many of the sounds reported seem more likely to have a cochlear origin than a physiological extra-auditory source.

Thus, it seems likely that there can be a real disorder of hearing and yet the audiogram appears totally normal. Some of these cases may well have been caused by noise. Nevertheless, one can still only rarely make a diagnosis of noise-induced tinnitus without evidence of noise damage in the puretone audiogram.

Severity

As with any body disorder that may be compensable, the monetary value will depend heavily on the degree of disability, handicap, or suffering caused. In the case of tinnitus, the distress it causes is only poorly assessed by measurements of its loudness. That is not to say that loudness is wholly unimportant because if, either spontaneously or as a result of treatment, the loudness is reduced, then the patient will be very pleased. Likewise, anything which makes the tinnitus louder will make it worse. But there are many other factors that influence the severity of tinnitus, many of them in the psychological domain (Erlandsson et al., 1992; Chapter 2; Lindberg et al., 1984; Tyler et al., 1992; Chapter 6).

With respect to the tinnitus sound itself, the actual nature of the sound may be important. Our tests may give some sort of indication on the pitch of the tinnitus, and in the infrequent cases of wholly tonal tinnitus, pitch matching may give a fairly accurate measurement and representation of the sound actually being heard (Tyler & Conrad-Armes, 1983b; Chapter 6). But, if pressed, the patient will almost always say that there is no external sound that quite resembles his tinnitus. Often he finds it almost impossible even to describe. Our tests may give some information on its pitch, loudness, and maskability, but they tell us virtually nothing about the actual quality of the sound. Some sounds seem to be inherently unpleasant, what might be called "dysphony." In this connection, we only have to think of the unpleasantness of the screech from a piece of chalk on a blackboard. This may not be very intense in terms of decibels, but is extremely unpleasant. In clinical assessment therefore, and in therapy of tinnitus, we have to be careful not to regard someone who is very upset by a not-very-loud tinnitus as psychologically overreacting (Coles & Baskill, 1996). The actual sound that is being heard may in fact be quite horrible.

What really matters though is the effect of the tinnitus on the person. This is important therapeutically too, as modern concepts of treatment of tinnitus, described as "tinnitus retraining therapy" (Jastreboff & Hazell, 1993; Jastreboff, 1998; Chapter 15), depend heavily on altering the person's reaction to their tinnitus. Thus, for a legal report, one has to get a careful description of the actual effects of the tinnitus on that individual. Initially, this should be done by nonleading questions: simply asking the person to describe his tinnitus and its effects on him. But some people are reticent or inarticulate, and leading questions will often be needed

to ascertain these effects and/or to elaborate the details. For instance, in a case where the tinnitus is causing difficulty in sleeping, one wants to know whether it is in getting to sleep or getting back to sleep after waking or both, about how long is each delay, and about how many nights of the week this occurs. The legal report has to distinguish between what is being said in answer to nonleading questions and to leading questions. A questionnaire could be used, but this is probably going too far in the direction of leading questions. A checklist along the lines of the list of tinnitus effects quoted in the literature, (Tyler & Baker, 1983) would be more appropriate.

The difficulty in all this is that we are largely dependent on what the claimant tells us. Consequently, we have to also make a general assessment of his apparent credibility. His "auditory honesty" can be checked by comparison of his volunteered audiometric thresholds with those obtained objectively by cortical electric response audiometry (Coles & Mason, 1984). His medical documents need to be checked to find out what help he may or may not have sought for this tinnitus. It would be difficult to believe a claimant describing severe effects of tinnitus if he had never bothered to go and see his doctor about it. But even then, we have to be careful and enquire whether there is any reason why he has not seen his doctor. The dismissive response to tinnitus by many doctors, including some otologists, if experienced by the claimant himself or by a colleague, friend, or relative, may make him feel that a visit to the doctor would be a waste of time.

As yet, there is no physical measurement that can tell us the severity of tinnitus. Simple mathematical scaling of severity by the claimant, for instance, from 1 to 10 or 1 to 100, is too subjective and lacking in detail. A detailed description of its effects is needed. These may then be summarized into one word, such as mild, moderate or severe. Sometimes a set sum of money is paid for "moderate" tinnitus, and more for "severe" tinnitus, but none at all for "mild" tinnitus.

Such a three-grade scale is often too restricting though, and it would be better to use a wider range of severity descriptors.

PROGNOSIS AND TREATMENT

In statutory compensation and contracted settlement schemes, the amount of compensation paid is usually a fixed sum with little or no scope for variation. But in common law almost any additional factor can be taken into account. There are three main additional issues in such cases.

Earning Capacity

Tinnitus can have a very severe effect on a person's life and this may include inability to work (Sinclair & Coles, 1995). The latter may result in a claim for compensation for actual loss of earnings, and expected further loss in the future. These factors have led to tinnitus sometimes receiving very much more compensation than hearing loss.

Prognosis

The courts will also attempt to make some allowance for the prognosis, perhaps reducing the amount of compensation if reduction of severity or recovery is to be expected. It is extremely difficult to make any predictions about the prognosis for tinnitus. The tendency is towards gradual habituation, but it is usually only partial (Coles et al., 1990). However, the very fact of having a claim pending is likely to delay habituation. Often it takes years before a case is finally settled and further habituation may thus be delayed or even prevented. The prognosis most usually given by the writer in a legal report is that the severity is not likely to change substantially.

Treatment

Sometimes a claim is made for "special damages," which means additional money to pay for treatment, such as by hearing aids, tinnitus maskers, and/or a long course of counseling. But in the writer's experience it is best to keep the legal aspects and therapeutic aspects apart. Naturally if the defense is being asked for money for treatment, it will expect that treatment to be carried out. It will then want to consider the results and, if the treatment is successful, reduce the compensation paid. But in view of the influence of psychological factors on tinnitus severity, having a legal case pending with all its frequent reminders of how bad the condition is, of how someone's negligence caused it to happen, and of other associated grievances are the very worst thing possible for the tinnitus. It is highly counterproductive to the most common aim of therapy, to enhance habituation. It is probably better therefore to try to get the case settled as it is, and estimate the prognosis as it would be if no special treatment was to be given. It is then up to the claimant whether or not to spend part of his award on treatment.

FEIGNING AND EXAGGERATION

Naturally, where there is financial advantage to be gained by falsification, some claimants will totally fabricate symptoms and others will tend to exaggerate their severity. The examiner must always keep in mind this strong motivation for feigning or exaggeration. There are several indicators that should make the examiner particularly suspicious, but as yet there are no objective tests that can prove or disapprove the presence of tinnitus, let alone measure its severity.

Some authorities use a set of guidelines for the assessment of the validity of tinnitus claims. As an example, there are those used by the United States Veterans Administration. According to Dobie (1993) they are as follows. The complaint of tinnitus must have been unsolicited, and should have been be recorded in the claimant's medical documents prior to the claim. The tinnitus must accompany a compensable level of hearing loss. The treatment history must include one or more attempts to alleviate the tinnitus. There must be evidence in support of any claim for personality change or sleep disorder. There has to be no contributory history of substance abuse. Complaints of tinnitus must be supported by statements from family or significant others. Dobie then goes on to say: "The ultimate assessment is, of course, made by the jury."

In the writer's opinion, these requirements are somewhat draconian and unlikely to be accepted under common law. In that, there are no assessment rules other than having to meet the balance of probabilities criterion as applied to diagnosis and degree of effect, sufficiency of causative noise and proof of negligence. On the whole judges, and probably juries too where applicable, tend to accept what the plaintiff says, basically believing him to be honest unless there is good reason to think otherwise. That is my own premise in dealing with such cases, but taking account of any warning signs of possible feigning, exaggeration, or other untruth.

Warning Signs of Feigned or Exaggerated Tinnitus

Perhaps the most valuable test is to check the claimant's "auditory honesty." This is done by comparing his volunteered audiogram with an objective audiogram obtained by electric response audiometry, either by the brain stem responses or preferably by the more tone-specific cortical or slow vertex ones. If, in a case of alleged NIHL, the volunteered threshold level at 500 Hz is over 25 dB HL (Coles & Mason, 1984) or 35 dB HL (Alberti et al., 1978) it is advisable to check the audiogram objectively. This is because when people exaggerate their hearing loss they usually adopt a certain loudness level of test signal as their apparent threshold, commonly at about 40 to 70 phons. The damaging effects of noise are greatest around 4 kHz and slightest at about 500 Hz.

But due to there being more loudness recruitment where the hearing loss is greater, the equal-loudness contoured audiogram becomes flattened (Coles & Mason, 1984), such that the objective/subjective test difference will be smallest around 4 kHz and largest at low frequencies. Objective tests at low frequencies are therefore likely to be more sensitive in detecting false results. If the honesty at audiometry is thereby impugned, how can one then accept as truthful what the plaintiff says about his tinnitus?

Someone with a troublesome tinnitus will certainly be able to describe it and its effects. Consequently, inability to do this is highly suspicious. When questioned about this, one claimant went on to admit that his trade union had told him to "be sure to tell Dr. Coles that you have tinnitus as well." But when I asked him to describe his tinnitus, it became evident that he did not even know what the word meant.

It has already been mentioned that a person with seriously troublesome tinnitus would normally be expected to have seen his doctor, unless there is some valid reason for not doing so.

Since tinnitus is a purely subjective phenomenon and dependent for its diagnosis and severity assessment on what the patient tells us, substantial discrepancies without reasonable explanation must cause suspicion. Examples include differences in the history as given to different people, or in test results from one occasion to another, or between the history given and the content of the claimant's medical documents. While generally believing what a patient tells us will tend to tip a diagnostic opinion or severity assessment over the criterion of "more probably than not," so any substantial evidence that the particular person is not to be relied on in some related respect may well lead us to feel that this legal criterion has not been met.

Some noise-induced tinnitus can be intermittent, but usually it is continuous. The history taken should identify the degree to which the tinnitus is usually present. Consequently, if it is said to be always present but it is not there when it comes to be tested, then this is suspicious.

If the tinnitus pitch is more than an octave below the highest test frequency at which he has no apparent noise-induced hearing loss, then it is unlike a noise-induced tinnitus and this finding should at least cause the examiner to take a hard look at the overall evidence. The pitch-matching test result could be right, and the tinnitus nothing to do with noise. On the other hand, pitch matching is not an easy task for the testee and its result may be spurious.

It is often said that the loudness of tinnitus is seldom matched by a sound at more than 15 dB SL (sensation level). This is true where the tinnitus loudness is measured using an ear and frequency of signal where there is substantial cochlear hearing loss. Because of loudness recruitment, a sound at 15 dB SL may in fact be quite loud (Tyler & Conrad-Armes, 1983a). The effective loudness level of the tinnitus may be up to 70 dB HL according to Coles and Baskill (1996), who used the method of Matsuhira et al. (1992) to convert loudness match data into readily understandable units of loudness level as if heard by a normally-hearing person. Such loudness levels can often be measured directly if one follows the test recommendation of Goodwin and Johnson (1980), to use the best-hearing frequency in either ear for loudness matching. That is, provided there is little or no hearing loss at that frequency. Then the loudness sensation level could be quite high, a lot higher than 15 dB SL. Thus, the results of tinnitus loudness matches when expressed in SL units depend greatly on how much hearing loss there is at the frequency and ear selected for the test. Nevertheless, if loudness matches are done at a frequency at which there is substantial cochlear hearing loss, the SL will only exceed 15 dB in 4 percent of cases (Meikle & Taylor-Walsh, 1984). If it is greater, the results are at least unusual and suspicious of exaggeration.

Likewise, having five or six loudness matches repeat to within 2 dB (see Vernon's "2 dB rule"; Vernon, 1996) may often be achievable where the test signals are delivered to an ear and at a frequency where there is a considerable degree of recruitment. In the absence of recruitment, the variability is usually much higher, perhaps with a variability range as large as 10 dB. Consequently repeatability measurements of tinnitus loudness, or of maskability, have to be interpreted with great caution (Chapter 6).

Measurements of tinnitus loudness and maskability, and their repeatability, are often regarded as being very relevant to the assessment of tinnitus and even for checking the validity of a person's claim to have tinnitus (Vernon, 1996). However, in the present author's opinion, these tests have major limitations and problems associated with them, such that he does not often use them and, if demanded by the lawyer, he largely discounts their results in his report. There have been a number of studies looking at the accuracy of these tests, but many of them have used carefully selected cases of tinnitus, for instance with just one tinnitus sound, often of tonal type, and unilateral. Moreover, the exact methodology of how the tests were carried out is often very incompletely described.

For legal purposes, it seems better to get an account of the actual effects of the tinnitus on the particular person, and of the degree to which everyday sounds and other activities may cause the tinnitus to be masked or not be noticed. Repeatability of loudness and maskability tests for purposes of checking validity of the tinnitus can occasionally be useful, but there are so many problems of methodology and interpretation, to say nothing of the difficulties for the person being tested, that a poor degree of repeatability cannot reliably be accepted as evidence of feigning or exaggeration. With respect to assessment of severity of the tinnitus, the results of tinnitus tests bear only a poor relation to its severity and intrusiveness in the person's everyday life (although for a contrasting viewpoint, see Chapter 6).

SUMMARY

Many types of injury can lead to compensation claims for tinnitus. The most common is tinnitus in association with noise-induced hearing loss, but claims also arise from acute acoustic trauma, head or ear injury, ear syringing, neck trauma, psychological trauma, pharmacological injury, and surgical injury. Tinnitus sometimes shows as the first symptom of an acoustic neuroma and failure to investigate an unexplained unilateral tinnitus may lead to litigation, if subsequently the tinnitus is found to be due to an acoustic neuroma.

It is important to distinguish between causes of tinnitus and triggers of its onset. Compensation claims may be directed to one or other or both, according to circumstances.

There are two main routes to compensation: statutory law and common law, the principal features of which are discussed. The factors involved in arriving at a diagnosis of noise-induced tinnitus are presented, much of which applies also to other forms of compensable tinnitus. Concerning the severity of tinnitus, it is concluded that a good history is far more important than any tests. Assessment has also to cover prognosis and treatment, and deal with the potential problem of feigned or exaggerated tinnitus.

REFERENCES

Alberti, P. W. (1987). Tinnitus in occupational hearing loss: Nosological aspects. *Journal of Otolaryngology, 16,* 34–35.

Alberti, P. W., Morgan P. P., & Czuba, I. (1978). Speech and pure-tone audiometry as a screen for exaggerated hearing loss in industrial claims. *Acta Otolaryngologica, 87,* 728–731.

Anonymous. (1981). Definition and classification of tinnitus. In D. Evered & G. Lawrenson (Eds.), *Tinnitus: CIBA Foundation Symposium 85* (pp. 300–302). London: Pitman.

Axelsson, A., & Barrenäs, M. L. (1992). Tinnitus in noise-induced hearing loss. In A.L. Dancer, D. Henderson, R. J. Salvi, & R. P. Hamernik (Eds.), *Noise-induced hearing loss* (pp. 269–276). St. Louis: Mosby.

Axelsson, A., & Sandh, A. (1985). Tinnitus in noise-induced hearing loss. *British Journal of Audiology, 19,* 271–276.

Baskill, J. L., & Coles, R. R. A. (1996). A two-year study of SOAEs in tinnitus clinic patients. In G. E. Reich & J. A. Vernon (Eds.), *Proceedings of the Fifth International Tinnitus Seminar, Portland, 1995* (pp. 31–37). Portland, OR: American Tinnitus Association.

Bohne, B. A., & Clark, W. W. (1982). Growth of hearing loss and cochlear lesion with increasing duration of noise exposure. In R. P. Hamernik, D. Henderson, & R. Salvi (Eds.), *New perspectives on noise-induced hearing loss* (pp. 283–302). New York: Raven.

Claussen, C. F., & Constantinescu, L. (1995). Tinitus in whiplash injury. *International Tinnitus Journal, 1,* 105–114.

Coles, R., Smith, P., & Davis, A. (1990). The relationships between noise-induced hearing loss and tinnitus and its management. In B. Berglund & T. Lindval (Eds.), *Noise as a public health problem: Vol. 4, New advances in noise research, Part 1* (pp. 87–112). Stockholm: Swedish Council for Building Research.

Coles, R. R. A. (1984). Epidemiology of tinnitus: (2) Demographic and clinical features. *Journal of Laryngology and Otology* (Suppl. 9), 195–202.

Coles, R. R. A. (1996). Compensable tinnitus from causes other than noise. In G. E. Reich & J. A. Vernon (Eds.), *Proceedings of the Fifth International Tinnitus Seminar, Portland, 1995* (pp. 367–382). Portland, OR: American Tinnitus Association.

Coles, R. R. A. (1997). Tinnitus. In S. D. G. Stephens (Vol. Ed.), *Scott-Brown's otolaryngology* (6th ed., vol. 2, pp. 2/18/1–34). Oxford: Butterworth Heinemann.

Coles, R. R. A., & Baskill, J. L. (1996). Absolute loudness of tinnitus: Tinnitus clinic data. In G. E. Reich & J. A. Vernon (Eds.), *Proceedings of the Fifth International Seminar, Portland, 1995* (pp. 135–141). Portland, OR: American Tinnitus Association.

Coles, R. R. A., & Mason, S. M. (1984). The results of cortical electric response audiometry in medico-legal investigations. *British Journal of Audiology, 18,* 71–78.

Coles, R. R. A., & Sood, S. K. (1988). Hyperacusis and phonophobia in tinnitus patients. *British Journal of Audiology, 22,* 228.

Cox, G. I. (1993). Intracanalicular acoustic neuromas: A conservative approach. *Clinical Otolaryngology, 18,* 153–154.

Davis, A. C., Coles, R. R. A., Smith, P. A., & Spencer, H. S. (1992). Factors influencing tinnitus report in Great Britain. In J. M. Aran & R. Dauman (Eds.), *Proceedings of the Fourth International Tinnitus Seminar, Bordeaux, 1991* (pp. 239–243). Amsterdam: Kugler.

Dineen, R., Doyle, J., Bench, J., & Perry, A. (in press). The influence of training on tinnitus perception: An evaluation 12 months after tinnitus management training. *British Journal of Audiology.*

Dobie, R. A. (1993). *Medical-legal evaluation of hearing loss.* New York: Van Nostrand.

Douek, E., & Reid, J. (1968). The diagnostic value of tinnitus pitch. *Journal of Laryngology and Otology, 82,* 1039–1042.

Erlandsson, S. L., Hallberg, L. R. M., & Axelsson, A. (1992). Psychological and audiological correlates to perceived tinnitus severity. *Audiology, 31,* 168–179.

Fowler, E. P. (1943). Control of head noises: Their illusions of loudness and of timbre. *Archives of Otolaryngology, 37,* 391–398.

Fowler, E. P., & Fowler, E. P. (1948). The emotional factor in tinnitus aurium. *Laryngoscope, 58,* 145–154.

Goodwin, P. E., & Johnson, R. M. (1980). The loudness of tinnitus. *Acta Otolaryngologica, 90,* 353–359.

Hallam, R. S., Rachman, S., & Hinchcliffe, R. (1984). Psychological aspects of tinnitus. In S. Rachman (Ed.), *Contributions to medical psychology* (Vol. 3, pp. 31–53). Oxford: Pergamon.

Hazell, J. W. P. (1996). Support for a neurophysiological model of tinnitus. In G. E. Reich & J. A. Vernon (Eds.), *Proceedings of the Fifth International Tinnitus Seminar, Portland, 1995* (pp. 51–57). Portland, OR: American Tinnitus Association.

Hazell, J. W. P., & Sheldrake, J. B. (1992). Hyperacusis and tinnitus. In J. M. Aran & R. Dauman (Eds.), *Tinnitus 91: Proceedings of the Fourth International Tinnitus Seminar, Bordeaux, 1991* (pp. 245–248). Amsterdam: Kugler.

Hazell, J. W. P., Wood, S. M., Cooper, H. R., Stephens, S. D. G., Corcoran, A. L., Coles, R. R. A., Baskill, J. L., & Sheldrake, J. B. (1985). A clinical study of tinnitus maskers. *British Journal of Audiology, 19,* 65–146.

Heller, M. F., & Bergman, M. (1953). Tinnitus aurium in normally hearing persons. *Annals of Otology, Rhinology and Laryngology, 62,* 72–83.

Hinchcliffe, R., & King, P. F. (1992). Medicolegal aspects of tinnitus. I: Medicolegal position and current state of knowledge. II: Features of tinnitus in various disorders. *Journal of Audiological Medicine, 1,* 38–58 and 59–78.

Jakes, S. C., Hallam, R. S., Chambers, C. & Hinchcliffe, R. (1986). Matched and self-reported loudness of tinnitus: Methods and sources of error. *Audiology, 25,* 92–100.

Jastreboff, P. J. (1990). Phantom auditory perception (tinnitus): Mechanisms of generation and perception. *Neuroscience Research, 8,* 221–254.

Jastreboff, P. J. (1996). Usefulness of the psychoacoustical characterisation of tinnitus. In G. E. Reich & J. A. Vernon (Eds.), *Proceedings of the Fifth International Tinnitus Seminar, Portland, 1995* (pp. 158–166). Portland, OR: American Tinnitus Association.

Jastreboff, P. J. (1998). Tinnitus. In G. Gates (Ed.), *Current therapy in otolaryngology—Head and neck surgery* (pp. 90–95). St Louis: Mosby.

Jastreboff, P. J., & Hazell, J. W. P. (1993). A neurophysiological approach to tinnitus: Clinical implications. *British Journal of Audiology, 27,* 7–17.

Jastreboff, P. J., Hazell, J. W. P., & Graham, R. L. (1994). Neurophysiological model of tinnitus: Dependence of the minimal masking level on treatment outcome. *Hearing Research, 80,* 216–232.

Jayarajan, V., Harris, N. D., Stevens, J. C., & Coles, R. R. A. (1995). Tinnitus following ear syringing. *Journal of Audiological Medicine, 4,* 85–96.

Lindberg, P., Lyttkens, L., Melin, L., & Scott, B. (1984). Tinnitus—Incidence and handicap. *Scandinavian Audiology, 13,* 287–291.

Man, A., & Naggan, L. (1981). Characteristics of tinnitus in acoustic trauma. *Audiology, 20,* 72–78.

Matsuhira, T., Yamashita, K., & Yasuda, M. (1992). Estimation of the loudness of tinnitus from matching tests. *British Journal of Audiology, 26,* 387–395.

McShane, D. P., Hyde, M. L., & Alberti, P. W. (1988). Tinnitus prevalence in industrial hearing loss compensation claimants. *Clinical Otolaryngology, 13,* 323–330.

Meikle, M. B., & Taylor-Walsh, E. (1984). Characterization of tinnitus and related observations in over 1,800 tinnitus clinic patients. *Journal of Laryngology and Otology* (Suppl. 9), 17–21.

Meikle, M. B., Vernon, J., & Johnson, R. M. (1984). The perceived severity of tinnitus: Some observations concerning a large population of tinnitus patients. *Otolaryngology—Head and Neck Surgery, 92,* 689–696.

Miller, J. J. (1985). *CRC handbook of ototoxicity.* Boca Raton: CRC Press.

Moffat, D. A., Baguley, D. M., Beynon, G. J., & da Cruz, M. (1998). Clinical acumen and vestibular schwannoma. *American Journal of Otology, 19,* 82–87.

Penner, M. J., Brauth, S., & Hood, L. (1981). The temporal course of the masking of tinnitus as a basis for inferring its origin. *Journal of Speech and Hearing Disorders, 24,* 257–261.

Sacher, A. (1927). Beitrag zur Lehre der professionellen Schwerhörigkeit. Die Taubheit der Kesselschmiede. *Monatsschrift fur Ohrenheslkunde unt Laringologie—Rhinologie, 61,* 337–359.

Sallustio, V., Portalina, P., Soleo, L., Cassano, F., Pesola, G., Lasorsa, G., Quaranta, N., & Salonna, I. (1998). Auditory dysfunction in occupational noise exposed workers. *Scandinavian Audiology* (Suppl. 27), 95–110.

Sharp, J. F., Wilson, J. F., Ross, L., & Barr-Hamilton, R. M. (1990). Ear wax removal: A survey of current practice. *British Medical Journal, 301,* 1251–1253.

Sheldrake, J. B., Jastreboff, P. J., & Hazell, J. W. P. (1996). Perspectives for total elimination of tinnitus perception. In G. E. Reich & J. A. Vernon (Eds.), *Proceedings of the Fifth International Tinnitus Seminar Portland, 1995* (pp. 531–536). Portland, OR: American Tinnitus Association.

Sinclair, A., & Coles, R. R. A. (1995). Hearing and vestibular disorders. In R. A. F. Cox, F. C. Edwards, & R. I. McCallum (Eds.), *Fitness for work* (2nd ed., pp. 60–87). Oxford University Press.

Smith, P. A. (1998). Hearing in young adults and the effect of social noise exposure. Personal communication on draft paper by P. A. Smith, A. C. Davis, M. E. Ferguson, & M. E. Lutman.

Stouffer, J. L., & Tyler, R. S. (1990). Characterization of tinnitus by tinnitus patients. *Journal of Speech and Hearing Disorders, 55,* 439–453.

Toglia, J. U. (1976). Acute flexion-extension injury of the neck. *Neurology, 26,* 808–814.

Tyler, R. S., Aran, J. M., & Dauman, R. (1992). Recent advances in tinnitus. *American Journal of Audiology, 1,* 36–44.

Tyler, R. S., & Baker, L. J. (1983). Difficulties experienced by tinnitus sufferers. *Journal of Speech and Hearing Disorders, 48,* 150–154.

Tyler, R. S., & Conrad-Armes, D. (1983a). The determination of tinnitus loudness considering the effect of recruitment. *Journal of Speech and Hearing Research, 26,* 59–72.

Tyler, R. S., & Conrad-Armes, D. (1983b). Tinnitus pitch: A comparison of three measurement methods. *British Journal of Audiology, 17,* 101–107.

Vernon, J. (1996). Is the claimed tinnitus real and is the claimed cause correct? In G. E. Reich & J. A. Vernon (Eds.), *Proceedings of the Fifth International Tinnitus Seminar, Portland, 1995* (pp. 395–396). Portland, OR: American Tinnitus Association.

World Health Organization. (1980). *International classification of impairments, disabilities and handicaps.* Geneva: World Health Organization.

World Health Organization. (1997). *International classification of impairments, activities and participation: Beta–1 draft for field trials, June 1997.* Geneva: World Health Organization.

CHAPTER 18

American Tinnitus Association and Self-Help Groups

Gloria E. Reich, Ph.D.

HISTORY OF ASSOCIATION

The American Tinnitus Association (ATA) has been a preeminent tinnitus organization since 1971 when it was founded by the late Dr. Charles Unice of Downey, California. Dr. Unice had tinnitus and recognized the need for an organization to raise money for supporting tinnitus research. During this time the primary goal of ATA has been to find a cure for tinnitus. The association has supported research studies to the extent of its financial ability and just recently has passed the million dollar mark in research funding.

Early in ATA's life, it became apparent that supporting research was not enough. People who had tinnitus and people who treated tinnitus patients called on the organization to provide them with current information about the problem and techniques for helping people who suffered from it. As a result, the association began in 1978 to conduct workshops, regional meetings, and seminars in which professionals and patients could come together to learn about tinnitus. In addition, the association has supported the efforts of other tinnitus experts to share their knowledge in workshops, lectures, seminars, and media articles and appearances. See Table 18-1.

In 1973, Dr. Unice and Dr. Jack Vernon, director of the Kresge Hearing Research Laboratory of the University of Oregon Medical School met. Dr. Vernon had been studying tinnitus and when news of his work reached Dr. Unice, Unice offered him the fledgling ATA. The Oregon Medical School agreed to sponsor ATA as an affiliated nonprofit association.

Soon after, ATA acquired its first National Chairman, the late Robert Hocks of Portland, Oregon. ATA was gathering momentum. There were, as yet, no employees but administrative assistance had arrived through loyal volunteers including ATA's executive director, Dr. Gloria Reich. ATA soon acquired a national scientific advisory board comprised of prominent professionals who were specialists in auditory disorders and research. Excellent news coverage during 1978 and 1979 increased inquiries dramatically.

By 1979, it became apparent that ATA needed to be able to manage itself and to

Table 18-1. History of the American Tinnitus Association

Year	Event	Outcome
1971	ATA was founded by Dr. Charles Unice	Birth of the only national organization devoted to the problem of tinnitus
1973	ATA moves to Oregon Health Sciences University	The organization has a home
1974	Bob Hocks becomes National Chairman	Portland businessman leads ATA's growth
1975	Gloria Reich volunteers to organize ATA	Organizes ATA and administers its programs
1976	National Advisory Board appointed	Prestigious counsel for policy and planning
1978	ATA goes on the road with professional workshops	Trains providers of tinnitus treatment
1979	ATA becomes incorporated as nonprofit association	Launched as a freestanding organization
1981	First tinnitus self-help group organized	Person-to-person support for tinnitus sufferers
1983	ATA joins National Voluntary Health Agencies	Financial support comes from Federal Employees and Military
1984	ATA develops new brochures for patient "handouts"	Supplements information brochure with specific helpful topics
1985	Chairman, Bob Hocks dies. Bob Johnson assumes the Chair	The torch is passed
1986	Gloria Reich writes to Ann Landers	Column spurs an unprecedented response of over 130,000 letters
1987	*Tinnitus Today*	Newsletter graduates to magazine format after thirteen years
1988	ATA moves to downtown Portland offices	Expansion of programs and services now possible
1990	Staff and board expand	Growth continues
1990	ATA conducts hyperacusis survey	Informational brochure developed
1992	ATA's Executive Board becomes national; advisors continue to provide counsel	Governance formalized
1995	ATA hosts Fifth International Tinnitus Seminar	Twenty-five countries represented at quadrennial meeting, proceedings published in book form
1996	ATA embarks on strategic planning and development	Long-range planning involves many segments; patients, volunteers, manufacturers, professionals
1997	EARS: ATA's Strategic Plan is implemented: Education, Advocacy, Research, Support and Organization	Meeting the goals of promoting relief, prevention, and an eventual cure for tinnitus
1998	ATA surpasses the million dollar mark in funding research; Support group leader, John Nichols writes to Dear Abby	Important findings come from ATA-funded studies; Dear Abby column brings over 40,000 inquiries
1999	Staff and Board expand; programs turn to prevention of tinnitus through hearing conservation	Growth continues; partnerships for program development are explored with corporations and sister organizations

hire people to carry out the tasks of running a large organization. Up until then all the work of the organization had been done by volunteers. The association became legally incorporated as a nonprofit organization, and was no longer under the guardianship of the Health Sciences Center of the University of Oregon. This step was made possible by support from many of the 33,000 people who had contacted ATA for help. Many of these people had become aware of ATA from an article in *Parade* magazine in 1978. ATA started on its mission of carrying out and supporting research and education about tinnitus.

At the end of the 1970s, Jack Vernon and Bob Hocks presented their tinnitus masker patent to ATA. Subsequently several manufacturers began turning out masking units for clinical fittings. The funds provided by the manufacturers during this time sustained ATA and made possible the publication of the ATA Newsletter. ATA sponsored workshops providing training in tinnitus management for more than 1,200 clinicians over a period of three years. Finally, there were specialists in tinnitus to whom ATA could refer the thousands of people who contacted the organization for help.

Opportunities for growth continued as celebrities and politicians began to speak out for tinnitus. Senator Mark Hatfield was the voice on one of ATA's earliest radio announcements as was William Christopher of *M*A*S*H*. Many celebrities have spoken about their tinnitus, either in the media or in public service announcements for ATA. These occurrences have always brought new inquiries to ATA from people who identified with the conditions described by their favorite personalities (see Table 18-2). ATA began to hear from more and more young people who had noise-induced tinnitus.

In 1983, ATA entered the federal fund raising campaign certified as a National Voluntary Health Agency. (The organization is now known as Community Health Charities.) This affiliation allows ATA to receive payroll donations from federal, state, and local government employees in all fifty states and federal installations overseas. ATA also participates in a number of non-United Way workplace health appeal programs.

The expansive growth brought about by the massive reply to the Ann Landers column signaled a new phase for ATA. By 1988, the office ATA occupied at the Oregon Health Sciences Center became so cramped that we moved the entire operation to a small office building in downtown Portland where ATA remains today.

The year 1992 saw ATA's executive board become national. This board is responsible for the governance of the organization. The board development committee considers applications for board service and elects members annually or to fill out partial terms. A board member serves for a three-year term which is renewable once. It relies on the Scientific Advisory Committee for medical and scientific direction. This committee elects its own members, subject to the approval of the board, for renewable four-year terms. (See Tables 18-3 and 18-4.)

ATA's founder, Dr. Charles Unice, died in 1993 without realizing his dream of curing tinnitus, but with a knowledge that the organization he had created was bringing information and help to millions. By 1990 ATA could no longer provide free publications to everyone who inquired about tinnitus. To receive the mailings people now had to make an annual contribution to the organization in support of the developing programs, which include education, support services and resources, and tinnitus research funding.

In 1994, board member, Phil Morton, presented the board with a plan that they adopted entitled "Mission 2000," which among other programs included finding a cure for tinnitus by the year 2005. This plan was eventually superceded by the Strategic Action Plan which will be explained next.

ATA set about confirming its mission and its direction by embarking on a strategic planning year in 1996. Through a series of focus

Table 18-2. Celebrity involvement with the American Tinnitus Association

Year	Celebrity	Event
1978	Senator Mark Hatfield	Becomes Honorary Board Member
1980	The Styx (Rock Musicians)	Donates Golden Record proceeds to research
1981	Lou Ferrigno (Actor, Star of *Incredible Hulk* TV Series)	Television public service announcement joint with Better Hearing Institute brings 5,000 telephone calls
1983	William Christopher (Actor, *M*A*S*H*), and Senator Mark Hatfield	Radio Public Service Announcements
1983	Dear Abby	20,000 letters arrive after mention in her column
1985	Tony Randall (Actor)	Television Public Service Announcements
1986	Ann Landers and Dear Abby	Mention in their columns brought more than 130,000 letters
1987	President Ronald Reagan	Tinnitus started from a gunshot in 1930s movie
1988	Al Unser, auto racing driver and Jeff Float, Olympic Gold Medalist	Television Public Service Announcements
1989	Portland Mayor Bud Clark	Proclaims Tinnitus and Better Hearing Month
1990	Crazy 8s, Musicians, Rock Group	Stars in tinnitus Public Service Announcements for Television
1990	Tony Randall and Senator Paul Simon	Testify before Senator Harkin's committee about tinnitus
1991	Jerry Stiller (Actor)	Actor interviewed about his tinnitus in the national media
1994	Barbra Streisand (Actress)	Speaks of her tinnitus and donates money for research
1995	William Shatner (Actor)	Public Service Announcements and testifies before Congress
1996	Tony Randall and Jerry Stiller	Public Service Announcements
1997	Rosalyn Carter (Former First Lady)	Media announcements of her tinnitus
1998	Charlton Heston (Actor) and William Shatner (Actor)	American Medical Review Video and "Silent Night" Christmas Ornament

groups, retreats, and personal interviews, every aspect of ATA's operation was evaluated to assure pursuit of the proper objectives and use of the correct methods to achieve the desired and appropriate results and to meet the expectations of ATA members. By spring 1997, this resulted in a more focused Mission Statement and the development of the official ATA Strategic Action Plan EARS (for the defined program priority areas of Education, Advocacy, Research, and Support), the strategic plan was approved and in place. The revised mission statement is: "To promote relief, prevention, and the eventual cure of tinnitus for the benefit of present and future generations."

The board of directors expanded its membership to ten with a goal of fifteen members

Table 18-3. Advisors to ATA: Name, year appointed, year resigned (or deceased)

Charles Unice, M.D.	1971	1978 (d. 1993)
David DeWeese, M.D.	1973	1990 (d.)
Del Clawson, U.S. House of Representatives	1971	1990
Robert Hocks (transfer to board of directors in 1979)	1973	1979
David Plant	1974	1978
Honorary: Mark O. Hatfield, U.S. Senator from Oregon	1978	
Bobby Alford, M.D.	1978	1980
Roger Boles, M.D.	1978	1981
Howard House, M.D.	1978	1985
Merle Lawrence, Ph.D.	1978	1988
Gunnar Proud, M.D.	1978	1991
Harold Tabb, M.D.	1978	1994
George Reed, M.D.	1978	1991
Robert M. Johnson, Ph.D.	1978	1999 (d.)
Robert Sandlin, Ph.D.	1980	
Jerry Northern, Ph.D.	1978	1997
Abe Shulman, M.D.	1980	
Jack Clemis, M.D.	1982	
John Emmett, M.D.	1982	
Chris Foster, M.D.	1982	
Francis Sooy, M.D.	1982	1986 (d.)
John House, M.D.	1985	
Honorary: Tony Randall	1985	
Gale W. Miller, M.D.	1988	
Gail Neely, M.D.	1988	
Richard Goode, M.D.	1988	1997
Mansfield Smith, M.D.	1988	
Alfred Weiss, M.D.	1990	1993
W. F. Sam Hopmeier (transfer to Exec. Board 1994)	1990	1994
Honorary: Tony Randall	1991	
Barbara Goldstein, Ph.D.	1992	
Robert Brummett, Ph.D.	1992	
Ronald Amedee, M.D.	1992	
Alexander J. Schleuning, II, M.D.	1994	
Robert A. Dobie, M.D. (Chairman 1998–)	1994	
William H. Martin, Ph.D.	1995	
Honorary: William Shatner	1995	
Robert Sweetow, Ph.D.	1997	
Pawel J. Jastreboff, Ph.D., Sc.D.	1997	
Gary Jacobson, Ph.D.	1997	

Table 18-4. ATA Board of Directors: Name, year appointed, year resigned (or deceased)

Bob Hocks	1979	1985 (d.)
Jack A. Vernon, Ph.D.	1979, 1997	1982
Gloria E. Reich, Ph.D.	1979, 1999	1997
Henry Breithaupt, Corporate Secretary (not board member)	1979	
Charles Unice, M.D.	1980	1982 (1993 d.)
Tom Wissbaum	1980	1994
Robert M. Johnson, Ph.D.	1985	1994 (1999 d.)
Jack Artz	1986	1988
Phil Morton	1988	1999
Dan Robert Hocks	1988	1996
Edmund (Buzz) Grossberg	1992	1998
Aaron Osherow	1992	1999
Timothy Sotos	1994, 1998	1996
Paul Meade	1996	
Stephen Nagler, M.D.	1997	
Megan Vidis	1997	
Sid Kleinman	1997	
James Chinnis, Ph.D.	1998	

in the next several years. The advisory committee expanded also to nineteen members. The ATA office has been enlarged. The computer and telephone systems were upgraded in anticipation of significant growth. That growth has begun with the more than 40,000 inquiries received in the spring of 1998 as a result of a letter to "Dear Abby" by one of ATA's support group leaders, John Nichols. The ATA staff also will grow over the next several years as income and program services expand.

PROGRAMS FOR PROFESSIONALS

From 1977 through 1980, educational workshops were presented nationwide. These workshops provided information and training to more than 1,200 professionals who were interested in the evaluation and management of tinnitus patients.

The year 1979 saw the beginnings of international communication among tinnitus researchers when the First International Tinnitus Seminar took place in New York City. The Proceedings from this and subsequent International Seminars have been published and widely cited as authoritative works about tinnitus. The International Tinnitus Study Group was established as the official organizer of the quadrennial seminars.

In 1981, Tinnitus research efforts were recognized when the prestigious chemical company, CIBA, devoted its 85th Symposium, held in London, England, to the topic of tinnitus. The published results became the first widely available tinnitus reference work.

Dr. Vernon's laboratory, funded by an NIH grant, continued with the development of masking techniques for relief of tinnitus, and with seed money from ATA began to develop the computerized Tinnitus Data Registry at the Oregon Tinnitus Clinic.

In 1983, research funding was continued for the Tinnitus Data Registry and a new grant was made for tinnitus research at the University of Iowa (see Chapter 6). In 1985, research grants were made for studies involving electrical stimulation for tinnitus relief, and for the effects of salicylates on tinnitus. Temporomandibular joint (TMJ) disorders were the subject of a tinnitus study funded in 1988 and in the same year a study was funded involving the drug Furosemide as a tinnitus treatment. Subsequent studies have been funded at various medical centers and universities in the United States and Canada and have involved the study of drugs to relieve tinnitus, psychological interventions for tinnitus relief, medical imaging techniques, and basic chemical actions that may have an effect on tinnitus, as well as studies to produce an objective testable model for hearing loss and tinnitus.

To date, ATA has expended over a million dollars for tinnitus research through the generous gifts and bequests of its members

(see Table 18-5). ATA has also encouraged other funding for tinnitus research by supporting the National Institute on Deafness and Other Communication Disorders, and by its relationships with other funding organizations such as Deafness Research Foundation.

Bob Hocks, ATA's first national chairman, died in 1985 and his family established a memorial research award. Winners of the ATA Hocks Memorial Award for outstanding work in the field of tinnitus were Dr. Jack Vernon, Director Emeritus of the Oregon Hearing Research Center (see Chapter 14); Dr. Jonathan Hazell, prominent researcher and clinician, London, England; Dr. John House, President of the House Institute, who recognized the psychological component of tinnitus in his 1970s studies of biofeedback; Abraham Shulman, M.D., Professor Emeritus at the State University of New York at Brooklyn, author, editor of the *International Tinnitus Journal*, and chairman of the first two International Tinnitus Seminars, in 1979 and 1983; Robert M. Johnson, Ph.D., research audiologist and Director of the Tinnitus Clinic at the Oregon Hearing Research Center; Pawel & Margaret Jastreboff, Ph.D., developers of an objective measure for tinnitus and tinnitus retraining therapy, at the Tinnitus Center and research laboratory at the University of Maryland at Baltimore (see Chapter 15); Ross R. A. Coles, M.D., retired British tinnitus expert whose epidemiology studies confirmed tinnitus prevalence worldwide; and Robert E. Brummett, Ph.D., retired pharmacologist whose work with ototoxic drugs helped shed light on drugs that might affect tinnitus.

Munster, Germany was the site of the Third International Tinnitus Seminar in 1987. There were more than 200 papers about tinnitus presented. The Fourth International Tinnitus Seminar was held in 1991 in Bordeaux, France. By then, tinnitus research was truly worldwide. When the Fifth International Tinnitus Seminar was hosted by ATA in Portland, Oregon, in 1995, scientists from twenty-five countries presented papers

Table 18-5. Tinnitus research funded by ATA since incorporation in 1979

Investigator	Institution	Topic	Amount	Date
Mary Meikle, Ph.D.	Oregon Hearing Research Center	Tinnitus data registry	12,000.	1980
Mary Meikle, Ph.D.	OHRC	Tinnitus data registry	11,309.	1984
Mary Meikle, Ph.D.	OHRC	Tinnitus data registry	12,500.	1985
Jack A. Vernon, Ph.D.	OHRC	Electrical suppression	20,000.	1985
Richard S. Tyler, Ph.D.	University of Iowa Hospitals	Binaural phase effects of masking	6,500.	1984
Jack A. Vernon, Ph.D.	OHRC	Electrical suppression	20,000.	1986
Mary Meikle, Ph.D.	OHRC	TDR	25,000.	1986
Mary Meikle, Ph.D.	OHRC	Continuing research	300.	1987
Ian M. Windmill, Ph.D.	University of Louisville, KY	Brain Mapping	8,684.	1987
Richard S. Tyler, Ph.D.	University of Iowa Hospitals	Binaural phase effects of masking	9,600.	1988
Douglas H. Morgan, D.D.S.	TMJ Foundation	TMJ and tinnitus	20,000.	1988
Jack A. Vernon, Ph.D.	OHRC	Electrical stimulation	12,250.	1989
Paul S. Guth, Ph.D.	Tulane University	Furosemide as a tinnitus treatment	10,000.	1989
Gary A. Jacobson, Ph.D.	Henry Ford Hospital, Detroit, MI	Magnetic resonance imaging	19,462.	1989
Robert W. Sweetow, Ph.D.	San Francisco Hearing and Speech Center	Maskers: effects of earmold design	7,500.	1990
Frank Marlow, M.D.	Temple University	Hypnosis as a tinnitus treatment	10,000.	1990
Wayne Briner, Ph.D.	House Ear Institute	Misoprostal, drug effects on tinnitus (Prostiglandin)	11,650.	1990
Donna Wayner, Ph.D.	Albany Medical Center	Cognitive-Therapy report and manual	4,500.	1991
Richard S. Tyler, Ph.D.	University of Iowa Hospitals	Masking	10,000.	1991
Robert A. Dobie, M.D.	University of Texas, San Antonio	Lasix (furosemide) for tinnitus	9,975.	1991
Mary Meikle, Ph.D.	OHRC	Spectral analyzer	9,540.	1992
Gary Jacobson, Ph.D.	Henry Ford Hospital	Attentional mechanisms of tinnitus	16,883.	1992
Carol A. Bauer, M.D.	University of Iowa Hospitals	To replicate animal model for tinnitus	6,600.	1992
Margaret M. Jastreboff, Ph.D.	University of Maryland at Baltimore	Tinnitus changes in the auditory pathways	15,000.	1993
Aage R. Møller, Ph.D.	University of Pittsburgh	Tinnitus mechanisms	10,068.	1993
Wayne Briner, Ph.D.	University of Nebraska	Anatomic basis for tinnitus	5,770.	1993
Pawel J. Jastreboff, Ph.D., Sc.D.	University of Maryland at Baltimore	Objective measures for tinnitus	20,000.	1993
Paul R. Kileny, Ph.D.	University of Michigan	Drug, trental for tinnitus	9,860.	1993
James A. Kaltenbach, Ph.D.	Wayne State University	Tinnitus and spontaneous cochlear activity	15,000.	1994

continues

Table 18-5. *continued*

Investigator	Institution	Topic	Amount	Date
Donald A. Godfrey, Ph.D.	Medical College of Ohio	Neurochemistry of cochlear samples (previous study with Kaltenbach)	10,000.	1994
Aage R. Møller, Ph.D.	University of Pittsburgh	Pathophysiology of tinnitus	15,000.	1994
Anthony T. Cacace, Ph.D.	Albany Medical College	Neuroanatomical localization of tinnitus	10,270.	1994
Pawel J. Jastreboff, Ph.D.	University of Maryland, Baltimore	Model for noise-induced tinnitus	100,000.	1995
Jos. J. Eggermont, Ph.D.	University of Calgary, Canada	Effects of salicylates and quinine on tinnitus	52,000.	1995
Aage Møller, Ph.D.	University of Pittsburgh	Tinnitus and neural plasticity in ascending auditory path	59,000.	1995
Donald Godfrey, Ph.D.	Medical College of Ohio	Neurochemistry in CN after high-intensity sound	25,000.	1995/1996
James Kaltenbach, Ph.D.	Wayne State	Changes spontaneous activity and neurochem CN	30,000.	1995/1996
Pawel Jastreboff, Ph.D.	University of Maryland	Mapping metabolic brain activity of tinnitus (Part II)	111,536.	1996/1997
Alan Lockwood, M.D.	SUNY Buffalo, with Richard Salvi, Ph.D.	Use of PET to localize tinnitus sites in brain	46,145.	1996/1997
Aage Møller, Ph.D.	University of Texas at Dallas	Pharmacological management and prevention of tinnitus with female sex hormone	51,000.	1997
Gary Jacobson, Ph.D.	Henry Ford Hospital, Detroit, MI	Influence of selective auditory attention on long latency aud. evok. pot. PI & NI components in patients with and without tinnitus	56,723.	1997
Xi Lin, Ph.D.	House Ear Institute	Cellular model for quinine-induced tinnitus	40,500.	1997
Curtin Mitchell, Ph.D.	OHRC	Masking curves and otoacoustic emissions in patients with and without tinnitus	35,300.	1997
Richard J. Hallworth, Ph.D.	University of Texas, San Antonio	Mechanisms of quinine induced tinnitus	16,000.	1997
Mary Meikle, Ph.D.	OHRC	Tinnitus data registry	30,000.	1998
Kejian Chen, Ph.D.	Medical College of Ohio	Spontaneous activity in dorsal cochlear nucleus	33,000.	1999
George Gerken, Ph.D.	University of Texas, Dallas	Auditory-evoked potentials in tinnitus, etc.	30,000.	1999
Mary Meikle, Ph.D.	OHRC	Tinnitus data registry	22,500.	1999
		TOTAL:	$1,108,940.	

about tinnitus. Future seminars will be held in Cambridge, the United Kingdom in 1999, and in Perth, Australia in 2002. See Figure 18-1.

ATA encourages professional societies to offer continuing education to their members about tinnitus. ATA has conducted workshops and sponsored sessions about tinnitus at various professional meetings, including the American Academy of Audiology, the American Academy of Otolaryngology—Head and Neck Surgery, and the International Hearing Society, to name a few. The International Tinnitus Forum meets annually to study tinnitus at the convention of the American Academy of Otolaryngology—Head and Neck Surgery. Courses about tinnitus are available at yearly meetings of audiologists, social workers, physicians, and hearing aid specialists. A tinnitus management workshop program has been carried on at the University of Iowa for several years under the leadership of Professor Richard Tyler.

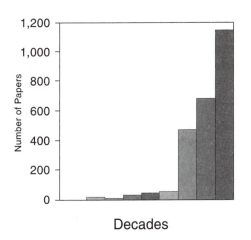

Before 1925	19
1925–1934	8
1935–1944	30
1945–1954	45
1955–1964	52
1965–1974	472
1975–1984	686
1985–1994	1155

Figure 18-1. Number of tinnitus papers by decade. ATA tinnitus bibliography

In 1996, a new program of regional meetings about tinnitus was initiated with the first two years' meetings in Chicago, Illinois; Baltimore, Maryland; Anaheim, California; and Oakland, California. These popular new meetings combined sessions for professionals earning continuing education credits with lectures and open forum sessions for laymen interested in learning more about their tinnitus. ATA's board shelved these programs in 1998 because of lack of available staff to organize them, and reinstituted the public forums in conjunction with regularly scheduled professional meetings that could be easily facilitated and fulfilled the public's desire to have an opportunity to question professionals who are tinnitus experts.

PROGRAMS TO HELP PATIENTS

By 1982 the tinnitus self-help movement had begun. ATA developed and made available guidelines and tips for people who wanted to get together to help themselves conquer their tinnitus. The first group was set in motion in Bergen County, New Jersey, by the late Dr. Trudy Drucker and the movement spread nationwide very quickly. ATA membership grew by over 6,000 during the first six months of 1982.

The First Tinnitus Self-Help Group Convention took place in Wycoff, New Jersey, in 1983 drawing hundreds to hear ATA's officers answer their many questions about tinnitus. "Tinnitus '90" a seminar of self-help group members drew more than 300 to Washington, DC, for a second convention. ATA's Fort Washington and Silver Springs tinnitus groups hosted that meeting, helped by committees from other east coast groups.

ATA sponsored its first series of TV PSAs focusing on hearing protection. Tony Randall, also an honorary ATA director, helped by starring in a series of PSAs about tinnitus. Gloria Reich appeared on the *McNeil-Lehrer News Hour* in a 1980 segment about tinnitus and the ATA. The tinnitus self-help groups now numbered over 150 and were spread throughout the United States and Canada. Guest appearances were made by ATA board members at self-help groups in California, Maryland, New York, and New Jersey.

In 1987, ATA joined a coalition of organizations concerned with hearing problems to further the progress of hearing research. Thousands of ATA members wrote letters to their legislators in support of bills to create a special institute for hearing problems within the National Institutes of Health. ATA, along with its local self-help groups, sponsored tinnitus public forums in New York City in March, in Washington, DC, in September, and a regional conference in Philadelphia, in October.

A pilot survey study of hyperacusis patients was conducted in 1990 and a hyperacusis brochure developed. In 1992, ATA conducted a Tinnitus Patient Survey similar to the one done in 1986 and printed the resulting information in a brochure. This survey was repeated in 1997. A Family Information Brochure was developed with the help of support group leaders. By 1993 ATA had expanded its contact with professionals by presenting programs and exhibits at meetings of groups concerned with the problems of aging, and at meetings of doctors in the specialty of family practice. A school program was developed to make young people aware of the need to protect their hearing

In 1997, a Public Awareness Survey was conducted which showed that about 16 percent of the population was aware of, and had an accurate definition for tinnitus. About 6 percent of the sample indicated they had tinnitus themselves and another 14 percent indicated they knew someone with the condition. A Professional Awareness Survey conducted in 1998 confirmed that almost all doctors and hearing clinicians could correctly define tinnitus but only about half of the sample indicated that they treated tinnitus patients. From 1 to 5 percent

of the samples offered that they have tinnitus although it was not a question on this survey.

Two regional meetings for laymen, which also provided continuing education credit for professionals, were organized by ATA in 1996 and 1997. These meetings drew more than 400 participants who heard about the latest in tinnitus treatments and who were able to participate in question and answer sessions with tinnitus experts.

New public service announcements emphasizing hearing protection featured the Crazy 8s Rock Group who said, "Hurt your ears and you'll never hear the end of it." In 1996, Tony Randall and Jerry Stiller filmed new video clips. These comedians, whose own tinnitus prompted them, created an amusing banter about the pronunciation of tinnitus. They compromised by calling it the "T" word. William Shatner, Captain Kirk of *Star Trek*, and ATA's newest honorary director, also made public service announcements and encouraged other celebrities with tinnitus to speak for ATA. In 1998 American Medical Review filmed a segment about ATA and tinnitus to be broadcast on Public Broadcasting System and other networks. The series is introduced by Charlton Heston and some footage featuring William Shatner is included in the segment as well as footage of patients being treated for tinnitus and information from ATA spokesmen. New public service announcements were also produced at this time.

Today, ATA provides services to more than 20,000 current supporters as well as providing tinnitus information to anyone who asks for it. ATA volunteers and staff also visit congressmen and senators in support of the National Institute on Deafness and other Communication Disorders at the National Institutes of Health. ATA has joined with other organizations from time to time to bring concerns about hearing to the attention of the government. See Table 18-6.

Table 18-6. International Tinnitus Support Associations

Country	Name	Address
AUSTRALIA	Australian Tinnitus Association NSW	P.O. Box 660, Woollahra NSW 2025, Australia
	Australian Tinnitus Association Victoria, Inc.	5 High Street Prahran, Victoria 3181, Australia
CANADA	Tinnitus Association of Canada	23 Ellis Park Road, Toronto ON M6S 2V4, Canada
ENGLAND	British Tinnitus Association	4th flr. White Bldg. Fitzalan Square, Sheffield S1 2AZ, United Kingdom
FRANCE	France Acouphene	La Varazelle, F-69510, Thurins, France
GERMANY	Deutsche Tinnitus Liga	Postfach 349, 42353 Wuppertal, Germany
NETHERLANDS	Comm Tinnitus NVVS	Verdiweg 305 Amersfoort NL 3816 KJ, Netherlands
INDIA	India Tinnitus Association	H12-33/H/I Ganesh Nagar, India Ramanthaput 500-013 Hyderabad
IRELAND	Irish Tinnitus Association	35 N Frederick St Dublin 1, Ireland
	Ulster Tinnitus Association	9 Glebe Gardens, Glengormley, BT36-6ED, Belfast, Ireland
NEW ZEALAND	New Zealand Tinnitus Association	P.O. Box 100734 NS Mail Ctr Auckland 10, New Zealand
NORWAY	Norwegian Tinnitus Committee	Landsforbund PB 5293 Majorstua 0303 Oslo, Norway
SPAIN	Aso de Personas Afectades Por Tinitus	Apartado De Correos #57 08320 El Masnou Barcelona, Spain
SWITZERLAND	Schweizerische Tinnitus-Liga	Ländliweg 12, Baden Ch-5400, Switzerland

ATA PUBLICATIONS

Informational brochures have been part of ATA since it moved to Oregon. The first two brochures were developed in the 1970s. The ATA brochure described the organization and included a return card for more information and membership. A version of that brochure still exists and is widely distributed. Another early brochure, "Information About Tinnitus," continues to be the most popular of all ATA brochures.

ATA also provides a range of brochures and publications designed to help the tinnitus patient. Topics covered include general information, noise, stress, first steps to take, information for the family, and tinnitus treatments. These are available both in English and in Spanish. A selection of books useful to the tinnitus sufferer, tapes, videos, and bibliography materials are also available. The list changes frequently as new items are added. A current list can be requested from ATA or found at the ATA website http:\\www.ata.org.

The tinnitus bibliography service, utilizing ATA's tinnitus reference files, today contains more than 3,200 tinnitus-specific citations. These citations are drawn from many sources, the principal one being Medline. Tinnitus has become a viable field of study in the research community. The following graph shows the dramatic increase in tinnitus publications during recent decades. Since 1994, an additional 858 papers have been listed in the bibliography, demonstrating that the increase continues.

WHY IS SELF-HELP FOR TINNITUS IMPORTANT?

Self-help group approaches are more flexible, less bureaucratic, and often more responsive to the individual problems of their clients than are the formal systems. They are clearly cost-effective and offer both concrete help to new members and an enhancement in self-esteem to those who turn their own experience into a valuable asset to be shared by others.

Self-help can provide constructive guidance to someone newly diagnosed with tinnitus. It can also relieve distress and provide hope for patients whose treatment has failed.

This quotation, attributed to J. Krishnamurti, from the Hull Tinnitus Self-Help Group publication, states it well. "In oneself lies the whole world and if you know how to look and learn then the door is there and the key is in your hand. Nobody on earth can give you either the key or the door to open, except yourself."

WHAT SELF-HELP GROUPS HAVE TO OFFER PATIENTS

Self-help is not a new approach to solving social problems. Spontaneous neighborliness has been a feature of society since its inception. In America, the early granges provided farmers with the benefit of cooperative efforts and early labor unions provided health and pension benefits for their members. Ethnic groups immigrating to the United States turned to each other for help. Since World War II, special purpose groups, often disease-specific, have emerged to provide services and support research to find cures. Several hundred thousand of these special-purpose groups exist in the United States today. The American Tinnitus Association has a commitment to support research and education and while not technically a self-help group, it performs that function for many of its members. It is the community-based self-help groups of ATA that truly provide support and encouragement on the local level. They are the hands and voices of ATA, extended across the country. Members share their concerns and provide mutual support and encouragement. And, these are true self-help groups in that each member knows the other as well as the leader.

In the 1960s and 1970s, academic interest in support groups increased and the earlier work involving leadership/followship, decision making, social influence, power, and problem solving became topics to study with these groups as well. Self-help groups were viewed as adjuncts to professional service, much as they are now. As rehabilitation services became more widespread, so did self-help groups. Often professional services were inadequate for the numbers of people who needed them, or sometimes they were perceived as being too costly. Most self-help group members are not in extremis. Their primary concern is in coping with problems of outlook and functioning and in dealing with family, friends, and employers. While these are real needs, people often cannot or do not wish to pay professionals for that service. As an individual's network of kinfolk becomes sparse due to job mobility and smaller families, the self-help group can fill an important social need. By the mid-1970s, a generally accepted definition of a self-help group evolved with five criteria (Lieberman & Borman, 1979):

1. Its purpose is to provide help and support for members and their problems.
2. The group is sanctioned by the members themselves rather than an external agency, although it is alright for such an agency to be initially involved.
3. It is a source of help relying on the skills and expertise of the members to provide that help. However, it may call upon professionals for information and guidance if desired.
4. It is composed of members who share a common experience.
5. It is controlled by the members.

Thousands of tinnitus sufferers in this country have found help through self-helping. The British Standing Conference for the Advancement of Counseling, 1969, provided a definition of counseling that certainly describes what frequently happens in the self-help arena.

> Counseling is a process through which one person helps another by purposeful conversation in an understanding atmosphere. It seeks to establish a helping relationship in which the one counseled can express his thoughts and feelings in such a way as to clarify his own situation, come to terms with some new experience, see his difficulty more objectively, and to face his problem with less anxiety and tension. *Its basic purpose is to assist the individual to make his own decisions from among the choices available to him.*

The onset of tinnitus is often met with panic followed by mad dashes to many doctors for answers. The fact that the answers received by new tinnitus sufferers are so often unsatisfactory raises its own questions. Is it because the tinnitus sufferer is anxious and worried and not able to focus closely on the patient/doctor dialogue? Is it because there are too many health professionals who are still in the dark about the treatments and causes of tinnitus? Or is it that the right questions are not being asked?

Tinnitus sufferers have really only one question: "How do I get rid of this noise in my head?", a question for which there could be hundreds of answers. The majority, however, are usually told that since nothing can be done they need to go home and live with it. But they are not told how to live with it, and their families are not told how to live with them. A recent study by Sanchez and Stephens (1997) builds on earlier work (Tyler & Baker, 1983) analyzing the complaint domains of tinnitus. The most common complaints fall into five areas; psychological, hearing, health, sleep, and situational. Its easy to see why many patients do not immediately consult a doctor about tinnitus. Only the domains of hearing and health would be likely to provoke an instant consultation. On the other hand, patients with vague and undefined complaints of sleep problems, situational problems or psychological problems might be perceived by the professional as a frustrating case to treat. Professionals sometimes view self-help as a threat, fearing lack of professional care for their patients, but more and more they are coming to realize what research has shown, that self-help members utilize the services of professionals more than do their general public counterparts. People who adjust the best are the ones who do as much for themselves as possible (Powell, 1987).

Many audiologists and hearing aid dispensers serve as support group facilitators because they have seen for themselves that the need is so great. These professionals recognize a person's fear of being alone with a chronic and incurable malady is the stuff depression (and sometimes suicide) is made of. Ear, Nose, and Throat specialists, audiologists, or hearing aid dealers may be the last or only professional point of contact for someone with tinnitus. Because the instillation of hope is of such significance to the well-being of their patient or client, we strongly encourage all health professionals to make one last referral—to the American Tinnitus Association. ATA's research efforts continue, and are growing, but for the moment, our self-help network can fill in the gaps for the tinnitus sufferer who is just trying to live with the noise. Until a cure is found, we want them to learn to live with it too. We just want them to live with it well.

ISSUES IN SELF-HELP GROUPS

One of the most important issues in learning to live with tinnitus is that of learning to ignore it. Some people naturally habituate to the sound of tinnitus, much as they learn to ignore the sound of their refrigerator or air conditioner. Others can be trained to ignore it. Another group may be comforted by substituting other sounds for the tinnitus. A few people will always hear their tinnitus and be bothered by it, either mildly or severely, but there are ways to help them too. What could happen in a poorly constituted self-help group is acquisition of a negative focus on tinnitus. A particularly disturbed patient who happens to be articulate and convincing could swing others to view their tinnitus as threatening. It is the job of the leader, either lay or professional, to be sensitive to these kinds of problems and head them off before they become critical.

While not necessarily a problem, there are people who are reticent to share their troubles with others. The problem then is for the leader of the group to gently draw the new person into the group and to make them feel comfortable. We often hear from people who arrived at their first tinnitus self-help group meeting desperate and left the meeting feeling calmer, sensing a safety

in numbers, feeling that they were really understood. They made contact with people who they could call during a personal down time. At the meeting, they observed others who had been where they were now, but who had managed to survive and get on with their lives. They had found coping role models. They also experienced the sharing of vital information, techniques, names of doctors, clinics, audiologists, and alternative therapies to try and to avoid (Hill, 1977). They learned that knowledge equals power, power equals control, and control contributes to relief. Psychologists sometimes refer to this phenomena as the role of learned resourcefulness. Because of the group, they had something to do, something to get ready for, something to take an active part in. They made friends. A group —a good one anyway—is usually greater than the sum of its parts.

Groups that are led by hearing health professionals, usually who also have tinnitus themselves, are particularly fortunate because these leaders can share techniques they have acquired in their professional training. They can, for example, use a rudimentary form of cognitive therapy (see Chapter 3) to help group members learn to cope with their tinnitus by changing the way they think about their tinnitus. The simple ABCs of cognitive therapy can take place in ordinary conversation (Greenberger & Padesky, 1995). For example, a person who is alone at night worries the tinnitus will become too loud to tolerate. The person may believe there is no escape from the internal noise and that it will drive them mad. Consequently the person is anxious, panicky, and feels helpless. The group leader, hearing this, might ask others how they handle worrying about tinnitus when they are alone and it is quiet. That will surely elicit ideas from others such as, "I turn on the radio and leave it on all night so that even if I wake up, I hear something other than my tinnitus." They might also comment that listening to music not only takes their mind off of the tinnitus, it also is a pleasant and soothing pastime. Someone might suggest a soothing hot beverage before going to bed. There are a myriad of activities by which people encourage restful sleep. The important thing here is that by taking charge of the situation, the person no longer needs to feel anxious, panicky, or helpless.

We all know that tinnitus cannot be abolished simply through positive thinking and from the therapists' view it is necessary to determine what the patient perceives as the greatest problem and attack it first. There are anecdoctal reports and even some scientific evidence to support various stress-relieving measures as a way of relieving tinnitus (Goebel, 1998). What is important to remember, however, is that someone can become very proficient at yoga, biofeedback, and other relaxation methods while still holding firmly to the root problem. What needs to be changed is the person's perception of the problem itself and of the options available for help. The patient who presents him or herself at the clinician's door with reasonable expectations for treatment, and with a positive attitude that has been acquired through membership in a self-help group, will be much easier to treat.

In a recent letter, one of our self-help coordinators told us of her feelings about working with her group and her involvement with ATA. "I feel good . . . Not only do I help myself, but I help others and it's so satisfying. I feel like I'm my own best medicine." Our self-help volunteers give time to their communities and help to people who are often in distress. They distribute our brochures by the thousands across the country, and attend local health meetings to discuss tinnitus and the services offered by ATA. They have let us know that ever since they asked for information about being part of our support network, their involvement with ATA has become very therapeutic. The appropriate health care and the best medicine often appear, it seems, when we ask the right questions—of our therapists and ourselves.

HOW TO START A LOCAL SELF-HELP GROUP

To start your own self-help group, contact ATA to receive a questionnaire for potential Self-Help Group facilitators. You will be provided a brochure with brief information about starting a group, ideas and suggestions for meetings, an explanation of the role of a group facilitator, and a listing of the present support network.

Once you make a committment to starting a group, you will receive more detailed instructions on the formation of a group, including how to recruit helpers, sample of a first meeting invitation, sample of a press release, how to find a meeting place, and other information ATA needs to help you get started.

Upon receipt of the date, time, and place of the first meeting ATA sends invitations to members within the identified local zipcodes area inviting them to attend.

Group leaders receive additional meeting announcements to distribute locally, back issues of *Good News*, the self-help newsletter published just for ATA group leaders, an ATA binder, brochures for the first meeting, and more suggestions about getting started.

Group leaders are expected to encourage membership in ATA and to regularly report the activities of their group to the ATA office. In turn, ATA provides ongoing information for the group along with leadership suggestions and tips. ATA helps the leaders to find speakers to address the group and tries to facilitate solutions for problems that may arise in the group setting.

SUMMARY

The American Tinnitus Association has always been about helping; helping to find a cure for tinnitus, helping counsel the people who have to endure the incessant sounds of tinnitus, and helping to develop better treatments so that the time between now and the time tinnitus is no more is not only a bearable time, but a time to be enjoyed and lived to the fullest.

Ralph Waldo Emerson stated it well when he said, "It is one of the most beautiful compensations of life that no man can sincerely try to help another without helping himself."

REFERENCES

CIBA Foundation Symposium 85, Tinnitus. (1981). D. Evered & G. Lawrenson (Eds.). Bath, UK: Pitman Press.

Goebel, G. (Ed.). (1998). *Tinnitus — Psychosomatic aspects of complex chronic tinnitus.* London, Quintessence Publishing.

Greenberger, Dennis, & Padesky, Christine A. (1995). *Mind over mood.* New York: The Guildford Press.

Hill, William Fawcett. (1977). *Learning thru discussion.* Beverly Hills: Sage Publications.

Lieberman, Morton A., Borman, and Leonard D., et al. (1979). *Self-help groups for coping with crisis.* San Francisco: Jossey-Bass Publishers.

Powell, Thomas J. (1987). *Self-help organizations and professional practice.* Silver Spring, MD: National Association of Social Workers.

Proceedings of the Fifth International Tinnitus Seminar. (1996). G. Reich & J. Vernon (Eds.). Portland, OR: American Tinnitus Association.

Proceedings of the First International Tinnitus Seminar, Tinnitus. (1981). Suppl. No. 4, *Journal of Laryngology and Otology,* A. Shulman (Ed.). Ashford, UK: Headley Brothers.

Proceedings of the Fourth International Tinnitus Seminar, Tinnitus 91. (1991). J.M. Aran & R. Dauman (Eds.). Amsterdam, The Netherlands: Kugler Publications.

Proceedings of the Second International Tinnitus Seminar. (1984). Suppl. No. 9, *Journal of Laryngology and Otology.* A. Shulman (Ed.). Ashford, UK: Headley Brothers.

Proceedings of the Third International Tinnitus Seminar. (1987). H. Feldmann (Ed.). Karlsruhe, Germany: Harsch Verlag.

Sanchez, Linnett, & Stephens, Dafydd. (1997). A tinnitus problem questionnaire in a clinic population. *Ear and Hearing,* Vol. 18, No. 3, 210–217.

Tyler, R. S., & Baker, L. J. (1983). Difficulties experienced by tinnitus sufferers. *Journal of Speech and Hearing Disorders, 48,* 150–154.

Appendix

PUBLICATIONS ABOUT TINNITUS AND RELATED ISSUES AVAILABLE FROM THE AMERICAN TINNITUS ASSOCIATION

This list changes frequently. For an up-to-date list, including prices, please call ATA (800) 634-8978, or FAX your request to ATA at (503) 248-0024, or e-mail to <http://tinnitus@ata.org>

Brochures

(In English)

American Tinnitus Association (Brochure about ATA with reply card)

Coping with the stress of tinnitus

If you have tinnitus *The First Steps to Take*

Information about tinnitus

Noise: Its effects on hearing and tinnitus

Understanding Tinnitus: Advice for family and friends

Tinnitus Treatments information for the professional

(In Spanish)

Manejando El Estres De Tinitus

Si Usted Tiene Tinitus—Los Primeros Pasos A Seguir

Informacion Sobre El Tinitus

Ruido Sus Efectos En La Audicion Tinitus

Informacion Sobre Tinitus Para La Familia

Tratamientos Para El Tinitus (informacion para el profesional)

Books & Journals

A Consumer Handbook on Hearing Loss & Hearing Aids—A Bridge to Healing Edited by Richard Carmen

Proceedings of the Fifth International Tinnitus Seminar 1995 Edited by Gloria Reich & Jack Vernon

Tinnitus: Treatment and Relief Edited by Jack Vernon

Tinnitus: What Is That Noise in My Head? by Joan Saunders

TMJ: The Self-Help Program by John Taddey

Tinnitus Today (sent to current donors quarterly at no charge). Back issues available.

Tapes, Videos, and Other Materials

Conversations with Drs. Vernon, Hazell, and Jastreboff (VHS, 8 min)

Informational Video (VHS, 2.5 min)

Tinnitus: Ringing in the Ears Lecture by Jack A. Vernon, Ph.D. (VHS, 60 min)

Sounds of Tinnitus (5 min. audio cassette tape)

Posters (various formats—call for details)

Prescription Pad (ATA referral form to give to patients or clients)

Tinnitus Bibliography—list of more than 3,000 tinnitus articles updated annually

CHAPTER 19

A History of Tinnitus

Dafydd Stephens

INTRODUCTION

Tinnitus, being essentially a reflection of abnormal function of the ear, has presumably occurred in man since his evolution. From the earliest written medical records we find that individuals have been consulting healers for help with this symptom. In this chapter, I shall endeavor to address the attitudes and approaches of such healers over the millennia towards the symptom and their subsequent approach adopted. It will be impossible to cover in detail all writings about tinnitus, even from a limited period of medical history. Instead, I shall concentrate on a number of representative writings, usually by well-known authors and authorities of the period that reflect the then-current attitudes towards the symptom. Detailed accounts of various aspects of the history of tinnitus may be found in a number of other publications including Stephens (1984, 1987) and Feldmann (1991).

In the English language, while some translations of early writers such as El Razi (Rhazes) quote two types of ear noises, "Tinnitus and Sonitus," only the former has found its way into general usage and is included in the Oxford Dictionary (1971). There it is described as having been introduced in Blanchard's Physician's Dictionary (2nd edition, 1693) in which tinnitus aurium is described as "a certain buzzing or tingling in the ears." It is derived from the Latin *tinnire*, to ring/tinkle. In the present chapter this one term will be applied to the conscious sound that originates in the head of its owner (without the voluntary origin obvious to that person) (after McFadden, 1982).

Other languages such as French, have a variety of terms; for example, "acouphènes," "bourdonnements" (buzzing), "sifflements" (whistling), "tintements" (ringing) and "tintouins" (unpleasant noise) (Guerrier & Mounier-Kuhn, 1980). More recently, workers in the field have tended to adopt one term covering all sounds, in this case, "acouphènes." Yet other languages, such as Welsh, have no specific word, with the most comprehensive English-Welsh dictionary (Griffiths & Jones, 1995) listing for tinnitus, "Cloch fach" (small bell) or "Canu yn y clust" (singing in the ear). Various Welsh patients, however, frequently use other terms such as "stwr" or "mwstwr" (noise) or "stêm yn y clust" (steam in the ear).

BABYLON

In ancient Babylon, medical treatments were inscribed on clay tablets, dating back to at least the seventh century B.C. A large collection of these are to be found in the British Museum where many were translated by Thompson (1931). Among those for diseases of the ears that he translated are some twenty-two for tinnitus of which eighteen are concerned with the ears singing, two with either the right or left ear speaking, and two with either the right or left ear whispering.

Five of the eighteen concerned with the ears singing involve a ghost, either "the hand of a ghost seizing on a man" (4) or "if a ghost seizes on a man" (1). The treatment in most cases includes a fumigation of the ears such as with seeds of juniper, seeds of laurel, horsehair, and so forth, together with incantations. Such incantations are generally relatively short: "wherever thou be may Ea restrain thee," but as illustrated elsewhere (Stephens, 1984, 1987) may be lengthy, involving ritual sets of numbers including seven times seven as, for example, in:

"O Seven heavens,
Seven earths,
Seven winds,
Seven hurricanes,
Seven fires,
Seven backs,
Seven sides;
By heaven be ye exorcised . . ."

The exorcism is complemented, for example with the insertion of the tooth of a female ibex, the horn of an ox into the ear, rituals compatible with the driving out of an evil spirit, which the priest/physician feels, has occupied the individual.

The question arises as to whether the priest/physician regarded all tinnitus as stemming from the individual being seized by a ghost. Certainly, this would seem to be true of all the "singing" tinnitus, for which there is no difference between the treatments of those specified as being caused by

a ghost and those not, and for which an individual ear is not indicated.

On the other hand, for "whispering" in the ears, for which the right and left ears are specified, the treatment is only recital of charm, possibly together with treatment with turmeric.

When the ears are said to "speak," again specified for the two ears separately, the treatment is one of purging, and with a good prognosis indicating in both cases that repeated purging over a period of seven days should lead to a recovery. This would tend to imply that while the physician sees one type of tinnitus to be an intractable symptom needing a psychological-religious treatment, in the other case a potentially treatable organic condition is found without any defined supernatural overlay.

In Babylon, spirit intrusion was considered to be the chief cause of disease. Such intrusion could take place as a result of lack of caution or fate, because of sin (for example, murder, adultery, theft, fraud) or as a result of sorcery (Sigerist, 1951). The body of physicians also included amongst them incantation priests to help with the exorcisms although there was also a major rational element to the treatments including various drugs and oils introduced into the ears, identical to those found repeatedly in different civilizations over the centuries.

CELSUS AND GRAECO-ROMAN MEDICINE

The two main themes of Graeco-Roman medicine stem from the Greek physicians Empedocles and Hippocrates of the fifth century B.C. Empedocles of Agrigento in Sicily (504–433 B.C.) introduced the concept of the four humors to medicine and Hippocrates of Kos (460–370 BC.) emphasized the importance of careful observation of the patient.

In Empedocles' concept, the body comprises cold, dry, moist and hot humors corresponding to earth, air, water, and fire (Figure 19-1). Health is maintained by a balance between these humors which are

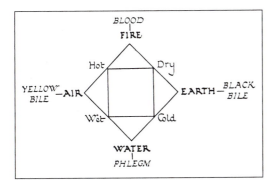

FIGURE 19-1. The four Elements in association with the four Humors and the four Qualities (from Singer, 1928)

represented in the body by combinations of these. Thus blood is hot and moist, phlegm is cold and moist, yellow bile hot and dry, and black bile cold and dry. In turn these are equivalent to the personality types sanguine, phlegmatic, choleric or melancholic. These can further be influenced by particular foods and various treatments such as purging, bleeding etc.

Such approaches, amalgamated with the more pragmatic but observational approaches of the Hippocratic corpus, which in itself incorporated the theory of humors, were the basis of the writings of the later Graeco-Roman writers. Within the corpus may be found the concept that tinnitus is related to air trapped within the ear.

One of the later writers was Aurelius Cornelius Celsus (25 B.C.–50 A.D.), a Roman nobleman rather than a physician himself, who compiled and translated treatises on medicine and other topics. His major contribution to medicine was entitled "De Medicina." In Book 6 of this he states: "Another class of lesion is that in which the ears produce a ringing noise within themselves and this also prevents them from perceiving sounds from without" (Spencer, 1938). He goes on to describe three types of tinnitus: due to a cold in the head, produced by diseases or prolonged pains of the head, and that which precedes the onset of serious illnesses such as epilepsy.

The tinnitus due to a cold in the head (otitis media?) was treated practically by get-

ting the patient to hold his breath until some "humors" froths out of the ear. The prognosis was regarded as good.

For the other two types, less amenable to treatment, the approach is more humorally based with nonfattening foods, exercise, rubbing, effusion, and gargling as well as introducing a variety of drops into the ear. A similar approach is applied to tinnitus without one of these causes and which is considered to be more sinister. For this, regulation of the diet must be prescribed with great care and the patient must abstain from wine.

Among other writers of this period Pliny (23–79 A.D.) described particular techniques based on folk medicine and Galen (130–200 A.D.), while repeating some of these approaches, also advocated the use of opium and mandrake as sedatives, apparently aware of the anxiety often found in tinnitus sufferers.

In Graeco-Roman medicine, the theoretical concept of the balance between the humors, equivalent to the Chinese concept of a balance between yin and yang, in order to obtain good health provided the theoretical underpinning of the medical approach. Medicine was practiced by physicians in the cities but by a variety of traditional healers in the more rural areas, and some of the collections of medical writing such as those of Celsus and Pliny owed much to both traditions. On top of this was the observational approach, often pragmatic, derived from the Hippocratic school and continued by the leading exponents of Roman medicine.

ISLAMIC AND MEDIEVAL MEDICINE

This period represents an extension of the basic premises of Graeco-Roman medicine with few significant changes in approach. Some writers, particularly Paul of Aegina (625-690 A.D.) bridged the gap but articulated treatments in similar ways. Thus he described the chronic noises as arising from thick and viscid humors and also reported the associated "increased sensibility" (phono-phobia or hyperacusis) that should be treated with castor, hemlock seeds, and vinegar (Adams, 1844).

The main contributions from Islamic medicine came from two Persians, El-Razi or Rhazes (850–923) and Ibn Sina or Avicenna (980–1034). El Razi separated sonitus and tinnitus but essentially advocated similar traditional treatments for both. Avicenna followed the earlier Graeco-Roman classification but further subdivided tinnitus into sonitus, tinnitus, and sibilus (whispering/ hissing).

Similar approaches persisted through medieval times and indeed up to the seventeenth century, with various additional approaches provided by, among others, Paracelsus (1493–1541) incorporating the doctrine of signatures (curing diseases by remedies resembling the part of the body being treated, such as cyclamen with ear-shaped leaves for ear disease), and replacing poly-pharmacy with the use of simple inorganic remedies.

A fairly representative and more traditional approach of medieval medicine is found in the writings of Gilbertus Anglicus (1180–1250) who provided with his "Compendium" of 1240, the first complete English medical text.

He devoted a section of this book to "Ringing in the Eris (Ears)," stating:

> Ringing in a man's ears, or other noise like blowing of horns, comes in diverse manners; otherwise of a great windy matter that is in the ear and moves up and down and all about therein and may not escape because of its boistrousness, and therefore there is a continual ringing and noise in the ears.

This concept of wind trapped in the ears giving rise to tinnitus was a common concept at this time and later was to lead to Jean Riolan (1580–1657) advocating trepanation of the mastoid to allow the escape of this wind. When put into practice, this procedure often had fatal consequences and was rapidly discontinued.

Gilbertus seems, however, to have regarded this type of tinnitus as of an insignificant cause and advocated no particular treatment. He did, however, follow the humoral theory for his other types of tinnitus due to a "viscous and corrupt humor," one that "comes of heat," one that "comes of cold," and one that "comes of feebleness of the ears."

That of a "viscous and corrupt humor" should first be treated by purging, the type of purging dependent on the humor. With a hot humor, purge the anger, if a cold humor, purge the melancholia. For tinnitus "coming of heat" the approach was one of eardrops based on the juice of bitter almonds—a therapy dating back to ancient Egypt.

Tinnitus caused by cold should be treated with drops of myrrh and castor, or alternatively radish or leek juice or woman's milk. Again, all these treatments date back several millennia. For that due to "feebleness of the ears," not discussed by earlier authors, he advocated the juice of wormwood mixed with warm vinegar.

Finally, he concluded with a general warning not to use "sharp and biting medicines" for the ears (Getz, 1981).

It may be seen that while this period extended over a millennium, there was little progress beyond what was available and known in late Roman times. The theoretical underpinning remained the theory of humors with increasing elaboration in the approaches to redressing the disbalance between these together with the first hints of a more pragmatic approach when such orthodoxy failed. While Paracelsus publicly burned the works of Galen and Avicenna together with the humoral concept, he also advocated the "doctrine of signatures" treating conditions with plants resembling the diseased organ, but at the same time did try to cut through the overcomplicated approaches of many of his predecessors. This inevitably led to more of his contemporaries and successors questioning established doctrines but not, however, coming up with major new concepts.

THE SEVENTEENTH CENTURY AND DUVERNEY

From the standpoint of tinnitus, the seventeenth century was notable for two events. The first was the publication of a number of theses on tinnitus (see Stephens, 1987), which drew together many of the earlier findings and views in a reasonably systematic manner. These were written in Latin from German Universities and generally had the title "Dissertationem de tinnitu aurium." The main authors of these are listed in Table 19-1.

The second important event was the publication by Guichard Joseph DuVerney of his Traité de L'ouie (1683) (Figure 19-2). This

Table 19-1. Early theses on tinnitus

Year	Author	University
1630	Zeidler	Leipzig
1667	Soheck	Jena
1669	Hartmann	Jena
1681	Krause	Jena
1694	Bolland	Jena
1699	Helbich	Altdorf
1706	Finckenau	Konigsberg
1770	Cartheuser	Frankfurt
1784	Schedel	Duisberg
1787	Liedenfrost	Duisberg

TRAITE'
DE
L'ORGANE
DE L'OUIE;
CONTENANT LA STRUCTURE,
les Ufages & les Maladies de toutes
les parties de l'Oreille.

Par M. Du Verney, *de l'Academie*
Royale des Sciences, Confeiller, Medecin
Ordinaire du Roy, & Profeffeur en
Anatomie & en Chirurgie au Iardin
Royal des Plantes.

A PARIS,
Chez ESTIENNE MICHALLET,
ruë S. Jacques à l'Image S. Paul.

M. DC. LXXXIII.
AVEC PRIVILEGE DE SA MAESTE'.

FIGURE 19-2. Title page of "Traité de l'organ de l'ouie" of DuVerney (1683)

was translated into Latin, German, Dutch and English and had a major impact on attitudes and approaches to diseases of the ear (Black, 1973). The first complete English edition was published as "A treatise of the organ of Hearing" in 1737, although part 3, including the section on tinnitus, had been published in translation as early as 1684 in Medicina Curiosa (Asherson, 1979).

One of the most comprehensive of the theses on tinnitus, that of Hartmann (1669), an inaugural medical thesis of the University of Jena in Germany, presented tinnitus as a disorder of the ear. Within this thesis, he accepted one view dating back to Greek times, *that it was caused by air trapped within the ear.* He divided the causes into:

Supernatural

Natural—related to: temperament, hereditary disposition, eunuchs

Non-natural—related to abnormal activity in the trapped air, stemming from cerebral, psychological and systematic causes

Preternatural—related to depression, hypochondriasis, and venereal diseases.

Within this he did not attempt to draw new conclusions, limiting his approach to drawing together the main part of existing knowledge in the field, much as Celsus had done a millennium and a half earlier.

On the other hand, DuVerney (1648–1730), working in Paris, brought a fresh new analytical approach to the field, refused to accept old concepts merely because they had been repeated and elaborated on over the centuries, and approached causation from a functional pragmatic standpoint. His approach to treatment was, however, traditional using remedies dating back to Classical and earlier times, including the comment that a woman's milk is better than any other milk to introduce into the ear to relieve otalgia.

However, his approach to tinnitus was one of regarding it as an example of depravation of hearing "rendering the ear sensible

of noises which are not in reality, or which are not external." This makes the ear less able to hear external sound.

He was scathing about the concept of tinnitus arising from implanted air, arguing rather that it arose either from vascular pulsation (a true sound) from disease of the ear (false sounds) and from disorders of the brain. He even argued that the last did not need to affect the ear directly, but could exert their influence directly on the nerves in the auditory pathway. Treatment was orientated towards the underlying lesion, whether it was vascular, aural, or in the brain. Brain disease included vertigo and epilepsy.

At this time we see, therefore, an increase in the interest in tinnitus, particularly in Germany, but one not associated with any major advances in its management or its theoretical basis. The concepts of DuVerney, however, studying in detail the anatomy of the ear (Figure 19-3) and the brain led to a rejection of earlier theoretical concepts and an approach regarding tinnitus merely as a manifestation of ear disease.

JEAN MARIE GASPARD ITARD

While almost a century and half elapsed between DuVerney's "Traité de l'organe de l'ouie" and Traité des Maladies de l'oreille et de l'audition" written by Itard in 1821, they represent part of a clear continuum in our thinking of ear disease in general and tinnitus in particular. Itard (1774–1838), like DuVerney, was not an orthodox otologist but rather an ex-military doctor who was a physician to the Institution Royale des Sourds-Muets in Paris and attempted to teach the "Enfant Sauvage," the wild boy of the woods, to talk.

He included tinnitus in his section on "Depravation of the ear," together with various dysacuses. He subdivided tinnitus into two major categories, those related to real sounds, objective tinnitus or somatosounds, that he called "true tinnitus" and those

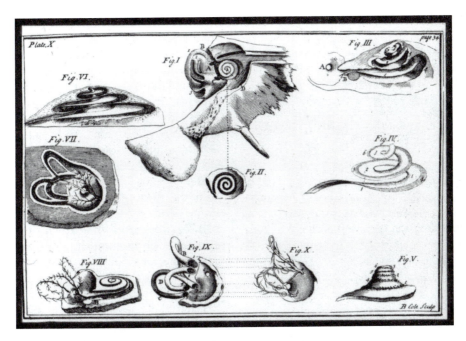

Figure 19-3. Anatomical drawings from DuVerney's English edition (1737)

without any acoustical basis ("false tinnitus"), but including "fantastic" sounds, possibly auditory hallucinations.

He next emphasized the importance of determining whether the tinnitus occurred alone (very rare) or was accompanied by hearing impairment. The latter group was further subdivided into those in which the tinnitus caused the hearing impairment and those in which they were independent, basing this division partly on the history of their onset and partly on suppressing the tinnitus by pressure on the carotid artery for several minutes! If the hearing loss disappears, then it was due to the tinnitus.

False tinnitus was divided into idiopathic, usually following noise exposure or acoustic trauma, or symptomatic related to other psychosomatic symptoms in "office workers, hypochondriacs and hysterical women."

He regarded tinnitus as "an extremely irksome discomfort which leads to a profound sadness in affected individuals. Of all symptoms, it is the one to which we habituate the least over time."

As with DuVerney, treatments were very traditional and dependent on the classification and origins of the symptom. However, he went on to state that, in all kinds of tinnitus, treatments fail against the stubbornness of the symptom. In this case, the aim should be to make the tinnitus less intolerable and he focused on what he regarded as the greatest consequence of tinnitus—sleep disturbance (Table 19-2). To overcome this he aimed to produce a variety of masking noises in the bedroom, ranging from a roaring fire to the sound of a mechanical organ. The choice of environmental masker was matched to the nature of the tinnitus, the most extreme mentioned among his case histories with one suggesting the lady concerned went to stay in a watermill, which was ultimately very successful.

This orientation towards managing the consequences of the tinnitus rather than the tinnitus itself, represented a major advance as well as an admission that most treatment was ineffective. He heralded a more modern approach to the problem which was mainly picked up and extended in the

Table 19-2. Jean Marie Gaspard Itard's thesis of tinnitus

"Il arrive bien souvent que le traitement le plus méthodique du bourdonnement, tant vrai que faux, lors méme qu'il n'est point ancien ni compliqué de surdité, échoue contre l'opiniâtreté de cette lésion acoustique. Il ne reste alors autre chose à faire qu'à le rendre moins insupportable, en lui ôtant de plus grand de ses inconvénients, celui de priver de sommeil ou de le troubler presque continuellement; je me suis avisé pour cela d'un expédient bien simple et qui manque rarement son effet, c'est de couvrir le bruit intérieur, réel ou imaginaire, par un bruit extérieur analogue et également continuel."

["It happens quite often that the most systematic treatment of tinnitus, whether of true or false tinnitus, even if it is neither long-standing nor complicated by deafness, fails against the obstinacy of this acoustical lesion. The only thing to do is to make it less unbearable, by removing its biggest inconvenience, that of sleep deprivation, or to interfere with it almost continuously; I recommend for that a simple technique which is rarely ineffective, that is by covering the internal noise, real or imaginary by an external noise, similar and equally continuous."]

---

twentieth century. The approach was, in some ways an observational one related to the principles of the Hippocratic School largely unencumbered by outdated theorizing. This could easily be incorporated with the rapidly developing concepts of medicine in the nineteenth century.

THE LATE NINETEENTH CENTURY

This was the time when major technological advances in medicine such as asepsis and anesthesia were beginning to be widely applied together with more sophisticated applications of electricity. Electricity had been used in the treatment of tinnitus from the time of Wibel (1768), who in his thesis "Casum aegroti auditi difficili" (Figure 19-4) stated "Finally the strength of static electricity is highly recommended for hearing problems and tinnitus, as may be shown by many examples."

Its application was elaborated by Grappengiesser (1802) (see Feldmann, 1987) who used voltaic cells, and by Brenner (1868). This was discussed further by MacNaughton Jones (1891) who supported Politzer's conclusion that "Galvanic treatment effects a lasting improvement . . . in the complete removal of subjective noises extremely rarely."

In the meantime, Toynbee (1815–1866), Wilde (1815–1876), and Kramer (1801–1875) had contributed much to advancing the science and understanding of ear disease. They had provided the foundations on which Politzer and his school in Vienna had been able to build.

What had happened to the approach to tinnitus? In reality, relatively little. Here I shall consider two writers who both acknowledged their debts to Politzer, MacNaughton Jones, who wrote the first book in English on tinnitus "Noises in the head and ears" in 1891 and Guiseppe Gradenigo (1859–1926) who did much to establish otology as a scientific discipline.

MacNaughton Jones' book, based on his presentation to the British Medical Association meeting in Birmingham in 1890, in some ways resembled the theses of the seventeenth century, being essentially a compendium of current knowledge, thought and treatment of tinnitus. He classified the tinnitus largely according to its site of origin within the auditory pathway (see Table 19-3) and treated it according to the underlying condition.

He did, however, very effectively pull together relevant information and provide a cogent approach to the assessment of the patient with tinnitus, including the effect of pressure on the neck. Interestingly, however, although he refers to the effect of meatal occlusion on the loudness of the tuning fork (Bing test) he made no remark on the effect of meatal occlusion on tinnitus loudness.

MacNaughton Jones even included a chapter on prognosis, listing conditions such as eustachian tube problems, therapeutic

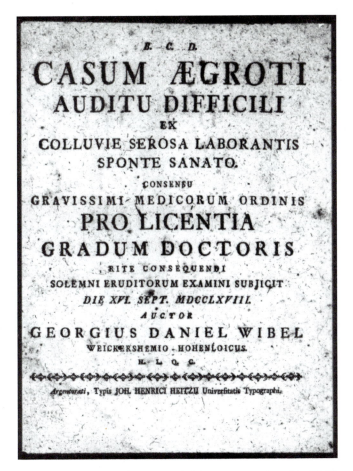

FIGURE 19-4. Title page of Wibel's "Casum negroti auditi difficili" (1768)

Table 19-3. MacNaughton Jones' Classification of Tinnitus (1891)

1. Impulses originating in the temporal lobe, or superior temporal gyrus, the cerebellum or the auditory nuclei.

2. Impulses due to irritation direct or reflected in any portion of the auditory nerve.

3. Impulses originating in the peripheral ends of the auditory nerve.

4. Irritations arising from interference with the intratympanic muscles.

5. Irritations transmitted by altered conditions of equilibration of air in the tympanic cavity.

6. Irritations due to disease in the middle ear and labyrinth.

7. Irritations arising in the external ear.

8. True aural hallucinations.

9. Therapeutic causes of tinnitus aurium.

causes, and labyrinthitis as having a good prognosis, whereas chronic Ménières's disorder, chronic middle ear disease, and labyrinthine trauma had a poor prognosis.

When describing various treatments, which largely followed current orthodoxy in their techniques, McNaughton Jones failed to discuss what he was treating should abolition of the tinnitus fail. He did, admittedly discuss some alternative therapies including massage, tapotement (gentle flicking) of the earlobe, counterirritation and electrical stimulation, but gave little indication as for which types of patients he considered these to be appropriate. Indeed, discussing electrical stimulation, on which he included a separate chapter based on the work of his friend James Cagney, he said "As regards Galvanism and its effects in tinnitus, I may say at once that personally it is a remedy I cannot strongly recommend and am not much in favor of."

Giuseppe Gradenigo (1859–1926) (Figure 19-5) was an important figure in Italian and European otology and made many contributions to the field of hearing and hearing disorders (Stephens et al., 1997). His writings on tinnitus were mainly restricted to sections in textbooks in Italian and German, but also included three brief papers on the topic. In these he certainly indicated his awareness of the psychological effects of the symptoms. Thus in 1890, he began "one of the most frequent and most tormenting symptoms . . . is noises in the ears." He went on to say that "in some cases it may lead to psychoses and even to suicide." In a case-report (Gradenigo, 1890) he described how the tinnitus can be aggravated by psychological factors, but also that the tinnitus in this case could in turn result in a psychological disturbance.

We thus see in the late nineteenth century a slow coming together of new ideas and approaches to tinnitus management using new technologies and also becoming aware of the psychological components. These established the foundations for much of the work that was to be extended particularly in the second half of the twentieth century.

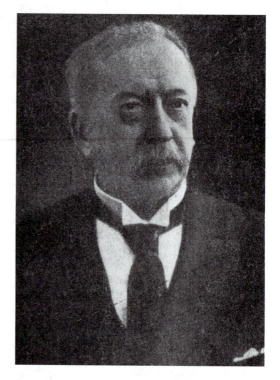

FIGURE 19-5. Giuseppe Gradenigo

THE FOWLERS AND THE BEGINNING OF MODERN APPROACH

The modern approach to tinnitus began effectively with the work of a father and son: Earl Prince Fowler (1873–1966) and Earl Prince Fowler Junior. Both were otologists, but the father was a great pioneer of audiometry, developing the Western Electric IA audiometer in 1922 with Wegel, and the alternate binaural loudness balance test in 1928. His son was more interested in the psychological aspects of audiovestibular disorders and particularly by Ménière's disorder.

Fowler Senior produced a series of papers on techniques of matching and masking tinnitus together with their clinical value from 1928 onwards, although his most important papers were a cluster of publications in the early 1940s. He divided tinnitus into: (1) Vibratory tinnitus (objective tinnitus/

somatosounds) and (2) Nonvibratory tinnitus, caused by "biochemical irritation of the auditory neural mechanism" (Fowler, 1943). Feldmann (1991) has discussed his contributions to tinnitus at some length. They are best summarized in Fowler Senior's 1941 paper "Tinnitus aurium in the light of recent research."

In this he:

■ Divided his tinnitus into vibratory and nonvibratory (see previous item no. 2).
■ Showed how loudness may be objectively estimated using a loudness balance technique.
■ Indicated that subjectively loud tinnitus is often matched to a low level stimulus.
■ Described a pitch-matching technique.
■ Indicated the maskability of tinnitus by broadband noise.
■ Demonstrated that loudness and pitch matches determine completely the maskability of tinnitus.
■ Demonstrated that tinnitus is always associated with some hearing loss.
■ Indicated that loudness and pitch determine the hearing loss derived from the tinnitus.
■ Discussed the auditory "fatigue" arising from the tinnitus.
■ Considered the mechanism of tinnitus generation.
■ Indicated that increases in tinnitus loudness are often associated with increase in pitch.
■ Pointed out that it is impossible to generate beats between the tinnitus tone and an externally generated tone.
■ Shown that sensorineural tinnitus does not follow normal acoustical perceptual behaviors and rarely has the timbre of a pure tone.
■ Considered the relevant neurophysiology and pathology.
■ Found it difficult to explain the masking of tinnitus in the context of current auditory theory.
■ Discussed the mechanism of bilateral tinnitus.

■ Indicated that sustained tinnitus is a sign of increasing or potential hearing loss.

It may be clearly seen from this that Fowler Senior had a very clear and modern view of tinnitus and described most of the behavioral techniques for its measurement which have been used since that time (see Chapter 6).

Fowler Junior made important contributions to the psychosomatic/somatopsychic consideration of hearing and balance disorders and applied Sheldon's concept of somatotypes (ectomorphs/endomorphs/mesomorphs) in this context. When he came together to write with his father (Fowler & Fowler, 1955), they managed to bring together their two approaches to tinnitus in a sophisticated patient-centered way. After discussing many of the behavioral traits associated with tinnitus including "evasiveness" and "ineffectiveness of reassurance," they drew together their approaches in a list of nine points in "How do we examine people who suffer from tinnitus?".

These are:

1. Listen attentively to their story and obtain a complete personal history, particularly concerning the symptoms of the present and past episodes possibly related to emotional strains at home and in the business world.
2. Obtain a real family history not only concerning disease but also the personality of siblings and immediate ancestors.
3. Examine carefully, not only otolaryngologically, but as a physician.
4. Measure the hearing capacity.
5. Measure the loudness and pitch of the tinnitus.
6. Estimate related aural symptoms—vertigo, nausea, and so on.
7. Examine carefully for nystagmus.
8. Tell the patient the results of your examination in a clear, confident, reassuring manner and outline what treatment and management is indicated and not indicated.

9. Explain simply and briefly the basic types of tinnitus and their pathophysiology . . . Impress on him that it is *not a delusion*, and that unless he was crazy before he saw you he probably will not be crazy afterwards.

CONCLUSIONS

We all have much to learn from our forebears. By paying attention to what they have done, we avoid repeating the mistakes that so many have made in the past that have led to lessons learned the hard way. Progress has broadly come from developing technology together with improving understanding of the mechanisms involved. Most patients, after a careful explanation, do not seek a cure, but rather a rational explanation of what may be causing their problem, in the light of current understanding. While we may have progressed from the seizure of the ears by ghosts and a dysbalance of the humors we have to admit that our successors may find some of our current ideas equally quaint.

However by reassurance, explanation, and using the techniques described by our forebears to give patients symptomatic relief, we can still alleviate the suffering of many of our patients and reduce the tinnitus to a minor annoyance.

REFERENCES

Adams, F. (1844). *The seven books of Paulus Aeginata.* London: Sydenham Society.

Asherson, N. (1979). Traité de l'organe de L'Ouie. *Journal of Laryngology and Otology* (Suppl. 2).

Black, J. W. (1973). A treatise of the organ of hearing by Guichard Joseph DuVerney. New York: AMS Press, Inc.

Campbell Thompson, R. (1931). Asyrian prescriptions for diseases of the ears. *Journal of the Royal Asiatic Society,* 1–25.

Feldmann, H. (1987). Electrical stimulation in suppressing of tinnitus—historical remarks. In H. Feldmann (Ed.), *Proceedings of the Third*

International Tinnitus Seminar (pp 394–399). Karlsruhe: Harsch.

Feldmann, H. (1991). History of tinnitus research. In A. Shulman (Ed.), *Tinnitus diagnosis/treatment* (pp 3–37). Philadelphia: Lea & Febiger.

Fowler, E. P. (1928). Marked deafened areas in normal ears. *Transactions of the American Otological Society, 18,* 262–275.

Fowler, E. P. (1941). Tinnitus aurium in the light of recent research. *Annals of Otology, 50,* 139–158.

Fowler, E. P. (1943). Control of head noises. *Archives of Otolaryngology, 37,* 391–398.

Fowler, E. P., & Fowler, Junior, E. P. (1955). Somatopsychic and psychosomatic factors in tinnitus, deafness, and vertigo. *Annals of Otology, 64,* 29–37.

Getz, F. M. (1981). A edition of the middle English Gilbertus Auglius found in Wellcome MS 537. Ph.D., University of Toronto.

Gradenigo, G. (1890). I rumori subiettivi di orecchio nell'otite interna. *Sordomuto,* 1–8.

Griffiths, B., & Jones, D. G. (1995). *Geiriadur yr Academi.* Cardiff: University of Wales Press.

Guerriér, Y., Mounier-Kuhn, P. (1980). *Histoire des maladies de l'oreille, du nez et de la gorge.* Paris: DaCosta.

Hartmann, M. (1669). *Dissertationem Inauguralem Medicam de Tinnitu Aurium.* Jena: Samuelis Krebsii.

Itard, J-M-G. (1821). *Traité des maladie de l'oreille et de l'audition.* Paris: Méquignon-Marvis.

MacNaughton Jones, H. (1891). Subjective noises in their head and ears. London: Baillière, Tindall and Cox.

McFadden, D. (1982). *Tinnitus: Facts, theories and treatments.* Washington, DC: National Academic Press.

Sigerist, H. E. (1951). *A history of medicine.* New York: Oxford University Press.

Singer, C. (1928). *A short history of medicine.* Oxford: Clarendon.

Spencer, W. G. (1938). Celsus—De Medicina. London: Heinemann.

Stephens, S. D. G. (1984). The treatment of tinnitus—A historical perspective. *Journal of Laryngology and Otology, 98,* 963–972.

Stephens, S. D. G. (1987). Historical aspects of tinnitus. In J. W. P. Hazell (Ed.), *Tinnitus* (pp. 1–19). Edinburgh: Churchill Livingstone.

Stephens, S. D. G., Orzan, E., & Galleti di San Cataldo, F. (1997). Giuseppe Gradenigo and his contributions to audiology. *Journal of Laryngology and Otology, 111,* 418–423.

INDEX

Note: Page numbers in **bold** type reference non-text information.